New Frontiers in Blood Cells Research and Hematology

New Frontiers in Blood Cells Research and Hematology

Editor: Brian Jenkins

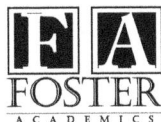

FA **FOSTER**
A C A D E M I C S

www.fosteracademics.com

www.fosteracademics.com

FA FOSTER
ACADEMICS

Cataloging-in-Publication Data

New frontiers in blood cells research and hematology / edited by Brian Jenkins.
    p. cm.
Includes bibliographical references and index.
ISBN 978-1-63242-558-4
1. Blood cells--Research. 2. Hematology. I. Jenkins, Brian.
QP94 .N49 2018
612.11--dc23

Foster Academics,
118-35 Queens Blvd., Suite 400,
Forest Hills, NY 11375, USA

ISBN 978-1-63242-558-4 (Hardback)

Contents

Preface...IX

Chapter 1   **Impact of Early Reoperation following Living-Donor Liver Transplantation
on Graft Survival**..1
Yoshikuni Kawaguchi, Yasuhiko Sugawara, Nobuhisa Akamatsu, Junichi Kaneko,
Tsuyoshi Hamada, Tomohiro Tanaka, Takeaki Ishizawa, Sumihito Tamura,
Taku Aoki, Yoshihiro Sakamoto, Kiyoshi Hasegawa, Norihiro Kokudo

Chapter 2   **Stage-Specific Binding Profiles of Cohesin in Resting and Activated B
Lymphocytes Suggest a Role for Cohesin in Immunoglobulin Class Switching
and Maturation**..9
Gamze Günal-Sadık, Maciej Paszkowski-Rogacz, Kalaimathy Singaravelu,
Andreas Beyer, Frank Buchholz, Rolf Jessberger

Chapter 3   **Leucocyte Telomere Length and Risk of Type 2 Diabetes Mellitus: New
Prospective Cohort Study and Literature-Based Meta-Analysis**........................18
Peter Willeit, Julia Raschenberger, Emma E. Heydon, Sotirios Tsimikas,
Margot Haun, Agnes Mayr, Siegfried Weger, Joseph L. Witztum,
Adam S. Butterworth, Johann Willeit, Florian Kronenberg, Stefan Kiechl

Chapter 4   ***Ex Vivo* Response to Histone Deacetylase (HDAC) Inhibitors of the HIV Long
Terminal Repeat (LTR) Derived from HIV-Infected Patients on
Antiretroviral Therapy**...27
Hao K. Lu, Lachlan R. Gray, Fiona Wightman, Paula Ellenberg, Gabriela Khoury,
Wan-Jung Cheng, Talia M. Mota, Steve Wesselingh, Paul R. Gorry,
Paul U. Cameron, Melissa J. Churchill, Sharon R. Lewin

Chapter 5   **The Long-Term Effects of Pitavastatin on Blood Lipids and Platelet Activation
Markers in Stroke Patients: Impact of the Homocysteine Level**........................36
Hideki Sugimoto, Shingo Konno, Nobuatsu Nomoto, Hiroshi Nakazora,
Mayumi Murata, Hisao Kitazono, Tomomi Imamura, Masashi Inoue,
Miyuki Sasaki, Akihisa Fuse, Wataru Hagiwara, Mari Kobayashi, Toshiki Fujioka

Chapter 6   **Spatiotemporal Characterization of a Fibrin Clot using Quantitative Phase
Imaging**..42
Rajshekhar Gannavarpu, Basanta Bhaduri, Krishnarao Tangella, Gabriel Popescu

Chapter 7   **Presence of Neutrophil Extracellular Traps and Citrullinated Histone H3 in
the Bloodstream of Critically Ill Patients**..49
Tomoya Hirose, Shigeto Hamaguchi, Naoya Matsumoto, Taro Irisawa,
Masafumi Seki, Osamu Tasaki, Hideo Hosotsubo, Norihisa Yamamoto,
Kouji Yamamoto, Yukihiro Akeda, Kazunori Oishi, Kazunori Tomono,
Takeshi Shimazu

Chapter 8   **Induced Differentiation of Human Myeloid Leukemia Cells into M2
Macrophages by Combined Treatment with Retinoic Acid and 1α,25-
Dihydroxyvitamin D$_3$**..58
Hiromichi Takahashi, Yoshihiro Hatta, Noriyoshi Iriyama, Yuichiro Hasegawa,
Hikaru Uchida, Masaru Nakagawa, Makoto Makishima, Jin Takeuchi,
Masami Takei

Chapter 9   **Prognostic Significance of Neutrophil Lymphocyte Ratio in Patients with Gastric Cancer**...67
Xi Zhang, Wei Zhang, Li-jin Feng

Chapter 10   **Hematopoietic Stem/Progenitor Cell Sources to Generate Reticulocytes for *Plasmodium vivax* Culture**..74
Florian Noulin, Javed Karim Manesia, Anna Rosanas-Urgell, Annette Erhart,
Céline Borlon, Jan Van Den Abbeele, Umberto d'Alessandro,
Catherine M. Verfaillie

Chapter 11   **Defects in the Acquisition of Tumor-Killing Capability of CD8⁺ Cytotoxic T Cells in Streptozotocin-Induced Diabetic Mice**...81
Shu-Ching Chen, Yu-Chia Su, Ya-Ting Lu, Patrick Chow-In Ko, Pei-Yu Chang,
Hung-Ju Lin, Hong-Nerng Ho, Yo-Ping Lai

Chapter 12   **Vancomycin Dosing in Neutropenic Patients**...89
Michiel B. Haeseker, Sander Croes, Cees Neef, Cathrien A. Bruggeman,
Leo M. L. Stolk, Annelies Verbon

Chapter 13   **High Levels of Soluble Ctla-4 are Present in Anti-Mitochondrial Antibody Positive, but not in Antibody Negative Patients with Primary Biliary Cirrhosis**..96
Daniele Saverino, Giampaola Pesce, Princey Antola, Brunetta Porcelli,
Ignazio Brusca, Danilo Villalta, Marilina Tampoia, Renato Tozzoli, Elio Tonutti,
Maria Grazia Alessio, Marcello Bagnasco, Nicola Bizzaro

Chapter 14   **Differential Antigen Expression Profile Predicts Immunoreactive Subset of Advanced Ovarian Cancers**...103
Kevin H. Eng, Takemasa Tsuji

Chapter 15   **Assessment of CD4+ T Cell Responses to Glutamic Acid Decarboxylase 65 using DQ8 Tetramers Reveals a Pathogenic Role of GAD65 121–140 and GAD65 250–266 in T1D Development**...112
I-Ting Chow, Junbao Yang, Theresa J. Gates, Eddie A. James, Duy T. Mai,
Carla Greenbaum, William W. Kwok

Chapter 16   **Increased CD112 Expression in Methylcholanthrene-Induced Tumors in CD155-Deficient Mice**...121
Yoko Nagumo, Akiko Iguchi-Manaka, Yumi Yamashita-Kanemaru, Fumie Abe,
Günter Bernhardt, Akira Shibuya, Kazuko Shibuya

Chapter 17   **Peripheral CD4⁺ T Cell Cytokine Responses following Human Challenge and Re-Challenge with *Campylobacter jejuni***...128
Kelly A. Fimlaid, Janet C. Lindow, David R. Tribble, Janice Y. Bunn,
Alexander C. Maue, Beth D. Kirkpatrick

Chapter 18   **Peroxisome Proliferator-Activated Receptor γ Deficiency in T Cells Accelerates Chronic Rejection by Influencing the Differentiation of CD4+ T Cells and Alternatively Activated Macrophages**...136
Xiaofan Huang, Lingyun Ren, Ping Ye, Chao Cheng, Jie Wu, Sihua Wang,
Yuan Sun, Zheng Liu, Aini Xie, Jiahong Xia

Chapter 19   **Tumor Induced Hepatic Myeloid Derived Suppressor Cells can Cause Moderate Liver Damage**...**145**
Tobias Eggert, José Medina-Echeverz, Tamar Kapanadze, Michael J. Kruhlak, Firouzeh Korangy, Tim F. Greten

Chapter 20   **The Ratio of Circulating Regulatory T Cells (Tregs)/Th17 Cells is Associated with Acute Allograft Rejection in Liver Transplantation**.......................**154**
Ying Wang, Min Zhang, Zhen-Wen Liu, Wei-Guo Ren, Yan-Chao Shi, Yan-Ling Sun, Hong-Bo Wang, Lei Jin, Fu-Sheng Wang, Ming Shi

Chapter 21   **Pharmacological Inhibition of the Chemokine CXCL16 Diminishes Liver Macrophage Infiltration and Steatohepatitis in Chronic Hepatic Injury**...................**161**
Alexander Wehr, Christer Baeck, Florian Ulmer, Nikolaus Gassler, Kanishka Hittatiya, Tom Luedde, Ulf Peter Neumann, Christian Trautwein, Frank Tacke

Chapter 22   **Longitudinal Analysis of T and B Cell Phenotype and Function in Renal Transplant Recipients with or without Rituximab Induction Therapy**...................**170**
Elena G. Kamburova, Hans J. P. M. Koenen, Martijn W. F. van den Hoogen, Marije C. Baas, Irma Joosten, Luuk B. Hilbrands

Chapter 23   **Fingolimod Increases CD39-Expressing Regulatory T Cells in Multiple Sclerosis Patients**...**178**
Nathalie Muls, Hong Anh Dang, Christian J. M. Sindic, Vincent van Pesch

Chapter 24   **BDC12-4.1 T-Cell Receptor Transgenic Insulin-Specific CD4 T Cells are Resistant to *In Vitro* Differentiation into Functional Foxp3+ T Regulatory Cells**.........**185**
Ghanashyam Sarikonda, Georgia Fousteri, Sowbarnika Sachithanantham, Jacqueline F. Miller, Amy Dave, Therese Juntti, Ken T. Coppieters, Matthias von Herrath

Chapter 25   **The C-Type Lectin OCILRP2 Costimulates EL4 T Cell Activation via the DAP12-Raf-MAP Kinase Pathway**...**191**
Qiang Lou, Wei Zhang, Guangchao Liu, Yuanfang Ma

Chapter 26   **Coincident Pre-Diabetes is Associated with Dysregulated Cytokine Responses in Pulmonary Tuberculosis**...**200**
Nathella Pavan Kumar, Vaithilingam V. Banurekha, Dina Nair, Rathinam Sridhar, Hardy Kornfeld, Thomas B. Nutman, Subash Babu

Chapter 27   **Effects of Increased Von Willebrand Factor Levels on Primary Hemostasis in Thrombocytopenic Patients with Liver Cirrhosis**...................................**208**
Andreas Wannhoff, Oliver J. Müller, Kilian Friedrich, Christian Rupp, Petra Klöters-Plachky, Yvonne Leopold, Maik Brune, Mirja Senner, Karl-Heinz Weiss, Wolfgang Stremmel, Peter Schemmer, Hugo A. Katus, Daniel N. Gotthardt

Permissions

List of Contributors

Index

Preface

Over the recent decade, advancements and applications have progressed exponentially. This has led to the increased interest in this field and projects are being conducted to enhance knowledge. The main objective of this book is to present some of the critical challenges and provide insights into possible solutions. This book will answer the varied questions that arise in the field and also provide an increased scope for furthering studies.

The branch of medicine which is concerned with the study of blood and diseases related to it is known as hematology. Some of the diseases that occur in the blood are leukemia, myelofibrosis, multiple myeloma, anemia and polycythemia. Bone marrow transplantation is the stem cell therapy that is very commonly used in diseases related to the blood. It is mainly used to treat cancer. The various advancements in blood cell research and hematology are glanced at in this book and their applications as well as ramifications are looked at in detail. This book will prove to be immensely beneficial to students and researchers in this field.

I hope that this book, with its visionary approach, will be a valuable addition and will promote interest among readers. Each of the authors has provided their extraordinary competence in their specific fields by providing different perspectives as they come from diverse nations and regions. I thank them for their contributions.

Editor

Impact of Early Reoperation following Living-Donor Liver Transplantation on Graft Survival

Yoshikuni Kawaguchi[1], Yasuhiko Sugawara[1]*, Nobuhisa Akamatsu[1], Junichi Kaneko[1], Tsuyoshi Hamada[3], Tomohiro Tanaka[2], Takeaki Ishizawa[1], Sumihito Tamura[1], Taku Aoki[1], Yoshihiro Sakamoto[1], Kiyoshi Hasegawa[1], Norihiro Kokudo[1]

1 Artificial Organ and Transplantation Surgery Division, Department of Surgery, Graduate School of Medicine, University of Tokyo, Tokyo, Japan, 2 Organ Transplantation Service, University of Tokyo, Tokyo, Japan, 3 Department of Gastroenterology, Graduate School of Medicine, University of Tokyo, Tokyo, Japan

Abstract

Background: The reoperation rate remains high after liver transplantation and the impact of reoperation on graft and recipient outcome is unclear. The aim of our study is to *evaluate the impact of early reoperation following living-donor liver transplantation* (LDLT) on graft and recipient survival.

Methods: Recipients that underwent LDLT (n = 111) at the University of Tokyo Hospital between January 2007 and December 2012 were divided into two groups, a reoperation group (n = 27) and a non-reoperation group (n = 84), and case-control study was conducted.

Results: Early reoperation was performed in 27 recipients (24.3%). Mean time [standard deviation] from LDLT to reoperation was 10 [9.4] days. Female sex, Child-Pugh class C, Non-HCV etiology, fulminant hepatitis, and the amount of intraoperative fresh frozen plasma administered were identified as possibly predictive variables, among which females and the amount of FFP were identified as independent risk factors for early reoperation by multivariable analysis. The 3-, and 6- month graft survival rates were 88.9% (95%confidential intervals [CI], 70.7–96.4), and 85.2% (95%CI, 66.5–94.3), respectively, in the reoperation group (n = 27), and 95.2% (95%CI, 88.0–98.2), and 92.9% (95%CI, 85.0–96.8), respectively, in the non-reoperation group (the log-rank test, p = 0.31). The 12- and 36- month overall survival rates were 96.3% (95%CI, 77.9–99.5), and 88.3% (95%CI, 69.3–96.2), respectively, in the reoperation group, and 89.3% (95%CI, 80.7–94.3) and 88.0% (95%CI, 79.2–93.4), respectively, in the non-reoperation group (the log-rank test, p = 0.59).

Conclusions: Observed graft survival for the recipients who underwent reoperation was lower compared to those who did not undergo reoperation, though the result was not significantly different. Recipient overall survival with reoperation was comparable to that without reoperation. The present findings enhance the importance of vigilant surveillance for postoperative complication and surgical rescue at an early postoperative stage in the LDLT setting.

Editor: Guy Brock, University of Louisville, United States of America

Funding: This work was supported by a Grant-in-aid for Scientific Research from the Ministry of Education, Culture, Sports, Science and Technology of Japan and from the Ministry of Health, Labor and Welfare of Japan (AIDS Research). The funders had no role in study design, data collection and analysis, decision to publish, or preparation of the manuscript.

Competing Interests: The authors have declared that no competing interests exist.

* Email: yasusugatky@yahoo.co.jp

Introduction

Continuous advances in surgical techniques, postoperative management, and immunosuppression have improved the safety of liver transplantation (LT) and patient survival [1–5]. In fact, overall survival rates in the later period of experience are reportedly better than those in the earlier period [6]. The Japanese Liver Transplantation Society reported overall survival rates for deceased-donor LT (DDLT) (n = 98) of 80.5% at 1 year, 77.8% at 3 years, and 76.0% at 5 years, and overall survival rates for living-donor LT (LDLT) (n = 6097) of 83.4% at 1 year, 79.3% at 3 years, and 76.9% at 5 years based on the data from 1998 to 2010 [7]. Similar survival rates are reported in Europe (83% at 1

year, and 71% at 5 years [1995–2000]) [8] and the United States (83.3% at 1 year [2002–2004], and 67.4% at 5 years [1997–2000]) [9].

Despite improved graft and recipient survival, the reoperation rate among LT recipients remains high, ranging from 9.2% to 34% [10–13], compared to that for liver resection, which ranges from 2.5% to 10.9% [14–16]. While several studies about the post-LT complication rates, including early reoperation, have been reported, there are few reports of the factors associated with early reoperation and the influence of early reoperation on LT recipient outcome. Recent reports indicate that early reoperation is a risk factor for impaired recipient outcome in both LDLT [12] and DDLT [10] recipients.

In the present study, we conducted a retrospective analysis investigating the incidence and cause of early reoperation, the factors associated with early reoperation, and the impact of early reoperation on graft and recipient survival among 111 consecutive adult LDLT recipients.

Patients and Methods

Patients

Between January 1996 and December 2012, 500 patients, including 77 pediatric patients, underwent LDLT at the University of Tokyo Hospital. Considering the technical standardization and establishment of criteria for reoperation, 111 consecutive adult LDLT cases between January 2007 and December 2012 were the subjects of the present study. The clinical records of these patients were retrospectively reviewed. The data of blood tests were based on the results in recipients' admission for the transplantation. All operations and reoperations were performed after obtaining informed consent from the patients and approval by the local ethics committee of the University of Tokyo.

Graft selection criteria and surgical treatment

The indication for LDLT and the type of liver graft were determined according to the ratio of the remnant liver volume to the total liver volume in living donors, and that of the graft volume to the standard liver volume (SLV) [17] in recipients [4]. Briefly, 40% of the recipient SLV was the minimum requirement for the graft and the donor remnant liver volume needed to be over 30% of total liver volume of the donor. Our detailed donor selection criteria and surgical procedures for both the donor and recipient are described elsewhere [18].

Postoperative management

All recipients were transferred to the intensive care unit with respirator support after the initial LDLT procedure. Recipients with an uneventful course were transferred to the surgical ward around postoperative day (POD) 5.

Routine postoperative investigations were as follows; blood tests (complete blood count, biochemical measurements, and coagulation profiles) were performed three or four times daily until POD 3, and twice daily between POD 4 and POD 14, chest and abdominal radiographs were examined twice daily until POD 3 and once daily between POD 4 and POD 14, Doppler ultrasonography to examine flow in the graft vessels was performed at least twice daily until POD 14 to detect abnormal flow in the hepatic artery/portal vein/hepatic vein, thrombi in the graft vessels, and intraabdominal fluid collection.

Indications for blood transfusions were as follows: red blood cell concentrate if the hemoglobin level or hematocrit was less than 6 g/dL and 15%, respectively, FFP if the prothrombin time-international normalized ratio (PT-INR) was greater than 2.00, and platelet concentrate if the platelet count was less than $3.0 \times 10^4/\mu L$.

The basic immunosuppression regimen consisted of tacrolimus and steroids for all recipients, and the doses of each drug were gradually tapered for 6 months after LDLT. Our detailed protocol of immunosuppression is described elsewhere [2].

Anticoagulation regimen after LDLT

To prevent early vascular thrombosis, anticoagulation therapy was started just after transplantation and continued until POD 14 in all recipients. The regimen was started with dalteparin (25 IU/kg/d), which was administered until POD 2. On POD 3, the anticoagulant drug was changed to heparin (unfractionated heparin sodium, 5000 U/d), the dose of which was adjusted to achieve a targeted activated clotting time of between 130 and 160 seconds.

Definitions for early reoperation and early graft loss

Early reoperation in our study was defined as surgical intervention after LDLT between just after transplant and the day of initial discharge. Early graft loss was defined as graft loss occurring within 6 months after LDLT.

Indications for early reoperation after LDLT

Indications for early reoperation were generally divided into three categories, postoperative bleeding, vessel flow problems, and biliary complications. Reoperation for postoperative bleeding was indicated for recipients with postoperative bleeding with hemodynamic instability, hemorrhage above Grade B defined by International Study Group of Liver Surgery [19], or suspected intraabdominal hematoma infection. Vessel flow problems included hepatic arterial thrombosis, portal venous thrombosis, and decreased or hepatofugal portal flow developing during the early postoperative period, all which were detected by Doppler US. Biliary complications, which we initially attempted to treat with interventional strategies, were indicated for early reoperation in cases with massive biliary leakage resulting in biliary peritonitis or biliary obstruction with intrahepatic biliary dilatation just after LDLT.

Ethics Statement

All LDLTs were performed after individually obtaining informed consent from recipients and donors. LDLT program at the University of Tokyo Hospital has been approved by its Institutional Review Board, and all aspects of the procedures have been conducted according to the principles expressed in the Declaration of Helsinki. The current human subject research was approved as project number G3515 by Graduate School of Medicine and Faculty of Medicine, the University of Tokyo Research Ethics Committee and Human Genome, Gene Analysis Research Ethics Committee. All subjects have been properly instructed and participated by signing the appropriate informed consent paperwork. In the preparation of this manuscript, all efforts have been made to protect patient privacy and anonymity.

Statistical analysis

Continuous variables are expressed as mean values (with standard deviations). Categorical variables are expressed as number (%), and were compared between groups using Fisher's exact test or the chi-square test, as appropriate. Graft and overall survival were measured from the time of LT. Survival curves were constructed using the Kaplan-Meier method, and compared using the log-rank test. Factors with $p<0.10$ in a Cox proportional hazard model as a univariable analysis were considered potential risk factors and were further analyzed in a multivariable Cox model. Hazard ratios (HR) and 95% confidential intervals (CI) were calculated for each factor. A p value of less than 0.05 was considered to indicate statistical significance. Statistical analysis was performed with JMP software (version 9.0; SAS Institute Inc., Cary, NC).

Results

Patient characteristics

The characteristics of the 111 consecutive patients are summarized in Table 1. The cohort included 50 males and 61 females (male:female, reoperation group; 7: 20, non-reoperation group; 43: 41). Mean [standard deviation (SD)] age was 51 [12] years (reoperation group; 49.9 [13.2] years, non-reoperation group; 50.7 [11.6] years). Mean [SD] Child-Pugh score was 9.3 [1.9] (reoperation group; 9.6 [1.9], non-reoperation group 9.1 [1.9]) and the mean [SD] model for end-stage liver disease score was 16.8 [7.3] (reoperation group; 17.6 [7.0], non-reoperation group; 16.6 [7.4]). There was no significant difference in the indications between the reoperation group and the non-reoperation group (Table 2). The indications for LT were liver cirrhosis caused by hepatitis C virus infection (reoperation group vs. non-reoperation group, 5 [18.5%] vs. 32 [38.1%], p = 0.052), liver cirrhosis caused by hepatitis B virus infection (2 [7.4%] vs. 13 [15.5%], p = 0.35), primary biliary cirrhosis (5 [18.5%] vs. 15 [17.8%], p>0.99), primary sclerosing cholangitis (5 [18.5%] vs. 15 [17.8%], p>0.99), alcoholic cirrhosis (2 [7.4%] vs. 5 [6.0%], p = 0.68), biliary atresia (1 [3.7%] vs. 2 [2.4%], p = 0.57), autoimmune hepatitis (1 [3.7%] vs. 2 [2.4%], p = 0.57), fulminant hepatitis (6 [22.3%] vs. 7 [8.3%], p = 0.07), and others (5 [18.5%] vs. 2 [2.4%]).

Profiles of early reoperation

Early reoperations after LDLT (reoperation group) were performed in 27 recipients (24.3%) on POD 10 [9.4]. Among them, 19 cases (70.4%) were performed within 10 days after LDLT and 5 cases (18.5%) required multiple reoperations. Table 3 lists the reasons for reoperation, which comprised mainly postoperative bleeding (n = 13, 48%), vessel problems (n = 8, 30%), and biliary complications (n = 5, 19%). One recipient underwent reoperation for strangulated bowel obstruction. Early graft loss subsequent to early reoperation occurred in 4 cases. Two recipients had graft loss subsequent to reoperation for portal venous thrombosis and simultaneous hepatic artery and portal venous thrombosis, and both underwent successful retransplantation. The remaining two recipients underwent reoperation for biliary problems, one for severe biliary leakage and the other for biliary stricture with severe cholangitis, both of which finally resulted in graft loss; only one recipient was saved by retransplantation.

Table 1. Characteristics of reoperation and non-reoperation cases after LDLT.

Variables			Total (n = 111)	Reoperation Group (n = 27, 24.3%)	Non-reoperation Group (n = 84, 75.7%)
Recipient factors					
	Age, y*		50.5 [12.0]	49.9 [13.2]	50.7 [11.6]
	Sex (female), n (%)		61 (55.0)	20 (74.1)	41 (48.8)
	Child-Pugh score, pts*		9.3 [1.9]	9.6 [1.9]	9.1 [1.9]
	MELD score, pts*		16.8 [7.3]	17.6 [7.0]	16.6 [7.4]
	Preoperative status (hospitalized), n (%)		5 (4.5)	1 (3.7)	4 (4.8)
	Preoperative blood data*				
		Albumin level, g/dL	2.9 [0.4]	2.8 [0.3]	2.9 [0.5]
		Serum creatinine, mg/dL	0.8 [0.5]	0.8 [0.3]	0.8 [0.6]
		Total bilirubin, mg/dL	8.9 [9.1]	8.9 [8.5]	9.0 [9.4]
		PT-INR	1.51 [0.68]	1.60 [0.46]	1.49 [0.74]
		Platelet count, $\times 10^4/\mu L$	8.8 [6.5]	8.9 [7.3]	8.7 [6.2]
Donors factors					
	Age, years*		39.6 [12.7]	38.6 [13.5]	39.6 [12.5]
	Sex (female), n (%)		60 (54.1)	15 (55.6)	45 (53.6)
	Graft type (LL: RL:PS)		40: 67: 4	12: 14: 1	28: 53: 3
	GV/SLV, %		45.4 [9.7]	45.5 [11.1]	45.4 [9.3]
	GV, g		528 [126]	504 [129]	536 [125]
Operative factors*					
	Operative time, min		788 [132]	801 [206]	783[99]
	Operative blood loss, L		5.5 [7.9]	7.7 [15.2]	4.8 [2.7]
	Transfusion				
		Red blood cell concentrate, U	9.5 [12.3]	13.6 [22.2]	8.2 [6.2]
		Fresh frozen plasma, U	21.2 [19.2]	29.8 [33.8]	18.4 [9.8]
		Platelet concentrate, U	24.6 [19.7]	25.9 [24.5]	24.2 [18.1]
	Biliary reconstruction, duct-to-duct, n (%)		99 (89.2)	25 (92.6)	74 (88.1)

Abbreviations: LDLT, living-donor liver transplantation; LL, left lobe; MELD, model for end-stage liver disease; PT-INR, international normalized ratio of prothrombin time; PS, posterior sector; RL, right lobe; GV, graft volume; SLV, standard liver volume.* mean [standard deviation].

Table 2. Comparison of primary disease between reoperation and non-reoperation cases after LDLT.

Variables	Total (n = 111)	Reoperation Group (n = 27, 24.3%)	Non-reoperation Group (n = 84, 75.7%)	p value
Liver cirrhosis-HCV	37 (33.4)	5 (18.5)	32 (38.1)	0.052
Liver cirrhosis-HBV	15 (13.5)	2 (7.4)	13 (15.5)	0.35
PBC	20 (18.1)	5 (18.5)	15 (17.8)	>0.99
PSC	6 (5.4)	0 (0)	6 (7.1)	0.33
Alcoholic cirrhosis	7 (6.3)	2 (7.4)	5 (6.0)	0.68
Biliary atresia	3 (2.7)	1 (3.7)	2 (2.4)	0.57
Autoimmune hepatitis	3 (2.7)	1 (3.7)	2 (2.4)	0.57
Fulminant hepatitis	13 (11.6)	6 (22.3)	7 (8.3)	0.07
Others	7 (6.3)	5 (18.5)	2 (2.4)	N.A.

Abbreviations: HCV, hepatitis C virus; HBV, hepatitis B virus; PBC, primary biliary cirrhosis, PBC; PSC, Primary sclerosing cholangitis; LDLT, living-donor liver transplantation; N.A., not applicable. n (%).

Risk factors for early reoperation

The results of analyses to identify risk factors for early reoperation in a Cox proportional hazard model were shown in Table 4. Recipient female sex (hazards ratio [HR] 2.63, 95% confidential intervals [CI] 1.17–6.72, p = 0.02), Child-Pugh class C (HR 2.27, 95% CI 1.04–5.29, p = 0.04), Non-HCV etiology (HR 2.44, 95%CI 1.00–7.28, p = 0.05), fulminant hepatitis (HR 2.78, 95%CI 1.02–6.49, p = 0.05), and the amount of fresh frozen plasma (FFP) administered (HR 1.01, 95% CI 1.00–1.02, p = 0.04) were demonstrated to be potential risk factors for early reoperation with p<0.10 in the univariable Cox model. Subsequent multivariable Cox model revealed that female sex (HR 2.90, 95% CI 1.18–8.27, p = 0.02) and the amount of FFP (HR 1.02, 95%CI 1.00–1.03, p = 0.03) were independent risk factors for early reoperation.

Graft and recipient survival in each group

Among the present cohort, early graft loss occurred in 10 cases, 4 in the reoperation group and 6 in the non-reoperation group. Mean follow-up time was 48.2 [25.9] months in the reoperation group and 50.6 [24.1] months in the non-reoperation group (p = 0.679). The 3-, 6-, 12-, and 36- month graft survival rates were 88.9% (95%CI, 70.7–96.4), 85.2%, (95%CI, 66.5–94.3), 85.2% (95%CI, 66.5–94.3), and 77.1% (95%CI, 57.4–89.4), respectively, in the reoperation group (n = 27), and 95.2% (95%CI, 88.0–98.2), 92.9% (95%CI, 85.0–96.8), 89.3% (95%CI, 80.7–94.3), and 88.1% (95%CI, 79.2–93.4), respectively, in the non-reoperation group (n = 84). The 1- and 3-year overall survival rates were 96.3% (95%CI, 77.9–99.5), and 88.3% (95%CI, 69.3–96.2), respectively, in the reoperation group, and 89.3% (95%CI,

Table 3. Reasons of reoperation after LDLT.

Variables		Number of cases (n = 27)	Early graft loss, n (%)
Postoperative bleeding		13	
	Graft surface	4	0
	Diaphragm	3	0
	Hepatic artery	3	0
	Hilar plate	1	0
	Drain insertion site	1	0
	Undetected	1	0
Vessels		8	
	HAT	2	0
	PVT	3	1(33)
	Simultaneous HAT and PVT	1	1(100)
	Regurgitant portal flow	1	0
	The portal steal phenomenon in APOLT	1	0
Biliary tract		5	
	Biliary peritonitis	4	1 (25)
	Biliary stenosis	1	1 (100)
Others		1	
	Incarcerated obstruction of the jejunum	1	0

Abbreviations: LDLT, living-donor liver transplantation; HAT, hepatic artery thrombosis; PVT, portal vein thrombosis; APOLT, auxiliary partial orthotopic liver transplantation.

Table 4. Univariable and multivariable Cox proportional hazards model analysis to identify risk factors for early reoperation.

Variables		Univariable analysis			Multivariable analysis		
		HR	95% CI	p value	HR	95% CI	p value
Recipient factors							
	Age, years	0.99	0.97–1.03	0.72			
	Sex, female	2.63	1.17–6.72	0.02	2.90	1.18–8.27	0.02
	Child-Pugh, C vs A, B	2.27	1.04–5.29	0.04	1.47	0.61–3.67	0.39
	MELD score	1.01	0.96–1.06	0.57			
Preoperative blood data							
	Albumin level, g/dL	0.87	0.37–1.99	0.75			
	Serum creatinine, mg/dL	0.71	0.22–1.47	0.43			
	Total bilirubin, mg/dL	1.00	0.95–1.04	0.97			
	PT-INR	1.17	0.67–1.62	0.50			
	Platelet count, $\times 10^4/\mu L$	1.00	0.94–1.06	0.87			
Primary disease							
	Non-HCV vs others	2.44	1.00–7.28	0.05	1.59	0.60–4.98	0.37
	Fulminant hepatitis vs others	2.78	1.02–6.49	0.05	2.44	0.84–6.45	0.10
Donors factors							
	Age, years	0.99	0.96–1.02	0.69			
	Sex, female	1.15	0.40–1.86	0.72			
	GV/SLV, %	1.00	0.96–1.04	0.87			
	GV, g	1.00	0.99–1.00	0.18			
Operative factors							
	Operative time, min	1.00	1.00–1.003	0.58			
	Operative blood loss, L	1.00	1.00–1.00004	0.16			
Transfusion							
	RCC, U	1.02	1.00–1.03	0.10			
	FFP, U	1.01	1.00–1.02	0.04			
	PC, U	1.00	0.98–1.02	0.74			
	Biliary duct-to-duct	1.61	0.48–9.98	0.49	1.02	1.00–1.03	0.03

Abbreviations: LDLT, living-donor liver transplantation; MELD, model for end-stage liver disease; PT-INR, international normalized ratio of prothrombin time; GV, graft volume; SLV, standard liver volume; RCC, red blood cell concentrate; FFP, fresh frozen plasma; PC, platelet concentration.

80.7–94.3) and 88.0% (95%CI, 79.2–93.4), respectively, in the non-reoperation group. Graft and recipient survival did not differ significantly between groups (the log-rank test, p = 0.31, and 0.59, respectively) (Figure 1). A multivariable Cox proportional hazards model was applied to evaluate the risk of early reoperation for graft survival adjusting for other potential risk factors (female sex; HR 2.67, 95%CI 1.02–8.27, p = 0.05, GV/SLV; HR 1.05, 95%CI 1.00–1.09, p = 0.06) (Table 5). Reoperation was not a significant risk factor for graft survival (HR 1.28, 95% CI 0.45–3.29, p = 0.63). No significant risk factors for overall survival were identified in a Cox proportional hazards model. The duration of postoperative hospital stay was significantly longer in the reoperation group than in non-reoperation group (99 [117] vs. 52 [29]; p<0.01).

Discussion

In the present study, 24% (27/111) of LDLT recipients required early reoperation, comparable to previous reports [10–12]. The causes of reoperation, most of which were categorized as postoperative bleeding, vascular complications, and biliary complications, were also consistent with those in previous reports [10–12]. Early reoperation places additional surgical stress on each recipient, which may theoretically have a negative impact on both the graft and recipient. Previous reports have indicated an impaired graft/overall survival rate of recipients with early reoperation [10,12]. In the current study, early reoperation also tended to lead decreased graft survival rate. However, overall survival rates for recipients who underwent reoperation were comparable to those who did not, and therefore, our results

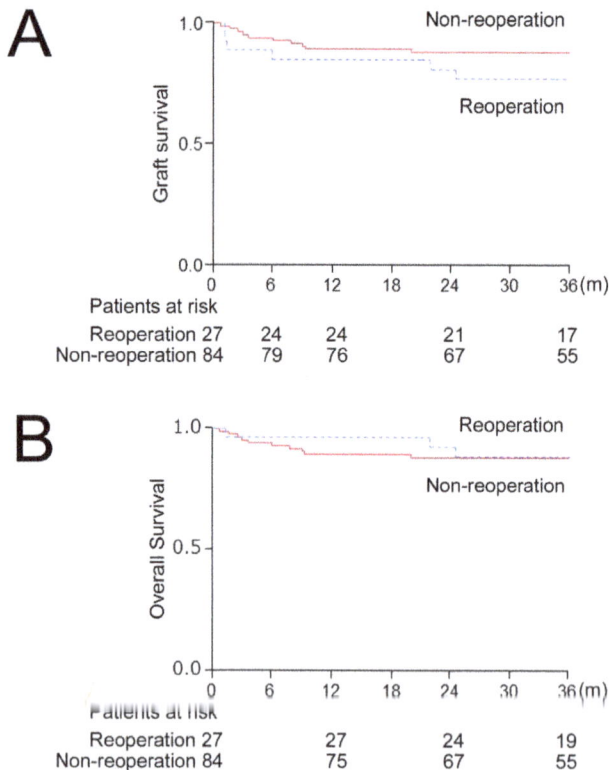

Figure 1. Graft and overall survival. (A) Graft survival rates for the reoperation group and the non-reoperation group. p = 0.31(the log-rank test). **(B)** Overall survival rates for the reoperation group and the non-reoperation group. p = 0.59 (the log-rank test).

enhance the importance of vigilant surveillance for early postoperative complication and early surgical rescue.

The reoperation rate after LT is reported to be high, ranging from 9.2% to 34% [10–13], while the reoperation rate after liver resection is reported to be as low as 2.5% to 10.9% [14–16]. In fact, at our institute, reoperations were performed for only 3 cases (2.7%) among 111 corresponding donors for biliary leakage (2 cases, 1.8%) and postoperative bleeding (1 case, 0.9%). The reasons for the increased rate of reoperation after LT could be attributed to poor recipient preoperative condition with hepatic failure, the administration of particular drugs such as immuno-suppressants and anticoagulants, and the need for meticulous vessel reconstructions, including the hepatic vein, hepatic artery, portal vein, and bile duct [20–22]. The reoperation rate is reported to be even higher for LDLT than for DDLT [11,20,23].

Regarding risk factors for early reoperation, female sex, Child-Pugh class C, Non-HCV etiology, fulminant hepatitis, and the amount of intraoperative FFP administered were identified as possibly predictive variables, among which female sex and the amount of intraoperative FFP were identified as independent risk factors by multivariable analysis. Hendriks et al. [10] and Kappa et al. [13] reported that intraoperative blood loss predicted early reoperation. Child-Pugh class C and the amount of intraoperative FFP, which represent poor recipient liver function and have been associated with poor recipient outcome [24,25], can reasonably be associated with early reoperation after liver transplantation, although, to the best of our knowledge, this is the first report demonstrating a higher early reoperation rate in more seriously ill recipients. Although there is no previous reports supporting the reason for female sex as a predictive risk factors of reoperation in liver transplantation, in the setting of coronary stenting, there is the preponderance of evidence supporting that female had increased risk of in-hospital death and complications [26,27]. One possible reason in our study is that female recipient has significant smaller body and graft size in comparison with male (body height; female vs male, 156.6 [7.1] cm vs 170.5 [5.9] cm, p<0.01, body weight; 52.8 [8.4] kg vs 69.1 [9.9] kg, p<0.01, and graft size; 486.6 [127.7] g vs 579.4 [105.0] g, p<0.01), which might indicate the possible technical complications in smaller vessel reconstructions as reported in liver transplantation in children [28].

One concern for patients with liver failure and LT recipients is hemostatic balance [29]. While routine laboratory tests of these patients show bleeding diathesis, they are actually in hemostatic balance, because both pro- and antihemostatic factors are affected, the latter of which are not well reflected in routine coagulation testing [30]. This balance, however, can easily be tipped toward a hypo- or hypercoagulable state [31]. Our results demonstrating the high incidence of postoperative hemorrhage and vessel thrombosis as the cause for reoperation despite close monitoring with heparin administration, are representative of this situation. Further studies to investigate the ideal balance of coagulability are needed to reduce the incidence of early reoperation after LDLT.

Recently, Yoshiya et al. [12] of the Kyushu group and Hendriks et al. [10] reported that early reoperation was significantly associated with poor graft and/or recipient survival after LDLT and DDLT, respectively. In the present study, observed graft survival for the recipients who underwent reoperation was also lower compared to those who did not, though the result was not significantly different. Overall survival in the reoperation group was comparable to that in the non-reoperation group (Figure 1). These results in our study imply the importance of vigilant surveillance for early complications and early surgical interventions to improve graft/overall survival of recipients. However, the

Table 5. Univariable and multivariable Cox proportional hazards model analysis for graft survival.

Variables		Univariable analysis			Multivariable analysis		
		HR	95% CI	p value	HR	95% CI	p value
Reoperation		1.54	0.54–3.89	0.40	1.28	0.45–3.29	0.63
Recipient factors							
Age, years		0.99	0.96–1.03	0.51			
Sex, female		2.67	1.02–8.27	0.05	2.54	0.95–7.94	0.06
Child-Pugh, C vs A, B		1.00	0.40–2.50	0.99			
MELD score		1.05	0.99–1.11	0.14			
Preoperative blood data							
	Albumin level, g/dL	0.92	0.33–2.44	0.87			
	Serum creatinine, mg/dL	1.36	0.66–2.12	0.34			
	Total bilirubin, mg/dL	1.03	0.98–1.07	0.28			
	PT-INR	1.23	0.69–1.70	0.40			
	Platelet count, $\times10^4/\mu L$	1.01	0.93–1.07	0.86			
Primary disease							
	Non-HCV vs others	1.11	0.32–2.28	0.83			
	Fulminant hepatitis vs others	2.37	0.67–6.53	0.16			
Donors factors							
Age, years		0.95	0.38–2.38	0.90			
Sex, female		1.15	0.40–1.86	0.72			
GV/SLV, %		1.05	1.00–1.09	0.06	1.04	1.00–1.09	0.06
GV, g		1.00	1.00–1.004	0.70			
Operative factors							
Operative time, min		1.00	1.00–1.002	0.61			
Operative blood loss, L		1.00	1.00–1.00003	0.40			
Transfusion							
	RCC, U	0.99	0.92–1.02	0.60			
	FFP, U	1.00	0.96–1.01	0.85			
	PC, U	0.99	0.97–1.02	0.64			
Biliary duct-to-duct		0.65	0.21–2.77	0.51			

Abbreviations: LDLT, living-donor liver transplantation; MELD, model for end-stage liver disease; PT-INR, international normalized ratio of prothrombin time; GV, graft volume; SLV, standard liver volume; RCC, red blood cell concentrate; FFP, fresh frozen plasma; PC, platelet concentration.

different results between our study (4 early graft losses [14.8%] in 27 recipients with reoperation) and the Kyushu group study (10 graft losses [34.5%] in 26 recipients with reoperation) need further investigation. The learning curve, as suggested by Kyushu group, as well as the radiologic and hematologic assays used to detect early complications, and differences in the criteria for reoperation might partially explain the discrepancy.

The main limitations of our study are its retrospective nature, the small number of cases, and biases caused by learning curves of surgical techniques and postoperative management. The early reoperation group was a small inhomogenous cohort with various causes for reoperation, which may make the data inadequate to support the findings with a multivariable analysis. Further analyses with a large number of patients in a well-designed multicenter study are needed to clarify the impact of early reoperation on outcome.

In conclusion, observed graft survival for the recipients who underwent reoperation was lower compared to those who did not undergo reoperation, though the result was not significantly different. Recipient overall survival with reoperation was comparable to that without reoperation. Independent risk factors for reoperation were recipient female sex and the amount of intraoperative FFP in our study. The present findings enhance the importance of vigilant surveillance for early postoperative complication and early surgical rescue at a postoperative period in the LDLT setting.

Supporting Information

Checklist S1 This study was conducted based on the STROBE statement.

Author Contributions

Conceived and designed the experiments: YK Y. Sugawara. Performed the experiments: NA JK TH TT. Analyzed the data: TI ST TA Y. Sakamoto. Contributed reagents/materials/analysis tools: KH. Wrote the paper: YK Y. Sugawara NK.

References

1. Starzl TE, Klintmalm GB, Porter KA, Iwatsuki S, Schroter GP (1981) Liver transplantation with use of cyclosporin a and prednisone. N Engl J Med 305: 266–269.
2. Sugawara Y, Makuuchi M, Kaneko J, Ohkubo T, Imamura H, et al. (2002) Correlation between optimal tacrolimus doses and the graft weight in living donor liver transplantation. Clin Transplant 16: 102–106.
3. Sugawara Y, Makuuchi M, Akamatsu N, Kishi Y, Niiya T, et al. (2004) Refinement of venous reconstruction using cryopreserved veins in right liver grafts. Liver Transpl 10: 541–547.
4. Kokudo N, Sugawara Y, Imamura H, Sano K, Makuuchi M (2005) Tailoring the type of donor hepatectomy for adult living donor liver transplantation. Am J Transplant 5: 1694–1703.
5. Pomposelli JJ, Verbesey J, Simpson MA, Lewis WD, Gordon FD, et al. (2006) Improved survival after live donor adult liver transplantation (LDALT) using right lobe grafts: program experience and lessons learned. Am J Transplant 6: 589–598.
6. Jain A, Reyes J, Kashyap R, Dodson SF, Demetris AJ, et al. (2000) Long-term survival after liver transplantation in 4,000 consecutive patients at a single center. Ann Surg 232: 490–500.
7. (2010) Liver transplantation in Japan: registry by the Japanese Liver Transplantation Society. Jap J Transpl 46: 524–536.
8. Adam R, McMaster P, O'Grady JG, Castaing D, Klempnauer JL, et al. (2003) Evolution of liver transplantation in Europe: report of the European Liver Transplant Registry. Liver Transpl 9: 1231–1243.
9. The Organ Procurement and Transplantation Network. http://optn.transplant.hrsa.gov/accessed on 2014 July 14.
10. Hendriks HG, van der Meer J, de Wolf JT, Peeters PM, Porte RJ, et al. (2005) Intraoperative blood transfusion requirement is the main determinant of early surgical re-intervention after orthotopic liver transplantation. Transpl Int 17: 673–679.
11. Freise CE, Gillespie BW, Koffron AJ, Lok AS, Pruett TL, et al. (2008) Recipient morbidity after living and deceased donor liver transplantation: findings from the A2ALL Retrospective Cohort Study. Am J Transplant 8: 2569–2579.
12. Yoshiya S, Shirabe K, Kimura K, Yoshizumi T, Ikegami T, et al. (2012) The Causes, Risk Factors, and Outcomes of Early Relaparotomy After Living-Donor Liver Transplantation. Transplantation Journal 94: 947–952.
13. Kappa SF, Gorden DL, Davidson MA, Wright JK, Guillamondegui OD (2010) Intraoperative blood loss predicts hemorrhage-related reoperation after orthotopic liver transplantation. Am Surg 76: 969–973.
14. Schroeder RA, Marroquin CE, Bute BP, Khuri S, Henderson WG, et al. (2006) Predictive indices of morbidity and mortality after liver resection. Ann Surg 243: 373–379.
15. Barbas AS, Turley RS, Mallipeddi MK, Lidsky ME, Reddy SK, et al. (2013) Examining reoperation and readmission after hepatic surgery. J Am Coll Surg 216: 915–923.
16. Imamura H, Seyama Y, Kokudo N, Maema A, Sugawara Y, et al. (2003) One thousand fifty-six hepatectomies without mortality in 8 years. Arch Surg 138: 1198–1206; discussion 1206.
17. Urata K, Kawasaki S, Matsunami H, Hashikura Y, Ikegami T, et al. (1995) Calculation of child and adult standard liver volume for liver transplantation. Hepatology 21: 1317–1321.
18. Sugawara Y, Makuuchi M, Kaneko J, Ohkubo T, Matsui Y, et al. (2003) Living-donor liver transplantation in adults: Tokyo University experience. J Hepato-biliary Pancreat Surg 10: 1–4.
19. Rahbari NN, Garden OJ, Padbury R, Maddern G, Koch M, et al. (2011) Post-hepatectomy haemorrhage: a definition and grading by the International Study Group of Liver Surgery (ISGLS). HPB (Oxford) 13: 528–535.
20. Duailibi DF, Ribeiro MA Jr (2010) Biliary complications following deceased and living donor liver transplantation. Transplant Proc 42: 517–520.
21. Soong RS, Chan KM, Chou HS, Wu TJ, Lee CF, et al. (2012) The risk factors for early infection in adult living donor liver transplantation recipients. Transplant Proc 44: 784–786.
22. Arshad F, Lisman T, Porte RJ (2013) Hypercoagulability as a contributor to thrombotic complications in the liver transplant recipient. Liver Int 33: 820–827.
23. Khalaf H (2010) Vascular complications after deceased and living donor liver transplantation: a single-center experience. Transplant Proc 42: 865–870.
24. Onaca NN, Levy MF, Sanchez EQ, Chinnakotla S, Fasola CG, et al. (2003) A correlation between the pretransplantation MELD score and mortality in the first two years after liver transplantation. Liver Transpl 9: 117–123.
25. Kamath PS, Wiesner RH, Malinchoc M, Kremers W, Therneau TM, et al. (2001) A model to predict survival in patients with end-stage liver disease. Hepatology 33: 464–470.
26. Anderson ML, Peterson ED, Brennan JM, Rao SV, Dai D, et al. (2012) Short- and long-term outcomes of coronary stenting in women versus men: results from the National Cardiovascular Data Registry Centers for Medicare & Medicaid services cohort. Circulation 126: 2190–2199.
27. Peterson ED, Lansky AJ, Kramer J, Anstrom K, Lanzilotta MJ (2001) Effect of gender on the outcomes of contemporary percutaneous coronary intervention. Am J Cardiol 88: 359–364.
28. Sanada Y, Wakiya T, Hishikawa S, Hirata Y, Yamada N, et al. (2013) Risk factors and treatments for hepatic arterial complications in pediatric living donor liver transplantation. J Hepatobiliary Pancreat Sci.
29. Lisman T, Caldwell SH, Burroughs AK, Northup PG, Senzolo M, et al. (2010) Hemostasis and thrombosis in patients with liver disease: the ups and downs. J Hepatol 53: 362–371.
30. Tripodi A, Primignani M, Chantarangkul V, Dell'Era A, Clerici M, et al. (2009) An imbalance of pro- vs anti-coagulation factors in plasma from patients with cirrhosis. Gastroenterology 137: 2105–2111.
31. Lisman T, Porte RJ (2009) Hepatic artery thrombosis after liver transplantation: more than just a surgical complication? Transpl Int 22: 162–164.

Stage-Specific Binding Profiles of Cohesin in Resting and Activated B Lymphocytes Suggest a Role for Cohesin in Immunoglobulin Class Switching and Maturation

Gamze Günal-Sadık[1], Maciej Paszkowski-Rogacz[2], Kalaimathy Singaravelu[3], Andreas Beyer[3,4], Frank Buchholz[2], Rolf Jessberger[1]*

Institute of Physiological Chemistry, Faculty of Medicine Carl Gustav Carus, Dresden University of Technology, Dresden, Germany, **2** Department of Medical Systems Biology, University Hospital and Medical Faculty Carl Gustav Carus, Dresden University of Technology, Dresden, Germany, **3** Cellular Networks and Systems Biology, Biotechnology Center, Dresden University of Technology, Dresden, Germany, **4** CECAD, Universität zu Köln, Köln, Germany

Abstract

The immunoglobulin heavy chain locus (Igh) features higher-order chromosomal interactions to facilitate stage-specific assembly of the Ig molecule. Cohesin, a ring-like protein complex required for sister chromatid cohesion, shapes chromosome architecture and chromatin interactions important for transcriptional regulation and often acts together with CTCF. Cohesin is likely involved in B cell activation and Ig class switch recombination. Hence, binding profiles of cohesin in resting mature murine splenic B lymphocytes and at two stages after cell activation were elucidated by chromatin immunoprecipitation and deep sequencing. Comparative genomic analysis revealed cohesin extensively changes its binding to transcriptional control elements after 48 h of stimulation with LPS/IL-4. Cohesin was clearly underrepresented at switch regions regardless of their activation status, suggesting that switch regions need to be cohesin-poor. Specific binding changes of cohesin at B-cell specific gene loci *Pax5* and *Blimp-1* indicate new cohesin-dependent regulatory pathways. Together with conserved cohesin/CTCF sites at the *Igh* 3′RR, a prominent cohesin/CTCF binding site was revealed near the 3′ end of Cα where PolII localizes to 3′ enhancers. Our study shows that cohesin likely regulates B cell activation and maturation, including Ig class switching.

Editor: Brian P. Chadwick, Florida State University, United States of America

Funding: This work was supported by the SFB655 (DFG) to RJ and FB, the TUD "Support-the-best" program to FB, and by the EU (SyBoSS FP7-242129) to AB. The funders had no role in study design, data collection and analysis, decision to publish, or preparation of the manuscript.

Competing Interests: The authors have declared that no competing interests exist.

* Email: Rolf.Jessberger@tu-dresden.de

Introduction

Cohesin is a chromosome-associated multi-protein complex, conserved from yeast to man, is essential for sister chromatid cohesion, and is involved in DNA repair and recombination (for recent reviews on cohesin see [1,2,3,4,5,6]. The somatic cohesin complex is composed of two members of the Structural Maintenance of Chromosomes family of proteins, SMC1 and SMC3, the kleisin RAD21, and either protein SA1 or SA2. SMC1 and SMC3 polypeptides form a V-shape heterodimer, linked at the central hinge domains of the two SMCs. The kleisin connects the ATPase heads of the two SMC proteins, thereby forming a ring-like structure, with which the SA protein associates. This ring or multiple rings connects two double-stranded DNA molecules.

In addition to its role in sister chromatid cohesion, the cohesin protein complex facilitates several kinds of chromatin interactions, some of which are cell type-specific [7,8,9,10,11]. Cohesin/CTCF co-localisation also aids transcriptional regulation and insulation [12,13]. Cohesin regulates transcription through physical interaction with the mediator complex and juxtaposing enhancer and promoter regions during transcription [14,15]. In T cells, Rad21

deficiency led to reduced promoter-enhancer looping at the TCRa locus associated with transcriptional changes [16].

Throughout B cell development, the immunoglobulin heavy chain (IgH) locus undergoes various conformational changes such as locus compaction to assure stage-specific assembly of Ig molecule [17,18]. These conformational changes are facilitated by transcription factors, including YY1 and PAX5, and other chromatin-binding factors (Jhunjhunwala et al., 2008). EBF1 is another transcription factor that modulates B cell fate and is a downstream target of AID [19,20]. Recent studies revealed that the co-localization of cohesin and CTCF at the variable *Igh* segments affects the usage of V gene segments during V(D)J recombination in pre B cells. Cohesin and CTCF facilitate long-range interactions between the V genes, the Eμ enhancer and some 3′ cohesin/CTCF binding sites [21,22].

Mature B cells perform class switch recombination (CSR) upon antigen stimulation to diversify a constant antigen specificity into different effector functions by changing the constant region of the Ig molecule [23]. Following the introduction of double-strand breaks at switch (S) regions, located upstream of each Ig constant region, a DNA-loop is formed between the donor and acceptor S regions. The intervening DNA is excised and both ends are repaired by a mechanism involving the non-homologous end-joining pathway. Initiation of CSR requires transcription of the enzyme activation-induced deaminase (AID), which is essential for introducing DSBs at or near S regions. The *Igh* locus becomes accessible for AID when non-coding germ-line transcription (GLT) occurs at the specific S region to act as the target of CSR. GLT starts at intronic (I) promoters 5′ of the S regions. GLT requires long-range interactions between the common Eμ locus enhancer at the 5′, the respective I promoter, and the 3′ regulatory regions (3′RR) of the *Igh* locus [23].

Initiation of germline transcription, formation of double strand breaks at the switch (S) regions, and maintenance of synapsis between the donor and acceptor S regions likely require long-range chromosomal interactions within the Ig heavy chain locus [23,24]. How these interactions are facilitated and regulated, and which factors are involved remains to be elucidated. Since cohesin topologically links two DNA molecules such as sister chromatids or intrachromosomally, cohesin is a candidate to facilitate these processes or to restrict them to the proper chromosomal regions. Initial evidence for a role of cohesin in regulating Ig class switch recombination in a B cell line was presented very recently [25].

To elucidate a potential role of cohesin in Ig class switching in primary B cells we investigated the association of cohesin before, during, and at a late stage of Ig class switching of murine splenic B cells. We used chromatin immuno precipitation (ChIP) of the cohesin subunit RAD21 followed by deep sequencing and determined binding profiles of cohesin that are stage- and region-specific.

Results

Cohesin associates with the Igh locus in a stage-specific manner

To obtain insights into the potential role of cohesin during CSR, we traced the differential binding of the cohesin subunit RAD21 to chromatin in purified B cells, which were left unstimulated (day 0) or were stimulated with IL-4 and LPS to induce the switch to IgG1. The B cells were analyzed at 48 h and at 96 h after induction of Ig class switching. Up to 21% of B220-positive B cells expressed IgG1 on the cell surface after 96 h of stimulation (Fig S1). At 96 h, typically app. 22% of the cells express the plasma cell marker syndecan (CD138). IgG1 positive B cells were purified and enriched by negative selection to eliminate chromatin derived from cells that did not switch after 96 h hours of stimulation (Fig. S1).

Peak calling and analysis of RAD21 ChIP-Seq data revealed that cohesin binds to B cell chromatin in a stage-specific manner. Peak calling with a stringent cut-off criteria of 0.05 false discovery rate (FDR) identified 5687 cohesin binding sites in resting B cells (Fig. 1A), and 5547 binding sites in cells stimulated for 48 h with LPS and IL-4. The 96 h-stimulated B cells revealed 12803 binding sites for cohesin, implying either that cohesin binding to chromatin is more abundant in B cells stimulated for 96 h, or that the 96 h culture was more uniform, which may have resulted in a better signal-to-noise ratio and thus higher confidence peak calling. Nevertheless, the distribution of peaks clearly changed between resting, 48 h and 96 h stimulated cells.

We analyzed three biological replicates. Each replicate consisted of purified B cells pooled from 12 mice. Between all three time points 2383 sites were shared, and 140 sites were unique to the resting state. The 48 h time point yielded 2120 unique cohesin sites, and 6985 sites were only present in 96 h-stimulated cells. We conclude that cohesin occupancy significantly differs before,

during and at a late stage of LPS/IL-4 induced B cell activation and Ig class switching.

Extensive changes of cohesin binding at gene expression control regions

Since cohesin contributes to the control of gene expression and since the induction of Ig class switching involves B cell activation and specific changes in gene expression, we analyzed the cohesin binding sites specific for either time point for their potential association with transcription. Cohesin association with transcriptional elements was determined using RefSeq gene annotations through cis-regulatory element annotation system (CEAS) [26]. We compared binding of cohesin to a selected region to the average genome-wide binding.

In resting B cells, cohesin significantly (p<0.0001) binds about 4-fold more frequently to promoter regions at a distance of <1 kb, <2 kb and <3 kb from the start site than to average genomic regions (Fig. 1B). Within coding exons, however, cohesin was not enriched. Cohesin was found app. 2-fold more frequently at downstream regions of genes and app. 5-fold more frequently at 5′UTRs, but underrepresented at the 3′UTR.

At day 2 this pattern completely changed. There was no enrichment or depletion for cohesin at any of the promoter or downstream regions, nor at the 5′UTRs. Thus, upon induction of Ig class switching cohesin became redistributed to a genomic average at these loci. The underrepresentation of cohesin at 3′UTRs was maintained, but the coding exons became depleted of cohesin.

At the late 96 h time point, a cohesin pattern was re-established that largely reflected that of resting B cells. The differences were not as succinct, but cohesin was enriched app. 2-fold at promoter and downstream regions and at the 5′UTR. Cohesin was mildly enriched at coding exons. The only large difference to resting cells is in 3′UTRs, which are less bound by cohesin in resting B cells, but cohesin-enriched in B cells at day 4.

This data suggest a very significant reshuffling of cohesin at genes and their transcriptional control elements when B cells become activated and switch their Ig class.

Cohesin is underrepresented at switch regions

It remains largely elusive how remote S regions are brought into physical proximity and how the synapsis between donor and acceptor S regions is maintained through CSR. S regions have not yet been analyzed with respect to cohesin association. To determine whether cohesin may be involved in establishment and/or maintenance of S/S synapsis, we searched for cohesin enrichment at S regions at the three time points. We measured the RAD21 reads at the centers of Sμ and Sγ1 and at increasing distance from these centers. The reads were normalized to input control. Based on this, the enrichment plots were generated to show the cohesin representation at and next to the S regions (Fig. 2). To validate the approach, a random peak was chosen to display the enrichment around this peak's center. Our analysis revealed that cohesin is under-represented for up to >10-fold at S regions in resting and at both time points after activation of class switching (Fig. 2B). At the latter two time points, cohesin was even further reduced compared to resting B cells. Similar results were obtained for the Sγ2a region, indicating that lower cohesin binding is not specific to the Sμ and Sγ1 regions. Like at Sμ and Sγ1, there was even less cohesin bound after B cell activation although Sγ2a does not undergo switch recombination. Since S regions thus feature a cohesin-poor environment, we speculate that facilitation of Sμ/Sx region synapsis by cohesin is rather unlikely.

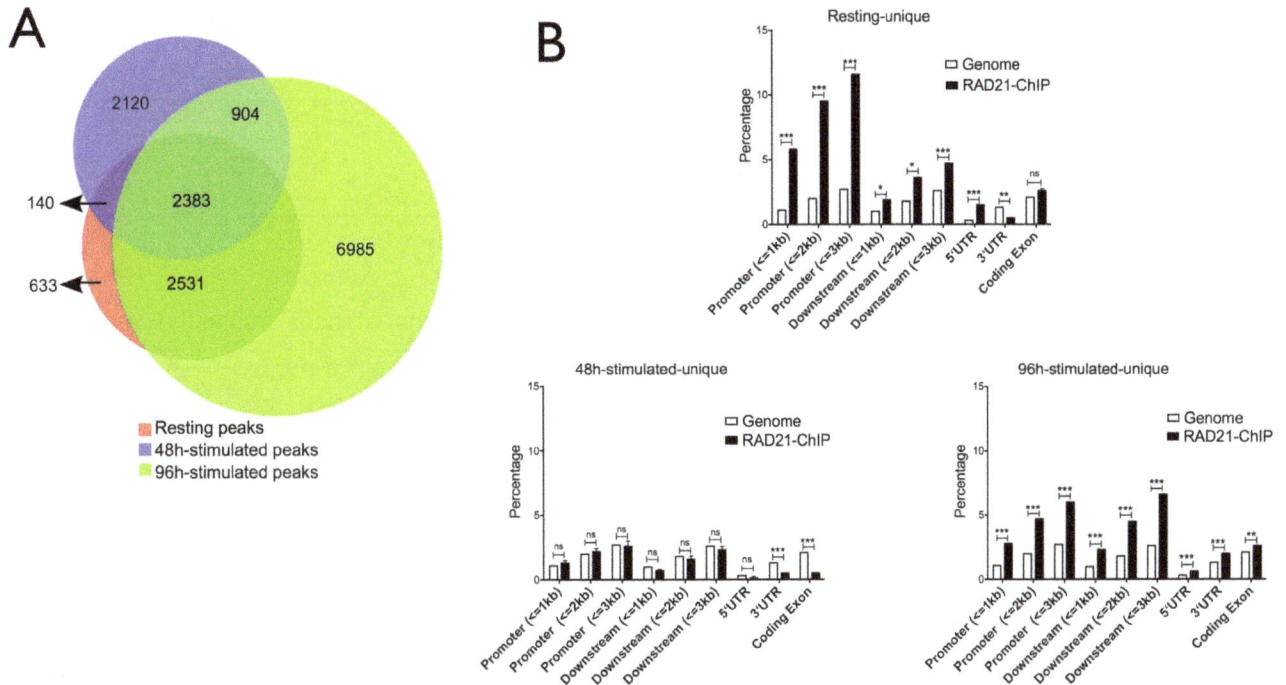

Figure 1. Cohesin binding sites. (A) Overlapping peaks of cohesin binding in cells with or without stimulation. Venn diagrams depict unique and common binding sites for cohesin in three different ChIP conditions based on 3 replicates, each using purified B cells pooled from 12 mice. Resting B cells: cohesin binding sites in the resting state. 48 h-stimulated B cells: binding sites detected after 48 hour stimulation of LPS and IL-4. 96 h-stimulate B cells: binding sites detected after 96 hours of stimulation with LPS and IL-4. (B) Enrichment of chromosomal features of ChIP regions. Cohesin peaks were aligned to RefSeq gene annotations by the use of CEAS tool. Each graph is based on sites unique to the indicated time point. Significance determined by one-sided binominal test. Asterisks represent p-values; ***: p<0.0001, **: p<0.001, ns: p>0.05.

Cohesin binds to shared and unique sites at the Igh locus

RAD21 cohesin binds to CTCF sites in proB cells and it is likely that cohesin and CTCF facilitate V(D)J recombination by modulating long-range interactions in pro-B cells [9,19]. To start elucidating whether cohesin may play a similar role in class switch recombination, we traced the genome wide differential binding of cohesin at the *Igh* locus.

To test the potential impact of cohesin binding on class switch recombination, in particular transcription associated to CSR, cohesin binding sites at the *Igh* locus were investigated and potential co-binding of cohesin with CTCF, PolII and B cell transcription factors PAX5 and EBF1 analyzed [20,27,28].

Publicly available ChIP-Seq raw data were processed and used for comparison. We first analyzed differential binding of cohesin, CTCF in *Rag1$^{-/-}$* pro-B cells and EBF1 in resting splenic mature B cells (Table S1).

Our analysis revealed that the *Igh* locus enhancer Eμ, which is shown to be in physical proximity of the 3′RR region, is bound by cohesin neither in pro-B cells nor in mature B cells (Fig. S2) [21]. CTCF is enriched (please consider the scale, adjusted to the very strong 3′ CTCF signals) at the Eμ enhancer in mature B cells, implying that the Eμ-3′RR interaction might be facilitated via CTCF at these sites but not by cohesin binding, suggesting a cohesin-independent action of CTCF. Co-localization of EBF1 and PolII at Eμ provides further evidence for Eμ enhancer activity in mature B cells.

Since frequent cohesin binding was observed at the 3′RR (Fig. S2), we analyzed this in more detail. The 3′ end of the murine *Igh* locus contains four quasi-palindromic DNAseI hypersensitive sites

(HS3a, HS1,2, HS3b and HS4) that are required for CSR [29]. Downstream of HS1-4 localizes another subset of hypersensitive sites (HS5-7) that possess conserved, overlapping CTCF and cohesin binding sites [30]. The deletion of HS5-7 region had no effect on CSR [31].

In addition to the common cohesin/CTCF sites at the 3′ end of the *Igh* locus, we identified a rather novel cohesin/CTCF site towards the 3′ end of the intronic α constant region (intronic Cα-iCα), which overlaps with the initiation of PolII enrichment in activated mature B cells (Fig. 3). This site was only very recently described in an activated B cell line [25]. PolII enrichment indicates the active transcription through HS1-4 DNAseI hypersensitive sites and the novel cohesin/CTCF site marks the initiation of this transcription. We hypothesize that this stage-specific cohesin/CTCF site is likely to be necessary for the transcription of 3′ enhancer units that are critical for class switch recombination. Transcription factors EBF1 and PAX5 bind to HS5-7 only at one site, 3RR2 (Fig. 3 and Fig. S3).

In addition to 3′ cohesin binding events, a prominent cohesin binding site (5′HS) at the 5′ flanking region of *Igh* is observed (Fig. S4). This site corresponds to a hypersensitive site located in an intronic region of the neighboring 5′ gene, *Zfp386* [32]. This 5′HS is bound by CTCF in pro- and mature B cells, but cohesin binding is present only in mature B cells. Cohesin is diminished at day 2 when the B cells undergo class switching and re-appears at day 4. EBF1 is not present at this site, although RNA PolII shows a moderate peak. Although an *Igh*-regulatory role has previously been suggested for this HS site, the site was shown to have no effect on CSR or on VDJ recombination [32,33].

A

B

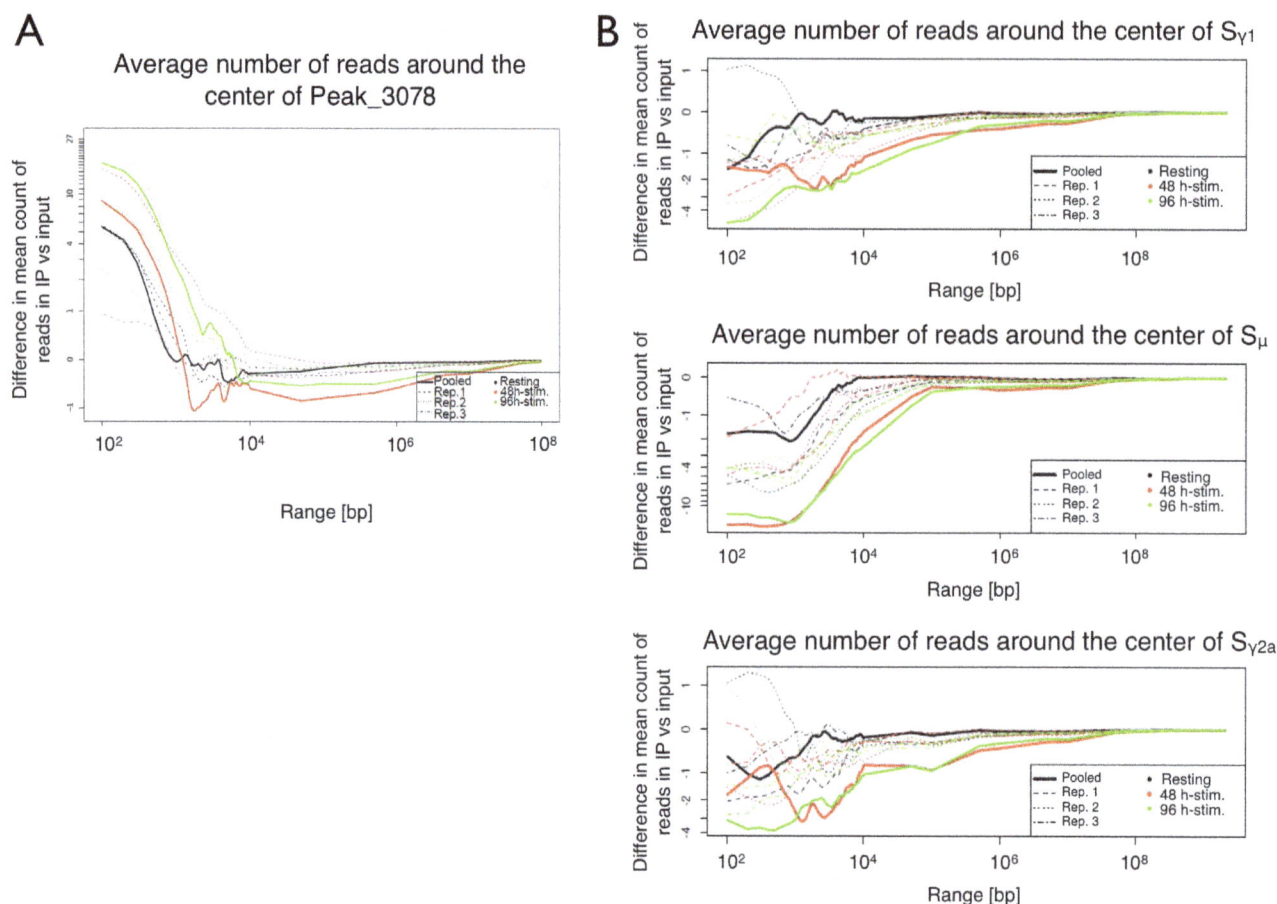

Figure 2. Cohesin representation at S regions. (A) A prominent MACS peak used as control (Peak 3078). (B) Counts of immunoprecipitated fragments within the S regions are plotted against the center of S regions. The coordinates of the regions under investigation: Peak 3078: chr12: 114384401-114384577; Sμ: chr12:114663654-114662317; Sγ1: chr12:114576873-114571615; Sγ2a: chr12:114530197-114533786.

Changes of cohesin binding patterns at B cell-relevant gene loci

Since cohesin regulates transcription we also analyzed stage-specific cohesin binding changes at gene loci of particular importance for B cell biology.

Binding changes of cohesin at the *Aicda* locus are of interest with respect to a potential role of cohesin in modulation of CSR, since stage-specific expression of AID is indispensible for CSR. We determined shared CTCF/cohesin sites (Fig. S5) that are present in the first intron (site a), the last exon (site c) and in the second intron (site b) of the AID gene. The first intron (site a) contains low amounts of CTCF and cohesin, but it is specific to mature B cells. However, sites a and b were not detected as statistically significant cohesin peaks with the applied 0.05 FDR cut-off, although at a slightly less stringent cut-off they were. The CTCF enrichments at those sites were significant (Fig. S5). Cohesin was not enriched at the *Aicda* gene in 48 h-stimulated B cells.

The expression of B cell master regulator PAX5 is diminished as B cells differentiate into plasma cells upon completion of class switching [34]. Therefore, we investigated differential binding of cohesin at the *Pax5* gene locus (Fig. 4A).

Correlation of CTCF, cohesin and EBF1 binding is often observed at sites of PolII enrichment (Fig. 4A and data not shown). One EBF1 binding site, site b, is enriched by cohesin and CTCF both in pro- and and mature B cells, whereas the upstream EBF1

site, site a, is enriched only for CTCF and only in mature B cells. This site corresponds to the TSS with high levels of PolII. These two EBF1 sites (a and b) are suggestive of a promoter-enhancer interaction since site b is identified as a cis-regulatory site important for B-cell specific Pax5 expression [35]. Cohesin binding at site number c appears only in switched B cells and is intronic. This site is also bound by CTCF. Site number d represents a site conserved for CTCF, but not for cohesin. Cohesin binding at this site is observed only after 96 hour of stimulation. Those two cohesin binding events might suggest a role for turning off *Pax5* gene expression as B cells express IgG1 on the cell surface and become plasma cells.

The transition of splenic mature B cells into plasma cells is modulated by the transcription factor BLIMP-1 (B lymphocyte-induced maturation protein-1). BLIMP-1 is expressed in plasma cells and in a subset of germinal center B cells [36]. Forced expression of Blimp-1 drives mature B cells to plasma cell stage [37]. Therefore, we addressed binding changes of cohesin at the Blimp-1 gene, *Prdm1*, upon stimulation of the cells. The *Prdm1* promoter contains a binding site for CTCF and cohesin specific for mature B cells (Fig. 4B, site b). Around 2 kb upstream of the promoter another cohesin/CTCF site specific for mature B cells (Fig. 4B, site a) is present. At both sites, cohesin binding is reduced 48 h after initiation of stimulation. Moreover, cohesin binds frequently to a CTCF site (Fig. 4B, site c) in the second intron of *Prdm1* gene only after 96 hours of stimulation. Binding kinetics of

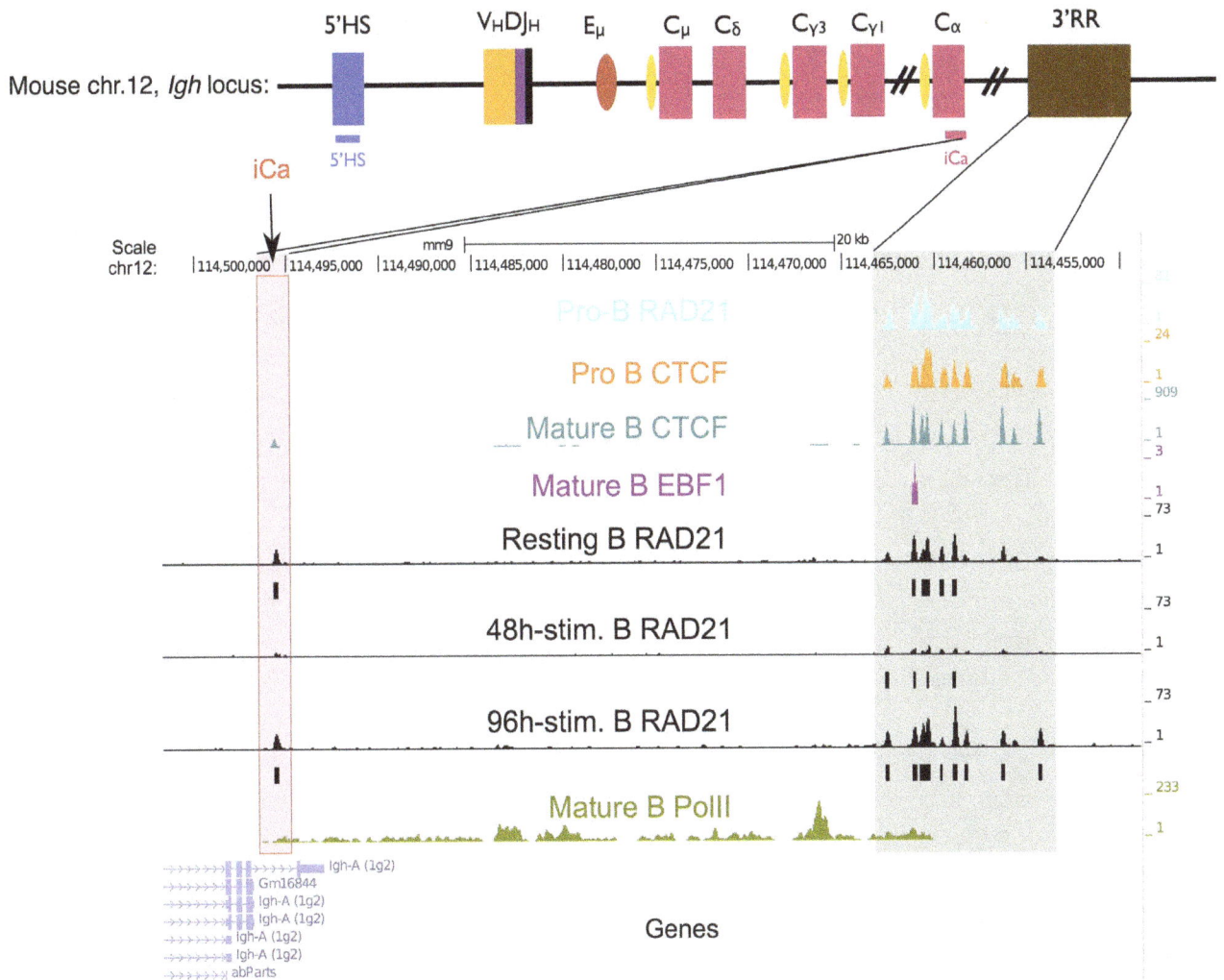

Figure 3. Shared and common binding events at the Igh locus. A stage-specific cohesin/CTCF site (iCa) is shown together with 3′ RR cohesin/CTCF sites.

cohesin at this CTCF site might be critical for higher *Prdm1* expression levels necessary for plasma cell identity. We conclude that cohesin binds to *Pax5* and *Prdm1* gene loci in a stage-specific manner and therefore cohesin is likely to regulate chromosomal interactions for the regulation of expression of these genes.

Discussion

Given that cohesin regulates distinct molecular events, i.e. transcription and recombination, we directed our analysis to identify cohesin's potential roles in late B cell maturation and B cell class switch recombination and used primary mouse splenic B cells for these analyses. By performing ChIP-seq, we revealed that cohesin is enriched at sites of transcription in resting and 96 h-switch-stimulated B cells, but not in 48 h-stimulated B cells. Cohesin association to transcriptional sites implies that cohesin acts in regulation of transcription, probably by facilitation of promoter-enhancer interactions and/or RNA polII binding to those sites. Upon stimulation for 48 h, cohesin associated less with transcriptional elements. Such a pattern could be explained by the fact that during class switch recombination cells undergo several rounds of division. Presence of 5547 high-confidence cohesin

binding sites in 48 h-stimulated B cells indicates that cohesin binding greatly changes upon stimulation for CSR. Since at this time point of stimulation the cells are highly activated and undergo extensive of proliferation, an overall reduction of heterochromatin and of cohesin binding to chromatin may be expected.

Our analysis reveals that cohesin is much underrepresented at S regions. Cohesin is less represented at S regions than in the flanking regions, contrary to a recent finding that suggests cohesin is associated with Sμ, although not Sγ1, upon switch-activation [25]. The difference may be explained in several ways. We have performed a more detailed analysis of the S and S-flanking regions. Our strategy of having biological replicates, which are then pooled at the stage of mapping the reads to the mouse genome, boosts signal to noise ratio and consequently increases predictive power of the peak calling algorithm. Claudepierre et al did not apply such a strategy. The use of different antibodies may also contribute somewhat to the difference. Claudepierre et al. have used an anti SMC3 antibody and thus an antibody recognizing the core SMC heterodimer of cohesin. We have used an anti RAD21 antibody and thus have targeted the much more labile kleisin subunit of cohesin, and thus those cohesin complexes

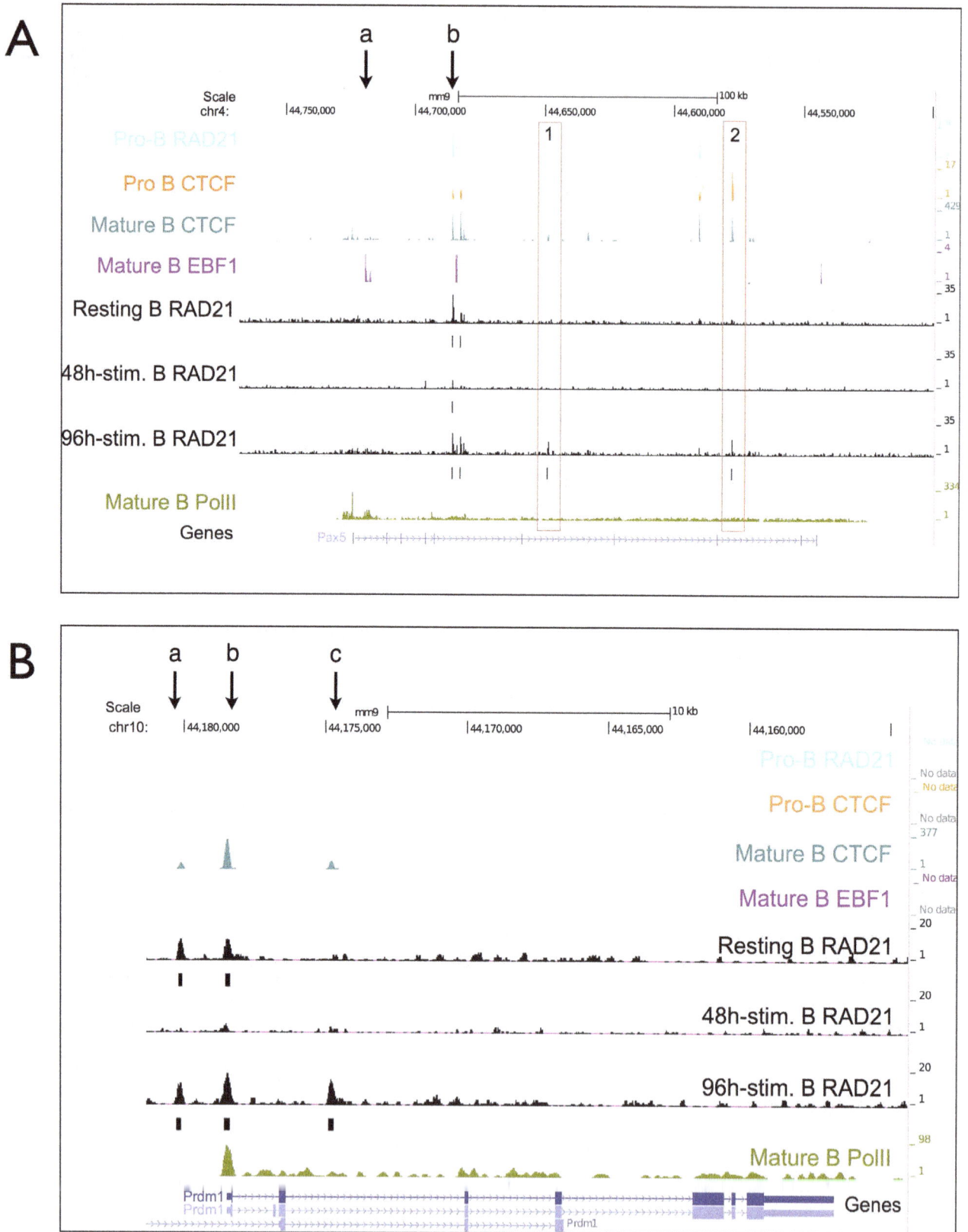

Figure 4. Binding profiles at the Pax5 and Prdm1 gene loci. (A) Binding profiles at the Pax5 gene locus. ChIP-seq profiles of RAD21, CTCF, EBF1 and PolII binding at the Pax5 gene. (B) Binding profiles at the Prdm1 gene locus - ChIP-seq profiles of RAD21, CTCF, EBF1 and PolII binding at the Blimp-1 gene.

that are truly bound to chromatin as fully intact cohesin complexes.

Our findings implicate that the cohesin-free nature of S regions is not specific for those S regions undergoing recombination but also seen at S regions that are not made accessible to recombination by GLT. If this is true, besides other processes like mis-regulation of AID expression, also the largely cohesin-free status of S regions may contribute to the high levels of oncogenic translocations occurring at the *Igh* locus [38]. Although cohesin is targeted to silenced chromatin in yeast, cohesin is not enriched at sites of convergent transcription in mammals [7,39]. Therefore such underrepresentation of cohesin as seen in S regions could be distinct from other known functions of cohesin in gene regulation. Knock-down of cohesin subunits in the CH12 B cell line impaired CSR but not S region transcription, implying that cohesin plays a more global role in modulation of CSR [25]. Additionally, B cells derived from Cornelia de Lange Syndrome patients show increased microhomology-based end joining during CSR, suggesting that cohesin, and its loading factor NIPBL, are necessary for non-homologous end joining during CSR [40].

Our findings demonstrate that the iCa binding site is only enriched by cohesin and CTCF, once the cells reach mature B cell stage. iCa contains a CTCF-binding motif and PolII binding is initiated there only in mature, activated B cells. PolII is enriched at the genomic region between iCa and 3′RR CTCF/cohesin binding sites. Between the last exon of Cα and 3′ CTCF/cohesin sites, a set of DNAse hypersensitive area act as enhancers for class switch recombination (HS3a, HS1,2, HS3b and HS4). Combined deletion of these enhancers blocks switching to all isotypes [41]. Given that cohesin sits at the 3′ Cα site only at the mature stage, and that this site overlaps to the region where PolII enrichment starts, an important role of cohesin/CTCF interplay for the control of 3′ enhancer activity could be anticipated. Molecular approaches to snap-shot chromatin interactions at a given time, i.e. chromosome conformation capture, could provide further evidence for cohesin's impact in the regulation of 3′ enhancer transcription which is indispensable for switch recombination.

We did not detect cohesin/CTCF binding at the Blimp1 (*Prdm1*) gene in proB cells. The *Prdm1* promoter is bound by cohesin and CTCF only in mature B cells. Interestingly, one site of intronic cohesin/CTCF enrichment is observed only after 96 h of stimulation. One can assume that this site is only bound by cohesin as Blimp1 expression increases to drive switched B cells to become plasma cells, i.e. CD138+ cells, which are present at the 96 h time point. We also revealed two stage-specific cohesin/CTCF binding events at the *Pax5* gene body activated only after 96 h of stimulation, implying these a role for the termination of PAX5 transcription, which is necessary for plasma cell differentiation. One of these cohesin sites coincides with a conserved CTCF site. However, the second cohesin site is enriched for CTCF only in mature, activated B cells. Possible interactions, including those regions at the *Pax5* locus should be further addressed to clarify a potential role for these sites in diminishing PAX5 expression upon plasma cell differentiation.

Together, these data indicate potential candidate regions of regulation, suggested by cohesin binding changes upon switch-stimulation. As patients with mutations in cohesin loading factor NIPBL reveal high levels of Ig isotype deficiency [42], learning about the stage-specific binding events at the *Igh* locus and at B-cell related genes, i.e. *Pax5* and *Prdm1* will open new avenues to understanding how cohesin contributes to regulation of B cell maturation, isotype switching and associated events.

Materials and Methods

Cell preparation and culture conditions

C57BL/6J wild-type (wt) mice were obtained from the Jackson Laboratories and maintained under pathogen-free conditions in the animal facility of the Medical Faculty Carl Gustav Carus. The experiments were performed under approval by the Animal Welfare Committee of the State of Saxony (permission number 24-9168.24-1/2010/25). Mice were used for tissue removal only under euthanasia conditions approved by the Animal Welfare Committee of the Technische Universität Dresden. Euthanasia was performed using carbon dioxide anesthesia. Splenic B cells were isolated from 8- to 10-week-old C57BL/6J mice. The spleen was dissected from the mouse, meshed on a 40 μm nylon mesh and resuspended in culture medium Hybridoma-SFM (12045-084, InVitrogen), supplemented with 10% FCS, 100 U/ml penicillin, 100 U/ml streptomycin and 5×10^{-5} M ß-mercaptoethanol. B cell cultures were prepared using B cells purified on MACS columns according to the manufacturers instructions (130-090-862, Miltenyi Biotec). For the switch to IgG1, purified B cells were cultured at a cell density of 3×10^5 cells/ml in complete culture medium supplemented with 50 μg/ml LPS (L6511, Sigma) and 2 ng/ml mouse recombinant IL-4 (404ML, R&D Systems).

Flow cytometry

B cells were washed with PBS supplemented with 2 mM EDTA and 0.5% BSA followed by staining with anti-mouse B220 antibody conjugated with Pacific Blue (103230, BioLegend) and anti-mouse IgG1 antibody conjugated with APC (406609, BioLegend). Stained cells were incubated for 20 minutes on ice and were washed twice. Cell surface staining measurements were carried out with BD LSR II Flow Cytometer and data plots were generated using FlowJo software.

Quantitative Real-Time PCR

Conventional polymerase chain reactions (PCRs) were performed using Dream Taq DNA polymerase and buffers according to manufacturer's instructions (EP0713, Fermentas). Quantitative PCRs were performed using the Rotor Gene SYBR Green PCR kit supplied from Qiagen (204074) in a Rotor Gene 3000 real-time PCR cycler, and comparative quantification analyses of PCR products and melt curve analyses were carried out using the Rotor Gene software.

Chromatin immunoprecipitation (ChIP) and deep sequencing

B cells were cross-linked with 1% formaldehyde at room temperature for 10 minutes and cross-linking was quenched by 125 mM glycine. Cells were lysed in SDS lysis buffer (1% SDS, 10 mM EDTA, 50 mM Tris-HCl, pH 8.1) and the chromatin was sonicated to an average fragment length of 500 base pairs (bp) using a Branson Sonifier 450. Sonicated chromatin was pre-cleared and incubated with 2 μg of anti-RAD21 antibody (ab992, Abcam), 4 μl anti-CTCF (07729, Millipore), 2 μg anti-PAX5 (sc-1974, Santa Cruz) and 1 μg anti-IgG (sc-2027, Santa Cruz) overnight. The complexes were washed with increasing salt stringency and cross-links were reversed in the presence of 0.2 M NaCl at 65°C for 6 hours. Proteinase K treatment was carried out in the presence of 10 μM EDTA, 40 μM Tris-HCl, pH 6.5 and 20 μg Proteinase K. DNA fragments were recovered with phenol-chloroform extraction following one chloroform extraction. DNA was precipitated with 2 volumes of ethanol, 1/3 volumes of 7.5 M ammonium acetate and 20 μg glycogen with an overnight incubation at −20°C. Precipitated DNA was washed with 70% Ethanol to remove excess salt and DNA was resuspended in 30 µl TE buffer supplemented with 0.3 µg RNAseA. A ChIP-Seq library was prepared by the Deep Sequencing Facility of the Biotechnology Center/SFB655 of Dresden University of Technology. Immunoprecipitated fragments were end-repaired with NEBnext End Repair Module (NEB) and purified by using Agencourt Ampure XP - beads (Beckman Coulter) and A-tailed using the NEBnext dA-Tailing Module according to manufacturers' instructions. After purification, adaptors were ligated (Adaptor-Oligo 1: 5'ACACTCTT-TCCCTACACGACGCTCTTCCGATCT-3', Adaptor-Oligo 2: 5'-P-GATCGGAAGAGCACACGTCTGAACTCCAGTCAC-3') by using 1x NEBnext Quick Ligation Buffer (NEB), 10x excess of DNA Adaptors, 5 µl Quick T4 DNA Ligase (NEB) at 50 µl total volume. Large-scale amplification of library constructs was performed by using the PCR Enrich Adaptor Ligated cDNA Library module (NEB). Fragment length selection was carried out by agarose gel electrophoresis and concentrations were determined by using Qubit dsDNA HS Assay Kit (Invitrogen).

Genome-wide analyses of RAD21 ChIP-seq

Alignment of RAD21 ChIP-Seq reads to reference mouse genome assembly mm9 was performed using the Bowtie 2 version 0.12.8 (Langmead et al. 2009) with the "–very-sensitive" option. From each set of aligned reads, a subset of 7 million unique positions was randomly selected for further processing and, additionally, IP and control samples from biological replicates were merged to form additional "pooled" samples. Binding site detection in each set of biological replicates and pooled samples was done with the MACS 2 peak calling software (Yong Zhang et al. 2008) with 0.05 FDR used as a cut-off value, and with standard parameters for shifting model calculations. Binding site overlaps between different sample sets were calculated with BEDTools utilities (Quinlan & Hall 2010). Genome-wide analysis of enrichment of chromosomal features and chromosomal distribution of ChIP regions were determined using CEAS package (Shin et al. 2009) provided by Galaxy/Cistrome platform http://cistrome.org/ap (Giardine et al. 2005). Genome mapping of RAD21 binding regions and publicly available ChIP-seq data were visualized using the University of California Santa Cruz (UCSC) Genome Browser interface (Kent et al. 2002).

The GEO accession number is GSE61443 and can be accessed at http://www.ncbi.nlm.nih.gov/geo/query/acc.cgi?token=glwd cwgcrjgfzid&acc=GSE61443

ChIP-Seq data comparison

All the ChIP-seq data listed in Table S1 was processed using the following computational pipeline. Adapter sequences, quality of raw reads, sequence duplication levels and over-represented sequences were analyzed using FastQC. Adapter sequences were removed and reads were trimmed using the FastX Toolkit (Patel & Jain 2012) such that the quality criteria of quality value per base (Phred score) was at least 35 and the read length was at least

17 bp. Raw reads were mapped to the mouse genome (mm9), using Bowtie 2 version 0.12.8 (Langmead et al. 2009) with 17 bp seed length with a maximum of two allowed mismatches. SAMtools (H. Li et al. 2009) was used to create BAM files. Peak calling was done using MACS (Yong Zhang et al. 2008) for transcription factors with 0.0001 p-value cutoff. Qeseq (Micsinai et al. 2012) was used for PolII binding data with 0.001 p-value cutoff.

Supporting Information

Figure S1 (A) Scheme of purification of IgG1-positive and -negative B cells. (B) FACS profiles of resting B cells and B cells stimulated for 48 or 96 h. At 48 h, 2.7% of the cells were IgG1-positive. The IgG1-positive and -negative fractions are shown for the 96 h time point, where the IgG1-negative fraction contained 0.5% IgG1-positive cells, and the IgG1-positive fraction contained 65%. Many cells in the IgG1-negative gate of this fraction also started to express IgG1 as they shifted in fluorescence towards the IgG1-positive gate.

Figure S2 **ChIP-Seq profile of binding factors around the Eµ and 3'RR.** Binding profile of RAD21, CTCF, EBF1 and PolII in pro- and/or in mature B cells. The highest enrichment of PolII marks the locus enhancer Eµ. The highest cohesin-CTCF colocalization marks the cohesin/CTCF bound to 3'RR. Genes depict UCSC Gene annotations. ChIPSeq data plots are generated by using data obtained in this study and from publicly available sources mentioned in Table S1.

Figure S3 **Binding of factors at Igh locus cohesin sites.** (A) Scheme of the Igh locus binding events under investigation. (B) Enrichment of RAD21, CTCF, and PAX5 at cohesin binding sites in resting B cells were quantified by ChIP-qPCR.

Figure S4 **Mature B cell-specific cohesin/CTCF site corresponds to the 5' flanking gene of Igh locus.** ChIP-Seq data plot indicates a mature B cell specific binding of cohesin subunit RAD21 at the HS region located at the 5' of *Igh* locus.

Figure S5 **Binding profile at the Aicda gene locus.** ChIP-seq profiles of RAD21, CTCF, EBF1 and PolII binding at *Aicda*.

Table S1 **ChIP-seq data sets used for comparison studies.**

Author Contributions

Conceived and designed the experiments: GGS AB FB RJ. Performed the experiments: GGS MPR KS. Analyzed the data: GGS MPR KS AB FB RJ. Contributed reagents/materials/analysis tools: MPR KS AB FB. Wrote the paper: GGS MPR KS AB FB RJ.

References

1. Botran JM, Tadaachi A, Schmitz J (2008) The cohesin complex and its roles in chromosome biology. Genes Dev 22: 3089–3114.
2. Jessberger R (2009) Cohesin's dual role in the DNA damage response: repair and checkpoint activation. EMBO J 28: 2491–2493.
3. Nasmyth K (2011) Cohesin: a catenase with separate entry and exit gates? Nat Cell Biol 13: 1170–1177.
4. Nasmyth K, Haering CH (2009) Cohesin: its roles and mechanisms. Annu Rev Genet 43: 525–558.
5. Haering CH, Jessberger R (2012) Cohesin in determining chromosome architecture. Exp Cell Res 318: 1386–1393.
6. Élison JG, Haering T (2012) Chromosomal resolution: a cohesin releasing network and beyond. Chromosoma 119: 459–467.
7. Peric-Hupkes D, van Steensel B (2008) Linking cohesin to gene regulation. Cell 132: 925–928.
8. Feeney KM, Wasson CW, Parish JL (2010) Cohesin: a regulator of genome integrity and gene expression. Biochem J 428: 147–161.
9. Degner SC, Wong TP, Jankevicius G, Feeney AJ (2009) Cutting edge: Developmental stage-specific recruitment of cohesin to CTCF sites throughout immunoglobulin loci during B lymphocyte development. J Immunol 182: 44–48.

10. Schmidt D, Schwalie PC, Ross-Innes CS, Hurtado A, Brown GD, et al. (2010) A CTCF-independent role for cohesin in tissue-specific transcription. Genome Res 20: 578–588.

11. Hou C, Dale R, Dean A (2010) Cell type specificity of chromatin organization mediated by CTCF and cohesin. Proc Natl Acad Sci U S A 107: 3651–3656.

12. Parelho V, Hadjur S, Spivakov M, Leleu M, Sauer S, et al. (2008) Cohesins functionally associate with CTCF on mammalian chromosome arms. Cell 132: 422–433.

13. Wendt KS, Yoshida K, Itoh T, Bando M, Koch B, et al. (2008) Cohesin mediates transcriptional insulation by CCCTC-binding factor. Nature 451: 796–801.

14. Kagey MH, Newman JJ, Bilodeau S, Zhan Y, Orlando DA, et al. (2010) Mediator and cohesin connect gene expression and chromatin architecture. Nature 467: 430–435.

15. Nitzsche A, Paszkowski-Rogacz M, Matarese F, Janssen-Megens EM, Hubner NC, et al. (2011) RAD21 cooperates with pluripotency transcription factors in the maintenance of embryonic stem cell identity. PLoS One 6: e19470.

16. Seitan VC, Hao B, Tachibana-Konwalski K, Lavagnolli T, Mira-Bontenbal H, et al. (2011) A role for cohesin in T-cell-receptor rearrangement and thymocyte differentiation. Nature 476: 467–471.

17. Guo C, Gerasimova T, Hao H, Ivanova I, Chakraborty T, et al. (2011) Two forms of loops generate the chromatin conformation of the immunoglobulin heavy-chain gene locus. Cell 147: 332–343.

18. Meffre E, Casellas R, Nussenzweig MC (2000) Antibody regulation of B cell development. Nat Immunol 1: 379–385.

19. Guo C, Yoon HS, Franklin A, Jain S, Ebert A, et al. (2011) CTCF-binding elements mediate control of V(D)J recombination. Nature 477: 424–430.

20. Yamane A, Resch W, Kuo N, Kuchen S, Li Z, et al. (2011) Deep-sequencing identification of the genomic targets of the cytidine deaminase AID and its cofactor RPA in B lymphocytes. Nat Immunol 12: 62–69.

21. Jhunjhunwala S, van Zelm MC, Peak MM, Cutchin S, Riblet R, et al. (2008) The 3D structure of the immunoglobulin heavy-chain locus: implications for long-range genomic interactions. Cell 133: 265–279.

22. Chaumeil J, Skok JA (2012) The role of CTCF in regulating V(D)J recombination. Curr Opin Immunol 24: 153–159.

23. Stavnezer J, Guikema JE, Schrader CE (2008) Mechanism and regulation of class switch recombination. Annu Rev Immunol 26: 261–292.

24. Wuerffel R, Wang L, Grigera F, Manis J, Selsing E, et al. (2007) S-S synapsis during class switch recombination is promoted by distantly located transcriptional elements and activation-induced deaminase. Immunity 27: 711–722.

25. Thomas-Claudepierre AS, Schiavo E, Heyer V, Fournier M, Page A, et al. (2013) The cohesin complex regulates immunoglobulin class switch recombination. J Exp Med 210: 2495–2502.

26. Shin H, Liu T, Manrai AK, Liu XS (2009) CEAS: cis-regulatory element annotation system. Bioinformatics 25: 2605–2606.

27. Gyory I, Boller S, Nechanitzky R, Mandel E, Pott S, et al. (2012) Transcription factor Ebf1 regulates differentiation stage-specific signaling, proliferation, and survival of B cells. Genes Dev 26: 668–682.

28. Degner SC, Verma-Gaur J, Wong TP, Bossen C, Iverson GM, et al. (2011) CCCTC-binding factor (CTCF) and cohesin influence the genomic architecture of the Igh locus and antisense transcription in pro-B cells. Proc Natl Acad Sci U S A 108: 9566–9571.

29. Rouaud P, Vincent-Fabert C, Fiancette R, Cogne M, Pinaud E, et al. (2012) Enhancers located in heavy chain regulatory region (hs3a, hs1,2, hs3b, and hs4) are dispensable for diversity of VDJ recombination. J Biol Chem 287: 8356–8360.

30. Chatterjee S, Ju Z, Hassan R, Volpi SA, Emelyanov AV, et al. (2011) Dynamic changes in binding of immunoglobulin heavy chain 3' regulatory region to protein factors during class switching. J Biol Chem 286: 29303–29312.

31. Volpi SA, Verma-Gaur J, Hassan R, Ju Z, Roa S, et al. (2012) Germline deletion of Igh 3' regulatory region elements hs 5, 6, 7 (hs5-7) affects B cell-specific regulation, rearrangement, and insulation of the Igh locus. J Immunol 188: 2556–2566.

32. Pawlitzky I, Angeles CV, Siegel AM, Stanton ML, Riblet R, et al. (2006) Identification of a candidate regulatory element within the 5' flanking region of the mouse Igh locus defined by pro-B cell-specific hypersensitivity associated with binding of PU.1, Pax5, and E2A. J Immunol 176: 6839–6851.

33. Perlot T, Pawlitzky I, Manis JP, Zarrin AA, Brodeur PH, et al. (2010) Analysis of mice lacking DNaseI hypersensitive sites at the 5' end of the IgH locus. PLoS One 5: e13992.

34. Nera KP, Kohonen P, Narvi E, Peippo A, Mustonen L, et al. (2006) Loss of Pax5 promotes plasma cell differentiation. Immunity 24: 283–293.

35. Decker T, Pasca di Magliano M, McManus S, Sun Q, Bonifer C, et al. (2009) Stepwise activation of enhancer and promoter regions of the B cell commitment gene Pax5 in early lymphopoiesis. Immunity 30: 508–520.

36. Shaffer AL, Lin KI, Kuo TC, Yu X, Hurt EM, et al. (2002) Blimp-1 orchestrates plasma cell differentiation by extinguishing the mature B cell gene expression program. Immunity 17: 51–62.

37. Schliephake DE, Schimpl A (1996) Blimp-1 overcomes the block in IgM secretion in lipopolysaccharide/anti-mu F(ab')2-co-stimulated B lymphocytes. Eur J Immunol 26: 268–271.

38. Ramiro AR, Jankovic M, Callen E, Difilippantonio S, Chen HT, et al. (2006) Role of genomic instability and p53 in AID-induced c-myc-Igh translocations. Nature 440: 105–109.

39. Donze D, Adams CR, Rine J, Kamakaka RT (1999) The boundaries of the silenced HMR domain in Saccharomyces cerevisiae. Genes Dev 13: 698–708.

40. Enervald E, Du L, Visnes T, Bjorkman A, Lindgren E, et al. (2013) A regulatory role for the cohesin loader NIPBL in nonhomologous end joining during immunoglobulin class switch recombination. J Exp Med 210: 2503–2513.

41. Vincent-Fabert C, Fiancette R, Pinaud E, Truffinet V, Cogne N, et al. (2010) Genomic deletion of the whole IgH 3' regulatory region (hs3a, hs1,2, hs3b, and hs4) dramatically affects class switch recombination and Ig secretion to all isotypes. Blood 116: 1895–1898.

42. Jyonouchi S, Orange J, Sullivan KE, Krantz I, Deardorff M (2013) Immunologic features of cornelia de lange syndrome. Pediatrics 132: e484–489.

Leucocyte Telomere Length and Risk of Type 2 Diabetes Mellitus: New Prospective Cohort Study and Literature-Based Meta-Analysis

Peter Willeit[1,2*⑨], Julia Raschenberger[3⑨], Emma E. Heydon[2], Sotirios Tsimikas[4], Margot Haun[3], Agnes Mayr[5], Siegfried Weger[6], Joseph L. Witztum[4], Adam S. Butterworth[2], Johann Willeit[1], Florian Kronenberg[3], Stefan Kiechl[1*]

1 Department of Neurology, Innsbruck Medical University, Innsbruck, Austria, 2 Department of Public Health and Primary Care, University of Cambridge, Cambridge, United Kingdom, 3 Division of Genetic Epidemiology, Innsbruck Medical University, Innsbruck, Austria, 4 Department of Medicine, University of California San Diego, La Jolla, United States of America, 5 Department of Laboratory Medicine, Bruneck Hospital, Bruneck, Italy, 6 Department of Internal Medicine, Bruneck Hospital, Bruneck, Italy

Abstract

Background: Short telomeres have been linked to various age-related diseases. We aimed to assess the association of telomere length with incident type 2 diabetes mellitus (T2DM) in prospective cohort studies.

Methods: Leucocyte relative telomere length (RTL) was measured using quantitative polymerase chain reaction in 684 participants of the prospective population-based Bruneck Study (1995 baseline), with repeat RTL measurements performed in 2005 (n = 558) and 2010 (n = 479). Hazard ratios for T2DM were calculated across quartiles of baseline RTL using Cox regression models adjusted for age, sex, body-mass index, smoking, socio-economic status, physical activity, alcohol consumption, high-density lipoprotein cholesterol, log high-sensitivity C-reactive protein, and waist-hip ratio. Separate analyses corrected hazard ratios for within-person variability using multivariate regression calibration of repeated measurements. To contextualise findings, we systematically sought PubMed, Web of Science and EMBASE for relevant articles and pooled results using random-effects meta-analysis.

Results: Over 15 years of follow-up, 44 out of 606 participants free of diabetes at baseline developed incident T2DM. The adjusted hazard ratio for T2DM comparing the bottom vs. the top quartile of baseline RTL (i.e. shortest vs. longest) was 2.00 (95% confidence interval: 0.90 to 4.49; P = 0.091), and 2.31 comparing the bottom quartile vs. the remainder (1.21 to 4.41; P = 0.011). The corresponding hazard ratios corrected for within-person RTL variability were 3.22 (1.27 to 8.14; P = 0.014) and 2.86 (1.45 to 5.65; P = 0.003). In a random-effects meta-analysis of three prospective cohort studies involving 6,991 participants and 2,011 incident T2DM events, the pooled relative risk was 1.31 (1.07 to 1.60; P = 0.010; I^2 = 69%).

Conclusions/Interpretation: Low RTL is independently associated with the risk of incident T2DM. To avoid regression dilution biases in observed associations of RTL with disease risk, future studies should implement methods correcting for within-person variability in RTL. The causal role of short telomeres in T2DM development remains to be determined.

Editor: Arthur J. Lustig, Tulane University Health Sciences Center, United States of America

Funding: This project was funded by a grant of the 'Tiroler Wissenschaftsfonds', Austria. The Bruneck Study was supported by the 'Pustertaler Verein zur Prävention von Herz- und Hirngefaesserkrankungen, Gesundheitsbezirk Bruneck' and the 'Assessorat für Gesundheit', Province of Bolzano, Italy. The funders had no role in study design, data collection and analysis, decision to publish, or preparation of the manuscript.

Competing Interests: The authors have declared that no competing interests exist.

* Email: pwilleit@outlook.com (PW); stefan.kiechl@i-med.ac.at (SK)

⑨ These authors contributed equally to this work.

Introduction

Telomeres are the extreme ends of eukaryotic chromosomes, stabilising and protecting the chromosome from degradation [1,2]. Telomeres shorten with each cellular division, accelerated by inflammation and oxidative stress, and, below a critical length, the apoptotic programme of the cell is induced [1,3].

Short telomeres are associated with increased risk of several age-related diseases [2] such as cardiovascular diseases [4–8] and cancer [9–11]. It has been suggested that biological ageing reflected by telomere length is also related to the development of type 2 diabetes (T2DM) [12]. Proposed pathophysiological mechanisms include a reduction in beta-cell mass [13], impaired insulin secretion [14] and adipocyte insulin resistance elicited by cellular senescence [15]. On the other hand, diabetic patients suffer from elevated levels of oxidative stress [16], which in turn leads to telomere attrition [17]. To disentangle these two effects and establish a temporal relationship, it is crucial to investigate the association of telomere length with risk of new-onset T2DM in studies with a prospective design. In such studies, telomere length is assessed before the diabetes diagnosis (although subclinical prediabetic changes may already be present). Furthermore, because telomere length fluctuates considerably over time [18–27], studies are needed that take into account the within-person variability of telomere length. Such analyses use repeated measurements instead of single baseline measurements to predict "long-term average" telomere length and therefore help estimate the "true" aetiological association with T2DM risk.

Our aims were three-fold. First, to assess the association of baseline leucocyte relative telomere length (RTL) with new-onset T2DM in the prospective population-based Bruneck Study. Second, to correct association estimates for long-term within-person variability of RTL. Third, to contextualise findings in a literature-based meta-analysis of all prospective evidence available to date.

Material and Methods

The Bruneck Study

The Bruneck Study is a prospective, population-based survey conducted in 1,000 individuals aged 40 to 79 years (125 per sex and decade of life). In 1990, participants were randomly selected from the inhabitants of the town of Bruneck (South Tyrol, Italy) and were examined every five years between 1990 and 2010 [5,10,19,28,29]. Participation rates exceeded 90% at all surveys. In the present study, we used leucocyte RTL measurements available from the surveys in 1995, 2005 and 2010 (n = 684, 558, and 479, respectively). Full medical records were available for review for all individuals, including those who did not participate in or died during follow up (100% follow up for clinical endpoints). The study protocol was approved by the local ethic committee of Bolzano ('Comitato etico del comprensorio sanitario di Bolzano'; approval number 28–2010). All participants gave informed written informed consent before taking part and the study complies with the Declaration of Helsinki.

Clinical history and examination at baseline

We assessed risk factors by validated standard procedures as previously described [5,28]. Waist and hip circumferences were assessed with a plastic tape measure at the levels of the umbilicus and the greater trochanters respectively. We defined socioeconomic status on a three-category scale (low, medium or high) on the basis of information about occupational status and educational level of the person with the highest income in the household. High socioeconomic status was assumed if the participant had ≥12 years of education or an occupation with an average monthly income ≥$2,000 (baseline salary before tax). Low socioeconomic status was defined by ≤8 years of education or an average monthly income ≤$1,000. Physical activity was assessed using the validated Baeke Score [30]. Oxidation-specific biomarkers and other laboratory parameters were measured as previously described [31]. HbA1c was quantified using high performance liquid chromatography (DCCT-aligned assay). We estimated the degree of insulin resistance by homeostasis model assessment (HOMA-IR) using the formula fasting plasma glucose in mmol/l × fasting serum insulin in mU/l divided by 22.5 [32], with higher HOMA-IR values indicating higher insulin resistance. LDL cholesterol was estimated using the Friedewald equation [33].

Measurement of leucocyte telomere length

Genomic DNA from the Bruneck Study blood samples was extracted from frozen EDTA-blood samples with the Invisorb Blood Universal Kit. DNA concentrations were measured with the Tecan NanoQuant infinite M200. Samples were normalised in 96-well microtiter plates. Leucocyte RTL was measured in a single laboratory by a single person within a short time period using a quantitative polymerase chain reaction (qPCR) approach developed by Cawthon [34] to measure T/S-ratios. The protocol was modified with regard to control samples and data processing as recently described [35]. T/S-ratios are proportional to individual telomere length. The composition of singleplex PCRs for telomere (T) and housekeeping gene (S) PCRs was identical. DNA samples were run in 15 µl reactions containing 1× Quantifast TM SYBR Green PCR mastermix (Qiagen), 10 ng of DNA, 1 µM of telomere primer or 250 nm of housekeeping gene 36B4 primer. The primer sequences (5′→3′) were: tel1b CGGTTTGTTTGG-GTTTGGGTTTGGGTTTGGGTTTGGGTT; tel2b GGCTT-GCCTTACCCTTACCCTTACCCTTACCCTTACCCT; 36B4u CAGCAAGTGGGAAGGTGTAATCC; 36B4d CCCATTCTA-TCATCAACGGGTACAA [5]. Each qPCR was carried out in 384-well format which was vertically segmented in two parts: one for the telomeres (T) and one for the housekeeping gene 36B4 (S). Each qPCR plate contained the standard DNA, a quality control (commercially available DNA-Human Genomic DNA, Roche), and a non-template control. All samples, standards, and controls were analysed in quadruplicate. All sample transfers and dilution steps were performed with a Tecan robotic workstation. Relative qPCR was carried out on an Applied Biosystems Taqman Fast Real-Time PCR 7900HT System. The thermal cycling began with the initial polymerase activation step (10 min at 95°C) and was followed by 40 cycles of 95°C for 15 s, 60°C for 1 min. The relative quantities were determined by the efficiency correction method [36], which does not require calibration curves and includes the individual real-time PCR efficiencies. Efficiencies were computed for all replicates of each sample. To check PCR data for outliers, the coefficients of variation (intra-assay CVs) were assessed for the Ct-values and the efficiency-values of quadruplicates in each gene. All single outlying values (CV>5%) were removed from further analyses. Further details were already published before [35]. Although RTL of samples from 1995 and 2005 was already measured before [5,10], we reanalysed all samples of all time points together with the newly extracted samples from 2010 to avoid a measurement error over the time period. In addition, RTL measurement of samples of the same participant of all available time points were positioned on the same 384-well qPCR plate. After each qPCR run a melting curve analysis was performed to verify the specificity and identity of the products. The inter-assay coefficient of variation of T/S-ratios of the quality control, which was positioned on each 384-well plate (a total of 37 plates), was 11.8%. The laboratory personnel who performed the RTL measurements were blinded to the participants' status and outcome.

Definition of type 2 diabetes mellitus

We established the diagnosis of T2DM according to the 1997 American Diabetes Association criteria (fasting glucose ≥126 mg/dl, i.e. ≥7 mmol/l) or when the subjects had a clinical diagnosis of T2DM and received anti-diabetic treatment [37]. Impaired fasting glucose was defined as a fasting glucose level of 100 to <126 mg/dl (i.e. 5.6 to <7.0 mmol/l). Self-reported T2DM status was confirmed by reviewing the medical records of the subject's general practitioners and Bruneck Hospital. A major strength of the Bruneck Study is that virtually all participants living in the

Characteristic	Mean (SD) or n (%)	Standardised mean difference (95% CI) in RTL per SD increase or compared to reference group

Questionnaire-based and anthropometric measures

Age, years	63 (11)	-0.22 (-0.30, -0.15)***
Sex		
Male	335 (49%)	[Reference]
Female	349 (51%)	0.11 (-0.04, 0.25)
Body mass index, kg/m²	26 (4)	0.01 (-0.06, 0.08)
Current smoker		
Never/Ex	551 (81%)	[Reference]
Current	133 (19%)	-0.16 (-0.35, 0.03)
Socioeconomic status		
Low	412 (60%)	[Reference]
Middle	156 (23%)	-0.02 (-0.21, 0.17)
High	116 (17%)	0.12 (-0.08, 0.33)
Physical activity, Baeke score	2.4 (0.9)	-0.03 (-0.11, 0.05)
Alcohol consumption, g/d	23 (31)	-0.08 (-0.17, 0.01)

Lipid markers

HDL cholesterol, mg/dl	59 (17)	-0.04 (-0.11, 0.04)
LDL cholesterol, mg/dl	144 (38)	0.05 (-0.03, 0.12)
Log Lp(a), mg/dl	2.5 (1.4)	-0.02 (-0.09, 0.05)

Markers of inflammation

Log hsCRP, mg/l	-1.7 (1.0)	0.07 (-0.01, 0.14)
Fibrinogen, mg/dl	290 (78)	0.05 (-0.02, 0.13)
Leukocyte count per µl	6457 (1713)	-0.06 (-0.13, 0.01)
Log IL-6, ng/l	1.4 (1.0)	0.02 (-0.05, 0.10)
alpha1-Antitrypsin, mg/dl	200 (37)	-0.00 (-0.08, 0.07)

Markers of oxidative stress

Log OxPL/apoB, RLU	8.8 (0.9)	0.04 (-0.03, 0.12)
Log OxPL/apoB, ratio	-2.6 (0.9)	0.04 (-0.03, 0.12)
MDA-LDL IgG, RLU	9.6 (0.5)	0.02 (-0.05, 0.10)
MDA-LDL IgM, RLU	9.6 (0.5)	0.03 (-0.04, 0.11)
Cu-OxLDL IgG, RLU	9.0 (0.5)	0.04 (-0.04, 0.11)
Cu-OxLDL IgM, RLU	8.3 (0.6)	0.04 (-0.04, 0.12)
ApoB-IC IgG, RLU	7006 (3843)	-0.00 (-0.08, 0.07)
ApoB-IC IgM, RLU	5112 (2796)	0.04 (-0.04, 0.11)
Ferritin, ng/ml	136 (172)	-0.02 (-0.10, 0.05)
Ceruloplasmin, mg/dl	27 (5)	0.07 (-0.01, 0.15)
Uric acid, mg/dl	4.7 (1.3)	0.02 (-0.06, 0.10)

Markers of dysglycaemia

Fasting plasma glucose, mg/dl	102 (25)	-0.01 (-0.08, 0.07)
Urine glucose, mg/dl	116 (60)	-0.05 (-0.12, 0.03)
Log HOMA-IR	1.1 (0.6)	-0.03 (-0.10, 0.05)
HbA1c, %	5.8 (3.7)	-0.00 (-0.07, 0.07)

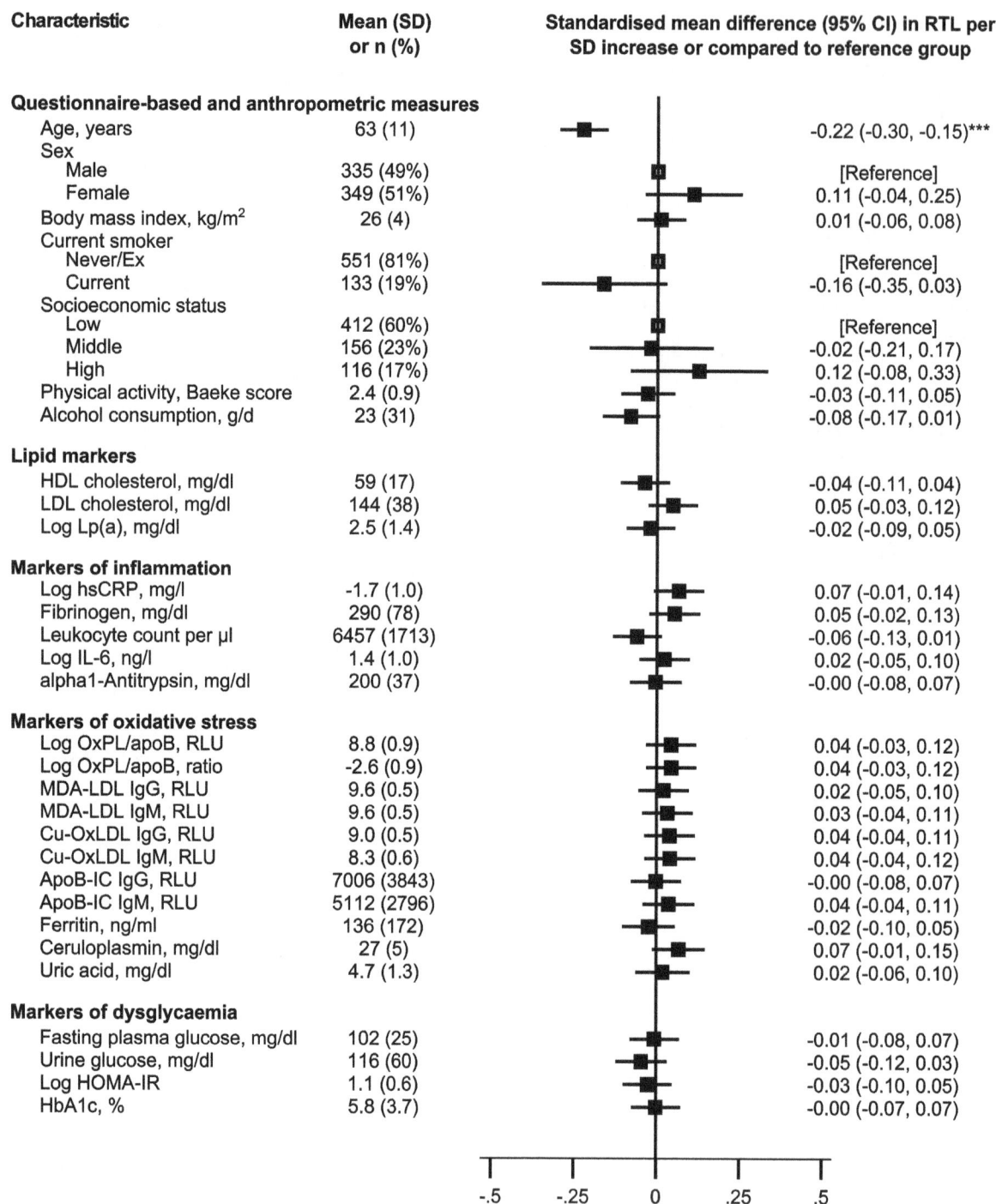

Axis: -.5   -.25   0   .25   .5

Figure 1. Baseline characteristics of the Bruneck Study population and their cross-sectional association with leucocyte relative telomere length (1995, n = 684). Standardised mean differences in leucocyte relative telomere length were adjusted for age and sex. Asterisks indicate level of statistical significance: *P≤0.05; **P≤0.01; ***P≤0.001. The mean (SD) of HbA1c was 5.8% (3.7%) in DCCT-derived units and 40 mmol/mol (17 mmol/mol) in SI units. Abbreviations: ApoB, apolipoprotein B; ApoB-IC, apoB-immune complexes; CI, confidence interval; Cu-OxLDL, copper-oxidised low-density lipoprotein; HbA1c, glycated haemoglobin; HDL, high-density lipoprotein; HOMA-IR, homeostatic model assessment of insulin resistance; hsCRP, high-sensitivity C-reactive protein; IgG, immunoglobulin G; IgM, immunoglobulin M; LDL, low-density lipoprotein; RTL, relative telomere length; MDA, malondialdehyde; OxPL/apoB, oxidised phospholipids on apolipoprotein B-100; SD, standard deviation; RLU, relative light unit; SMD, standardised mean difference; WHR, waist-hip ratio.

survey area are referred to the same hospital and the network existing between hospital and practitioners allows retrieval of full medical information. There were no cases of type 1 diabetes mellitus in this cohort.

Literature-based meta-analysis

Prospective studies of the association of telomere length with the risk of incident T2DM were sought using the databases PubMed, Web of Science and EMBASE. The search strategy combined

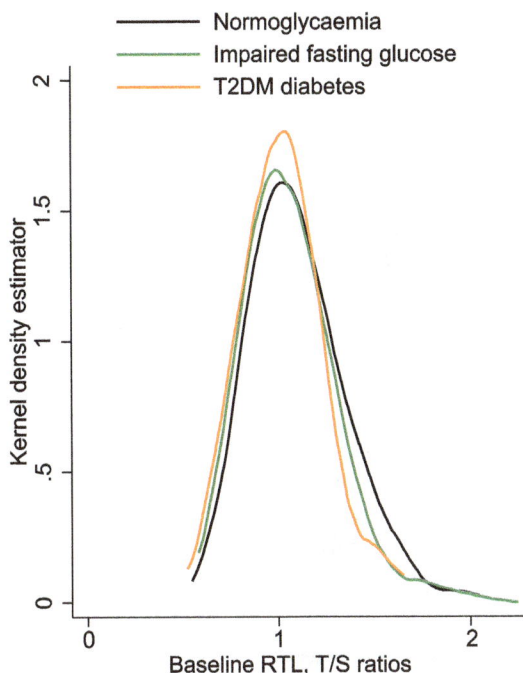

Figure 2. Distribution of baseline leucocyte relative telomere length in the Bruneck Study according to different disease states (1995, n = 684). Abbreviations: RTL, relative telomere length; T2DM, type 2 diabetes mellitus. There were 390 participants with normoglycaemia, 216 participants with impaired fasting glucose, and 78 participants with a clinical diagnosis of T2DM.

keywords related to the exposure of interest ("telomere" or "telomeres"), the outcome ("diabetes") and the study design ("cohort" or "prospective" or "longitudinal" or "hazard" or "risk" or "odds"). We included articles published before March 26th 2014 and applied no language restrictions. We scanned the reference lists of identified studies and reviews for any additional relevant articles. Because of their vulnerability to reverse causation biases, retrospective case-control studies were excluded from the meta-analysis (whereas nested case-control studies conducted within prospective cohort studies were included). Study level characteristics and participant characteristics were extracted using a standardised data extraction form, including information on: geographic location, population source, year of baseline survey, number of participants, mean age and age range, percentage of males, telomere length assay method, number of incident T2DM cases, duration of follow-up, and reported measures of association (i.e. hazard ratios, odds ratios, or other measures of relative risk) with corresponding confidence intervals and degree of adjustment for confounders. If studies had reported measures of association for different degree of adjustment, the most adjusted estimate was used in the meta-analysis. We assessed the quality of the included studies with the Newcastle-Ottawa scale, a quality score ranging from zero to nine points [38].

Statistical analysis

The statistical analysis was conducted according to a pre-specified analysis plan. Continuous variables were summarised as means (standard deviations) or medians (interquartile ranges), and dichotomous variables as numbers (percentages). Cross-sectional associations between RTL and other participant characteristics were determined using unadjusted and age- and sex-adjusted linear regression. To quantify within-person variability of RTL, regression dilution ratios were calculated using information from all available RTL measurements in 1995, 2005 and 2010 [39].

Table 1. Association of leucocyte relative telomere length with incident type 2 diabetes mellitus in the Bruneck Study (n = 606, 44 events).

Exposure/adjustment	Quartile 1 (Longest RTL)	Quartile 2	Quartile 3	Quartile 4 (Shortest RTL)	Quartile 4 vs. remainder
Baseline RTL					
Median (range) of RTL, T/S ratios	1.35 (1.21–3.87)	1.13 (1.05–1.21)	0.98 (0.92–1.05)	0.82 (0.52–0.91)	
Incidence rate of T2DM per 1,000 person-years	5.2 (2.9, 9.4)	3.1 (1.4, 6.9)	5.4 (3.0, 9.8)	10.6 (6.5, 17.2)	
Hazard ratio for T2DM (95% CI)					
Adjusted for age and sex	1.00 [Reference]	0.58 (0.22, 1.58)	0.95 (0.41, 2.22)	1.89 (0.85, 4.18)	2.21 (1.17, 4.16)*
Plus BMI, smoking, SES, and physical activity	1.00 [Reference]	0.57 (0.21, 1.56)	0.96 (0.41, 2.24)	1.89 (0.85, 4.21)	2.22 (1.17, 4.21)*
Plus alcohol consumption, HDL-C, log hsCRP, and WHR	1.00 [Reference]	0.58 (0.21, 1.58)	0.99 (0.42, 2.32)	2.00 (0.90, 4.49)	2.31 (1.21, 4.41)*
Long-term average RTL					
Median (range) of RTL, T/S ratios	1.29 (1.18–2.94)	1.12 (1.06–1.18)	1.02 (0.97–1.06)	0.89 (0.63–0.96)	
Incidence rate of T2DM per 1,000 person-years	3.6 (1.8, 7.3)	5.0 (2.7, 9.4)	4.5 (2.3, 8.6)	12.2 (7.6, 19.6)	
Hazard ratio for T2DM (95% CI)					
Adjusted for age and sex	1.00 [Reference]	1.36 (0.53, 3.45)	1.16 (0.44, 3.05)	3.24 (1.29, 8.15)*	2.76 (1.41, 5.41)**
Plus BMI, smoking, SES, and physical activity	1.00 [Reference]	1.24 (0.48, 3.20)	1.10 (0.41, 2.92)	3.05 (1.21, 7.70)*	2.73 (1.39, 5.36)**
Plus alcohol consumption, HDL-C, log hsCRP, and WHR	1.00 [Reference]	1.25 (0.49, 3.23)	1.11 (0.42, 2.94)	3.22 (1.27, 8.14)*	2.86 (1.45, 5.65)**

Asterisks indicate level of statistical significance: *$P \leq 0.05$; **$P \leq 0.01$; ***$P \leq 0.001$. Abbreviations: BMI, body mass index; HDL-C, high density lipoprotein cholesterol; hsCRP; high-sensitivity C-reactive protein; RTL, relative telomere length; SES, socio-economic status; T2DM, type 2 diabetes mellitus; WHR, waist-hip ratio. Participants with a baseline history of type 2 diabetes mellitus were excluded from the analysis (n = 78).

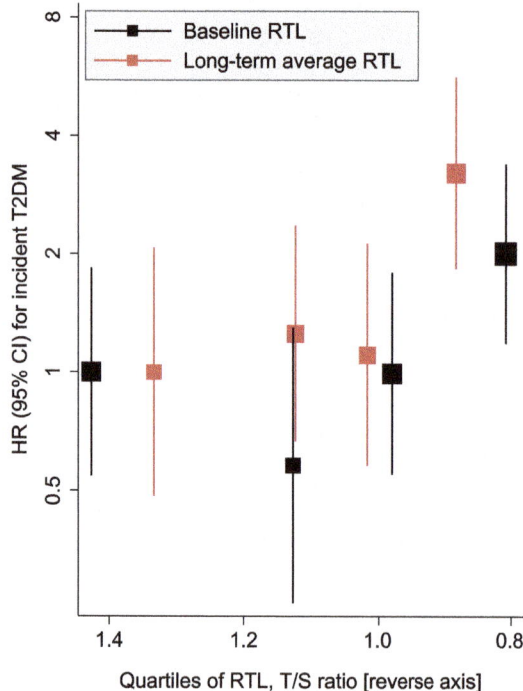

Figure 3. Association of leucocyte relative telomere length an risk of type 2 diabetes mellitus in the Bruneck Study (n = 606, 44 events over follow-up 1995–2010). Cox models were adjusted for age, sex, body mass index, smoking, socio-economic status, physical activity, alcohol consumption, high density lipoprotein cholesterol, log high-sensitivity C-reactive protein, and waist-hip ratio. Abbreviations: CI, confidence interval; HR, hazard ratio; RTL, relative telomere length; T2DM, type 2 diabetes mellitus.

Regression dilution ratios can range from 0 to 1, with 1 indicating absence of within-person variability. Long-term average RTL was estimated by multivariate linear-mixed regression calibration model that allowed for a random intercept at the participant level [40].

The time-to-event analysis excluded participants with baseline T2DM. Person-years of follow-up were accrued from the baseline in 1995 until diagnosis of T2DM, death or October 1, 2010, whichever came first. Cox proportional hazard models were used to assess the association between RTL and T2DM incidence. Following a previous report of a possible threshold effect in associations of RTL with T2DM risk [41], we categorised study participants into groups of RTL quartiles and compared T2DM risk across these groups. The analyses were progressively adjusted for age, sex, body mass index, smoking, socio-economic status, physical activity, alcohol consumption, high-density lipoprotein cholesterol, log high-sensitivity C-reactive protein, and waist-hip ratio. The proportional hazards assumption was tested and confirmed using Schoenfeld residuals. To assess effect modification by sex, subsidiary analyses used interaction term between sex and RTL quartiles and tested for interaction with a likelihood ratio test. For the literature-based meta-analysis, we did not need to rescale published relative risks (RRs), because all eligible studies reported RRs on the same scale, i.e. for a comparison of extreme RTL quartiles. Hazard ratios (HRs) and odds ratios (ORs) were assumed to approximate the same measure of RR. Reported RRs were pooled using random-effects meta-analysis. Heterogeneity between studies was quantified using the I^2 statistic and tested by a standard χ^2 test [42]. Potential publication and small-study bias was

formally assessed using Egger's test [43]. All analyses were conducted with Stata 12.0. A two-sided P value ≤0.05 was considered statistically significant. The presentation of results follows the recommendations by the STROBE and PRISMA guidelines (see **Checklists S1** and **S2**).

Results

Baseline characteristics

The median RTL at baseline was 1.05 T/S ratios (interquartile range: 0.92–1.21). **Figure 1** summarises baseline characteristics of the study population (n = 684). The mean age of study participants was 63 years (SD, 11) and 49% were men. The multivariable adjusted regression dilution ratio of RTL was 0.68 (95% confidence interval: 0.61 to 0.76). We investigated the age- and sex-adjusted cross-sectional association at baseline between several characteristics and standardised RTL (**Figure 1**). The strongest association was observed with age. On average, every one standard deviation older age (11 years) was associated with 0.22 shorter standardised RTL (−0.30 to −0.15; P = 2×10^{-9}). There was no significant correlation of RTL with other parameters, including markers of inflammation, oxidative stress and hyperglycaemia (all P>0.05).

We further investigated whether baseline RTL differed according to baseline T2DM status (**Figure 2**). We observed no significant difference in RTL across the groups of normoglycaemic participants (n = 390), participants with impaired fasting glucose levels (n = 216), and participants with a clinical diagnosis of T2DM (n = 78) (P$_{trend}$ = 0.346).

Association of leucocyte telomere length with risk of incident type 2 diabetes mellitus

The Cox regression analyses excluded 78 participants with a baseline diagnosis of T2DM. Between 1995 and 2010, 44 of the 606 individuals in the study population developed T2DM (incidence rate, 5.8 per 1,000 person years [4.3 to 7.8]). **Table 1** compares T2DM risk across quartiles of decreasing RTL. In a comparison of the bottom vs. top quartile of baseline RTL, the age- and sex-adjusted HR was 1.89 (0.85 to 4.18; P = 0.116). The most adjusted model yielded a HR of 2.00 (0.90 to 4.49; P = 0.091). In a comparison of the bottom quartile of baseline RTL vs. the remainder, the respective HRs were 2.21 (1.17 to 4.16; P = 0.015) and 2.31 (1.21 to 4.41; P = 0.011). **Table 1** also shows analyses using long-term average RTL. In the most adjusted model, participants in the bottom quartile of long-term average RTL had a HR of 3.22 (1.27, to 8.14; P = 0.014) compared with the top RTL quartile and 2.86 (1.45 to 5.65; P = 0.002) compared with all other quartiles. We observed that increases in T2DM risk were confined to the bottom RTL quartile (particularly when using long-term average RTL), in line with a possible threshold effect (**Figure 3**). Results were similar in analyses that excluded the first five years of follow-up (data not shown). There was no evidence for differential associations in women and men (likelihood-ratio tests for interaction: P = 0.776 for baseline RTL; P = 0.571 for long-term average RTL).

Subsidiary analysis evaluated the association of a baseline diagnosis of T2DM with RTL change over 15 years. There was no significant difference in RTL dynamics according to baseline T2DM status (mean standardised RTL change in participants with vs. without T2DM at baseline [95% confidence interval]: −0.068 [−0.450 to 0.314]; P = 0.727). This analysis had limited power because it included only 400 study participants with RTL measurements available both in 1995 and 2010, of which only 20 had T2DM at baseline.

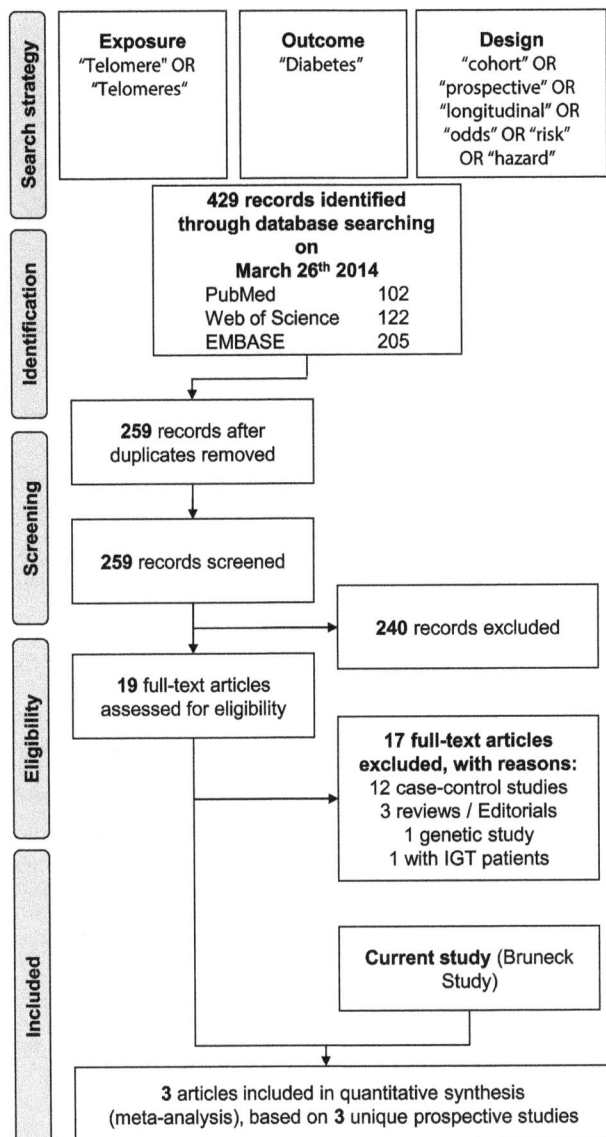

Figure 4. Study flow diagram of the literature-based meta-analysis. The figure is based on the 2009 PRISMA flow diagram template (available from http://www.prisma-statement.org/statement. htm).

Literature-based meta-analysis

Our literature search retrieved 429 records (**Figure 4**). We excluded 170 duplicate records and 240 records on the basis of their title and abstract. We carefully checked the full-text of the remaining 19 records and excluded a further 17 articles, including 12 case-control studies and 1 study that selectively recruited participants with impaired glucose tolerance [44]. Finally, together with the Bruneck Study, we identified three relevant prospective studies eligible for inclusion in the literature-based meta-analysis [41,45].

The characteristics of the three studies are summarised in **Figure 5**. The Strong Heart Family Study is a multigenerational study of American Indian families in four states of the USA, which recorded 292 incident T2DM events over a mean of 5.5 years (defined according to the 1997 American Diabetes Association criteria) [41]. The observational arm of the Women's Health

Initiative used a nested case-control analysis that included 1,675 incident cases of T2DM (defined based on self-report or T2DM hospitalisation) [45]. Overall, information from the three studies was available on 6,991 participants and 2,011 incident T2DM events recorded over a weighted mean of 6.6 years. Baseline age of participants ranged from 14 to 93 years; 18% were male. The reported multivariable adjusted RRs for T2DM were quantitatively similar in the Bruneck Study and the Strong Heart Family Study (**Figure 5**). The pooled RR for all three studies was 1.31 (1.07 to 1.60; P = 0.010) for a comparison of the bottom vs. the top quartile of baseline RTL. Between-study heterogeneity was moderate with an I^2 of 69% (0% to 91%) (**Figure 5**). There was no evidence of publication bias (P = 0.460). We could not calculate a pooled RR corrected for long-term variability, because such an estimate was only available for the Bruneck Study.

Discussion

In the present report, we demonstrate a significant positive association between shorter leucocyte telomeres and T2DM risk. In the Bruneck Study, the increase in risk appeared to be confined to the bottom quartile of RTL (i.e. participants with the shortest RTL) and was particularly evident in analyses correcting for long-term variability in RTL. In a pooled analysis of published reports from three prospective cohort studies, we estimated that people in the bottom RTL quartile had a 31% (7 to 60%) higher risk of developing T2DM than those in the longest RTL quartile.

RTL is a dynamic measure that may decrease but also increase over time [18–27]. Possible sources of variability in measured RTL include the (i) cumulative effect of environmental and behavioural exposures, (ii) varying telomerase activity, (iii) stress-induced repopulation of peripheral blood by recently dividing hematopoietic bone marrow cells, (iv) shifts in the cellular composition of peripheral blood leucocytes (differential blood count) and release of leucocyte subpopulations during acute infections [46,47] (i.e. "true variation"), and (v) measurement error. Previous epidemiological studies on RTL and T2DM risk have not been able to correct for RTL variability, potentially yielding biased estimates. The Bruneck study, which made such a correction on the basis of up to three repeated measurements taken over a follow-up time of 15 years, indicates an independent association of shorter telomeres with T2DM, of greater magnitude than previously reported. The within-person variability of RTL was comparable to that of commonly measured cardio-metabolic risk markers, such as blood pressure or high-sensitivity C-reactive protein. It was lower than previously reported [19] because we further optimised our technique for RTL quantification, including consistent DNA extraction method and re-measurement in quadruplicate.

Previous studies have suggested a possible threshold effect of associations of RTL with age-related diseases, including T2DM [41]. Our study independently confirms this hypothesis, demonstrating an elevation in T2DM risk only in the quartile of participants with the shortest telomeres. As suggested by Zhao *et al.* [41], one intriguing biological explanation for this finding could be the crossing of the "Hayflick limit" [3], beyond which cells cease to divide and undergo apoptosis. Furthermore, several pieces of evidence support that short telomeres play an important role in T2DM pathogenesis, rather than being an epiphenomenon of a pre-diabetic metabolic state. In mice, deletion of the telomerase RNA component (TERC) lowers the replication capacity of beta-cells and thereby leads to a reduced islet mass and failure to produce adequate amounts of insulin in response to glucose stimulation and high fat diet [13]. It has also been proposed that short telomeres impede insulin secretion through inhibition of

Study name	Location	Population source	n	Age range, years	% of males	NOS scale	No. of T2DM events	Length of follow-up, years	Level of adjustment*	Relative risk (95% CI) for T2DM comparing the bottom vs. the top quartile of leukocyte RTL
Bruneck Study	Italy	Population register	606	45-84	49	9	44	15.0†	■■■■■■ +2	2.00 (0.90, 4.49)
Strong Heart Family Study	USA	American Indian families	2328	14-93	40	8	292	5.5‡	■■■□□□□ +3	1.83 (1.26, 2.66)
WHI Observational Study	USA	Population register$	4057	50-79	0	6	1675	6.0†	■ x ■■□■■ +3	1.08 (0.84, 1.38)
Overall			6991	14-93	18		2011	6.6		1.31 (1.07, 1.60) [P=0.010] I^2=69%

(adjustment sub-columns: Age, Sex, Body mass index, Smoking, SES, Physical activity, Alcohol consumption, Further adjustment; forest plot axis: .5 1 2 4 8)

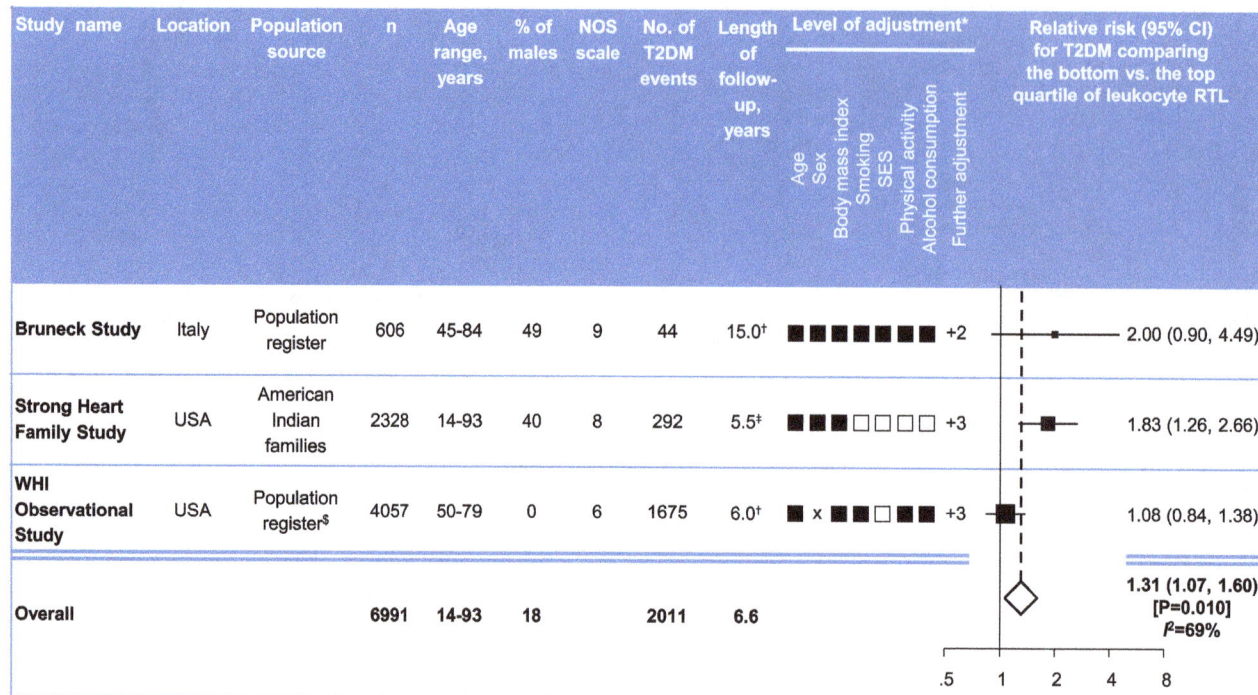

Figure 5. Description and meta-analysis of published data from three prospective cohort studies on the association of short telomeres and risk of type 2 diabetes mellitus. Published relative risks were pooled by random-effects meta-analysis. In the Bruneck Study and the Strong Heart Family Study, type 2 diabetes was defined according to the 1997 American Diabetes Association criteria. In the WHI Observational Study, diabetes was defined based on self-report and hospitalisation for type 2 diabetes. All three studies measured telomere length with a quantitative polymerase chain reaction technique. *Reported relative risks were additionally adjusted for two variables in the Bruneck Study (HDL cholesterol and log hsCRP), three variables in the Strong Heart Family Study (age^2, fasting glucose, total triglycerides), and three variables in the Women's Health Initiative Observational Study (date of blood collection, clinical centre, hormone therapy). †Max. ‡Mean. $The Women's Health Initiative Observational Study involved postmenopausal women who proved to be ineligible or unwilling to be randomised as part of the Women's Health Initiative Clinical Trial. Abbreviations: CI, confidence interval; NOS, Newcastle-Ottawa Scale for assessing the quality of nonrandomised studies in meta-analyses; T2DM, type 2 diabetes mellitus; WHI, Women's Health Initiative.

calcium-mediated exocytosis [14]. In adipocytes, cellular senescence leads to insulin resistance, which is reversible by inhibition of p53 activity [15]. In a study of 22,715 women and 1,445 incident T2DM events, Zee et al. have shown that genetic variants related to telomere pathways are associated with T2DM risk [48]. On the other hand, evidence suggests that diabetes has a marked impact on telomere length dynamics. High levels of oxidative stress observed in diabetes patients [16] accelerate telomere attrition because the high guanine content of telomeres makes them particularly vulnerable to reactive oxygen species [17]. Xu et al. demonstrated that new-borns have significantly shorter telomeres if their mother suffered from gestational diabetes [49]. However, the Nurses' Health Study has quantified genetic predisposition to T2DM with a risk score combining 36 genetic variants and ruled out a strong causal impact of T2DM on telomere dynamics (although the study was powered to only detect effects of ≥9% explained variability) [50].

To place our findings in context of the currently available epidemiological literature, we performed a systematic literature review and meta-analysis of the available published evidence from prospective cohort studies on the topic. The pooled RR for a comparison of bottom vs. top quartiles of telomere length (i.e. shortest vs. longest) involving data from 6,991 participants and 2,011 incident T2DM cases was 1.31 (1.07 to 1.60). In contrast to an earlier meta-analysis [12], we excluded articles reporting on case-control studies, thereby limiting the effect of reverse causation biases in our analysis. However, because the present evaluation

was based on observational studies, we cannot fully exclude the possibility that our estimates are confounded by other factors or the consequence of the often extended lag time between manifestation and diagnosis of T2DM.

Our study has several strengths. First, the Bruneck Study is representative of the general population (with a recruitment process using municipal registers and with a response rate>90%). It therefore crucially expands our knowledge from select populations (i.e. populations from specific ethnic backgrounds or other non-representative samples) to the healthy general community. Second, the Bruneck cohort is extremely well-characterised with 100% follow-up over 15 years and high-quality ascertainment of both clinical endpoints and potential confounders. The detailed characterisation of the study participants helped us estimate independent associations adjusted for a large panel of proposed risk markers for T2DM, including adiposity measures, smoking, social class, and physical activity. Third, the present study had a prospective design and used rigorous baseline examinations to exclude all individuals with T2DM at baseline, thereby minimising any reverse causation biases. Supplementary analyses that excluded the first five years of follow-up yielded qualitatively similar results. Fourth, to enhance validity of the measurement, we extracted all available DNA samples with the same DNA extraction kit. Although samples taken in 1995 and 2005 had been previously analysed [5,10], samples from all three time points were reanalysed simultaneously to avoid a measurement error over the time period. In addition, a bias according to the ascertainment of RTL on different qPCR plates was avoided by positioning the available DNA samples from a single individual from different time points side by side on the same plate. To maximise accuracy, RTL measurements were performed in quadruplicate, in an intensively standardised and automated manner, and within a short period of time by personnel blinded to the characteristics and outcome of the study participants. We have demonstrated previously that RTL measurement using qPCR, as performed in the Bruneck Study, is highly correlated with measurement of absolute telomere length using a Southern Blot technique (r = 0.765) [5]. Fifth, we were able to model long-term average RTL and provide effect estimates for T2DM corrected for fluctuations in RTL over time. Finally, we performed a comprehensive literature review and combined data from previously published prospective studies.

Our study also has potential limitations. First, the Bruneck Study population was entirely Caucasian and therefore findings are only generalizable to this ethnicity. Previous investigations by the Nurses' Health Study on differences by ethnicity (Caucasian, African Americans, Hispanic, and Asian) have shown generally comparable associations of RTL with T2DM incidence [45]. Second, telomere length was measured in circulating blood leucocytes only. More precise assessments and comparisons of telomere length in different tissues (e.g. liver, muscle, adipose tissue, and pancreas) would be helpful to better understand the role of telomeres in disease development but, clearly, this is not feasible in large population studies. Third, the number of incident T2DM events was low in the Bruneck Study limiting our ability to conduct more detailed investigations (e.g. extensive subgroup analyses), although major findings were independently confirmed in the literature-based meta-analysis. Fourth, the meta-analyses of published data used single baseline measurements of RTL to study the association with subsequent T2DM. Our analysis of RTL

reproducibility over up to 15 years suggests that previous studies could have substantially underestimated potential associations with T2DM. Finally, because the present evidence is limited to observational studies in primarily adult populations, no judgement on the causal involvement of telomere length in T2DM can be made on the basis of the present report.

Conclusion

Low RTL is independently associated with the risk of incident T2DM. To avoid regression dilution bias in observed associations of RTL with disease risk, future studies should implement methods correcting for within-person variability in RTL. Whether there is a causal involvement of telomeres in T2DM development remains to be determined.

Supporting Information

Checklist S1 STROBE Statement—Checklist of items that should be included in reports of cohort studies.

Checklist S2 PRISMA 2009 Checklist.

File S1 Underlying data for Figure 1, 3 and 5.

Author Contributions

Conceived and designed the experiments: PW AM SW JW FK SK. Performed the experiments: JR ST MH JLW FK. Analyzed the data: PW. Wrote the paper: PW JR EEH ST MH AM SW JLW ASB JW FK SK. Collected data on baseline characteristics and disease incidence of the Bruneck Study participants: PW AM SW JW SK.

References

1. Blackburn EH (1991) Structure and function of telomeres. Nature 350: 569–573.
2. Calado RT, Young NS (2009) Telomere diseases. N Engl J Med 361: 2353–2365.
3. Hayflick L (1965) The limited in vitro lifetime of human diploid cell strains. Exp Cell Res 37: 614–636.
4. Weischer M, Bojesen SE, Cawthon RM, Freiberg JJ, Tybjærg-Hansen A, et al. (2012) Short telomere length, myocardial infarction, ischemic heart disease, and early death. Arterioscler Thromb Vasc Biol 32: 822–829.
5. Willeit P, Willeit J, Brandstätter A, Ehrlenbach S, Mayr A, et al. (2010) Cellular aging reflected by leucocyte telomere length predicts advanced atherosclerosis and cardiovascular disease risk. Arterioscler Thromb Vasc Biol 30: 1649–1656.
6. Zee RY, Michaud SE, Germer S, Ridker PM (2009) Association of shorter mean telomere length with risk of incident myocardial infarction: a prospective, nested case-control approach. Clin Chim Acta 403: 139–141.
7. Brouilette SW, Moore JS, McMahon AD, Thompson JR, Ford I, et al. (2007) Telomere length, risk of coronary heart disease, and statin treatment in the West of Scotland Primary Prevention Study: a nested case-control study. Lancet 369: 107–114.
8. Haycock PC, Heydon EE, Kaptoge S, Butterworth AS, Thompson A, et al. (2014) Leucocyte telomere length and risk of cardiovascular disease: systematic review and meta-analysis. BMJ 349: g4227.
9. Wentzensen IM, Mirabello L, Pfeiffer RM, Savage SA (2011) The association of telomere length and cancer: a meta-analysis. Cancer Epidemiol Biomarkers Prev 20: 1238–1250.
10. Willeit P, Willeit J, Mayr A, Weger S, Oberhollenzer F, et al. (2010) Telomere length and risk of incident cancer and cancer mortality. JAMA 304: 69–75.
11. Ma H, Zhou Z, Wei S, Liu Z, Pooley KA, et al. (2011) Shortened telomere length is associated with increased risk of cancer: a meta-analysis. PLoS One 6: e20466.
12. Zhao J, Miao K, Wang H, Ding H, Wang DW (2013) Association between telomere length and type 2 diabetes mellitus: a meta-analysis. PLoS One 8: e79993.
13. Kuhlow D, Florian S, von Figura G, Weimer S, Schulz N, et al. (2010) Telomerase deficiency impairs glucose metabolism and insulin secretion. Aging (Albany NY) 2: 650–658.
14. Guo N, Parry EM, Li LS, Kembou F, Lauder N, et al. (2011) Short telomeres compromise β-cell signaling and survival. PLoS One 6: e17858.
15. Minamino T, Orimo M, Shimizu I, Kunieda T, Yokoyama M, et al. (2009) A crucial role for adipose tissue p53 in the regulation of insulin resistance. Nat Med 15: 1082–1087.
16. Roberts CK, Sindhu KK (2009) Oxidative stress and metabolic syndrome. Life Sci 84: 705–712.
17. Houben JM, Moonen HJ, van Schooten FJ, Hageman GJ (2008) Telomere length assessment: biomarker of chronic oxidative stress? Free Radic Biol Med 44: 235–246.
18. Weischer M, Bojesen SE, Nordestgaard BG (2014) Telomere shortening unrelated to smoking, body weight, physical activity, and alcohol intake: 4,576 general population individuals with repeat measurements 10 years apart. PLoS Genet 10: e1004191.
19. Willeit P, Willeit J, Kloss-Brandstätter A, Kronenberg F, Kiechl S (2011) Fifteen-year follow-up of association between telomere length and incident cancer and cancer mortality. JAMA 306: 42–44.
20. Svenson U, Nordfjäll K, Baird D, Roger L, Osterman P, et al. (2011) Blood cell telomere length is a dynamic feature. PLoS One 6: e21485.
21. Huzen J, Wong LS, van Veldhuisen DJ, Samani NJ, Zwinderman AH, et al. (2014) Telomere length loss due to smoking and metabolic traits. J Intern Med 275: 155–163.
22. Rehkopf DH, Dow WH, Rosero-Bixby L, Lin J, Epel ES, et al. (2014) Seasonal variation of peripheral blood leukocyte telomere length in Costa Rica: A population-based observational study. Am J Hum Biol 26: 367–375.
23. Epel ES, Merkin SS, Cawthon R, Blackburn EH, Adler NE, et al. (2009) The rate of leukocyte telomere shortening predicts mortality from cardiovascular disease in elderly men. Aging (Albany NY) 1: 81–88.
24. Nordfjäll K, Svenson U, Norrback KF, Adolfsson R, Lenner P, et al. (2009) The individual blood cell telomere attrition rate is telomere length dependent. PLoS Genet 5: e1000375.
25. Aviv A, Chen W, Gardner JP, Kimura M, Brimacombe M, et al. (2009) Leukocyte telomere dynamics: longitudinal findings among young adults in the Bogalusa Heart Study. Am J Epidemiol 169: 323–329.
26. Chen W, Kimura M, Kim S, Cao X, Srinivasan SR, et al. (2011) Longitudinal versus cross-sectional evaluations of leukocyte telomere length dynamics: age-dependent telomere shortening is the rule. J Gerontol A Biol Sci Med Sci 66: 312–319.

27. Farzaneh-Far R, Lin J, Epel E, Lapham K, Blackburn E, et al. (2010) Telomere length trajectory and its determinants in persons with coronary artery disease: longitudinal findings from the heart and soul study. PLoS One 5: e8612.

28. Kiechl S, Lorenz E, Reindl M, Wiedermann CJ, Oberhollenzer F, et al. (2002) Toll-like receptor 4 polymorphisms and atherogenesis. N Engl J Med 347: 185–192.

29. Kloss-Brandstätter A, Willeit P, Lamina C, Kiechl S, Kronenberg F (2010) Correlation between baseline telomere length and shortening over time–spurious or true? Int J Epidemiol 40: 840–841.

30. Baecke JA, Burema J, Frijters JE (1982) A short questionnaire for the measurement of habitual physical activity in epidemiological studies. Am J Clin Nutr 36: 936–942.

31. Tsimikas S, Willeit P, Willeit J, Santer P, Mayr M, et al. (2012) Oxidation-specific biomarkers, prospective 15-year cardiovascular and stroke outcomes, and net reclassification of cardiovascular events. J Am Coll Cardiol 60: 2218–2229.

32. Bonora E, Targher G, Alberiche M, Bonadonna RC, Saggiani F, et al. (2000) Homeostasis model assessment closely mirrors the glucose clamp technique in the assessment of insulin sensitivity: studies in subjects with various degrees of glucose tolerance and insulin sensitivity. Diabetes Care 23: 57–63.

33. Friedewald WT, Levy RI, Fredrickson DS (1972) Estimation of the concentration of low-density lipoprotein cholesterol in plasma, without use of the preparative ultracentrifuge. Clin Chem 18: 499–502.

34. Cawthon RM (2002) Telomere measurement by quantitative PCR. Nucleic Acids Res 30: e47.

35. Raschenberger J, Kollerits B, Hammerer-Lercher A, Rantner B, Stadler M, et al. (2013) The association of relative telomere length with symptomatic peripheral arterial disease: results from the CAVASIC study. Atherosclerosis 229: 469–474.

36. Pfaffl MW (2001) A new mathematical model for relative quantification in real-time RT-PCR. Nucleic Acids Res 29: e45.

37. Genuth S, Alberti KG, Bennett P, Buse J, Defronzo R, et al. (2003) Follow-up report on the diagnosis of diabetes mellitus. Diabetes Care 26: 3160–3167.

38. Wells G, Shea B, Peterson J, Welch V, Losos M, et al. (2000) The Newcastle-Ottawa Scale (NOS) for assessing the quality of nonrandomised studies in meta-analyses. Available: http://www.ohri.ca/programs/clinical_epidemiology/oxford.htm. Accessed 12 May 2014.

39. Wood AM, White I, Thompson SG, Lewington S, Danesh J (2006) Regression dilution methods for meta-analysis: assessing long-term variability in plasma fibrinogen among 27,247 adults in 15 prospective studies. Int J Epidemiol 35: 1570–1578.

40. Fibrinogen Studies Collaboration (2009) Correcting for multivariate measurement error by regression calibration in meta-analyses of epidemiological studies. Stat Med 28: 1067–1092.

41. Zhao J, Zhu Y, Lin J, Matsuguchi T, Blackburn E, et al. (2014) Short leukocyte telomere length predicts risk of diabetes in american indians: the strong heart family study. Diabetes 63: 354–362.

42. Higgins JP, Thompson SG, Deeks JJ, Altman DG (2003) Measuring inconsistency in meta-analyses. BMJ 327: 557–560.

43. Egger M, Smith GD, Schneider M, Minder C (1997) Bias in meta-analysis detected by a simple, graphical test. BMJ 315: 629–634.

44. Hovatta I, de Mello VD, Kananen L, Lindström J, Eriksson JG, et al. (2012) Leukocyte telomere length in the Finnish Diabetes Prevention Study. PLoS One 7: e34948.

45. You NC, Chen BH, Song Y, Lu X, Chen Y, et al. (2012) A prospective study of leukocyte telomere length and risk of type 2 diabetes in postmenopausal women. Diabetes 61: 2998–3004.

46. Cohen S, Janicki-Deverts D, Turner RB, Casselbrant ML, Li-Korotky HS, et al. (2013) Association between telomere length and experimentally induced upper respiratory viral infection in healthy adults. JAMA 309: 699–705.

47. Lin J, Epel E, Cheon J, Kroenke C, Sinclair E, et al. (2010) Analyses and comparisons of telomerase activity and telomere length in human T and B cells: insights for epidemiology of telomere maintenance. J Immunol Methods 352: 71–80.

48. Zee RY, Ridker PM, Chasman DI (2011) Genetic variants of 11 telomere-pathway gene loci and the risk of incident type 2 diabetes mellitus: the Women's Genome Health Study. Atherosclerosis 218: 144–146.

49. Xu J, Ye J, Wu Y, Zhang H, Luo Q, et al. (2014) Reduced fetal telomere length in gestational diabetes. PLoS One 9: e86161.

50. Du M, Prescott J, Cornelis MC, Hankinson SE, Giovannucci E, et al. (2013) Genetic predisposition to higher body mass index or type 2 diabetes and leukocyte telomere length in the Nurses' Health Study. PLoS One 8: e52240.

Ex Vivo Response to Histone Deacetylase (HDAC) Inhibitors of the HIV Long Terminal Repeat (LTR) Derived from HIV-Infected Patients on Antiretroviral Therapy

Hao K. Lu[1,2], **Lachlan R. Gray**[1,2], **Fiona Wightman**[1,2], **Paula Ellenberg**[1,2], **Gabriela Khoury**[1,2], **Wan-Jung Cheng**[2], **Talia M. Mota**[1,2,3], **Steve Wesselingh**[2,4], **Paul R. Gorry**[1,2,3], **Paul U. Cameron**[1,2,5], **Melissa J. Churchill**[2,6,7,9], **Sharon R. Lewin**[1,2,5,8]*,9

1 Department of Infectious Diseases, Monash University, Melbourne, Victoria, Australia, 2 Centre for Biomedical Research, Burnet Institute, Melbourne, Victoria, Australia, 3 Department of Microbiology and Immunology, University of Melbourne, Melbourne, Victoria, Australia, 4 South Australian Health and Medical Research Institute, Adelaide, Australia, 5 Infectious Disease Unit, Alfred Hospital, Melbourne, Victoria, Australia, 6 Department of Microbiology, Monash University, Clayton, Victoria, Australia, 7 Department of Medicine, Monash University, Clayton, Victoria, Australia, 8 Peter Doherty Institute, Melbourne University, Melbourne, Victoria, Australia

Abstract

Histone deacetylase inhibitors (HDACi) can induce human immunodeficiency virus (HIV) transcription from the HIV long terminal repeat (LTR). However, *ex vivo* and *in vivo* responses to HDACi are variable and the activity of HDACi in cells other than T-cells have not been well characterised. Here, we developed a novel assay to determine the activity of HDACi on patient-derived HIV LTRs in different cell types. HIV LTRs from integrated virus were amplified using triple-nested Alu-PCR from total memory CD4+ T-cells (CD45RO+) isolated from HIV-infected patients prior to and following suppressive antiretroviral therapy. NL4-3 or patient-derived HIV LTRs were cloned into the chromatin forming episomal vector pCEP4, and the effect of HDACi investigated in the astrocyte and epithelial cell lines SVG and HeLa, respectively. There were no significant differences in the sequence of the HIV LTRs isolated from CD4+ T-cells prior to and after 18 months of combination antiretroviral therapy (cART). We found that in both cell lines, the HDACi panobinostat, trichostatin A, vorinostat and entinostat activated patient-derived HIV LTRs to similar levels seen with NL4-3 and all patient derived isolates had similar sensitivity to maximum HDACi stimulation. We observed a marked difference in the maximum fold induction of luciferase by HDACi in HeLa and SVG, suggesting that the effect of HDACi may be influenced by the cellular environment. Finally, we observed significant synergy in activation of the LTR with vorinostat and the viral protein Tat. Together, our results suggest that the LTR sequence of integrated virus is not a major determinant of a functional response to an HDACi.

Editor: Fatah Kashanchi, George Mason University, United States of America

Funding: This work was supported by an Australian National Health and Medical Research Council (NHMRC) project grant 1009533 and 1051093; the National Institutes of Health, USA (NIMH100594) and the Division of AIDS, National Institute of Allergy and Infectious Disease, US National Institutes of Health (Delaney AIDS Research Enterprise, DARE; U19AI096109). S.R.L. is an NHMRC senior practitioner fellow. P.R.G is supported by an Australian Research Council Future Fellowship (FT2). L.R.G was supported by a NHMRC Early Career Fellowship (GNT0606967). G.K. is a recipient of an NHMRC Dora Lush biomedical post-graduate scholarship (579719). The funders had no role in study design, data collection and analysis, decision to publish, or preparation of the manuscript.

* Email: sharon.lewin@unimelb.edu.au

9 These authors contributed equally to this work.

Introduction

Despite the substantial reduction in morbidity and mortality following combination antiretroviral therapy (cART), current treatments do not cure HIV and treatment is required life-long. The major reason why cART cannot cure HIV is the persistence of HIV in resting memory and naïve CD4+ T-cells [1,2]. One strategy currently being pursued to eliminate latently infected cells is to stimulate virus production from latency [3].

Histone deacetylase inhibitors (HDACi) can activate HIV production efficiently in nearly all latently infected cell lines [4–9]. In contrast, in primary CD4+ T-cell models of latency, the capacity of an HDACi to activate virus production from a latent

provirus is variable –depending on the model used [10]. Using resting CD4+ T-cells from HIV-infected patients on cART *ex vivo*, the HDACi vorinsotat induced virus production in 50–80% of patients, in both the absence [11] or presence [8,12] of activated feeder cells. More recently, where virus production from patient cells was measured by RT-PCR in the absence of feeder cells, there was minimal virus production with vorinostat compared to the more potent HDACi romidepsin [9]. When using a reporter cell line to measure infection, other studies have shown minimal virus production following stimulation with all HDACi relative to maximal stimulation with a mitogen such as PMA and ionomycin [13]. Finally, when vorinostat and panobinostat were given to HIV-infected patients on ART, a variable response in activation of

Table 1. Primers and triple-nested Alu-LTR-PCR conditions.

	Primer	Sequence	PCR Condition
Round 1	Alu1	TCCCAGCTACTGGGGAGGCTGAGG	94°C for 10 minutes, 20 cycles of (94°C for 15 seconds, 56°C for 15 seconds and 72°C for 2 minutes), final extension at 72°C for 7 minutes
	Alu2	GCCTCCCAAAGTGCTGGGATTACAG	
	5′LTRf2	GCCACTTTTTAAAAGAAAAGGGGGACT	
Round 2	5′LTRf2	GCCACTTTTTAAAAGAAAAGGGGGACT	94°C for 10 minutes, 35 cycles of (94°C for 15 seconds, 51°C for 15 seconds and 72°C for 1 minutes), final extension at 72°C for 7 minutes
	3′nLTR#2	AAAAGGGTCTGAGGGATCTCT	
Round 3	5′KpnI-LTRf3	GGGGTACCAAAGGGGGACTGAAGGGCTAATTC	94°C for 10 minutes, 35 cycles of (94°C for 15 seconds, 52°C for 15 seconds and 72°C for 1 minutes), final extension at 72°C for 7 minutes
	3′nLTR#3	ACGGGCACACACTACTTGAA	

latent HIV has been observed in multiple studies [12,14,15]. Taken together these studies demonstrate a far more variable response of patient derived cells to treatment with HDACi *ex vivo* compared to models that are infected with laboratory strains of HIV.

It is likely that latent proviruses *in vivo*, may have variable sensitivity to stimulation with an HDACi. Factors such as sequence of the HIV LTR, the surrounding chromatin environment, the specific integration site or the cellular environment may all potentially play a role. Here, we found that the HIV LTR sequence isolated from T cells was not a factor in determining an *ex vivo* response to HDACi but that the capacity of an HDACi in inducing HIV transcription was dependent on the cell type examined with maximal LTR transcription observed in an epithelial cell line. Finally, the potency of the HDACi vorinostat was significantly enhanced in the presence of the viral protein Tat.

Materials and Methods

Patient recruitment

HIV-infected, cART naïve patients (n = 4) who were initiating cART were recruited at the Alfred Hospital, Melbourne. This was a sub-study of a previously reported prospective observational study [2]. Fifty millilitres of blood were collected at baseline and at 6, 12, 18, 24, and up to 60 months after initiation of cART. The parent study and sub-study were both approved by the Alfred hospital ethics committee (114/05) and written informed consent was obtained from all participants.

Isolation of the integrated HIV LTR from CD4+ T-cells

Total memory T-cells from HIV-infected patients, defined as CD4+CD45RO+CD28+, were isolated by flow cytometry sorting using anti-CD4-fluorescein isothiocyanate (FITC), anti-CD28-PE-cyanine dye (Cy5) and anti-CD45RO-allophycocyanin (APC; Becton Dickinson, San Jose, CA). Cells were lysed for PCR analysis using PCR lysis buffer (0.002% Triton X100, 0.002% SDS, 100 mM Tris.HCl (pH 8), 1 mM EDTA with freshly added Proteinase K 0.8 mg/ml). The DNA lysate was serially diluted using 1 in 10 dilutions and between 12 and 24 replicates from each

dilution were added to a first round PCR mix containing 0.2 μM of Alu1, Alu2 and 5′LTRf2 primers (Table 1) in ImmoMix PCR premix (Bioline, London, UK). The PCR was performed using conditions described in Table 1. Two microliters of the first-round product were then added to a second-round PCR mix containing 0.2 μM 5′LTRf2 and 3′nLTR#2 primers in ImmoMix PCR premix (Table 1). Subsequently, two microliters of the second-round product were then added to a third-round PCR mix containing 0.2 μM 5′KpnI-LTRf3 and 3′nLTR#3 primers in ImmoMix PCR premix (Table 1). The resulting products of the first round PCR were Alu-LTR, LTR-Alu, Alu-Alu with varying length, depending on the distance of the integrated LTR to the closest Alu. The second and third round PCRs then preferentially amplify the integrated LTR sequence. PCR products were analysed by 1% agarose gel electrophoresis. The dilution that yielded a PCR product in <30% of replicates, was assumed to contain one amplifiable template per reaction more than 80% of the time, according to a Poisson distribution [16]. Using ACH2 cells (NIH AIDS Reagent Program [17]), a T-cell line that contains a single integrated copy of HIV, we determined that the lower limit of detection was <2 copies of HIV DNA per well. PCR products were sequenced and hypermutated LTRs (G->A) were identified using the software Hypermut (http://www.hiv.lanl.gov/content/sequence/HYPERMUT/hypermut.html). Hypermutated LTRs were removed from further analyses. A phylogenetic tree was constructed using the neighbour-joining method with CLC Workbench software (Version 6, CLC Bio, Aarhus, Denmark), with bootstrapping resampling done with 100 replicates. The consensus NL4-3 sequence was used for comparison with patient samples.

Cells lines and cytotoxicity assay

The SVG astrocyte cell line [18] was cultured in Minimum Essential Medium (MEM) with Earle's salts supplemented with 10% heat-inactivated fetal bovine serum (HI-FBS), 1× penicillin-streptomycin-glutamine (PSG) (Invitrogen, Carlsbad, CA). The HeLa cell line (ATCC) was cultured in MEM containing 10% HI-FBS and 1× PSG.

Each cell line was treated with varying concentrations of trichostatin A (TSA; Sigma), vorinostat [suberoylhydroxamic acid (SAHA)], panobinostat (LBH589) and entinostat (MS-275; all from Selleck Chemicals, Houston, TX) for 24 hours and toxicity was assessed with the MTS colorimetric assay according to manufacturer's instructions (Promega, Madison, WI). Experiments were performed in triplicate and the cytotoxic concentration 50 (CC$_{50}$) values were generated using GraphPad Prism software (Version 6, Graphpad, La Jolla, CA).

Cloning of HIV LTR into pCEP4

The plasmid pCEP4 (Invitrogen) was digested with SalI (NEB Biolabs, Ipswich, MA) to remove the entire existing promoter region, the multiple cloning site and the SV40 poly A sequence (Fig 1). The plasmid was then blunt ended and a fragment of the Δ-57/-4 HIV [19] LTR-pGL3 plasmid spanning the entire LTR and including the luciferase gene [20] was digested with Acc65I/ BamHI and cloned into pCEP4. To clone the patient LTRs into pCEP4, patient-derived LTRs and the Δ-57/-4 HIV LTR-pCEP4 vector were both digested with Acc65I and HindIII according to the manufacturer's instructions (NEB Biolabs). The digested LTRs and pCEP4 vector were ligated using T4 DNA Ligase (NEB Biolabs). Correctly inserted clones were initially screened by colony-PCR and later confirmed by restriction digest using SalI (NEB Biolabs).

The pCEP4 plasmid contains an Epstein-Barr virus nuclear antigen protein (EBNA-1) to allow for extrachromosomal replication in mammalian cells [21]. Importantly, any genes cloned into pCEP4 are susceptible to post-transcriptional modifications such as methylation [21,22], which is important for our study.

Transfection of cells with pCEP4

HeLa (3,000 cells/well) or SVG (5,000 cells/well) cells were seeded overnight into a 96-well flat-bottom plate. The following day, media was replaced with 100 μL of cell media without antibiotics and transfected with 50 μL of pre-mixed Lipofectamine 2000 (Invitrogen) contain 200 ng/well of patient-derived or NL4-3 LTR-pCEP4 according to the manufacturer's instructions (Invitrogen). In some experiments, cells were also co-transfected with 4 ng/well of pTargeT-HxB2-Tat vector [20]. After 4 hours, cell culture media was replaced with fresh culture media containing antibiotics and incubated for another 20 hours. Subsequently, various doses of panobinostat, trichostatin A, vorinostat and entinostat; or phorbyl myristoacetate (PMA [20 ng/ml]; Sigma St. Louis, MO) were added for 24 hours. Cells were then lysed in 1× Luciferase Assay Buffer (Promega, Madison, WI) and the transcriptional activity of the LTR was measured by quantifying luciferase expression using the Luciferase Assay System (Promega) according to manufacturer's instructions. Luminescence was measured using a FLUOStar Optima microplate reader (BMG Labtech, Ortenberg, Germany).

To determine the transfection efficiency, HeLa or SVG were transfected as above with pEGFP-N1 (Clontech, Mountain View, CA), a GFP-expressing plasmid, and the percentage of cells expressing GFP was analysed 24 hours after transfection.

Quantification of HDAC proteins

To determine the expression level of HDAC 1, 2, 3 and 4 proteins in HeLa and SVG, five million cells were lysed in RIPA lysis buffer (Thermo Scientific, Rockford, IL), containing 1% Halt protease inhibitor cocktail (Thermo Scientific). Protein concentration was determined using a Bradford protein assay (Bio-Rad, Hercules, CA). Twenty microgram of total proteins were loaded onto a 10% SDS PAGE, transferred onto a PVDF membrane and

sequentially probed with rabbit anti-HDAC1, 2 and 4 and goat anti-HDAC3 (Santa Cruz Biotechnology, Dallas, TX). HDAC proteins were detected using Alexa Fluor 680-conjugated goat anti-rabbit or donkey anti-goat secondary antibodies (Cell Signaling Technology, Danvers, MA) and imaged on an Odyssey fluorescent reader (LI-COR, Lincoln, NE).

Statistical analysis

The potency of HDACi in each cell line was analysed using one-way analysis of variance (ANOVA) with Tukey post-test. The potency of HDACi between different cell lines was measured using a Student's t-test. The synergistic effects of vorinostat with PMA or Tat co-transfection was analysed using a Student's t-test where the combined effect of vorinostat + PMA or vorinostat + Tat was compared to the sum effect of the individual treatments (GraphPad Prism 6, LA Jolla, CA).

Results

HIV LTRs sequences isolated from memory CD4+ T-cells show no significant changes following cART

To investigate whether there was selection or evolution of the HIV LTR following suppressive cART, integrated HIV LTR from memory CD4+ T-cells from HIV infected patients prior to and after suppressive cART were cloned and sequenced. The clinical details of these patients (n = 4) are summarised in Table 2. Sequence analysis of the integrated HIV LTRs showed no compartmentalisation between viral sequences in memory CD4+ T-cells prior to and following 18–24 months (Fig 2, P4–6) or up to 60 months of suppressive cART (Fig 2, P1).

Patient-derived HIV LTRs are responsive to reactivation by all HDACi

To characterise the ex vivo response of patient derived HIV LTR to HDACi, we first determined the cytotoxicity of each HDACi in each cell line. In the SVG astrocyte cell line, cytotoxicity assays showed that the HDACi panobinostat (CC$_{50}$: 77 nM) was the most toxic followed by trichostatin A (CC$_{50}$: 482 nM), entinostat (CC$_{50}$: ~5296 nM) and vorinostat (CC$_{50}$: 6864 nM) (Fig 3A–I).

We then determined the dose response of individual HDACi on the HIV LTR using the pCEP4 plasmid that contained wild-type NL4-3 LTR. The pCEP4 plasmid forms a mini chromatin structure following transfection [23], which does not integrate into the host genome. This approach therefore allowed us to examine the effects of HDACi independent of integration site.

Following transfection of NL4-3 LTR-pCEP4 into SVG cells and treatment with various doses of HDACi, we quantified luciferase activity. Treatment with PMA (20 ng/ml) and co-transfection with Tat (4 ng) were used as positive controls and induced an increase in luciferase activity of 2.3 ± 0.3 and a 45.0 ± 1 fold above the media-treated sample, respectively. Panobinostat (50 nM), trichostatin A (250 nM), vorinostat (5 μM) and entinostat (5 μM) induced an increase in luciferase activity above the media-treated sample of 17.4 ± 2.6, 17.7 ± 3.3, 25.8 ± 1.7 and 26.8 ± 3.2 fold respectively (Fig 3A–II; n = 3). These concentrations of HDACi were used in subsequent experiments in SVG as they were shown to induce the maximal response from NL4-3 LTR-pCEP4 but were below the CC$_{50}$ value.

Patient-derived LTRs isolated prior to and following cART were ligated into pCEP4 as described above. We found that the patient derived LTRs had similar sensitivity to HDACi as seen with NL4-3 LTR-pCEP4 with a mean ± SE fold increase in luciferase above untreated control following panobinostat

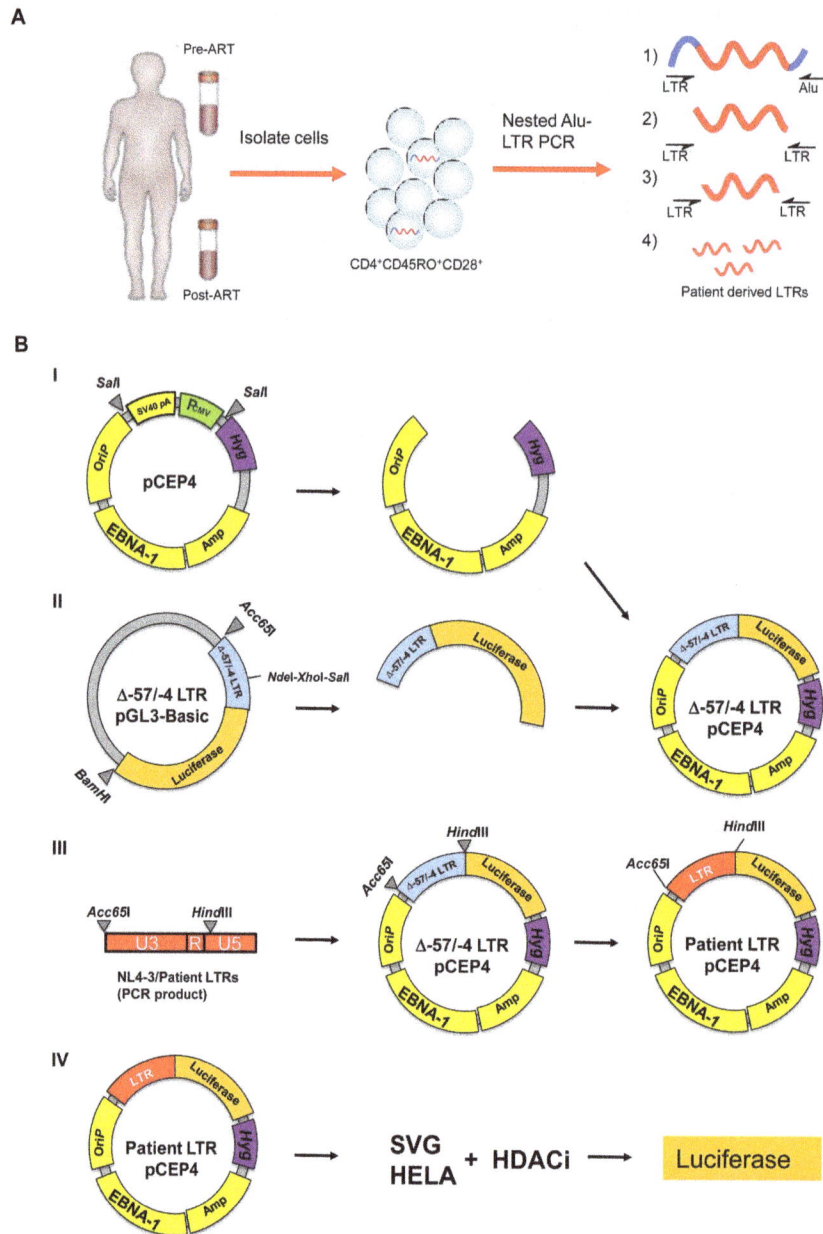

Figure 1. Cloning of patient-derived HIV LTRs into pCEP4. (A) Total memory T cells from HIV-infected individuals were isolated from blood collected prior to or after receiving cART. The integrated HIV LTRs from these cells were isolated by triple nested Alu-LTR PCR. (B)(I) The plasmid pCEP4 was digested with *Sal*I to remove the entire PCMV promoter region and the SV40 poly A sequences. (II) DNA sequence of the Δ-57/-4 HIV LTR and the luciferase gene was generated by digestion of the Δ-57/-4 LTR pGL3-Basic vector [20] and ligated into pCEP4. (III) Patient-derived HIV LTRs were cloned into the Δ-57/-4 LTR-pCEP4 vector using the *Acc65*I and *Hind*III sites. (IV) Patient LTR pCEP4 was transfected into SVG and HeLa cell lines; the activity of various HDACi on LTR transcription was measured by quantification of luciferase activity.

(23.8±2.7), trichostatin A (22.4±0.8), vorinostat (26.4±3) and entinostat (25.9±3.9) (Fig 3A–III, n = 9). There was no significant difference in the maximum fold luciferase induction between HDACi at the concentrations tested. LTRs derived from patients while on suppressive cART were also sensitive to reactivation by all HDACi (Fig 3A–III). To confirm that we were not missing subtle differences between patient-derived LTRs following stimulation with lower concentration of HDACi rather than maximal stimulation, we also evaluated the response of three patient derived LTRs to a wide range of HDACi concentrations and again found

no significant differences between the patient derived LTRs which all had similar EC50 to the wild type LTR (Figure S1).

Most LTRs showed a greater responsiveness to Tat than to treatment with HDACi (range 2.2-160 fold above untreated control). We identified one clone that was highly sensitive to reactivation by Tat (P4BL1) and a clone that was resistant to Tat-mediated transactivation (P6BL6). There were no obvious mutations of the LTR at the NF-kB, SP1 or TATA sites [24,25] that may have rendered this clone resistant to tat-mediated transactivation.

Table 2. Patient characteristics.

Patient ID	Age* (yrs)	Study sample (time on ART)	VL (RNA copies/ml)	CD4 count (cell/µl)
P1	43	BL	3700	27
		(60 months)	<50	183
P4	71	BL	100000	71
		(18 months)	<50	397
P5	41	BL	100000	118
		(24 months)	<50	792
P6	41	BL	71700	129
		(18 months)	<50	297

BL, Baseline; VL, viral load in plasma; * age at recruitment ie BL.

The same experiments were then performed in HeLa cells (Fig 3B–I to III) where the CC_{50} for each HDACi was similar to what we found with SVG (Fig 3B–I). In the HeLa cell line, the maximal fold induction of luciferase from patient-derived LTRs (n = 4) by panobinostat (622±35 fold increase) and vorinostat (660±59 fold increase) were significantly greater compared to trichostatin A (288±37 fold increase; p = 0.004), but was not significantly greater than entinostat (522± fold increase) (Fig 3B–III).

Significantly greater response of the HIV LTR to HDACi in the HeLa compared to SVG cell lines

We observed similar levels of luciferase in HeLa compared to SVG following stimulation with Tat (approximately a 40 fold increase) but significantly higher levels of luciferase activity following stimulation by each of the HDACi in HeLa (Fig 3C). The differences in the maximum fold induction of HDACi in SVG

and HeLa cells were unlikely to be attributed to the expression of the HDAC proteins 1–4 which were similar in the two cell lines (Figure S2A) or efficiency of transfection given that we observed similar transfection efficiency in both cell types when using an expressed green fluorescent protein (GFP) reporter plasmid (Figure S2B).

Vorinostat synergises with Tat to increase transcription of HIV LTRs

Given that the transactivation activity of Tat is tightly regulated by post-translational modification such as acetylation and methylation [26–28], we next investigated whether there was a synergistic response of the LTR to Tat and an HDACi. Using NL4-3 LTR-pCEP4 transfected into the SVG cell line, we showed that vorinostat significantly enhanced the transactivation activity of Tat by up to 2.7 fold (Fig 4A). This synergistic effect was also observed using two patient-derived LTRs (P4T3 and P5T4, n = 3).

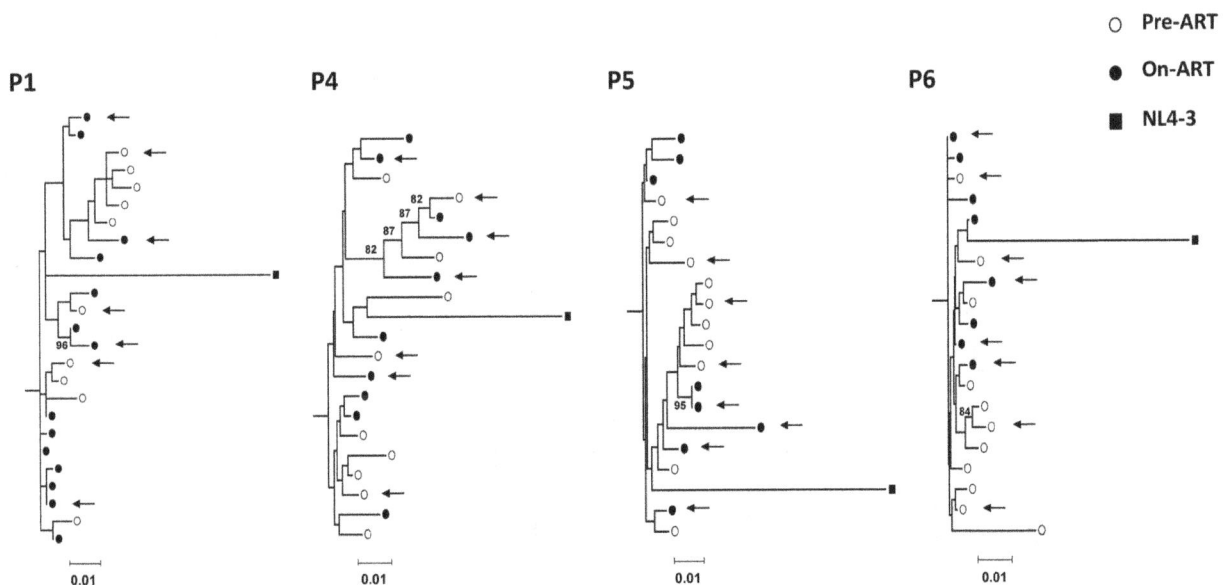

Figure 2. Phylogenetic analyses of DNA sequences derived from integrated virus in CD4+ memory T-cells. Phylogenetic trees were constructed using a neighbour-joining method with sequences from nucleotide 6 to 548 of the LTR derived from memory CD4+ T-cells prior to the initiation of cART (*open symbols*), after at least 18 months of cART (*closed symbols*) in four participants and the consensus sequence from NL4-3 (square symbol). Arrows indicate clones selected at random for cloning into pCEP4. Scale-bars indicate genetic distance (e.g., 0.01 = 1% genetic distance). Bootstrap values of >75 are shown on branches. All hypermutated clones (P<0.05 analysed on Hypermut V2.0) were excluded from the analysis.

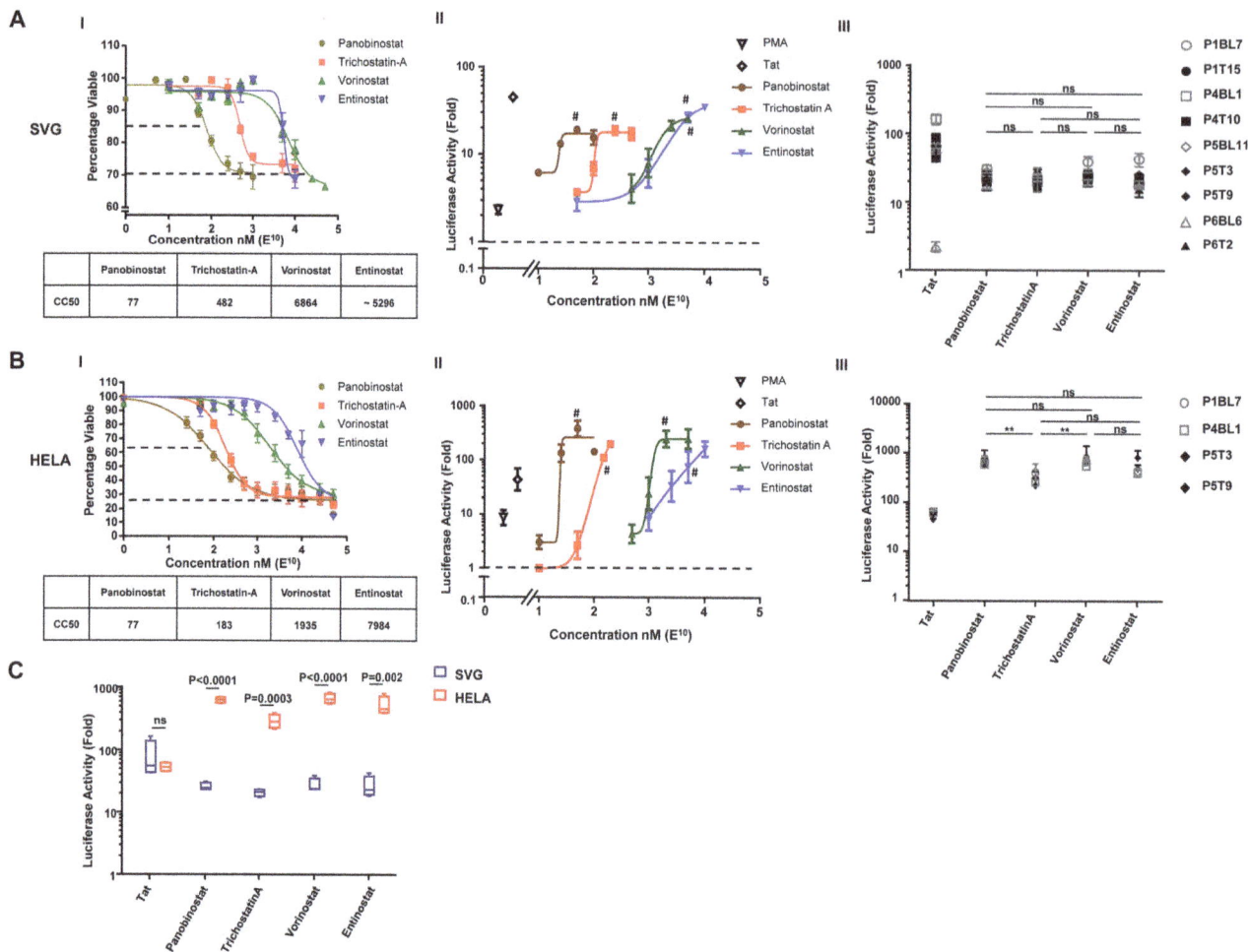

Figure 3. *Ex vivo* **response of patient-derived HIV LTRs to HDACi in A. SVG and B. HeLa cell lines.** (I) Each cell line was incubated with different concentrations of HDACi for 24 hr and toxicity was measured by the MTS assay. The cytotoxic concentration 50 (CC_{50}) for each drug is shown. (II) SVG or HeLa cells were transiently transfected with the wild-type NL4-3 LTR- pCEP4 and treated with various concentrations of HDACi for 24 hr. Co-transfection with Tat (4 ng) or incubation with PMA (20 nM) were used as positive controls. The activity of the LTR was measured as the fold change in luciferase compared to the untreated sample. # indicates doses of individual HDACi that were closest to the CC_{50} and induced the largest fold change increase in luciferase activity. (III) Luciferase expression following transfection of pCEP4 containing LTR sequences isolated from total memory CD4[+] T-cells prior to or after cART and treated with the optimal dose of HDACi. (C) Comparison of the luciferase expression in HeLa (red) and SVG (blue) following transfection of pCEP4 containing LTR sequences from (B III) and treated with the optimal dose of HDACi. Boxes represent the median, 25th and 75th percentiles and error bars the 10th and 90th percentiles. Ns = not statistically significant.

We also investigated the effects of HDACi on APOBEC3G induced hypermutated LTRs (defined as a G to A mutation [29]) given that up to ~1/3 of noninduced proviruses are hypermutated [30]. Despite failing to be activated by Tat alone, these hypermutated sequences were sensitive to reactivation by vorinostat (Fig 4B) and co-stimulation of cells with vorinostat and Tat significantly enhanced the level of luciferase production by up to 7.3-fold (Fig 4B, n = 3).

Finally, given that previous studies have shown that HDACi synergise with prostratin (an NF-κB/PKC activator [31,32]); we wanted to determine whether this synergism could be demonstrated in this model. Using PMA to activate PKC, we showed that vorinostat and PMA increased the transcriptional activity of NL4-3 LTR-pCEP4 by 1.5 fold (Fig 4C); however, there was no significant synergism between HDACi and PMA using patient-derived HIV LTRs in this model.

Discussion

HDACi are now being evaluated in HIV-infected patients on suppressive cART as a strategy to eliminate latently infected cells. The response of resting CD4[+] T-cells from HIV-infected patients on cART to HDACi stimulation is variable both *in vivo* and *ex vivo* but the mechanism for this variable response is currently unclear. Here we demonstrate that the HDACi panobinostat, trichostatin A, vorinostat and entinostat can induce transcription from the majority of HIV LTRs isolated from memory CD4[+] T-cells from HIV infected patients on suppressive cART. Furthermore, there were no differences in response to HDACi from HIV LTRs isolated from patients prior to or after treatment with cART. The main factor that determined the magnitude of response to HDACi stimulation was the cellular environment with a maximal fold induction of luciferase observed in the HeLa cell line.

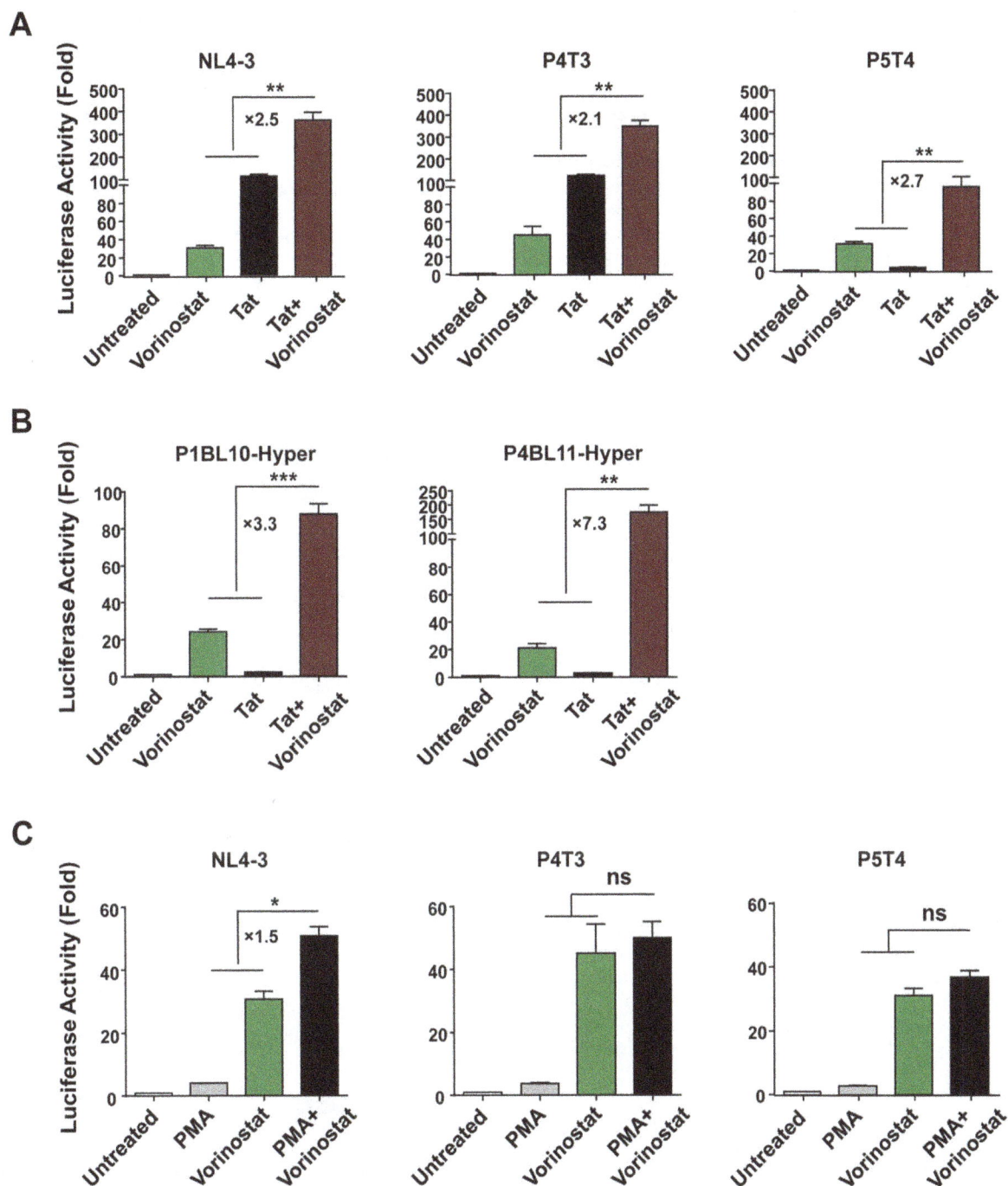

Figure 4. Vorinostat synergises with Tat and not PMA to increase transcription of the HIV LTR. SVG cells were transiently transfected with pCEP4 plasmid containing either NL4-3 or patient-derived HIV LTRs and luciferase activity was quantified following treatment with vorinostat (5 μM) and co-transfection with Tat using (A) non-mutated or (B) hypermutated ($P<0.05$ analysed on Hypermut V2.0) patient-derived HIV LTRs. (C) luciferase activity was quantified following stimulation of non-mutated patient-derived LTRs with vorinostat and PMA (20 ng/ml). Error bars represent standard error of the mean of three independent experiments. * $P<0.05$, ** $P<0.01$ and *** $P<0.001$. ns = not statistically significant.

HDACi are subdivided into different classes based on their biochemical structure. Trichostatin A and panobinostat are both hydroxamic acids, whereas vorinostat is a suberoylanilide hydroxamic acid and entinostat is a benzamide derivative [3,33,34]. Slight differences in the chemical structure of the various HDACi may affect the way they interact with host histone acetyltransferases and transcription factors. Additionally, panobinostat, trichos-

tatin A and vorinostat are pan-HDACi, whilst entinostat specifically inhibits HDAC1 and 3 [35]. We showed that both vorinostat and panobinostat induced a similar magnitude of luciferase expression when tested at concentrations below the CC_{50}. However, panobinostat was substantially more potent (> 100 fold) as described in multiple previous studies using $CD4^+$ T-cells from HIV-infected patients on cART [13,36], a primary T-cell model of HIV latency [36,37] or latently infected cell lines [38], which all showed a significantly lower EC50 of panobinostat compared to vorinostat. The maximum fold response, using concentrations of HDACi that were within the therapeutic range *in vivo* [39] was clearly not dependent on the sequence of the LTR.

The maximum fold increase in luciferase expression induced by HDACi varied significantly between the two cell lines tested, even though there were similar responses to Tat. The differences in response to HDACi between these cell lines were not explained by differential expression of HDACs in these cells or transfection efficiency (Figure S2). The SVG cell line was originally derived from a primary glial cell that is less activated and has lower replication rate and capacity [18] compared to the HeLa cell, a cervical cancer cell, which has a doubling time of approximately 18–24 hours [40]. As most transcription factors are increased in replicating cells or with activation [41], one might expect the transcriptional activity of an SVG to be lower than HeLa, which was indeed what we observed. It is also possible that these two cell lines may differ in other key factors required for transcription of HIV including recruitment of HDAC and histone acetyltransferases to the LTR, and/or the concentration of critical proteins such as positive transcription elongation factor b (P-TEFb) and its association with the inhibitory complex comprising of HEXIM1 and 7SK snRNP [31,42–44]. Phosphorylation of P-TEFb by vorinostat has recently been demonstrated and may also differ between the two cell lines tested in this study [45].

We observed clear synergy between Tat and the HDACi vorinostat – even with LTR sequences that had minimal responsiveness to Tat alone. The activity of Tat is tightly regulated by post-translation modification processes such as acetylation specifically at lysine 28 (K28) and K50/52 [26,27,46]. It is possible that vorinostat is capable of modifying Tat's function via acetylation of these key residues. Indeed, synergism between trichostatin A and Tat has previously been reported, and was dependent on lysine residues at K28 and K50 [46]. This synergistic interaction with Tat should be further exploited to increase the activity of HDACi in driving HIV transcription.

Finally, we found that all HDACi tested in this study could activate transcription from the HIV LTRs even when there was evidence of hypermutation. Although these hypermutated LTRs are unlikely to contribute to production of replication competent virus [29], the fact that these hypermutants were sensitive to reactivation by a HDACi could be of biological significance especially if protein produced from these viruses could also stimulate HIV-specific T-cells responses [9].

This is the first study to evaluate the effectiveness of HDACi to activate patient derived LTR sequences *ex vivo* in cells other than T cells. The study highlights the impact of the cellular environment on the ability of HDACi to activate transcription and is important for understanding the use of HDACi in cure strategies. However our approach has several limitations. First, the pCEP system although forming mini chromatin, doesn't integrate into the host genome. It is possible that the nucleosome positioning of these LTRs may therefore be different to what has been observed in HIV-infected cells from patients. However, we believe there are several reasons to expect they would be similar. First, our

patient-derived LTR-pCEP4 constructs included all the sequences normally required for integration and nucleosome positioning [47]. Second, it has been shown that nuc-0, 1, 2 are strictly formed at specific positions regardless of the site of virus integration in the host gene [47,48], suggesting it is the sequence of the LTR that confer nucleosome formation and not the surrounding host or plasmid sequences. However, we recognise that the epigenetic environment of host DNA will also influence the activity of HDACi *in vivo* and the use of an integrating vector with patient derived LTRs would be of interest. These experiments are currently being performed.

In conclusion, we have developed an *ex vivo* model to assess the response of patient derived LTRs to different HDACi. We have shown that changes in the HIV LTR sequence did not translate into differences in sensitivity to activation of transcription by an HDACi. Using concentrations of HDACi close to the CC_{50}, similar maximum fold activation was observed for a panel of HDACi. Therefore, we propose that other factors such as the site of integration and the surrounding epigenetic environment are likely to be relevant in determining the variable response of latently infected cells to stimulation with an HDACi.

Supporting Information

Figure S1   Dose response of HDACi on the activity of patient-derived HIV LTRs. HeLa cells was transiently transfected with three patient-derived LTR-pCEP4 and treated with various concentrations of HDACi for 24 hours. The activity of the LTR was measured as the fold change in luciferase compared to the untreated sample. All patient-LTRs produced a similar pattern of response to HDACi compared with the NL4-3 LTR from Figure 3A-II. Error bars represent standard deviation of two independent experiments.

Figure S2   Expression of HDACs proteins and transfection efficiency of HeLa and SVG cells. (A) Total cell lysate (20 μg) from HeLa and SVG were probed with antibodies to HDAC1, 2, 3 and 4 and detected by Western blotting. GAPDH was used as a control for equal protein loading. (B) HeLa (left) and SVG cells (right) were transfected with a GFP-expressing plasmid (solid line) or control plasmid (broken line) for 24 hours and expression of GFP was analysed by flow cytometry. Histogram is a representative of two experiments with similar GFP expression.

Acknowledgments

The authors gratefully acknowledge the contribution to this work of the Victorian Operational Infrastructure Support Program received by the Burnet Institute.

Author Contributions

Conceived and designed the experiments: HKL LRG SW PRG PUC MJC SRL PE. Performed the experiments: HKL. Analyzed the data: HKL LRG WJC MJC. Contributed reagents/materials/analysis tools: LRG FW GK WJC MJC SRL. Wrote the paper: HKL LRG FW GK TMM PRG PUC MJC SRL PE.

References

1. Siliciano JD, Kajdas J, Finzi D, Quinn TC, Chadwick K, et al. (2003) Long-term follow-up studies confirm the stability of the latent reservoir for HIV-1 in resting CD4+ T cells. Nature medicine 9: 727–728.

2. Wightman F, Solomon A, Khoury G, Green JA, Gray L, et al. (2010) Both CD31(+) and CD31(-) naive CD4(+) T cells are persistent HIV type 1-infected reservoirs in individuals receiving antiretroviral therapy. The Journal of infectious diseases 202: 1738–1748.

3. Wightman F, Ellenberg P, Churchill M, Lewin SR (2012) HDAC inhibitors in HIV. Immunology and cell biology 90: 47–54.

4. Ylisastigui L, Archin NM, Lehrman G, Bosch RJ, Margolis DM (2004) Coaxing HIV-1 from resting CD4 T cells: histone deacetylase inhibition allows latent viral expression. AIDS 18: 1101–1108.

5. Shehu-Xhilaga M, Rhodes D, Wightman F, Liu HB, Solomon A, et al. (2009) The novel histone deacetylase inhibitors metacept-1 and metacept-3 potently increase HIV-1 transcription in latently infected cells. AIDS 23: 2047–2050.

6. Savarino A, Mai A, Norelli S, El Daker S, Valente S, et al. (2009) "Shock and kill" effects of class I-selective histone deacetylase inhibitors in combination with the glutathione synthesis inhibitor buthionine sulfoximine in cell line models for HIV-1 quiescence. Retrovirology 6: 52.

7. Keedy KS, Archin NM, Gates AT, Espeseth A, Hazuda DJ, et al. (2009) A limited group of class I histone deacetylases acts to repress human immunodeficiency virus type 1 expression. Journal of virology 83: 4749–4756.

8. Archin NM, Keedy KS, Espeseth A, Dang H, Hazuda DJ, et al. (2009) Expression of latent human immunodeficiency type 1 is induced by novel and selective histone deacetylase inhibitors. AIDS 23: 1799–1806.

9. Cillo AR, Sobolewski MD, Bosch RJ, Fyne E, Piatak M Jr, et al. (2014) Quantification of HIV-1 latency reversal in resting CD4+ T cells from patients on suppressive antiretroviral therapy. Proceedings of the National Academy of Sciences of the United States of America.

10. Spina CA, Anderson J, Archin NM, Bosque A, Chan J, et al. (2013) An in-depth comparison of latent HIV-1 reactivation in multiple cell model systems and resting CD4+ T cells from aviremic patients. PLoS pathogens 9: e1003834.

11. Bouchat S, Gatot JS, Kabeya K, Cardona C, Colin L, et al. (2012) Histone methyltransferase inhibitors induce HIV-1 recovery in resting CD4+ T cells from HIV-1-infected HAART-treated patients. AIDS 26: 1473–1482.

12. Archin NM, Liberty AL, Kashuba AD, Choudhary SK, Kuruc JD, et al. (2012) Administration of vorinostat disrupts HIV-1 latency in patients on antiretroviral therapy. Nature 487: 482–485.

13. Bullen CK, Laird GM, Durand CM, Siliciano JD, Siliciano RF (2014) New ex vivo approaches distinguish effective and ineffective single agents for reversing HIV-1 latency in vivo. Nature medicine 20: 425–429.

14. Rasmussen TA, Tolstrup M, Brinkmann CR, Olesen R, Erikstrup C, el al. (2014) Panobinostat, a histone deacetylase inhibitor, for latent-virus reactivation in HIV-infected patients on suppressive antiretroviral therapy: a phase 1/2, single group, clinical trial. Lancet 1: e13–e21.

15. Elliott JH, Wightman F, Solomon AE, Ghneim K, Ahlers J, et al. (2014) Activation of HIV Transcription with Short-course Vorinostat in HIV-infected Patients on Suppressive Antiretroviral Therapy. PLoS pathogens. In Press

16. Salazar-Gonzalez JF, Bailes E, Pham KT, Salazar MG, Guffey MB, et al. (2008) Deciphering human immunodeficiency virus type 1 transmission and early envelope diversification by single-genome amplification and sequencing. Journal of virology 82: 3952–3970.

17. Clouse KA, Powell D, Washington I, Poli G, Strebel K, et al. (1989) Monokine regulation of human immunodeficiency virus-1 expression in a chronically infected human T cell clone. Journal of immunology 142: 431–438.

18. Major EO, Miller AE, Mourrain P, Traub RG, de Widt E, et al. (1985) Establishment of a line of human fetal glial cells that supports JC virus multiplication. Proceedings of the National Academy of Sciences of the United States of America 82: 1257–1261.

19. Zeichner SL, Kim JY, Alwine JC (1991) Linker-scanning mutational analysis of the transcriptional activity of the human immunodeficiency virus type 1 long terminal repeat. Journal of virology 65: 2436–2444.

20. Gray LR, Cowley D, Crespan E, Welsh C, Mackenzie C, et al. (2013) Reduced basal transcriptional activity of central nervous system-derived HIV type 1 long terminal repeats. AIDS Res Hum Retroviruses 29: 365–370.

21. Einav Y, Shistik E, Shenfeld M, Simons AH, Melton DW, et al. (2003) Replication and episomal maintenance of Epstein-Barr virus-based vectors in mouse embryonal fibroblasts enable synthetic lethality screens. Mol Cancer Ther 2: 1121–1128.

22. Zhu H, Geiman TM, Xi S, Jiang Q, Schmidtmann A, et al. (2006) Lsh is involved in de novo methylation of DNA. The EMBO journal 25: 335–345.

23. Hodin TL, Najrana T, Yates JL (2013) Efficient Replication of Epstein-Barr Virus-Derived Plasmids Requires Tethering by EBNA1 to Host Chromosomes. Journal of virology 87: 13020–13028.

24. Berkhout B, Jeang KT (1992) Functional roles for the TATA promoter and enhancers in basal and Tat-induced expression of the human immunodeficiency virus type 1 long terminal repeat. Journal of virology 66: 139–149.

25. Kamine J, Subramanian T, Chinnadurai G (1993) Activation of a heterologous promoter by human immunodeficiency virus type 1 Tat requires Sp1 and is distinct from the mode of activation by acidic transcriptional activators. Journal of virology 67: 6828–6834.

26. Kumar S, Maiti S (2013) The Effect of N-acetylation and N-methylation of Lysine Residue of Tat Peptide on its Interaction with HIV-1 TAR RNA. PLoS one 8: e77595.

27. He M, Zhang L, Wang X, Huo L, Sun L, et al. (2013) Systematic Analysis of the Functions of Lysine Acetylation in the Regulation of Tat Activity. PloS one 8: e67186.

28. Sakane N, Kwon HS, Pagans S, Kaehlcke K, Mizusawa Y, et al. (2011) Activation of HIV transcription by the viral Tat protein requires a demethylation step mediated by lysine-specific demethylase 1 (LSD1/KDM1). PLoS pathogens 7: e1002184.

29. Yu Q, Konig R, Pillai S, Chiles K, Kearney M, et al. (2004) Single-strand specificity of APOBEC3G accounts for minus-strand deamination of the HIV genome. Nat Struct Mol Biol 11: 435–442.

30. Ho YC, Shan L, Hosmane NN, Wang J, Laskey SB, et al. (2013) Replication-competent Noninduced Proviruses in the Latent Reservoir Increase Barrier to HIV-1 Cure. Cell 155: 540–551.

31. Bartholomeeusen K, Fujinaga K, Xiang Y, Peterlin BM (2013) Histone deacetylase inhibitors (HDACis) that release the positive transcription elongation factor b (P-TEFb) from its inhibitory complex also activate HIV transcription. The Journal of biological chemistry 288: 14400–14407.

32. Burnett JC, Lim KI, Calafi A, Rossi JJ, Schaffer DV, et al. (2010) Combinatorial latency reactivation for HIV-1 subtypes and variants. Journal of virology 84: 5958–5974.

33. Bolden JE, Peart MJ, Johnstone RW (2006) Anticancer activities of histone deacetylase inhibitors. Nature reviews Drug discovery 5: 769–784.

34. Finnin MS, Donigian JR, Cohen A, Richon VM, Rifkind RA, et al. (1999) Structures of a histone deacetylase homologue bound to the TSA and SAHA inhibitors. Nature 401: 188–193.

35. Khan N, Jeffers M, Kumar S, Hackett C, Boldog F, et al. (2008) Determination of the class and isoform selectivity of small-molecule histone deacetylase inhibitors. The Biochemical journal 409: 581–589.

36. Wei DG, Chiang V, Fyne E, Balakrishnan M, Barnes T, et al. (2014) Histone Deacetylase Inhibitor Romidepsin Induces HIV Expression in CD4 T Cells from Patients on Suppressive Antiretroviral Therapy at Concentrations Achieved by Clinical Dosing. PLoS pathogens 10: e1004071.

37. Shan L, Xing S, Yang HC, Zhang H, Margolick JB, et al. (2014) Unique characteristics of histone deacetylase inhibitors in reactivation of latent HIV-1 in Bcl-2-transduced primary resting CD4+ T cells. J Antimicrob Chemother 69: 28–33.

38. Rasmussen TA, Schmeltz Sogaard O, Brinkmann C, Wightman F, Lewin SR, et al. (2013) Comparison of HDAC inhibitors in clinical development: effect on HIV production in latently infected cells and T-cell activation. Hum Vaccin Immunother 9: 993–1001.

39. Wightman F, Lu HK, Solomon AE, Saleh S, Harman AN, et al. (2013) Entinostat is a histone deacetylase inhibitor selective for class 1 histone deacetylases and activates HIV production from latently infected primary T cells. AIDS 27: 2853–2862.

40. Kato TA, Tsuda A, Uesaka M, Fujimori A, Kamada T, et al. (2011) In vitro characterization of cells derived from chordoma cell line U-CH1 following treatment with X-rays, heavy ions and chemotherapeutic drugs. Radiat Oncol 6: 116.

41. Marelli-Berg FM, Fu H, Mauro C (2012) Molecular mechanisms of metabolic reprogramming in proliferating cells: implications for T-cell-mediated immunity. Immunology 136: 363–369.

42. Barboric M, Yik JH, Czudnochowski N, Yang Z, Chen R, et al. (2007) Tat competes with HEXIM1 to increase the active pool of P-TEFb for HIV-1 transcription. Nucleic Acids Res 35: 2003–2012.

43. Barboric M, Lenasi T (2010) Kick-sTARting HIV-1 transcription elongation by 7SK snRNP deporTATion. Nat Struct Mol Biol 17: 928–930.

44. Contreras X, Schweneker M, Chen CS, McCune JM, Deeks SG, et al. (2009) Suberoylanilide hydroxamic acid reactivates HIV from latently infected cells. The Journal of biological chemistry 284: 6782–6789.

45. Ramakrishnan R, Liu H, Rice AP (2014) SAHA (Vorinostat) Induces CDK9 Thr-186 (T-Loop) Phosphorylation in Resting CD4 T Cells: Implications for Reactivation of Latent HIV. AIDS Res Hum Retroviruses.

46. Kiernan RE, Vanhulle C, Schiltz L, Adam E, Xiao H, et al. (1999) HIV-1 tat transcriptional activity is regulated by acetylation. The EMBO journal 18: 6106–6118.

47. Van Lint C, Emiliani S, Ott M, Verdin E (1996) Transcriptional activation and chromatin remodeling of the HIV-1 promoter in response to histone acetylation. The EMBO journal 15: 1112–1120.

48. Verdin E, Paras P Jr, Van Lint C (1993) Chromatin disruption in the promoter of human immunodeficiency virus type 1 during transcriptional activation. The EMBO journal 12: 3249–3259.

5

The Long-Term Effects of Pitavastatin on Blood Lipids and Platelet Activation Markers in Stroke Patients: Impact of the Homocysteine Level

Hideki Sugimoto*, Shingo Konno, Nobuatsu Nomoto, Hiroshi Nakazora, Mayumi Murata, Hisao Kitazono, Tomomi Imamura, Masashi Inoue, Miyuki Sasaki, Akihisa Fuse, Wataru Hagiwara, Mari Kobayashi, Toshiki Fujioka

Division of Neurology, Department of Internal Medicine, Toho University Ohashi, Tokyo, Japan

Abstract

To examine the impact of the plasma homocysteine level on the anti-atherosclerotic effects of pitavastatin treatment, we retrospectively examined 59 patients who had a history of stroke and had been prescribed pitavastatin for the treatment of dyslipidemia at the Neurology department of Toho University Ohashi Medical Center Hospital. The patients were classified into two groups according to their homocysteine levels. Carotid artery plaque progression was determined before and after pitavastatin treatment. Plasma levels of high-sensitivity C-reactive protein, platelet molecular markers, and von Willebrand factor were measured. Pitavastatin treatment had beneficial effects on the lipid profiles of these patients and slowed atherosclerosis progression. These effects were observed in both the high and low homocysteine groups. Proactive lipid intervention using pitavastatin may inhibit the progression of atherosclerosis and contribute to secondary prevention of stroke in high-risk patients. We conclude that this statin could inhibit progression at any stage of disease and should therefore be proactively administered to these patient groups, regardless of disease severity.

Editor: Thiruma V. Arumugam, National University of Singapore, Singapore

Funding: The authors received no specific funding for this work.

Competing Interests: The authors have declared that no competing interests exist.

* Email: sugi-h@oha.toho-u.ac.jp

Introduction

The prevention of recurrent stroke is extremely important after a transient ischemic attack or initial stroke, and antiplatelet drugs are administered prophylactically in many cases. Dyslipidemia is a risk factor for stroke, and higher low-density lipoprotein cholesterol (LDL-C) levels have been reported to increase the risk of stroke [1]. The American Heart Association/American Stroke Association guidelines [2] recommend proactive LDL-C management by statin administration to prevent stroke recurrence, and this has become the standard approach to the care of these patients. However, there is less evidence for the efficacy of dyslipidemia countermeasures for stroke prevention in Japan, as compared to other countries, and they may be insufficient in this country.

A higher ratio of LDL-C: high-density lipoprotein cholesterol (HDL-C) (L/H ratio) increases platelet activation and elevates the risk of thrombosis. In addition, the independent atherosclerosis promoting factor, homocysteine, is a marker that reflects the degree of progression of atherosclerosis from its early stages. The L/H ratio and the homocysteine level affect each other and promote progression of atherosclerosis. Conversely, progression of this disease would be expected to be inhibited on reduction of the L/H ratio. However, it is not known if drug efficacy is affected by the degree of disease progression.

We therefore conducted this study with the objective of assessing the anti-atherosclerotic effects of pitavastatin in secondary prevention stroke patients who were divided into a high homocysteine group and a low homocysteine group, as a marker of the degree of atherosclerosis progression.

The study was conducted by measuring inflammatory makers such as high-sensitivity C-reactive protein (hs-CRP), platelet molecular markers (β-thromboglobulin [βTG] and platelet factor 4 [PF4]), and vascular endothelium injury markers such as von Willebrand factor (vWF). βTG is a platelet-specific globulin that accounts for 10% of platelet α granule molecules. PF4 is a chemokine that is expressed specifically in megakaryocytes and contributes to inflammation and wound healing. βTG and PF4 accumulate in platelet α granules and are extremely important indicators of activation. vWF is produced in vascular endothelial cells and megakaryocytes. It facilitates platelet adhesion to damaged vascular subendothelial tissue and thus has an important role in primary hemostasis. Levels of CRP, βTG, PF4, and vWF before and after pitavastatin administration were compared retrospectively.

Materials and Methods

Study Population

The subjects of this retrospective survey were 59 patients with a history of stroke who were examined and administered 1–2 mg/

Table 1. Patient Samples.

		All	Group L	Group H
Sample size		59	16	16
Mean age (range)		66 years (45–89 years)	64.1 years (48–82)	68.7 years (48–89)
Gender	Male	35 (59.3%)	7 (43.8%)	11 (68.8%)
Stroke type	Lacunar stroke	45 (76.3%)	12 (75.0%)	10 (62.5%)
	Non-lacunar stroke	14 (23.7%)	4 (25.0%)	6 (37.5%)
Complications	Hypertension	27 (45.8%)	5 (31.3%)	10 (62.5%)
	Diabetes	6 (10.1%)	0 (0.0%)	2 (12.5%)
	Hyperuricemia	8 (13.6%)	2 (12.5%)	5 (31.3%)
Antiplatelet drugs	Aspirin	13 (22.0%)	5 (31.3%)	3 (18.8%)
	Aspirin, dihydroxyaluminum aminoacetate, magnesium carbonate	7 (11.9%)	1 (6.3%)	3 (18.8%)
	Sarpogrelate hydrochloride	9 (15.3%)	1 (6.3%)	5 (31.3%)
	Cilostazol	2 (3.4%)	0 (0.0%)	1 (6.3%)
	Clopidogrel sulfate	1 (1.7%)	1 (6.3%)	0 (0.0%)

day of pitavastatin for treatment of dyslipidemia at the Neurology department of Toho University Ohashi Medical Center Hospital between 2006 and 2011. This study was approved by the Toho University Ohashi Medical Center Institutional Review Board (Confirmation No. 12-35) and all patients gave written informed consent before they were enrolled in the study. The mean administration period was 19 months. Patients were divided into two groups, according to their homocysteine levels. Group H consisted of patients whose homocysteine level was above the median, and Group L consisted of patients whose homocysteine level was below the median.

Blood Sampling and Biochemical Assays

Blood was carefully drawn by a small number of skilled medical technicians to minimize the impact of this process on the platelet molecular markers. Total cholesterol (TC), HDL-C, triglycerides (TG), L/H ratio, non-HDL-C, homocysteine, βTG, PF4, vWF, and hs-CRP were measured before and after pitavastatin administration. LDL-C was calculated using the Friedewald equation. Non-HDL-C was calculated by subtracting HDL-C from TC. Plasma homocysteine levels were determined using the AxSYM immunoassay (Abbott Laboratories, Abbott Park, Ill.), according to the manufacturer's instructions. βTG and PF4 were measured in the plasma samples by the Asserachrom enzyme-linked immunoassay (ELISA) (β-TG, cat. no. 11875370011; PF4, cat. no. 11875353011, Roche Diagnostics). vWF was measured by ELISA as described previously [3]. Hs-CRP was analyzed on a Modular Analytics P800 using Tina-quant reagents (cat. no. 11972855, Roche Diagnostics). The numbers of patients where βTG, PF4, vWF, homocysteine, and hs-CRP were successfully measured before and after pitavastatin administration were 35, 35, 11, 32, and 43, respectively.

Carotid ultrasonography

Carotid ultrasonography was performed for each study subject. The mean intima-media thickness (IMT) of the common carotid artery was calculated as the mean value of the maximum IMT and those measured at points 1 cm before and after it. The mean of these values (mean IMT) was determined successfully in 14 patients before and after pitavastatin administration. The plaque

score was also determined in 13 subjects. Using the internal/external arterial bifurcation as a standard, the area from the distal side to the proximal side was segmented into four parts at 15-mm intervals. The plaque score was calculated from the sum of the max IMT of 1.1 mm or above on both the carotids.

Statistical Analysis

Data were analyzed by a one-sample t-test or Wilcoxon signed rank sum test, and analysis of variance (ANOVA) was used for inter-group testing. In all tests, a two-tailed significance level of 5% was used, and $p < 0.05$ was therefore considered to indicate a significant difference.

Results

Subject Demographics

Information relating to the 59 patients enrolled in this study is presented in Table 1. Antiplatelet drugs were administered to 28 patients and two antiplatelet drugs were used together in four individuals. No vitamin supplements were used by the patients during statin treatment. There were no significant differences between the parameters presented in Table 1 for the H and L homocysteine groups.

Changes in Serum Lipids after Pitavastatin Administration

Serum lipid levels (TC, LDL-C, HDL-C, TG, non-HDL-C, and L/H ratio) before and after pitavastatin administration are shown in Fig. 1. In all patients, significant improvements in their lipid profiles were seen after pitavastatin administration, with mean TC (± standard deviation, SD) decreasing from 227±44 mg/dL to 178±34 mg/dL ($p<0.0001$), LDL-C from 139±30 mg/dL to 93±28 mg/dL ($p<0.0001$), and TG from 155±95 mg/dL to 125±85 mg/dL ($p = 0.004$). Although not significant, HDL-C tended to increase, rising from 63±20 mg/dL to 67±19 mg/dL ($p = 0.1747$).

The L/H ratio decreased significantly from 2.4±0.9 to 1.5±0.6 ($p<0.0001$) during pitavastatin administration and non-HDL-C also decreased significantly from 167±35 mg/dL to 111±29 mg/dL ($p<0.0001$). No significant difference was observed between the H and L groups of subjects divided on the basis of the median

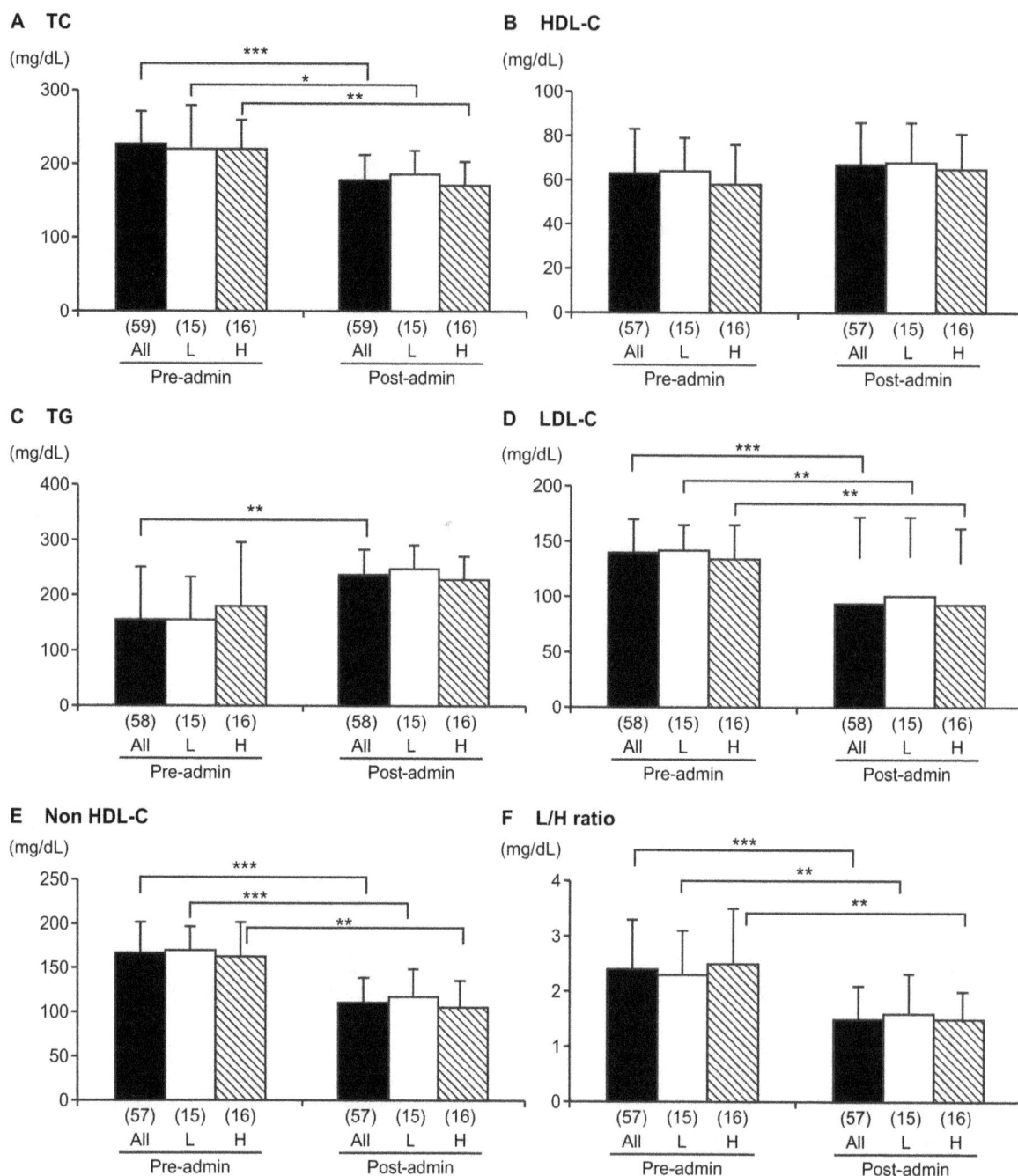

Figure 1. Lipid levels before and after pitavastatin treatment. The mean ± standard deviation is presented. H indicates the group with homocysteine values above the median (8.6 μmol/L), L indicates the group with homocysteine values <8.6 μmol/L. The number of subjects is indicated in parentheses. a) total cholesterol (TC), b) high-density lipoprotein cholesterol (HDL-C), c) triglyceride (TG), d) low-density lipoprotein cholesterol (LDL-C), e) non-HDL-C, and f) the L/H ratio. Pre- and post-pitavastatin values were compared as indicated by t-test or Wilcoxon signed-rank test (TG only). *$p<0.05$, **$p<0.01$, ***$p<0.001$.

homocysteine level, which was 8.6 μmol/L. Significant improvements in the lipid profiles of both subgroups were seen following pitavastatin administration, except for TG and HDL-C.

Effects of Pitavastatin on Markers in the Homocysteine Subgroups

The levels of hs-CRP, βTG, PF4, and vWF before and after pitavastatin administration are shown in Fig. 2 and Fig. 3.

Significant improvements in the levels of the inflammatory marker, hs-CRP, were seen after administration, as this decreased from 0.10±0.12 mg/dL to 0.06±0.07 mg/dL ($p<0.0001$, Fig. 2a). Both platelet molecular markers exhibited significant improvement, with βTG decreasing from 68±56 ng/dL to 44±32 ng/dL ($p=0.0049$, Fig. 2b), and PF4 decreasing from 22±27 ng/dL to 14±16 ng/dL ($p=0.012$, Fig. 2c). When subjects were divided into H and L groups based on their homocysteine level, no significant differences were observed in hs-CRP, βTG or PF4 before and after pitavastatin treatment, although a trend for βTG to decrease was seen in the L group.

There was no significant pitavastatin-related change in the level of vWF, which decreased from $152\pm32\%$ to $140\pm35\%$ ($p = 0.471$, Fig. 3a), although a significant increase in the activity of this endothelial marker was observed, from $117\pm32\%$ to $134\pm44\%$ ($p = 0.01$, Fig. 3b). No significant differences in vWF were observed between the H and L homocysteine groups.

Plaque Scores in the Homocysteine Subgroups

The mean IMT and plaque scores before and after administration in the H and L homocysteine groups are shown in Fig. 4. Mean IMT and plaque scores before pitavastatin administration tended to be higher in the H group, although these differences were not statistically significant ($p = 0.7$, $p = 0.11$, respectively). Mean IMT exhibited a decreasing trend in the H group, falling from a median value of 0.95 (0.70–1.11: first quartile–third quartile) mm before administration, to 0.90 (0.85–0.95) mm after administration. A similar decline was observed in the L group, from a median value of 0.85 (0.70–1.00) mm to 0.78 (0.63–1.28) mm, but neither of these differences were statistically significant. In the H group, plaque score shifted from a median value of 5.5 (4.40–11.75) before administration to 5.9 (2.40–8.80) after administration, and in the L group this was 2.8 (1.45–6.45) before, and 4.1 (3.00–9.90) after, pitavastatin administration.

Safety

No clinically problematic changes in laboratory test values or symptoms were seen throughout the pitavastatin administration period, and no adverse events were reported.

Discussion

In this study, we examined whether pitavastatin produced different effects in patients with advanced atherosclerosis and those

without, using homocysteine as an indicator. It has been reported that individuals with a high blood homocysteine concentration have an elevated risk for atherosclerotic disease and for death due to cerebro-cardiovascular disease [4]. Furthermore, in the Japanese population, elevated homocysteine level associated with an increased mean carotid artery IMT [5], and an association has also been reported with the risk for ischemic and lacunar stroke [6]. Homocysteine acts on vascular endothelial cells, amplifying the expression of 3-hydroxyl-3-methylglutaryl coenzyme A reductase, stimulating cholesterol production, and inhibiting nitric oxide production [7]. However, it has not yet been demonstrated that supplementation with folic acid and vitamins B6 and B12, which reduce homocysteine levels, can reduce the risk of stroke [8]. Previous studies reported that statins did not affect the homocysteine level [9] but partially inhibited homocysteine-mediated exacerbation of atherosclerosis [10], and showed that proactive lipid intervention using high doses of statins is critical for stroke prevention: however, only a few, studies have analyzed the efficacy of high dose statins for stroke prevention. The present study found no significant differences in the effects of pitavastatin administration on blood lipids, hs-CRP, platelet molecular markers, or vWF in the H and L homocysteine groups. We also considered the relationship between platelet molecular markers and homocysteine level. Since βTG tended to decrease after pitavastatin administration in the L group, pitavastatin may be more effective when started at the early stages of the disease, when relatively mild atherosclerotic changes are present. Pitavastatin was found to inhibit plaque progression, with no clear differences in the effect of this statin on the IMT and plaque scores in the H and L homocysteine groups. Antioxidant capacity has been reported to be weak in patients with high blood homocysteine concentrations [11], while lipid intervention using statins has direct anti-inflammatory [12] and antioxidant effects [13]. In the present study, our findings indicated that pitavastatin-related improvements in lipid profiles inhibited progression of atherosclerosis, even in patients at high risk of plaque progression.

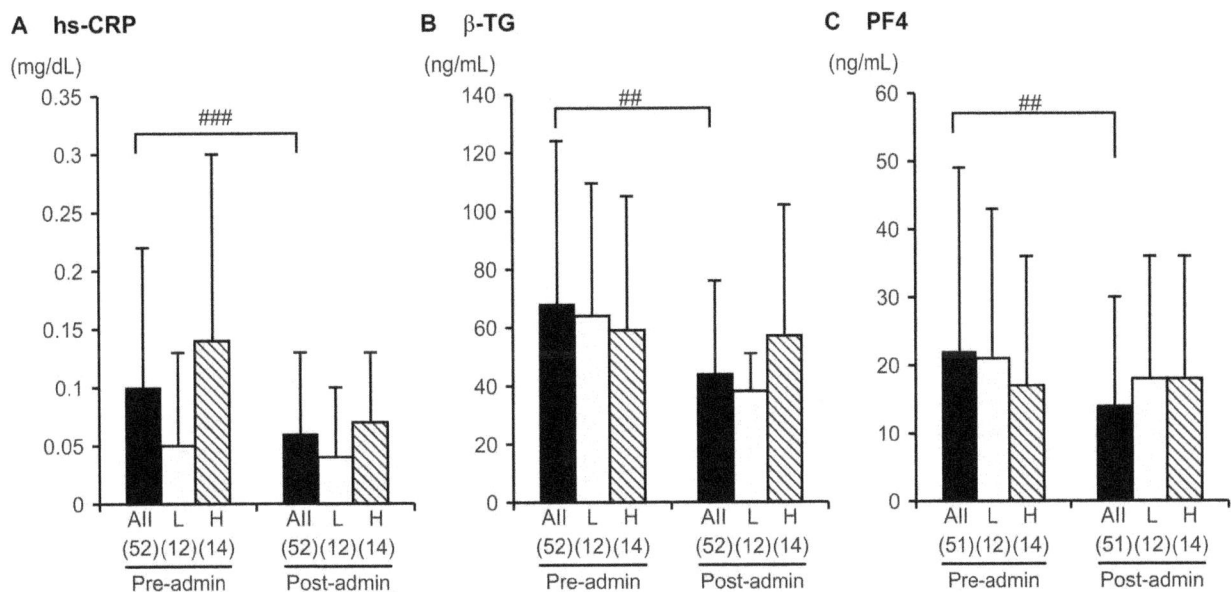

Figure 2. Inflammatory and platelet activity markers before and after pitavastatin treatment. Mean ± standard deviation is shown. H indicates the group with homocysteine values above the median (8.6 μmol/L), L indicates the group with homocysteine values <8.6 μmol/L. The number of subjects is indicated in parentheses. a) high-sensitivity C-reactive protein (hs-CRP), b) β-thromboglobulin (βTG), and c) platelet factor 4 (PF4). Pre- and post-pitavastatin values were compared by Wilcoxon signed-rank test. ##$p<0.01$, ###$p<0.001$.

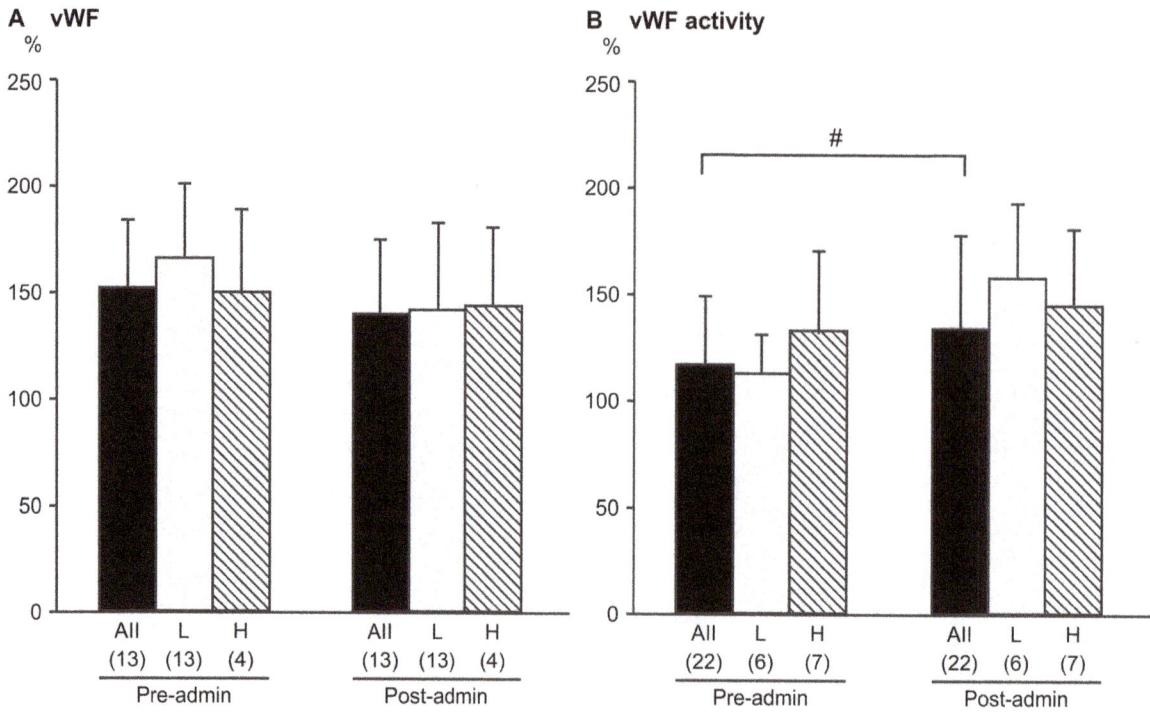

Figure 3. Levels and activity of von Willebrand factor (vWF) before and after pitavastatin treatment. Mean ± standard deviation is shown for a) vWF levels and b) vWF activity. H indicates the group with homocysteine values above the median (8.6 μmol/L), L indicates the group with homocysteine values <8.6 μmol/L. The number of subjects is indicated in parentheses. Pre- and post-pitavastatin values were compared using the Wilcoxon signed-rank test. #p<0.05

In contrast to the situation with cardiovascular disease, there is little evidence regarding the influence of lipid levels in primary and secondary stroke prevention, and LDL-C is not managed as stringently as it is in cardiovascular disease. Furthermore, in stroke patients with the complication of hypertension, blood pressure management is considered to be more important than lipid-lowering therapy and it is difficult to actually prevent stroke by lipid management alone. While the subjects of this study were extremely high-risk post-stroke patients, the fact that we observed an inhibition of carotid artery plaque progression following

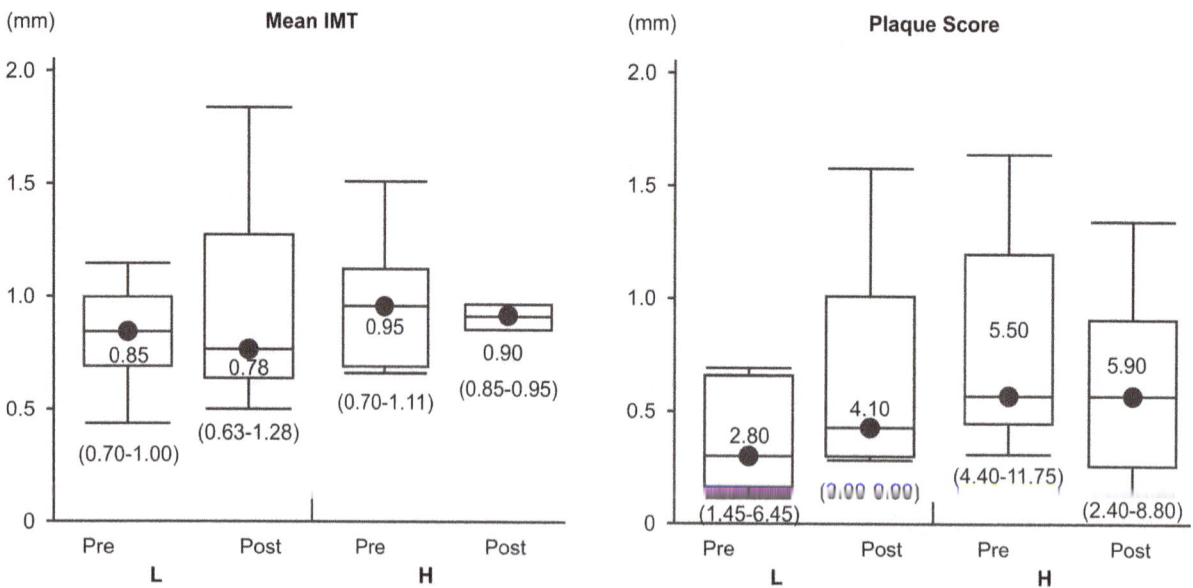

Figure 4. Intima-media thickness (IMT) and plaque scores before and after pitavastatin treatment. H indicates the group with homocysteine values above the median (8.6 μmol/L), and L indicates the group with homocysteine values <8.6 μmol/L. The median values and the range (first quartile to third quartile) are presented. Paired t-tests were performed but no significant differences were observed.

pitavastatin administration clearly indicated the importance of lipid management using statins in these patients.

Because the sample size was limited in this study, we could not investigate whether inhibition of plaque progression led to stroke prevention. We were also unable to ascertain the effect of pitavastatin administration on homocysteine levels. We hope to clarify these points by conducting a long-term large-scale study in the future.

Conclusions

Proactive lipid intervention using pitavastatin may inhibit progression of atherosclerosis and contribute to secondary prevention of stroke in high-risk patients. Although this intervention may be particularly useful at the early stages of the disease when homocysteine levels are low, we conclude that it could inhibit progression at any stage and should therefore be proactively administered to these patient groups, regardless of their disease severity.

Author Contributions

Conceived and designed the experiments: TF HS. Performed the experiments: HS SK NN HN MM HK TI MI MS AF WH MK. Analyzed the data: HS TF. Contributed reagents/materials/analysis tools: TF HS. Wrote the paper: HS.

References

1. Amarenco P, Labreuche J, Lavallée P, Touboul PJ (2004) Statins in stroke prevention and carotid atherosclerosis: systematic review and up-to-date meta-analysis. Stroke 35: 2902–2909.
2. Kernan WN, Ovbiagele B, Black HR, Bravata DM, Chimowitz MI, et al. (2014) Guidelines for the prevention of stroke in patients with stroke and transient ischemic attack: a guideline for healthcare professionals from the American Heart Association/American Stroke Association. Stroke 45: 2160–2236.
3. Cejka J (1982) Enzyme immunoassay for factor VIII-related antigen. Clin Chem 28: 1356–1358.
4. Cui R, Moriyama Y, Koike KA, Date C, Kikuchi S, et al. (2008) Serum total homocysteine concentrations and risk of mortality from stroke and coronary heart disease in Japanese: the JACC study. Atherosclerosis 198: 412–418.
5. Adachi H, Hirai Y, Fujiura Y, Matsuoka H, Satoh A, et al. (2002) Plasma homocysteine levels and atherosclerosis in Japan: epidemiological study by use of carotid ultrasonography. Stroke 33: 2177–2181.
6. Iso H, Moriyama Y, Sato S, Kitamura A, Tanigawa T, et al. (2004) Serum total homocysteine concentrations and risk of stroke and its subtypes in Japanese. Circulation 109: 2766–2772.
7. Li H, Lewis A, Brodsky S, Rieger R, Iden C, et al. (2002) Homocysteine induces 3-hydroxy-3-methylglutaryl coenzyme a reductase in vascular endothelial cells: a mechanism for development of atherosclerosis? Circulation 105: 1037–1043.
8. Lee M, Hong KS, Chang SC, Saver JL (2010) Efficacy of homocysteine-lowering therapy with folic acid in stroke prevention: a meta-analysis. Stroke 41: 1205–1212.
9. Milionis HJ, Papakostas J, Kakafika A, Chasiotis G, Seferiadis K, et al. (2003) Comparative effects of atorvastatin, simvastatin, and fenofibrate on serum homocysteine levels in patients with primary hyperlipidemia. J Clin Pharmacol 43: 825–830.
10. Lin CP, Chen YH, Lin WT, Leu HB, Liu TZ, et al. (2008) Direct effect of statins on homocysteine-induced endothelial adhesiveness: potential impact to human atherosclerosis. Eur J Clin Invest 38: 106–116.
11. Bogdanski P, Miller-Kasprzak E, Pupek-Musialik D, Jablecka A, Lacinski M, et al. (2012) Plasma total homocysteine is a determinant of carotid intima-media thickness and circulating endothelial progenitor cells in patients with newly diagnosed hypertension. Clin Chem Lab Med 50: 1107–1113.
12. Koshiyama H, Taniguchi A, Tanaka K, Kagimoto S, Fujioka Y, et al. (2008) Effects of pitavastatin on lipid profiles and high-sensitivity CRP in Japanese subjects with hypercholesterolemia: Kansai Investigation of Statin for Hyperlipidemic Intervention in Metabolism and Endocrinology (KISHIMEN) investigators. J Atheroscler Thromb 15: 345–350.
13. Maeda K, Yasunari K, Sato EF, Inoue M (2005) Enhanced oxidative stress in neutrophils from hyperlipidemic guinea pig. Atherosclerosis 181: 87–92.

6

Spatiotemporal Characterization of a Fibrin Clot Using Quantitative Phase Imaging

Rajshekhar Gannavarpu[1], Basanta Bhaduri[1], Krishnarao Tangella[2], Gabriel Popescu[1]*

1 Quantitative Light Imaging Laboratory, Department of Electrical and Computer Engineering, Beckman Institute for Advanced Science and Technology, University of Illinois at Urbana-Champaign, Urbana, Illinois, United States of America, **2** Department of Pathology, Christie Clinic, and University of Illinois at Urbana-Champaign, Urbana, Illinois, United States of America

Abstract

Studying the dynamics of fibrin clot formation and its morphology is an important problem in biology and has significant impact for several scientific and clinical applications. We present a label-free technique based on quantitative phase imaging to address this problem. Using quantitative phase information, we characterized fibrin polymerization in real-time and present a mathematical model describing the transition from liquid to gel state. By exploiting the inherent optical sectioning capability of our instrument, we measured the three-dimensional structure of the fibrin clot. From this data, we evaluated the fractal nature of the fibrin network and extracted the fractal dimension. Our non-invasive and speckle-free approach analyzes the clotting process without the need for external contrast agents.

Editor: Joseph Najbauer, University of Pécs Medical School, Hungary

Funding: National Science Foundation (grant CBET-1040462 MRI) (http://www.nsf.gov) and Swiss National Science Foundation (grant 146495) (http://www.snf.ch/en/Pages/default.aspx). The funders had no role in study design, data collection and analysis, decision to publish, or preparation of the manuscript.

Competing Interests: Gabriel Popescu has financial interest in Phi Optics, Inc., a company developing quantitative phase imaging technology for materials and life science applications, which, however, did not sponsor the research.

* Email: gpopescu@illinois.edu

Introduction

Fibrin is a biopolymer that constitutes the structural basis of the hemostatic plug, which prevents excessive blood loss upon vascular injury [1,2]. During blood coagulation, the protein *fibrinogen* in blood plasma is converted to *fibrin* by the action of thrombin [3,4]. As a result, a three-dimensional network or *gel* is formed, which comprises of entangled, branching fibrin fibers and binds the platelets to stop bleeding. In addition, this mesh anchors the neutrophils, macrophages, and fibroblasts to remove dead tissues and infectious agents during wound repair [4,5]. The fibrin structure has been associated with vascular disease [6], stroke [7], diabetes [8], and thromboembolic disorders [9,10]. In addition to clinical significance for hemostasis, fibrin can be used as scaffolding material for tissue engineering [11,12], for drug delivery [13,14], and in tissue patterning [15,16]. Thus, studying the dynamics of fibrin clot formation and its associated morphology is of great basic science and clinical significance.

The prominent techniques for analyzing fibrin network include scanning electron microscopy [17], atomic force microscopy [18,19], x-ray scattering [20,21], and neutron scattering [22,23]. Although these techniques provide high resolution detail, they involve bulky experimental configurations, require dedicated infrastructure, have low throughputs, and exhibit limited applicability to three-dimensional (3D) visualization of the fibrin structure. Alternatively, optical approaches have been proposed. Light scattering [24,25] is an important optical technique, which has been used for studying fibrin networks. Similarly, speckle characteristics of the scattered light have also been investigated for fibrin studies [26]. Due to limited optical sectioning provided by coherent illumination, the main limitation of these approaches is that they are not suitable for direct three-dimensional imaging of the fibrin network. Another class of optical techniques based on confocal fluorescence microscopy [27–30], deconvolution fluorescence microscopy [31], and total internal reflection fluorescence microscopy [32] have been proposed for studying the 3D structure and dynamics of fibrin polymerization. However, they rely on the addition of exogenous labeling agents to the specimen, which is subject to photobleaching and phototoxicity. Recently, differential interference contrast microscopy methods [33,34] and flow assay techniques [35] were proposed for label-free fibrin studies.

Here, we present a novel approach for assessing the spatiotemporal characteristics of a fibrin clot. Our approach relies on quantitative phase imaging (QPI), where we retrieve the fibrin clot structure via an interferometric measurement. Importantly, the nanoscale optical path length changes introduced by the clot result in observable phase shifts of the illumination field [36]. The imaging modality in our approach is based on spatial light interference microscopy (SLIM) [37,38], which has been applied previously for biological studies including red blood cell morphology [39], cell growth monitoring [40–42], cellular tomography [43] etc. Using QPI, we monitored the formation of a fibrin clot in real-time and analyzed the growth characteristics using the spatial power spectrum. We also measured the three-dimensional structure of the clot by capturing depth-resolved quantitative phase images and studied the associated fractal properties.

Methods

Ethics Statement

The studies have been performed in accordance with the procedure approved by the Institutional Review Board at University of Illinois at Urbana-Champaign (IRB Protocol Number: 10571). The blood sample used in this research project was procured after securing a signed general consent from the donor, which allows the specimen to be used for educational and research purposes.

Sample preparation

Human venous blood sample was collected in a trisodium citrate tube. The citrate acts an an anti-coagulant to prevent clotting before imaging. The whole blood was initially centrifuged at $1500\times g$ for about 5 minutes. Subsequently, we aspirated the top layered plasma, collected it in another microcentrifuge tube, and performed centrifugation for another 5 minutes at $1500\times g$. The double centrifugation was done to minimize the residual red blood cells and platelets. From the spun tube, the top layered plasma was collected for the experiment. A sample chamber was created by punching a hole in a double sided scotch tape and sticking one side of the tape onto a cover slip. Subsequently, we pipetted 3 μl of plasma into the chamber and added 0.5 μl of $CaCl_2$ (0.025 M, r^2 Diagnostics). Blood clotting is initiated by the addition of calcium, and is dependent upon the activation of FXII by glass (contact activation) [44,45]. Then, we sealed the top of the chamber using another cover slip to reduce evaporation, and transferred the sample to the SLIM setup for imaging.

Imaging and Image Processing

The imaging setup is shown in Fig. 1(A). Here, SLIM works as an add-on module to a commercial phase-contrast microscope (Zeiss Axio Observer Z1) with a 40X microscope objective (Zeiss, Ph 2, NA = 0.75). It relies on the spatial decomposition of the image field into its scattered and unscattered components. In addition to the conventional $\pi/2$ shift introduced in phase contrast microscopy, three phase shifts in increments of $\pi/2$ were introduced. The additional phase modulation was achieved by using a reflective liquid crystal phase modulator (LCPM, Boulder Nonlinear Systems). The LCPM is placed in the Fourier plane of the SLIM module. This plane is conjugate to the back focal plane of the microscope objective which contains the phase contrast ring. For effective control of the additional phase delay between the scattered and unscattered components, the active pattern on the LCPM is computed to precisely match the size and position of the phase contrast ring image. The 4f system formed by lens FL₁ (focal length $f_1 = 150$ mm) and lens FL₂ (focal length $f_2 = 200$ mm) provides additional magnification of f_2/f_1.

We used a scientific-grade complementary metal oxide semiconductor (sCMOS) camera (Andor Zyla) for capturing images. The camera records the superposition of the scattered field U_{sca} and unscattered field U_{ref}, as shown by the vectorial representation in Fig. 1(B). In the figure, $\Delta\phi$ is the phase difference between U_{ref} and U_{sca}, whereas ϕ is the phase of the image field, the quantity of interest in QPI. The four $\pi/2$ phase-shifted images can be represented as,

$$I_n(\mathbf{r}) = |U_{ref}(\mathbf{r})|^2 + |U_{sca}(\mathbf{r})|^2 + 2U_{ref}(\mathbf{r})U_{sca}(\mathbf{r})\cos[\Delta\phi(\mathbf{r}) + n\pi/2] \tag{1}$$

where $n \in [1,4]$. We can compute $\Delta\phi$ as,

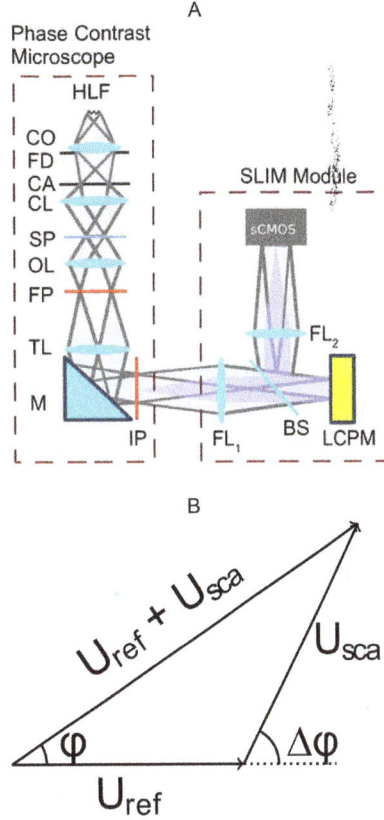

Figure 1. SLIM system. (A) Imaging setup. HLF: Halogen Lamp Filament, CO: Collector lens, FD: Field Diaphragm, CA: Condenser Annulus, CL: Condenser Lens, SP: Specimen, OL: Objective Lens, FP: Back Focal Plane of Objective, TL: Tube Lens, M: Mirror, IP: Image Plane, FL₁: Fourier Lens 1, FL₂: Fourier Lens 2, BS: Beam Splitter, LCPM: Liquid Crystal Phase Modulator. (B) Coherent superposition of scattered and unscattered waves.

$$\Delta\phi(\mathbf{r}) = \tan^{-1}\left[\frac{I_1(\mathbf{r}) - I_3(\mathbf{r})}{I_2(\mathbf{r}) - I_4(\mathbf{r})}\right] \tag{2}$$

Denoting β as the ratio of the amplitudes of the scattered and unscattered fields, i.e. $\beta(\mathbf{r}) = |U_{sca}(\mathbf{r})|/|U_{ref}(\mathbf{r})|$, the phase of the image field can be obtained as,

$$\phi(\mathbf{r}) = \frac{\beta(\mathbf{r})\cos[\Delta\phi(\mathbf{r})]}{1 + \beta(\mathbf{r})\sin[\Delta\phi(\mathbf{r})]} \tag{3}$$

The measured phase is dependent on the refractive index and thickness of the sample as

$$\phi(\mathbf{r}) = \frac{2\pi}{\lambda}\Delta n(\mathbf{r})h(\mathbf{r}) \tag{4}$$

where λ is the mean wavelength, $h(\mathbf{r})$ is the thickness and $\Delta n(\mathbf{r})$ is the refractive index difference between the sample and medium. As phase measurement is influenced by refractive index, it is important to minimize the transparent blood cells in the sample to

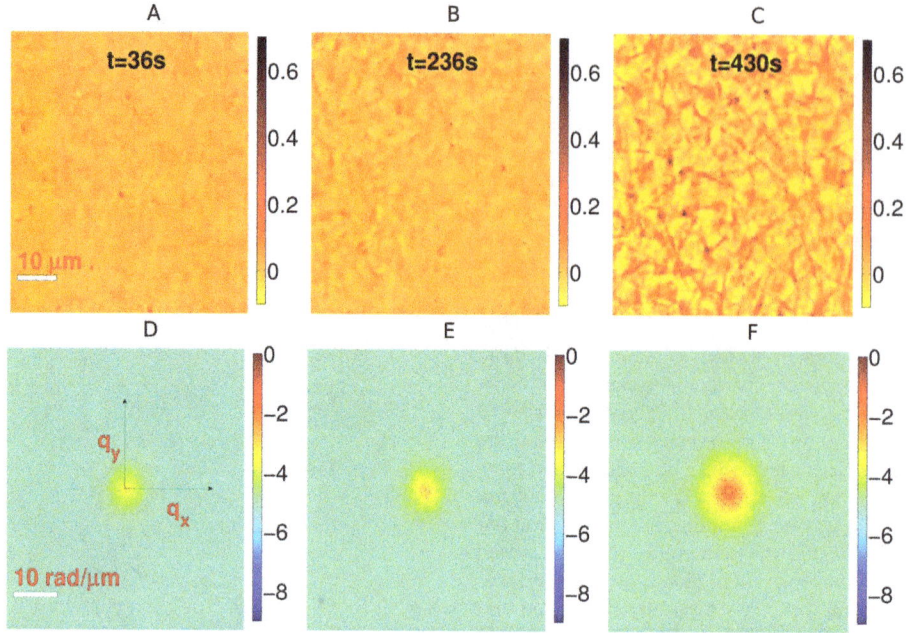

Figure 2. Fibrin clot formation. (A–C) illustrate the measured phase in radians at different time instants. (D–F) show the corresponding normalized log power spectra. On the top row, we see the evolution of a clot in time. This is accompanied by power spectrum broadening, shown on the bottom row.

clearly map the fibrin structure. More details about SLIM construction and working are reported elsewhere [38].

Power spectrum and fractal analysis

For analyzing the temporal dynamics of the fibrin clot, the 2D spatial power spectrum as a function of time was computed using the surface integral,

$$P_S(\mathbf{q},t) = |\int_S \phi(\mathbf{r},t)\exp[-i(\mathbf{q}\cdot\mathbf{r})]\mathrm{d}^2\mathbf{r}|^2, \qquad (5)$$

where $\mathbf{r}=(x,y)$ and $\mathbf{q}=(q_x,q_y)$, with q_x and q_y being angular spatial frequencies. Further, the spatial power spectrum was normalized by dividing the spectrum data by the maximum value. Subsequently, the radial average $P(q,t)$ is obtained by averaging the normalized $P_S(\mathbf{q},t)$ along $q=\sqrt{q_x^2+q_y^2}$.

For analyzing the three-dimensional structure of the fibrin network, the 3D spatial power spectrum was computed using the volume integral,

$$P_V(\mathbf{q}) = |\int_V \phi(\mathbf{r})\exp[-i(\mathbf{q}\cdot\mathbf{r})]\mathrm{d}^3\mathbf{r}|^2, \qquad (6)$$

where $\mathbf{r}=(x,y,z)$ and $\mathbf{q}=(q_x,q_y,q_z)$. Subsequently, the spherical average $P(q)$ was ascertained by averaging the normalized $P_V(\mathbf{q})$ along $q=\sqrt{q_x^2+q_y^2+q_z^2}$.

For fractal analysis of the 3D fibrin network, the spherically averaged spatial power spectrum $P(q)$ vs q was plotted on a log-log scale. The presence of a linear behavior on log-log scale, or equivalently a power law decay of the form $P(q)\propto q^{-\beta}$ is suggestive of the underlying fractal nature of the 3D network [46]. The decay exponent β was computed using a linear regression fit on the logarithmic scale. To quantify fractal

characteristics, the fractal dimension D_f was obtained from the decay exponent using $D_f\approx 4-\beta/2$ [46]. Fractal dimension can be considered to be a measure of compactness of the network in three-dimensional space.

All image processing tasks and mathematical operations were performed in MATLAB. The regression calculations were performed using MATLAB's built-in optimization routines.

Results

After initiating the clotting process, as discussed above, we obtained time-lapsed quantitative phase images at 1.2 Hz, each with a field of view (FOV) of approximately 60 μm × 60 μm. The quantitative phase maps at three different time instants are shown in Fig. 2. During the initial period of clotting, as shown in Fig. 2A, there is no significant spatial variation in phase. As clotting progresses, we observe that the fluctuations in refractive index, induced by fibrin polymerization, manifest as corresponding changes in the measured phase. This is evident from the phase maps at later time instants (Figs. 2B and C) where the emergence of a mesh structure is clearly visible. The growth of fibrin clot is also shown in Movie S1. Note that for dynamics studies, an important requirement is the temporal stability of the measuring system. SLIM offers such capability due to its robustness against temporal noise granted by the common-path geometry [37]. In addition, SLIM significantly reduces the speckle noise because of the broadband illumination. These features enable the assessment of dynamics of fibrin clot formation with high sensitivity.

To analyze the temporal evolution of the fibrin network, we used the spatial power spectrum of the quantitative phase map. The normalized power spectra (log scale) for the three quantitative phase maps, shown in Figs. 2A–C, are presented in Figs. 2D–F respectively. From these figures, we observe a distinct broadening of the power spectrum, as the clot forms. This can be attributed to the fact that the formation of an interconnected fibrin mesh is

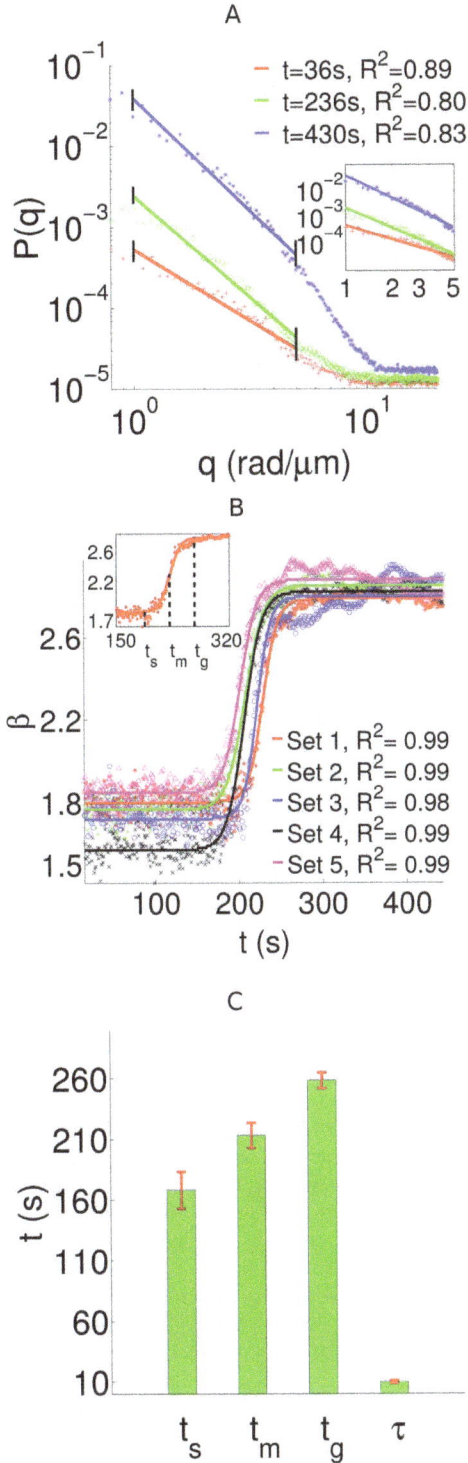

Figure 3. Fibrin temporal characteristics. (A) The radially averaged power spectra for different time instants on a log-log scale. For low q, these spectra exhibit a power law behavior, $P(q) \propto q^{-\beta}$, as confirmed by the linear fits (solid lines) on the log-log scale. This power law decay regime for the three time instants is shown in the inset. (B) The decay exponent β as a function of time t for five different datasets. The solid lines indicate sigmoidal fits. The inset shows a temporal interval of one dataset, where the two-stage behavior of fibrin polymerization is clearly evident. (C) The measured values of t_s, t_m, t_g and τ. The errorbars indicate the standard deviation.

accompanied by an increased spectral contribution to higher spatial frequencies. Hence, power spectrum of the quantitative phase carries important information about the growth characteristics of the fibrin network. This is clearly illustrated by the radially averaged power spectrum $P(q)$, as shown in Fig. 3A. Two important observations can be made from the plot: (1) for low q, the power spectrum varies linearly with q on log-log scale, which indicates a power law decay of the form $P(q) \propto q^{-\beta}$; (2) the decay exponent β varies with time as the fibrin polymerizes. Here, we are mainly interested in the low q region, as it corresponds to the large length scales at which fibrin fibers cross-link.

To quantify fibrin polymerization, we obtained time-lapsed quantitative phase images in different regions and computed the power spectrum decay exponent β as a function of time for each of these datasets. The temporal evolution of β is shown in Fig. 3B. Remarkably, the temporal response for each dataset shows a sigmoid shape, characterized by distinct lower and upper saturation values, along with an intermediate transition period. These observations reveal a two-stage dynamic behavior for fibrin polymerization, indicating the liquid to gel transition. Subsequently, we applied a sigmoidal fit for β as,

$$\beta(t) = \frac{a_1}{1 + \exp\left[-\frac{(t - t_m)}{\tau}\right]} + a_2, \qquad (7)$$

where a_1 is the response range which decides the upper plateau, a_2 indicates the lower plateau of the sigmoid, t_m is the time instant corresponding to the steepest growth rate, and τ is the time constant of the process, which controls the transition period from one stage to another. The sigmoidal fits, obtained using non-linear regression, are also shown in the figure. In particular, the figure inset illustrates the computed β and its fit for a dataset, where three temporal regimes are clearly visible, as follows. (1) The initial period of clotting characterized by $t \leq t_s$, when β has a lower plateau indicating minimal clot formation. (2) The intermediate period $t_s \leq t \leq t_g$ when β rises rapidly, which signifies the monomer (liquid) to polymer (gel) transition. (3) The saturation period $t \geq t_g$ when β reaches an upper plateau, indicating that the gel structure has formed. Here, t_g can be considered as an indicator of the *clotting* time [47]. To evaluate t_s and t_g, we considered the time instants at which β is below or above the upper and lower saturation values by 1% of the response range (see Text S1). The different temporal parameters characterizing the dynamics of fibrin polymerization are summarized in Fig. 3C. From these results, we can infer that QPI provides interesting insights into the dynamics of fibrin network formation. Interestingly, the observed two-level system is consistent with previously reported clotting behavior [47–49], where sigmoid growth characteristics were observed, and the clotting parameters were shown to be physiologically relevant [48].

Next, we studied the three-dimensional structure of the fibrin network. We obtained a z-stack of quantitative phase images by scanning a fully formed fibrin clot along the axial (depth) direction in steps of 0.1 μm at 6.6 Hz. As demonstrated recently, SLIM offers excellent optical sectioning due to broadband light, resulting in reliable tomographic reconstruction of transparent specimens [43]. We acquired a single 3D image (FOV approx. 60 μm × 60 μm × 25 μm) in 38 seconds, which underscores the high throughput of the system. By repeating the above procedure, we obtained ten different 3D phase maps of fibrin networks. Figure 4A illustrates the three-dimensional structure of one such fibrin network. The branching fibrin fibers and the inter-connected nodes are clearly visible in the figure. For better

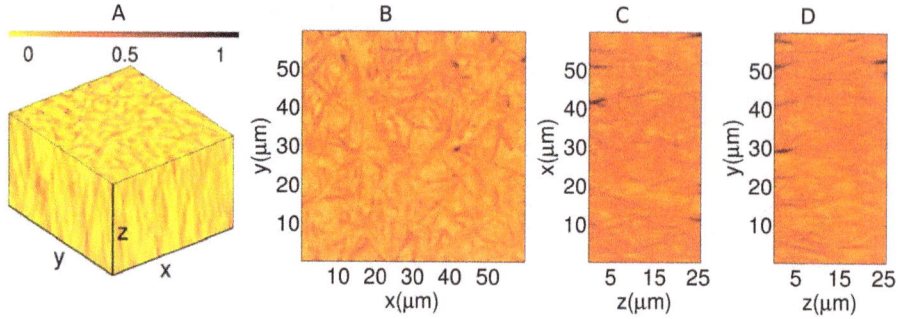

Figure 4. Three-dimensional clot imaging. (A) The 3D structure of fibrin network. The corresponding maximum value projections on the xy, xz, and yz planes are shown in (B), (C), and (D) respectively. The nodal points of the network are clearly visible. The colorbar indicates quantitative phase values in radians.

illustration, the depth-scanned quantitative phase images are also shown in Movie S2. The maximum value projections of the 3D quantitative phase image on the xy, xz and yz planes are shown in Figs. 4B–D respectively. Since the nodes indicate the cross-linking of several fibrin fibers, resulting in increased local density, these regions are characterized by large phase values. Hence, the maximum value projection maps shown here highlight the nodal

points of the network along the three dimensions and provide topological information about the fibrin gel.

Using the 3D QPI data, we obtained the spherically averaged spatial power spectrum for the different datasets. In Fig. 5A, we show the power spectrum plot for a particular dataset. The power spectrum plots for the other nine datasets are shown in Fig. S2. For all these data, at large length scales, we observed a power law decay behavior, which indicates the fractal nature of the fibrin clot. It is interesting to note that the fractal characteristics of the fibrin network have also been previously observed using neutron scattering [22] and clot rheology [50]. Using our technique, the measured values of the fractal dimension for the ten different sets are shown in Fig. 5B, resulting in $D_f = 2.09 \pm 0.03$ (mean $\pm$ standard deviation). The fractal dimension $D_f > 2$ is consistent with a surface fractal structure and indicates that the fibrin fibers exhibit rough surfaces at the observed length scales. Note that the fractal studies of the fibrin clot are important since fractal characteristics have been suggested as potential biomarkers for clotting related disorders [50].

Summary and Discussions

We demonstrated a novel approach based on quantitative phase imaging to study the fibrin network in a non-invasive and label-free manner. Using QPI and power spectrum analysis, we quantified the temporal evolution of a fibrin clot and presented a simple mathematical description of the two-stage growth characteristics of fibrin polymerization. The high throughput of our measurement system allows real-time monitoring of fibrin networks over large area. In addition, our system provides high temporal sensitivity for dynamics studies. Furthermore, we investigated the 3D structure of fibrin network and studied the associated fractal properties. For such studies, our technique provides full 3D imaging capability with good spatial sensitivity and non-requirement of exogenous markers.

For the current studies, we used blood plasma as the sample, which is mostly transparent, and free from residual blood cells. Even if stray platelets are present, their adverse effect on the accuracy of the spatio-temporal analysis would not be high. This is because of the much smaller platelet dimensions in contrast to the size of the branching fibrin network. Also, the effect of spherical averaging of the spatial power spectrum would mitigate the influence of phase variations induced by the platelets. Further, one can measure whole blood with our technique, provided an area devoid of cells is imaged, such as on a smear. In addition, slight dilution of the blood would be helpful to provide entire field of view without cells.

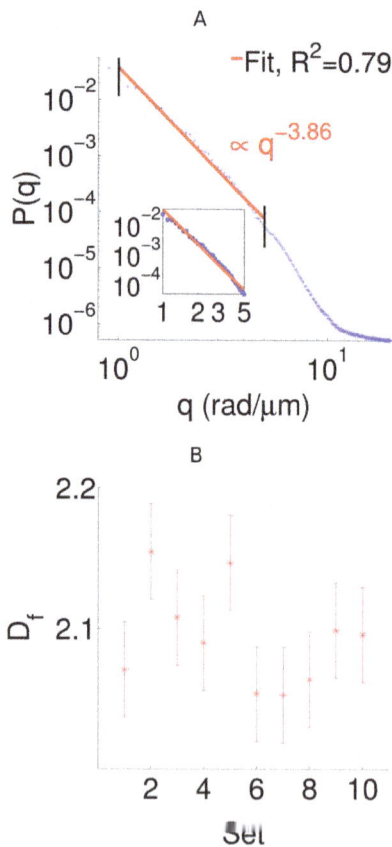

Figure 5. 3D structural characteristics of fibrin network. (A) Spherically averaged normalized 3D power spectrum for a dataset on the log-log scale. The inset shows the linear regime of the power spectrum indicating the fractal nature. The solid line represents the linear fit. (B) The computed fractal dimensions for different data sets. The errorbars indicate the standard deviation.

The QPI methodology opens up interesting possibilities for future research regarding fibrin clots. The fibrin microstructure could be explored by altering the concentrations of fibrinogen and calcium ions, and studying the corresponding effect on clot attributes such as the degree of crosslinking and lateral association, pore size etc. In addition, since our technique provides a full-field quantitative phase image without the need of pixel by pixel scanning, the spatial power spectrum analysis can be performed locally, by selecting a region of interest, instead of the whole image. This could provide important region-specific information such as the inhomogeneities within a clot structure. Another future research area is to investigate the temporal parameters associated with clot formation for pathological relevance by comparing healthy and unhealthy specimens.

To summarize, quantitative phase imaging offers several advantages for measuring clot characteristics, and exhibits great potential for fibrin related biological and clinical applications.

Supporting Information

Figure S1   Sigmoidal model of the decay exponent β as a function of time.

Figure S2   Spherically averaged normalized 3D power spectrum on a log-log scale for nine datasets in (A-I). The respective insets show the power law decay regions (linear regime on log-log scale) indicating the fractal nature. The solid lines represent linear fits.

Text S1   Description of sigmoid parmeters.

Movie S1   Temporal growth of a fibrin clot is monitored using quantitative phase imaging. The formation of a cross-linked fibrin mesh with time can be clearly observed. The colorbar indicates quantitative phase in radians.

Movie S2   Depth-scanned quantitative phase images of the fibrin clot. The 3D structure becomes evident as z is varied. The colorbar indicates quantitative phase in radians.

Acknowledgments

We thank Jongsik Kim for valuable suggestions on blood clotting.

Author Contributions

Conceived and designed the experiments: RG GP. Performed the experiments: RG BB. Analyzed the data: RG GP. Contributed reagents/materials/analysis tools: KT. Wrote the paper: RG BB KT GP.

References

1. Weisel JW (2005) Fibrinogen and fibrin. Adv Protein Chem 70: 247–299.
2. Van Cott E, Laposata M (2001) Coagulation. Laboratory Test Handbook 5th ed.: 327–358.
3. Wolberg AS (2007) Thrombin generation and fibrin clot structure. Blood Reviews 21: 131–142.
4. Mosesson M (2005) Fibrinogen and fibrin structure and functions. J Thromb Haemost 3: 1894–1904.
5. Laurens N, Koolwijk P, De Maat M (2006) Fibrin structure and wound healing. J Thromb Haemost 4: 932–939.
6. Mills JD, Ariens RA, Mansfield MW, Grant PJ (2002) Altered fibrin clot structure in the healthy relatives of patients with premature coronary artery disease. Circulation 106: 1938–1942.
7. Undas A, Podolec P, Zawilska K, Pieculewicz M, Jedlinski I, et al. (2009) Altered fibrin clot structure/function in patients with cryptogenic ischemic stroke. Stroke 40: 1499–1501.
8. Jorneskog G, Egberg N, Fagrell B, Fatah K, Hessel B, et al. (1996) Altered properties of the fibrin gel structure in patients with IDDM. Diabetologia 39: 1519–1523.
9. Undas A, Zawilska K, Ciesla-Dul M, Lehmann-Kopydlowska A, Skubiszak A, et al. (2009) Altered fibrin clot structure/function in patients with idiopathic venous thromboembolism and in their relatives. Blood 114: 4272–4278.
10. Undas A, Ariens RA (2011) Fibrin clot structure and function a role in the pathophysiology of arterial and venous thromboembolic diseases. Arterioscler Thromb Vasc Biol 31: e88–e99.
11. Osathanon T, Linnes ML, Rajachar RM, Ratner BD, Somerman MJ, et al. (2008) Microporous nanofibrous fibrin-based scaffolds for bone tissue engineering. Biomaterials 29: 4091–4099.
12. Janmey PA, Winer JP, Weisel JW (2009) Fibrin gels and their clinical and bioengineering applications. J R Soc Interface 6: 1–10.
13. Spicer PP, Mikos AG (2010) Fibrin glue as a drug delivery system. J Controlled Release 148: 49–55.
14. Martino MM, Briquez PS, Ranga A, Lutolf MP, Hubbell JA (2013) Heparin-binding domain of fibrin (ogen) binds growth factors and promotes tissue repair when incorporated within a synthetic matrix. Proc Natl Acad Sci USA 110: 4563–4568.
15. Matsumoto T, Sasaki JI, Alsberg E, Egusa H, Yatani H, et al. (2007) Three-dimensional cell and tissue patterning in a strained fibrin gel system. PLoS One 2: e1211.
16. Baranski JD, Chaturvedi RR, Stevens KR, Eyckmans J, Carvalho B, et al. (2013) Geometric control of vascular networks to enhance engineered tissue integration and function. Proc Natl Acad Sci USA 110: 7586–7591.
17. Ryan EA, Mockros LF, Weisel JW, Lorand L (1999) Structural origins of fibrin clot rheology. Biophys J 77: 2813–2826.
18. Liu W, Jawerth L, Sparks E, Falvo M, Hantgan R, et al. (2006) Fibrin fibers have extraordinary extensibility and elasticity. Science 313: 634–634.
19. Blinc A, Magdic J, Fric J, Musevic I (2000) Atomic force microscopy of fibrin networks and plasma clots during fibrinolysis. Fibrinolysis and Proteolysis 14: 288–299.
20. Doolittle RF (2003) Structural basis of the fibrinogen–fibrin transformation: contributions from x-ray crystallography. Blood Reviews 17: 33–41.
21. Yeromonahos C, Polack B, Caton F (2010) Nanostructure of the fibrin clot. Biophys J 99: 2018–2027.
22. Weigandt KM, Pozzo DC, Porcar L (2009) Structure of high density fibrin networks probed with neutron scattering and rheology. Soft Matter 5: 4321–4330.
23. Weigandt KM, Porcar L, Pozzo DC (2011) In situ neutron scattering study of structural transitions in fibrin networks under shear deformation. Soft Matter 7: 9992–10000.
24. Ferri F, Greco M, Arcovito G, De Spirito M, Rocco M (2002) Structure of fibrin gels studied by elastic light scattering techniques: dependence of fractal dimension, gel crossover length, fiber diameter, and fiber density on monomer concentration. Phys Rev E 66: 011913.
25. Ferri F, Greco M, Arcovito G, Bassi FA, De Spirito M, et al. (2001) Growth kinetics and structure of fibrin gels. Phys Rev E 63: 031401.
26. Tripathi MM, Hajjarian Z, Van Cott EM, Nadkarni SK (2014) Assessing blood coagulation status with laser speckle rheology. Biomedical Optics Express 5: 817–831.
27. Collet J, Park D, Lesty C, Soria J, Soria C, et al. (2000) Influence of fibrin network conformation and fibrin fiber diameter on fibrinolysis speed dynamic and structural approaches by confocal microscopy. Arterioscler Thromb Vasc Biol 20: 1354–1361.
28. Chernysh IN, Nagaswami C, Purohit PK, Weisel JW (2012) Fibrin clots are equilibrium polymers that can be remodeled without proteolytic digestion. Sci Rep 2: 879.
29. Magatti D, Molteni M, Cardinali B, Rocco M, Ferri F (2013) Modeling of fibrin gels based on confocal microscopy and light-scattering data. Biophys J 104: 1151–1159.
30. Münster S, Jawerth LM, Leslie BA, Weitz JI, Fabry B, et al. (2013) Strain history dependence of the nonlinear stress response of fibrin and collagen networks. Proc Natl Acad Sci USA 110: 12197–12202.
31. Chernysh IN, Weisel JW (2008) Dynamic imaging of fibrin network formation correlated with other measures of polymerization. Blood 111: 4854–4861.
32. Hategan A, Gersh KC, Safer D, Weisel JW (2013) Visualization of the dynamics of fibrin clot growth 1 molecule at a time by total internal reflection fluorescence microscopy. Blood 121: 1455–1458.
33. Baker SM, Phillips KG, McCarty OJ (2012) Development of a label-free imaging technique for the quantification of thrombus formation. Cellular and Molecular Bioengineering 5: 488–492.
34. Baker-Groberg SM, Phillips KG, McCarty OJ (2013) Quantification of volume, mass, and density of thrombus formation using brightfield and differential

interference contrast microscopy. Journal of Biomedical Optics 18: 016014–016014.

35. Neeves K, McCarty O, Reininger A, Sugimoto M, King M (2014) Flow-dependent thrombin and fibrin generation in vitro: opportunities for standardization: communication from SSC of the ISTH. Journal of Thrombosis and Haemostasis 12: 418–420.

36. Popescu G (2011) Quantitative phase imaging of cells and tissues. McGraw-Hill.

37. Wang Z, Millet L, Mir M, Ding H, Unarunotai S, et al. (2011) Spatial light interference microscopy (SLIM). Opt Express 19: 1016–1026.

38. Bhaduri B, Wickland D, Wang R, Chan V, Bashir R, et al. (2013) Cardiomyocyte imaging using real-time spatial light interference microscopy (SLIM). PLoS One 8.

39. Mir M, Tangella K, Popescu G (2011) Blood testing at the single cell level using quantitative phase and amplitude microscopy. Biomed Opt Express 2: 3259–3266.

40. Mir M, Wang Z, Shen Z, Bednarz M, Bashir R, et al. (2011) Optical measurement of cycle-dependent cell growth. Proc Natl Acad Sci USA 108: 13124–13129.

41. Mir M, Kim T, Majumder A, Xiang M, Wang R, et al. (2014) Label-free characterization of emerging human neuronal networks. Sci Rep 4: 4434.

42. Mir M, Bergamaschi A, Katzenellenbogen BS, Popescu G (2014) Highly sensitive quantitative imaging for monitoring single cancer cell growth kinetics and drug response. PloS One 9: e89000.

43. Kim T, Zhou R, Mir M, Babacan SD, Carney PS, et al. (2014) White-light diffraction tomography of unlabelled live cells. Nature Photonics 8: 256–263.

44. Colace TV, Tormoen GW, McCarty OJ, Diamond SL (2013) Microfluidics and coagulation biology. Annual Review of Biomedical Engineering 15: 283.

45. Woodruff RS, Sullenger B, Becker RC (2011) The many faces of the contact pathway and their role in thrombosis. Journal of Thrombosis and Thrombolysis 32: 9–20.

46. Persson B, Albohr O, Tartaglino U, Volokitin A, Tosatti E (2005) On the nature of surface roughness with application to contact mechanics, sealing, rubber friction and adhesion. Journal of Physics: Condensed Matter 17: R1.

47. Blombäck B, Okada M (1982) Fibrin gel structure and clotting time. Thrombosis Research 25: 51–70.

48. Baumann P, Jurgensen T, Heuck C (1989) Computerized analysis of the in vitro activation of the plasmatic clotting system. Pathophysiol Haemost Thromb 19: 309–321.

49. Vikinge TP, Hansson KM, Benesch J, Johansen K, Ra M, et al. (2000) Blood plasma coagulation studied by surface plasmon resonance. J Biomed Opt 5: 51–55.

50. Evans PA, Hawkins K, Morris RH, Thirumalai N, Munro R, et al. (2010) Gel point and fractal microstructure of incipient blood clots are significant new markers of hemostasis for healthy and anticoagulated blood. Blood 116: 3341–3346.

7

Presence of Neutrophil Extracellular Traps and Citrullinated Histone H3 in the Bloodstream of Critically Ill Patients

Tomoya Hirose[1]*[9][¶], Shigeto Hamaguchi[2][9][¶], Naoya Matsumoto[1], Taro Irisawa[1], Masafumi Seki[2], Osamu Tasaki[3], Hideo Hosotsubo[1], Norihisa Yamamoto[2], Kouji Yamamoto[4], Yukihiro Akeda[5], Kazunori Oishi[5], Kazunori Tomono[2], Takeshi Shimazu[1]

1 Department of Traumatology and Acute Critical Medicine, Osaka University Graduate School of Medicine, Osaka, Japan, 2 Division of Infection Control and Prevention, Osaka University Graduate School of Medicine, Osaka, Japan, 3 Department of Emergency Medicine, Unit of Clinical Medicine, Nagasaki University Graduate School of Biomedical Sciences, Nagasaki, Japan, 4 Department of Medical Innovation, Osaka University Hospital, Osaka, Japan, 5 International Research Center for Infectious Diseases, Research Institute for Microbial Diseases, Osaka University, Osaka, Japan

Abstract

Neutrophil extracellular traps (NETs), a newly identified immune mechanism, are induced by inflammatory stimuli. Modification by citrullination of histone H3 is thought to be involved in the in vitro formation of NETs. The purposes of this study were to evaluate whether NETs and citrullinated histone H3 (Cit-H3) are present in the bloodstream of critically ill patients and to identify correlations with clinical and biological parameters. Blood samples were collected from intubated patients at the time of ICU admission from April to June 2011. To identify NETs, DNA and histone H3 were visualized simultaneously by immunofluorescence in blood smears. Cit-H3 was detected using a specific antibody. We assessed relationships of the presence of NETs and Cit-H3 with the existence of bacteria in tracheal aspirate, SIRS, diagnosis, WBC count, and concentrations of IL-8, TNF-α, cf-DNA, lactate, and HMGB1. Forty-nine patients were included. The median of age was 66.0 (IQR: 52.5–76.0) years. The diagnoses included trauma (7, 14.3%), infection (14, 28.6%), resuscitation from cardiopulmonary arrest (8, 16.3%), acute poisoning (4, 8.1%), heart disease (4, 8.1%), brain stroke (8, 16.3%), heat stroke (2, 4.1%), and others (2, 4.1%). We identified NETs in 5 patients and Cit-H3 in 11 patients. NETs and/or Cit-H3 were observed more frequently in "the presence of bacteria in tracheal aspirate" group (11/22, 50.0%) than in "the absence of bacteria in tracheal aspirate" group (4/27, 14.8%) (p<.01). Multiple logistic regression analysis showed that only the presence of bacteria in tracheal aspirate was significantly associated with the presence of NETs and/or Cit-H3. The presence of bacteria in tracheal aspirate may be one important factor associated with NET formation. NETs may play a pivotal role in the biological defense against the dissemination of pathogens from the respiratory tract to the bloodstream in potentially infected patients.

Editor: Nades Palaniyar, The Hospital for Sick Children and The University of Toronto, Canada

Funding: This work was supported by a Grant-in-Aid for Scientific Research from the Ministry of Education, Culture, Sports, Science and Technology in Japan (no. 21390163, no. 25293366 and no. 25861718) and by ZENKYOREN (National Mutual Insurance Federation of Agricultural Cooperatives). The funders had no role in study design, data collection and analysis, decision to publish, or preparation of the manuscript.

Competing Interests: The authors have declared that no competing interests exist.

* Email: htomoya1979@hp-emerg.med.osaka-u.ac.jp

⑨ These authors contributed equally to this work.

¶ These authors are joint first authors on this work.

Introduction

Neutrophils play an important role as the first line of innate immune defense [1]. One function of neutrophils, called "neutrophil extracellular traps" (NETs), has been discovered recently. NETs are fibrous structures that are released extracellularly from activated neutrophils in response to infection and also the sterile inflammatory process [2–5]. This distinctive phenomenon was first reported by Brinkmann et al in 2004 [6]. The main components of NETs are deoxyribonucleic acid (DNA) and histones H1, H2A, H2B, H3, and H4; other components such as neutrophil elastase, myeloperoxidase, bactericidal/permeability-increasing protein, cathepsin G, lactoferrin, matrix metalloproteinase-9, peptidoglycan recognition proteins, pentraxin, and LL-37 have also been reported [5–11]. The type of active cell death involving the release of NETs is called NETosis [12], which differs from apoptosis and necrosis. Because formation of NETs does not require caspases and is not accompanied by DNA fragmentation, it is believed that this process is independent of apoptosis [12]. Despite several in vitro and animal experiments that have clearly shown the biological importance of NETs, little is known about the function of NETs in the human body [13,14].

Before the discovery of NETs, several studies reported on an increase in the concentration of circulating free DNA (cf-DNA) in the blood in various diseases including sepsis, trauma, stroke, autoimmune disorders, and several cancers [15–20]. This cf-DNA is thought to be derived from necrotic and/or apoptotic cells [21]. Recent articles have suggested that NETs and cf-DNA are related [15,16]. In these reports, cf-DNA was quantified directly in plasma, and the cf-DNA in plasma was treated the same as NETs in blood. However, it remains unknown whether cf-DNA is derived from NETs.

Citrullination of histone H3 is considered to be involved in NET formation in vitro. Neutrophils show highly decondensed nuclear chromatin structures during NETosis, and hypercitrullination of histone H3 by peptidylarginine deiminase 4 (PAD4) plays an important role in chromatin decondensation [14,22,23]. Inhibition of PAD4 prevents citrullination of H3 and NET formation [23]. Thus, measuring the presence of citrullinated histone H3 (Cit-H3) in conjunction with the presence of NETs may help clarify the kinetics of the response of NETs to systemic stress.

In preliminary studies, we recently identified NETs immuno-cytochemically in sputum and blood smear samples from intensive care unit (ICU) patients [24,25], whereas NETs could not be detected in blood smears from healthy volunteers [25].

In the present study, we used immunofluorescence to prospectively explore the existence of NETs and Cit-H3 in the blood of critically ill patients hospitalized in an ICU.

The respiratory tract is considered one of the most vulnerable places for bacterial invasion of the body, and NETs might start to be produced in response to pathogens before infection is completely apparent. Therefore, in this study we evaluated the presence of bacteria by Gram staining in tracheal aspirate as the preclinical stage of manifested infection to highlight its relationship with the induction of NETs in blood. The purpose of this study was to evaluate the relationships between NET or Cit-H3 and various clinical and biological parameters.

Materials and Methods

Patients and Setting

This study was a prospective observational study and was approved by the Ethics Committee of Osaka University Graduate School of Medicine. The institutional review board waived the need for informed consent. From April to June 2011, we examined blood samples collected from all patients who required intubation at the time of admission into the ICU of the Trauma and Acute Critical Care Center at the Osaka University Hospital (Osaka, Japan).

Evaluation of Clinical Background and Severity of Illness

Age, sex, Acute Physiological And Chronic Health Evaluation (APACHE) II score, and Sequential Organ Failure Assessment (SOFA) score were recorded at the time of admission. Systemic inflammatory response syndrome (SIRS) was diagnosed at the time of admission on the basis of the criteria for SIRS defined by the American College of Chest Physicians/Society of Critical Care Medicine Consensus [26]. At admission, the blood samples were analyzed to obtain the following laboratory data: white blood cell (WBC) count and concentrations of lactate, IL-8, TNF-α, HMGB1, and cf-DNA. WBC count was measured by an automated hematology analyzer (KX-21N; Sysmex, Hyogo, Japan). Lactate concentration was measured by a blood gas analyzer (ABL 835 Flex; Radiometer, Brønshøj, Denmark). The serum levels of IL-8 (R&D Systems, Minneapolis, MN, USA), TNF-α (R&D Systems), and HMGB1 (Shino-Test Corporation, Tokyo, Japan) were measured by enzyme-linked immunosorbent assay (ELISA) kits, and cf-DNA concentration was quantified

using the Quant-iT PicoGreen dsDNA Assay kit (Invitrogen, Carlsbad, CA, USA), according to the manufacturer's instructions.

Immunofluorescence Analysis to Identify the Presence of NETs and Cit-H3

For histological analysis, each blood sample collected at the time of admission to the ICU was immediately smeared in a thin layer on a glass slide. After drying, the specimens were stored at $-80°C$ until immunostaining was performed. We confirmed that this sample preparation method did not induce additional generation of NETs or citrullination of histone H3 using neutrophils isolated from healthy donors on the smear (Fig. S1). To identify NETs, DNA and histone H3, the main components in NETs, were visualized simultaneously by immunofluorescence, and Cit-H3 was also detected using a specific antibody as follows. The sample on the glass slide was fixed with 4% paraformaldehyde for 30 min, washed with phosphate-buffered saline (PBS) (pH 7.4), and then blocked with a solution containing 20% Block-Ace (Dainippon-Sumitomo Seiyaku, Osaka, Japan) and 0.005% saponin in PBS for 10 min. The samples were then incubated for 60 min with the primary antibody as follows: anti-human histone H3 mouse monoclonal antibody (diluted 1:100) (MABI0001; MAB Institute, Inc., Hokkaido, Japan) and anti-human Cit-H3 rabbit polyclonal antibody (1:100) (ab5103; Abcam, Cambridge, UK). After washing in PBS, each primary antibody was visualized using secondary antibodies coupled to 1:500 Alexa Fluor 546 goat anti-mouse IgG (Invitrogen) and 1:500 Alexa Fluor 488 goat anti-rabbit IgG (Invitrogen). The primary and secondary antibodies were diluted with 5% Block-Ace and 0.005% saponin in PBS. After incubation for 60 min with the secondary antibodies, the specimens were washed with PBS, and the DNA was stained with 4′,6-diamidino-2-phenylindole (DAPI; Invitrogen) in PBS for 5 min. All procedures were performed at room temperature. The specimens were analyzed using a confocal laser-scanning microscope (BZ-9000; Keyence Corporation; Osaka, Japan).

The validity of immunostaining was ensured by the negative results of control experiments in which whole mouse or rabbit IgG (Abcam) was used instead of primary antibodies or primary antibodies were omitted in the procedure (Fig. S2). In addition, neutrophils stimulated with phorbol myristate acetate from healthy donors were used as a positive control for immunostaining (Fig. S3).

In the preliminary experiments, string-like structure extending from the cell body, which was positive for DNA and histone, was exclusively also positive for neutrophil elastase (Fig. S4). Hence, we considered the extracellular component that is double-positive for DNA and H3 to be a NET. The production of NETs and the specific expression of the citrullination of histone H3 in neutrophils were confirmed using anti-CD66b antibody (Fig. 1). Diff-Quik staining revealed the presence of a variety of blood cells in the smears (Fig. S5).

For the purpose of estimating the presence of NETs and the occurrence of citrullination of histone H3 concurrently, triple staining for DNA, H3, and citrullinated H3 was performed in this study. Samples were considered negative for the presence of NETs or Cit-H3 if cells harboring NETs or Cit-H3 were not identified in 300 neutrophils by immunostaining. If at least one of NETs and Cit-H3 was positive in the smear according to the definition mentioned above, the corresponding patient was classified into the "NET- and/or Cit-H3-positive" group.

Detection of the presence of bacteria in tracheal aspirate

Aspiration is defined as the inhalation of oropharyngeal or gastric contents into the larynx and lower respiratory tract, and

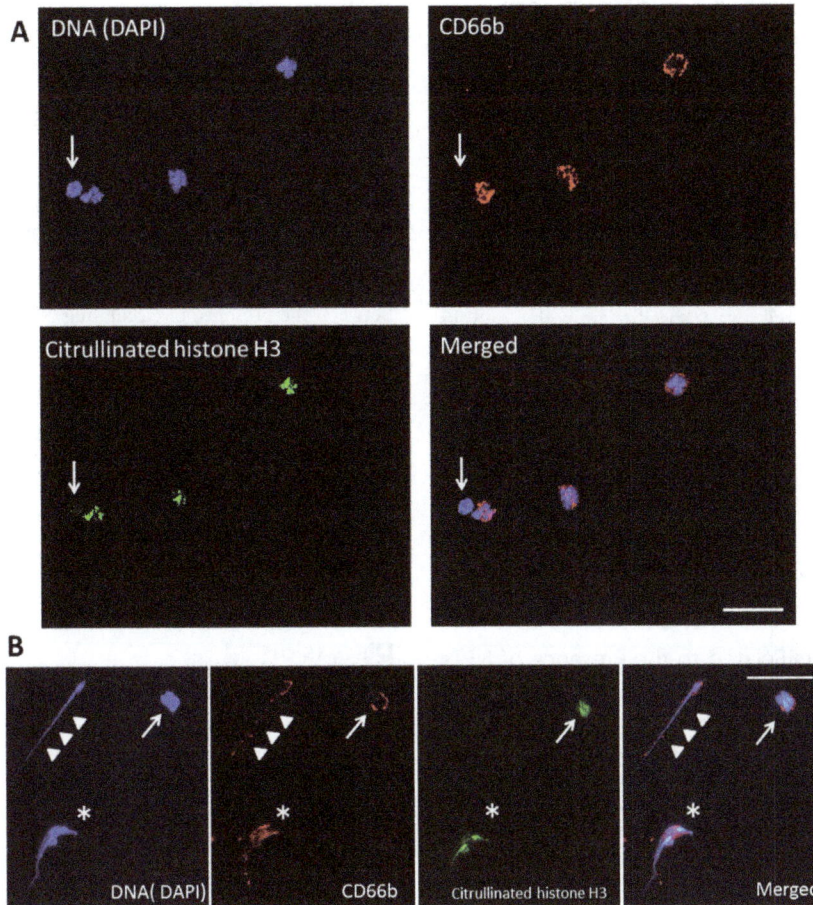

Figure 1. Representative images of immunostaining using anti-CD66b antibody in the blood smear sample from a critically ill patient. Triple staining by DAPI, anti-CD66b antibody, and anti-citrullinated histone H3 was performed using the blood smear sample obtained from a critically ill patient. A. The CD66b-positive cells were subjected to citrullination of histone H3 in their nuclei. Citrullination of histone H3 was not detected in the CD66b-negative cell (arrow). B. Arrow indicates the occurrence of citrullination of histone H3 in a neutrophil that had immunoreactivity against CD66b. Arrowheads indicate NETs stained with CD66b, whose appearance was of a string-like structure extending from the cell body. Asterisk indicates a neutrophil that was beginning to release NETs from its ruptured cell body. Interestingly, freshly produced NETs (asterisk) held immunoreactivity against citrullination of histone H3. In contrast, elongated NETs (arrowheads) were not stained with anti- citrullinated histone H3 antibody. Blue, DAPI; Red, CD66b; Green, citrullinated histone H3. (Magnification ×400). Scale bar; 50 μm.

aspiration pneumonia is an infectious process caused by the inhalation of oropharyngeal secretions that are colonized by pathogenic bacteria [27]. The presence of bacteria in tracheal aspirate by Gram staining is regarded as part of aspiration that favors the development of infection. In this study, we evaluated the presence of bacteria in tracheal aspirate as the preclinical stage of manifested infection. To screen for the presence of bacteria in tracheal aspirate, an aspirated sputum smear was also prepared independently from immunostaining at the time of each patient's admission to the ICU. For Gram staining, the smear was dried, stained with crystal violet (Merck KGaA, Darmstadt, Germany) followed by iodine (Merck KGaA), washed with 99.5% ethanol (Wako Pure Chemical Industries, Ltd., Osaka, Japan), and stained with Safranin (Merck KGaA). Images were captured on an optical microscope system (ECLIPSE 50i; Nikon Instruments Inc., Tokyo, Japan).

Statistical Analysis

Continuous variables are presented as the median and interquartile range (IQR). The Wilcoxon rank-sum test and Pearson's chi-square test were used to compare two patient groups.

Single and multiple logistic regression analyses were used to identify associations between the presence of NETs and/or Cit-H3 and the clinical and biological parameters studied. A p-value of $<$ .05 was considered significant. All statistical analyses were performed using JMP 9.0.2 (SAS Institute Inc., Cary, NC, USA) and reviewed by a statistician.

Results

Patient Characteristics

During the study period, 263 patients were admitted to the ICU; 49 of these 263 patients were intubated patients and were included in this study. We excluded patients with cardiopulmonary arrest (CPA) who could not be resuscitated on admission. The patients' characteristics are shown in Table 1. The study group comprised 29 men and 20 women with a median age of 66.0 (IQR, 52.5–76.0) years. The median APACHE II score was 18.0 (IQR, 12.5–21.5), and the median SOFA score was 5.0 (IQR, 4.0–8.0). Thirty-eight patients (77.6%) were diagnosed as having SIRS, and 22 patients (44.9%) were judged as positive for "the presence of bacteria in tracheal aspirate". Thirty-six patients (73.5%)

survived and 13 patients died. The ICU mortality rate of intubated patients during this study period was 26.5%. The median WBC count was 10,900/μL (IQR, 8215–14,915/μL). The diagnoses included trauma (n = 7, 14.3%), infection (n = 14, 28.6%), resuscitation from CPA (n = 8, 16.3%), acute poisoning (n = 4, 8.1%), heart disease (n = 4, 8.1%), brain stroke (n = 8, 16.3%), heat stroke (n = 2, 4.1%), and others (n = 2, 4.1%) (Table 2).

Presence of NETs and Cit-H3 in the Bloodstream

NETs were identified as extracellular string-like structures that were simultaneously immunoreactive for DNA and histone H3 (Fig. 2). Cit-H3 was detected by a specific antibody, and its presence was confirmed to be located inside lobulated nuclei and histone H3 (Fig. 3). In the blood smears surveyed in this study, we identified NETs in 5 patients and Cit-H3 in 11 patients (Table 2). Both NETs and Cit-H3 were identified concurrently in one patient with infection. We detected the presence of circulating NETs and/or Cit-H3-positive cells in samples from patients with infection (4/14, 28.6%), resuscitation from CPA (5/8, 62.5%), acute poisoning (1/4, 25.0%), brain stroke (3/8, 37.5%), and heat stroke (1/2, 50.0%). We found no NETs or Cit-H3-positive cells in samples from patients with trauma (0/7) or heart disease (0/4).

Identification of Factors Related to the Presence of NETs and Cit-H3 in the Bloodstream

We tried to identify the factors that are related to the presence of NETs or Cit-H3 in the bloodstream. We first examined clinical parameters recorded at the time of admission including age, APACHE II and SOFA scores, number of patients who presented with SIRS or with the presence of bacteria in tracheal aspirate, and biological parameters such as the total WBC count and concentrations of lactate, IL-8, TNF-α, HMGB1, and cf-DNA. We also recorded the number of survivors. We compared these variables between the patients positive or negative for NETs and/or Cit-H3. The results are shown in Table 3. Among the factors evaluated in this research, only "the presence of bacteria in tracheal aspirate" differed significantly between the NET- and/or Cit-H3-positive and -negative groups ($p<.01$, Wilcoxon rank-sum test and Pearson's chi-square test). The other factors were not significantly related to the presence of NETs and/or Cit-H3. In patients classified into two groups based on the presence or absence of bacteria in tracheal aspirate, the occurrence rate of NETs and/or Cit-H3 was significantly higher in "the presence of bacteria in tracheal aspirate" (BTA (+)) group (11/22, 50.0%) than

in "the absence of bacteria in tracheal aspirate" (BTA (−)) group (4/27, 14.8%) ($p<.01$) (Table S1). In patients with SIRS on admission, there was a trend toward greater expression of NETs and/or Cit-H3 ($p = .079$) (Table S2).

Logistic regression analysis was performed to identify the factors related to the presence of NETs and Cit-H3 in the bloodstream. The results of single logistic regression analysis of factors associated with the presence of NETs and Cit-H3 are shown in Table 4. Only BTA (+) at the time of intubation was a significant factor associated with the presence of NETs and Cit-H3 ($p = .0112$). Although there were indications of a trend toward an association between the presence of circulating NETs and/or Cit-H3 and the comorbid conditions of SIRS or elevated cf-DNA concentration ($p = .1093$ and.3003, respectively), these were not statistically significant. Table 5 shows the results of multiple logistic regression analysis of factors associated with the presence of NETs and/or Cit-H3 and model selection. Two methods of multiple regression analysis, backward and forward regression, yielded similar models. Again, "the presence of bacteria in tracheal aspirate" was the only factor that was significantly related to the presence of NETs and/or Cit-H3 in the bloodstream; the odds ratio for aspiration was 5.750.

Discussion

A series of in vitro and animal experiments have uncovered a suppressive function of NETs against the dissemination of microorganisms in blood by mechanical trapping and by exploiting coagulant function to segregate these microorganisms within the circulation [28,29]. However, direct evidence remains scarce in living human systems. In this clinical study of blood smears, we attempted to identify morphologically the presence of NETs and Cit-H3 in the bloodstream of critically ill patients at the time of admission to the ICU and to characterize the factors associated with the presence of NETs and Cit-H3.

Among the 49 enrolled patients, immunofluorescence analysis revealed blood-borne NETs in five patients (10.2%), Cit-H3 in 11 patients (22.4%), and NETs and/or Cit-H3 in 15 patients (30.6%) (Table 2). These data replicate the results of our previous preliminary study in which NETs were present in patients in a critical condition [25] and show for the first time, to our knowledge, the presence of Cit-H3 in circulating blood cells. Cit-H3-positive cells possessed a multi-segmented nucleus, and most were immunoreactive for CD66b (Fig. 1), suggesting that citrullination of histone H3 occurred exclusively in neutrophils.

Table 1. Patient characteristics.

Variable	Value
No. of patients (M/F)	49 (29/20)
Age (years, median, IQR)	66.0 (52.5–76.0)
APACHE II score (median, IQR)	18.0 (12.5–21.5)
SOFA score (median, IQR)	5 (4–8)
No. of patients with SIRS	48 (11.8%)
The presence of bacteria in tracheal aspirate	22 (44.9%)
No. of survivors	36 (73.5%)
WBC (median, IQR)	10,900 (8215–14,915)

During the study period, 263 patients were admitted to the ICU of whom 49 were intubated and were included in this study. We excluded patients with cardiopulmonary arrest who could not be resuscitated on admission. IQR: interquartile range, APACHE: Acute Physiological And Chronic Health Evaluation, SOFA: Sequential Organ Failure Assessment, SIRS: systemic inflammatory response syndrome, WBC: white blood cell.

Table 2. Diagnoses and the number of patients exhibiting neutrophil extracellular traps and citrullinated histone H3 in each diagnostic group.

Diagnosis	NET positive (n)	Cit-H3 positive (n)	NET and/or Cit-H3 positive (%)
Trauma (n = 7)	0	0	0/7 (0)
Infection (n = 14)	3	2	4/14 (28.6)
Resuscitated from cardiopulmonary arrest (n = 8)	2	3	5/8 (62.5)
Acute poisoning (n = 4)	0	1	1/4 (25.0)
Heart disease (n = 4)	0	0	0/4 (0)
Brain stroke (n = 8)	0	3	3/8 (37.5)
Heat stroke (n = 2)	0	1	1/2 (50.0)
Others (n = 2)	0	1	1/2 (50.0)
Total (n = 49)	5	11	15/49 (30.6)

In the blood smears surveyed in this study, we identified NETs in 5 patients and Cit-H3 in 11 patients. Both NETs and Cit-H3 were identified concurrently in one patient with infection. We found no NETs or Cit-H3-positive cells in samples from patients with trauma (0/7) or heart disease (0/4). NETs: neutrophil extracellular trap, Cit-H3: citrullinated histone H3.

Citrullination of histone H3 is considered an important process in the release of NETs through decondensation of chromatin [14,22,23]. Interestingly, the occurrence ratio of Cit-H3 was twice that of NETs. In vitro experiments imply that a substantial period of time is necessary to expel NETs extracellularly after the initiation of cell death by a stress stimulus [12,30,31]. However, it is still not clear how much time is required in vivo for NETs to appear intravascularly. The number of patients who exhibited circulating NETs in this study was lower than anticipated. We collected blood samples on admission to the ICU, and the timing might have been too early to detect NETs after the onset of a

critical illness. The 11 Cit-H3-positive patients could be considered to have been in an early stage of NET formation. The change in the appearance of NETs and Cit-H3 during the course of hospitalization should be studied. If it can be shown clinically that Cit-H3 expression is followed by NET formation, it might be important to evaluate Cit-H3 expression in the blood upon admission to an ICU.

Table 2 shows that NETs and Cit-H3 were detected in patients with infection, resuscitation from CPA, acute poisoning, brain stroke, or heat stroke; surprisingly, we could not detect NETs or Cit-H3 in patients with trauma or heart disease. NETs are formed

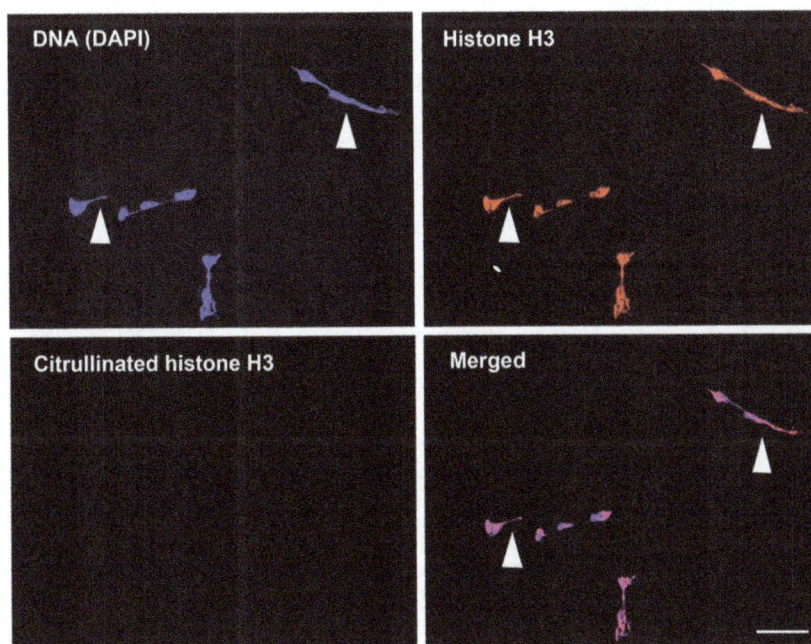

Figure 2. Representative images of immunofluorescence staining to detect neutrophil extracellular traps (NETs). NETs were visualized in the blood smear samples by immunocytochemistry and identified as extracellular string-like structures composed of chromatin (DNA and histone H3). NETs were present in the bloodstream of critically ill patients. Citrullination of histone H3 was not recognized in these images. In the blood smears surveyed in this study, we identified NETs in five patients (5/49, 10.2%). Blue, 4',6-diamidino-2-phenylindole (DAPI); red, histone H3; green, citrullinated histone H3. Arrowheads indicate the double-stained areas containing NETs (Magnification ×400). Scale bar; 50 μm.

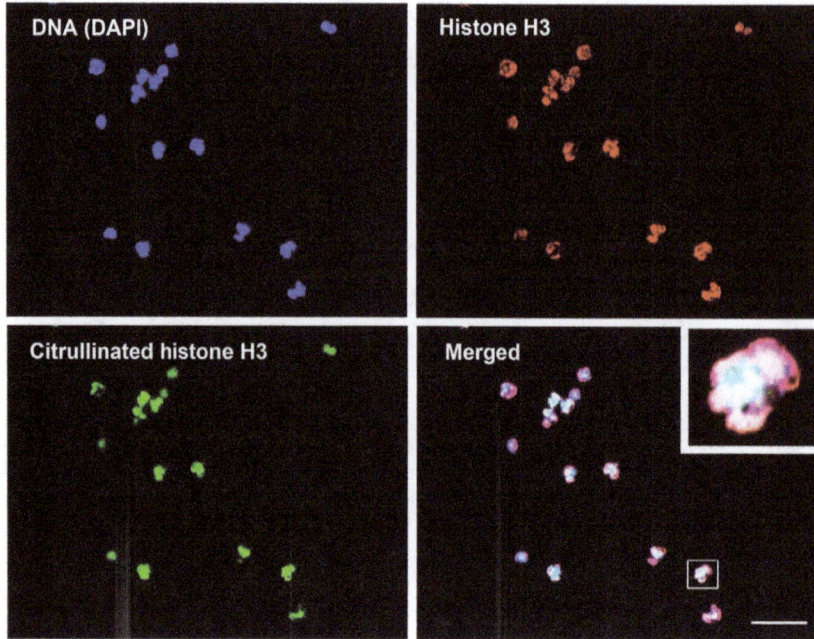

Figure 3. Representative images of immunofluorescence staining to detect citrullinated histone H3 (Cit-H3). Citrullination of histone H3, which is a critical enzymatic process to produce NETs through decondensation of chromatin, was visualized in the blood smear samples using anti-citrullinated histone H3 antibody by immunohistochemistry. Cit-H3 was present in the bloodstream of critically ill patients. The inset in the merged image is the magnified image of a representative cell (white rectangle) expressing citrullinated histone H3 in the nucleus. Neutrophil extracellular traps are not recognized here. In the blood smears surveyed in this study, we identified Cit-H3 in 11 patients (11/49, 22.4%). Blue, 4',6-diamidino-2-phenylindole (DAPI); red, histone H3; green, citrullinated histone H3 (Magnification ×400). Scale bar; 50 μm.

in response to various microorganisms and pathogens [14]. McDonald et al reported that NETs ensnare circulating bacteria and provide intravascular immunity that protects against bacterial dissemination during septic infection [29]. In this context, the presence of NETs and/or Cit-H3 in infected patients is to be expected. By contrast, trauma or heart disease patients were

Table 3. Comparison between patients positive and negative for neutrophil extracellular traps and/or citrullinated histone H3.

	NET and/or citrullinated histone H3		
	Positive	Negative	p
Number	15	34	
Age (years)	67.0 (49.0–78.0)	65.5 (56.8–75.3)	.8197
APACHE II score	20.0 (16.0–23.0)	17.5 (11.8–21.3)	.3171
SOFA score	6.0 (5.0–10.0)	5.0 (4.0–8.0)	.4062
Survivors (n)	10 (66.7%)	26 (76.5%)	.4737
SIRS patients (n)	14 (93.3%)	24 (70.6%)	.0786
The presence of bacteria in tracheal aspirate (n)	11 (73.3%)	11 (32.3%)	.0079
WBC count (/μl)	12,430 (8310.0–16510.0)	10,835 (8032.5–14307.5)	.5654
IL-8 (pg/mL)	57.6 (19.9–143.0)	65.3 (23.3–229.5)	.9136
TNF-α (pg/mL)	8.2 (6.2–21.6)	9.0 (4.8–16.3)	.9740
cf-DNA (ng/mL)	1038.3 (744.9–1329.7)	1072.7 (828.6–1770.7)	.6025
Lactate (mg/mL)	39 (11.0–71.0)	17.5 (13.0–56.0)	.3010
HMGB1 (ng/mL)	11.0 (6.8–21.5)	9.7 (5.9–16.3)	.5151

Among the factors evaluated to highlight the relation to the presence of NETs or Cit-H3 in the bloodstream, only "the presence of bacteria in tracheal aspirate" differed significantly between the NET- and/or Cit-H3-positive and -negative groups (p<.01). The other factors were not significantly related to the presence of NETs and/or Cit-H3. Continuous variables are presented as the median and IQR unless otherwise noted. The Wilcoxon rank-sum test and Pearson's chi-square test were used to compare two patient groups. NETs: neutrophil extracellular traps, Cit-H3: citrullinated histone H3, IQR: interquartile range, APACHE: Acute Physiological And Chronic Health Evaluation, SOFA: Sequential Organ Failure Assessment, SIRS: systemic inflammatory response syndrome, WBC: white blood cell, IL: interleukin, TNF: tumor necrosis factor, cf-DNA: circulating free DNA, HMGB1: high mobility group box-1.

Table 4. Results of single logistic regression analysis.

Variable	p
The presence of bacteria in tracheal aspirate	.0112
SIRS	.1093
cf-DNA	.3003
Lactate	.5476
WBC count	.7862
IL-8	.7875
TNF-α	.8321
HMGB1	.9439

Logistic regression analysis was performed to identify the factors related to the presence of NET and Cit-H3 in the bloodstream. Only "the presence of bacteria in tracheal aspirate" (+) at the time of intubation was a significant factor associated with the presence of NET and Cit-H3 ($p=.0112$). NETs: neutrophil extracellular traps, Cit-H3: citrullinated histone H3, SIRS: systemic inflammatory response syndrome, cf-DNA: circulating free DNA, WBC: white blood cell, IL: interleukin, TNF: tumor necrosis factor, HMGB1: high mobility group box-1.

transported to the hospital immediately after the onset of the condition, and there was no potential risk of infection on admission; this may explain why NETs and Cit-H3 were not detected in these patients.

Intriguingly, a high percentage (62.5%) of patients with CPA exhibited circulating NETs and/or Cit-H3. Acute poisoning, brain stroke, and heat stroke are clinical conditions that can cause disturbance of consciousness, which may induce aspiration. Adnet and Baud demonstrated that the risk of aspiration increases with the degree of unconsciousness (as measured by the Glasgow Coma Scale [GCS]) [32]. In the present study population, the GCS score on admission was significantly lower in the BTA (+) group than in the BTA (−) group (4 [IQR, 3–10.75] vs 13 [IQR, 7–14]; $p<.01$). Except for the infected patient group, the patients who exhibited NETs and/or Cit-H3 in their blood had a significantly lower GCS score on admission ($p=.0418$). We therefore investigated whether "the presence of bacteria in tracheal aspirate", which was represented as part of aspiration and as the presumable preclinical stage of manifested infection, was associated with the presence of NETs and/or Cit-H3, and found a significant association (odds ratio for aspiration, 5.750) (Tables 3–5). Bacteria drawn into the respiratory tract can induce epithelial injury, which provides an opportunity for bacterial translocation as well as leukocyte transmigration until completion of epithelial repair [33,34]. Concomitance of acid aspiration under impaired consciousness additionally enhances bacterial adherence to the epithelium [35]. Injured airway epithelium produces cytokines including IL-8 and alarmins such as HMGB1, both of which are representative inducers for NETs [36–39]. Next, bacteria and inflammatory

mediators infiltrating into the interstitial space secondary to epithelial injury will affect the endothelial integrity [40]. The presence of NETs in sputum following aspiration, a phenomenon that we reported previously [24], suggests breakdown of the epithelial barrier that is induced by local inflammation through direct contact between aspirated bacteria and epithelium or through activation of resident immune cells such as macrophages in the respiratory tract [41]. Such epithelial breakdown would allow influx of pathogens, pathogen-associated molecular patterns, cytokines, chemokines, and alarmins from the lumen of the respiratory tract into the circulation. These materials might stimulate the production of NETs intravenously to inhibit systemic invasion of bacteria. We assumed that NETs are induced in the respiratory tract to suppress bacterial dissemination leading to pneumonia and in the vessels to inhibit bacteremia against the invasion of bacteria into the blood and that even such colonization of bacteria in the respiratory tract could trigger citrullination of histone H3 to produce NETs in blood. Single logistic regression analyses of whether infection and/or BTA (+) associated with the presence of NETs and/or Cit-H3 produced an odds ratio of 7.312 (Table S3). These results suggest that induction of NETs systemically through the citrullination of histone H3 in blood maybe an initial response for protection against bacterial dissemination from latent respiratory infection.

Some researchers consider cf-DNA to be equivalent to NETs in the blood [15,16]. However, our results showed that the occurrence rate of NETs and/or Cit-H3 was not significantly associated with cf-DNA concentration ($p=.6025$) (Table 3). Although the number of patients was different due to sample limitations, additional analysis by MPO-DNA ELISA (Data S1) was also performed. As a result, there was no difference in the values between the group positive for (0.076 [IQR, 0.067–0.100]; n = 8) and the group negative for NET and/or citrullinated histone H3 (0.078 [IQR, 0.070–0.111]; n = 26). We reported recently that in patients with an acute respiratory infection, NETs became fragmented during recovery from infection [24], suggesting that NETs should also be digested in the blood with time. Our method using blood smear samples cannot detect NETs that harbor inside vessels or that are already degraded, whereas the method based on MPO-DNA ELISA might also measure neutrophil DNA fragments derived from necrosis or apoptosis and cannot detect NETs that are not truncated from the cell body. We consider that at the early phase of critical illness, i.e., when the production of NETs is just starting, the morphological approach has an advantage in being able to detect NETs that are still anchored to the cell body, in conjunction with the merit that identification of citrullination of histone H3 is possible at a stage prior to the release of NETs.

HMGB1 is a nuclear protein present in the nucleus of all nucleated cells. HMGB1 binds to DNA and acts as an inflammatory mediator once it is released extracellularly [42,43]. In this study, HMGB1 was significantly higher in SIRS patients

Table 5. Results of multiple logistic regression analysis of factors associated with the presence of neutrophil extracellular traps and/or citrullinated histone H3.

	Coeff (β)	p	OR	Lower	Upper
"the presence of bacteria in tracheal aspirate"	0.875	0.011	5.750	1.583	24.755

Two methods of multiple regression analysis, backward and forward regression, yielded similar models. "The presence of bacteria in tracheal aspirate" was the only factor that was significantly related to the presence of neutrophil extracellular traps and/or citrullinated histone H3 in the bloodstream. The odds ratio for aspiration was 5.750. Coeff (β): coefficient; OR: odds ratio, Lower: lower level of 95% confidence interval, Upper: upper level of 95% confidence interval.

than in non-SIRS patients (Table S2). Unexpectedly, however, HMGB1 was not a significant factor associated with the presence of NETs and/or Cit-H3 (Tables 3–5). NETs contain HMGB1 [44], and one possibility is that HMGB1 binding to NETs is not reflected in the amount of circulating HMGB1 measured by ELISA.

Although IL-8 and TNF-α are considered stimulatory factors that induce NET formation [14,39,45], they were not associated with the presence of NETs and/or Cit-H3 in this study (Tables 3–5). This negative result suggest the presence of an unknown complex regulatory mechanism for the production of NETs in vivo.

As limitations of this study, first, the sample size was small, and the patients were very heterogeneous. Second, we evaluated the presence of NETs and Cit-H3 and the associated factors in the bloodstream of critically ill patients only at admission. It should be investigated in the future how NETs are processed after the induction of NETosis in the circulation. It is presumable that NETs could be degraded by DNase, and the fragments would contribute partially to the formation of cf-DNA. Third, we did not rigorously quantify the amount of NETs and Cit-H3. The possibility of the degradation of NETs and the difficulty in detecting NETs, which are anchored in the vessels, might lead to underestimation of the presence of NETs in our method using blood smear samples. Further study is required to establish finer methods of quantification. We hope that future elucidation of the biological significance of NETs will lead to new strategies to treat critical illness by monitoring NET formation in blood.

Conclusions

The presence of NETs and Cit-H3 were identified immunocytochemically in the bloodstream of a subset of critically ill patients. "The presence of bacteria in tracheal aspirate" may be one important factor related to the presence of circulating NETs. NETs may play a pivotal role in biological defense in the bloodstream of infected and potentially infected patients.

Supporting Information

Figure S1 Representative images of immunostaining of isolated neutrophils that underwent drying and freezing steps before fixation. We tried to evaluate the influence of drying and freezing steps preceding paraformaldehyde fixation on the induction of NETs or citrullination of histone H3 in smear samples. For this, neutrophils separated by density gradient centrifugation from whole blood of a healthy donor were smeared on glass slides, dried, and frozen before fixation. At least through this method, the presence of NETs or citrullinated histone H3 was not identified in immunostaining. Blue, Hoechst 33342; Red, histone H3; Green, citrullinated histone H3 (left panels) or neutrophil elastase (right panels) (Magnification ×400). Scale bar; 50 μm.

Figure S2 Representative images of immunostaining for the negative control study using isotype control antibodies. To ensure accuracy for the immunoreactivity of primary antibodies against blood smear samples, whole mouse and rabbit IgG were used instead of primary antibodies in the immunostaining procedure. This control study resulted in negative signals for histone H3 and citrullinated histone H3. Blue, 4′,6-

diamidino-2-phenylindole (DAPI); Red, histone H3; Green, citrullinated histone H3. (Magnification ×200). Scale bar; 50 μm.

Figure S3 Representative images of immunostaining to detect citrullinated histone H3 (left panels) and neutrophil extracellular traps (NETs) (right panels) in the neutrophils from a healthy donor stimulated by phorbol myristate acetate. Neutrophils were isolated by density gradient centrifugation from the whole blood of a healthy donor and stimulated by phorbol myristate acetate. Citrullinated histone H3 and NETs were detected by immunohistochemistry using the same antibodies that were used against the smear samples collected from the critically ill patients. Blue, Hoechst 33342; Red, histone H3; Green, citrullinated histone H3 (left panels) or neutrophil elastase (right panels). (Magnification ×400). Scale bar; 50 μm.

Figure S4 Representative images of immunostaining to detect neutrophil extracellular traps (NETs) in the blood smear from a critically ill patient. The presence of circulating NETs was confirmed by immunohistochemistry using anti-neutrophil elastase antibody. String-like structures extending from the cell body (arrowheads) were composed of DNA and histone, and they contained neutrophil elastase. Blue, 4′,6-diamidino-2-phenylindole (DAPI); Red, histone H1; Green, Neutrophil elastase. (Magnification ×400). Scale bar; 50 μm.

Figure S5 Diff-Quik staining of a blood smear sample from the critically ill patient. Diff-Quik staining confirmed a subpopulation of cells other than neutrophils. (Magnification ×400). Scale bar; 50 μm.

Table S1 Comparison between patients presenting with and without "the presence of bacteria in tracheal aspirate". In patients classified into two groups based on the presence or absence of bacteria in tracheal aspirate, the rate of occurrence of NETs and/or Cit-H3 was significantly higher in "the presence of bacteria in tracheal aspirate" group (11/22, 50.0%) than in "the absence of bacteria in tracheal aspirate" group (4/27, 14.8%) ($p<.01$). Continuous variables are presented as the median and IQR unless otherwise noted. The Wilcoxon rank-sum test and Pearson's chi-square test were used to compare the two patient groups. NETs: neutrophil extracellular traps, Cit-H3: citrullinated histone H3, IQR: interquartile range, APACHE: Acute Physiological And Chronic Health Evaluation, SOFA: Sequential Organ Failure Assessment, SIRS: systemic inflammatory response syndrome, WBC: white blood cell, IL: interleukin, TNF: tumor necrosis factor, cf-DNA: circulating free DNA, HMGB1: high mobility group box-1.

Table S2 Comparison between patients with and without systemic inflammatory response syndrome. In patients with SIRS on admission, there was a trend toward greater expression of NETs and/or Cit-H3 ($p = .079$). Continuous variables are presented as the median and IQR unless otherwise noted. The Wilcoxon rank-sum test and Pearson's chi-square test were used to compare the two patient groups. NETs: neutrophil extracellular traps, Cit-H3: citrullinated histone H3, IQR: interquartile range, APACHE: Acute Physiological And Chronic Health Evaluation, SOFA: Sequential Organ Failure Assessment, SIRS: systemic inflammatory response syndrome,

WBC: white blood cell, IL: interleukin, TNF: tumor necrosis factor, cf-DNA: circulating free DNA, HMGB1: high mobility group box-1.

Table S3 Results of single logistic regression analysis of factors associated with the presence of neutrophil extracellular traps and/or citrullinated histone H3 according to the presence of infection and/or "the presence of bacteria in tracheal aspirate".

Single logistic regression analyses of whether infection and/or "the presence of bacteria in tracheal aspirate" were associated with the presence of NETs and/or Cit-H3 produced an odds ratio of 7.312. Coeff (β):

coefficient, OR: odds ratio, Lower: lower level of 95% confidence interval, Upper: upper level of 95% confidence interval.

Data S1 MPO-DNA ELISA.

Author Contributions

Conceived and designed the experiments: TH SH NM TI. Performed the experiments: TH SH NM TI HH NY. Analyzed the data: TH SH NM TI MS OT NY KY YA KO TS KT. Contributed reagents/materials/analysis tools: TH SH HH NY. Wrote the paper: TH SH NM.

References

1. Lekstrom-Himes JA, Gallin JI (2000) Immunodeficiency diseases caused by defects in phagocytes. New Engl J Med 343: 1703–1714.
2. Savchenko AS, Inoue A, Ohashi R, Jiang S, Hasegawa G, et al. (2011) Long pentraxin 3 (PTX3) expression and release by neutrophils in vitro and in ulcerative colitis. Pathol Int 61: 290–297.
3. Vitkov L, Klappacher M, Hannig M, Krautgartner WD (2009) Extracellular neutrophil traps in periodontitis. J Periodontal Res 44: 664–672.
4. Garcia-Romo GS, Caielli S, Vega B, Connolly J, Allantaz F, et al. (2011) Netting neutrophils are major inducers of type I IFN production in pediatric systemic lupus erythematosus. Sci Transl Med 3: 73ra20.
5. Kessenbrock K, Krumbholz M, Schonermarck U, Back W, Gross WL, et al. (2009) Netting neutrophils in autoimmune small-vessel vasculitis. Nat Med 15: 623–625.
6. Brinkmann V, Reichard U, Goosmann C, Fauler B, Uhlemann Y, et al. (2004) Neutrophil extracellular traps kill bacteria. Science 303: 1532–1535.
7. Jaillon S, Peri G, Delneste Y, Fremaux I, Doni A, et al. (2007) The humoral pattern recognition receptor PTX3 is stored in neutrophil granules and localizes in extracellular traps. J Exp Med 204: 793–804.
8. Curran CS, Demick KP, Mansfield JM (2006) Lactoferrin activates macrophages via TLR4-dependent and -independent signaling pathways. Cell Immunol 242: 23–30.
9. Zhang LT, Yao YM, Lu JQ, Yan XJ, Yu Y, et al. (2008) Recombinant bactericidal/permeability-increasing protein inhibits endotoxin-induced high-mobility group box 1 protein gene expression in sepsis. Shock 29: 278–284.
10. Urban CF, Ermert D, Schmid M, Abu-Abed U, Goosmann C, et al. (2009) Neutrophil extracellular traps contain calprotectin, a cytosolic protein complex involved in host defense against Candida albicans. PLoS Pathog 5: e1000639.
11. Cho JH, Fraser IP, Fukase K, Kusumoto S, Fujimoto Y, et al. (2005) Human peptidoglycan recognition protein S is an effector of neutrophil-mediated innate immunity. Blood 106: 2551–2558.
12. Fuchs TA, Abed U, Goosmann C, Hurwitz R, Schulze I, et al. (2007) Novel cell death program leads to neutrophil extracellular traps. J Cell Biol 176: 231–241.
13. Logters T, Margraf S, Altrichter J, Cinatl J, Mitzner S, et al. (2009) The clinical value of neutrophil extracellular traps. Med Microbiol Immunol 198: 211–219.
14. Remijsen Q, Kuijpers TW, Wirawan E, Lippens S, Vandenabeele P, et al. (2011) Dying for a cause: NETosis, mechanisms behind an antimicrobial cell death modality. Cell Death Differ 18: 581–588.
15. Margraf S, Logters T, Reipen J, Altrichter J, Scholz M, et al. (2008) Neutrophil-derived circulating free DNA (cf-DNA/NETs): A potential prognostic marker for posttraumatic development of inflammatory second hit and sepsis. Shock 30: 352–358.
16. Logters T, Paunel-Gorgulu A, Zilkens C, Altrichter J, Scholz M, et al. (2009) Diagnostic accuracy of neutrophil-derived circulating free DNA (cf-DNA/NETs) for septic arthritis. J Orthop Res 27: 1401–1407.
17. Thijssen MA, Swinkels DW, Ruers TJ, de Kok JB (2002) Difference between free circulating plasma and serum DNA in patients with colorectal liver metastases. Anticancer Res 22: 421–425.
18. Sozzi G, Conte D, Leon M, Ciricione R, Roz L, Ratcliffe C, et al. (2003) Quantification of free circulating DNA as a diagnostic marker in lung cancer. J Clin Oncol 21: 3902–3908.
19. Kamat AA, Bischoff FZ, Dang D, Baldwin MF, Han LY, et al. (2006) Circulating cell-free DNA: A novel biomarker for response to therapy in ovarian carcinoma. Cancer Biol Ther 5: 1369–1374.
20. Swarup V, Rajeswari MR (2007) Circulating (cell-free) nucleic acids—a promising, non-invasive tool for early detection of several human diseases. FEBS Lett 581: 795–799.
21. van der Vaart M, Pretorius PJ (2007) The origin of circulating free DNA. Clin Chem 53: 2215.
22. Neeli I, Khan SN, Radic M (2008) Histone deimination as a response to inflammatory stimuli in neutrophils. J Immunol 180: 1895–1902.
23. Wang Y, Li M, Stadler S, Correll S, Li P, et al. (2009) Histone hypercitrullination mediates chromatin decondensation and neutrophil extracellular trap formation. J Cell Biol 184: 205–213.
24. Hirose T, Hamaguchi S, Matsumoto N, Irisawa T, Seki M, et al. (2012) Dynamic changes in the expression of neutrophil extracellular traps in acute respiratory infections. Am J Respir Crit Care Med 185: 1130–1131.
25. Hamaguchi S, Hirose T, Akeda Y, Matsumoto N, Irisawa T, et al. (2013) Identification of neutrophil extracellular traps in blood of patients with systemic inflammatory response syndrome. J Int Med Res 41: 162–168.
26. Bone RC, Balk RA, Cerra FB, Dellinger RP, Fein AM, et al. (1992) Definitions for sepsis and organ failure and guidelines for the use of innovative therapies in sepsis. The ACCP/SCCM Consensus Conference Committee. American College of Chest Physicians/Society of Critical Care Medicine. Chest 101: 1644–1655.
27. Marik PE (2001) Aspiration pneumonitis and aspiration pneumonia. N Engl J Med 344: 665–671.
28. Massberg S, Grahl L, von Bruehl ML, Manukyan D, Pfeiler S, et al. (2010) Reciprocal coupling of coagulation and innate immunity via neutrophil serine proteases. Nat Med 16: 887–896.
29. McDonald B, Urrutia R, Yipp BG, Jenne CN, Kubes P (2012) Intravascular neutrophil extracellular traps capture bacteria from the bloodstream during sepsis. Cell Host Microbe 12: 324–333.
30. Yipp BG, Petri B, Salina D, Jenne CN, Scott BN, et al. (2012) Infection-induced NETosis is a dynamic process involving neutrophil multitasking in vivo. Nat Med 18: 1386–1393.
31. Brinkmann V, Zychlinsky A (2007) Beneficial suicide: Why neutrophils die to make NETs. Nat Rev Microbiol 5: 577–582.
32. Adnet F, Baud F (1996) Relation between Glasgow Coma Scale and aspiration pneumonia. Lancet 348: 123–124.
33. Evans SE, Xu Y, Tuvim MJ, Dickey BF (2010) Inducible innate resistance of lung epithelium to infection. Annu Rev Physiol 72: 413–435.
34. Sousa S, Lecuit M, Cossart P (2005) Microbial strategies to target, cross or disrupt epithelia. Curr Opin Cell Biol 17: 489–498.
35. Mitsushima H, Oishi K, Nagao T, Ichinose A, Senba M, et al. (2002) Acid aspiration induces bacterial pneumonia by enhanced bacterial adherence in mice. Microb Pathog 33: 203–210.
36. Hippenstiel S, Opitz B, Schmeck B, Suttorp N (2006) Lung epithelium as a sentinel and effector system in pneumonia-molecular mechanisms of pathogen recognition and signal transduction. Respir Res 7: 97.
37. Pittet JF, Koh H, Fang X, Iles K, Christiaans S, et al. (2013) HMGB1 accelerates alveolar epithelial repair via an IL-1beta- and alphavbeta6 integrin-dependent activation of TGF-beta1. PLoS One 8: e63907.
38. Tadie JM, Bae HB, Jiang S, Park DW, Bell CP, et al. (2013) HMGB1 promotes neutrophil extracellular trap formation through interactions with Toll-like receptor 4. Am J Physiol Lung Cell Mol Physiol 304: L342–L349.
39. Gupta AK, Hasler P, Holzgreve W, Gebhardt S, Hahn S (2005) Induction of neutrophil extracellular DNA lattices by placental microparticles and IL-8 and their presence in preeclampsia. Hum Immunol 66: 1146–1154.
40. Hiraiwa K, Van Eeden SF (2014) Nature and consequences of the systemic inflammatory response induced by lung inflammation. Lung Inflammation. Available: http://www.intechopen.com/books/lung-inflammation/nature-and-consequences-of-the-systemic-inflammatory-response-induced-by-lung-inflammation. Accessed 2014 Jul 4.
41. Hussell T, Bell TJ (2014) Alveolar macrophages: plasticity in a tissue-specific context. Nat Rev Immunol 14: 81–93.
42. Wang H, Bloom O, Zhang M, Vishnubhakat JM, Ombrellino M, et al. (1999) HMG-1 as a late mediator of endotoxin lethality in mice. Science 285: 248–251.
43. Wang H, Yang H, Tracey KJ (2004) Extracellular role of HMGB1 in inflammation and sepsis. J Intern Med 255: 320–331.
44. Mitroulis I, Kambas K, Chrysanthopoulou A, Skendros P, Apostolidou E, et al. (2011) Neutrophil extracellular trap formation is associated with IL-1beta and autophagy-related signaling in gout. PLoS One 6: e29318.
45. Gupta AK, Joshi MB, Philippova M, Erne P, Hasler P, et al. (2010) Activated endothelial cells induce neutrophil extracellular traps and are susceptible to NETosis-mediated cell death. FEBS Lett 584: 3193–3197.

Induced Differentiation of Human Myeloid Leukemia Cells into M2 Macrophages by Combined Treatment with Retinoic Acid and 1α,25-Dihydroxyvitamin D₃

Hiromichi Takahashi[1,2], Yoshihiro Hatta[2], Noriyoshi Iriyama[2], Yuichiro Hasegawa[1], Hikaru Uchida[1], Masaru Nakagawa[1,2], Makoto Makishima[1]*, Jin Takeuchi[2¤], Masami Takei[2]

1 Division of Biochemistry, Department of Biomedical Sciences, Nihon University School of Medicine, Tokyo, Japan, 2 Division of Hematology and Rheumatology, Department of Medicine, Nihon University School of Medicine, Tokyo, Japan

Abstract

Retinoids and 1α,25-dihydroxyvitamin D_3 (1,25(OH)$_2$D$_3$) induce differentiation of myeloid leukemia cells into granulocyte and macrophage lineages, respectively. All-*trans* retinoic acid (ATRA), which is effective in the treatment of acute promyelocytic leukemia, can induce differentiation of other types of myeloid leukemia cells, and combined treatment with retinoid and 1,25(OH)$_2$D$_3$ effectively enhances the differentiation of leukemia cells into macrophage-like cells. Recent work has classified macrophages into M1 and M2 types. In this study, we investigated the effect of combined treatment with retinoid and 1,25(OH)$_2$D$_3$ on differentiation of myeloid leukemia THP-1 and HL60 cells. 9-*cis* Retinoic acid (9cRA) plus 1,25(OH)$_2$D$_3$ inhibited proliferation of THP-1 and HL60 cells and increased myeloid differentiation markers including nitroblue tetrazolium reducing activity and expression of CD14 and CD11b. ATRA and the synthetic retinoic acid receptor agonist Am80 exhibited similar effects in combination with 1,25(OH)$_2$D$_3$ but less effectively than 9cRA, while the retinoid X receptor agonist HX630 was not effective. 9cRA plus 1,25(OH)$_2$D$_3$ effectively increased expression of M2 macrophage marker genes, such as *CD163*, *ARG1* and *IL10*, increased surface CD163 expression, and induced interleukin-10 secretion in myeloid leukemia cells, while 9cRA alone had weaker effects on these phenotypes and 1,25(OH)$_2$D$_3$ was not effective. Taken together, our results demonstrate selective induction of M2 macrophage markers in human myeloid leukemia cells by combined treatment with 9cRA and 1,25(OH)$_2$D$_3$.

Editor: R. Keith Reeves, Beth Israel Deaconess Medical Center, Harvard Medical School, United States of America

Funding: This work was supported by "Strategic Research Base Development" Program for Private Universities subsidized by MEXT (2008–2012) and funds from Nihon University School of Medicine. The funders had no role in study design, data collection and analysis, decision to publish, or preparation of the manuscript.

* Email: makishima.makoto@nihon-u.ac.jp

¤ Current address: Department of Internal Medicine, International University of Health and Welfare Shioya Hospital, Yaita, Tochigi, Japan

Introduction

Retinoids play roles in numerous biological functions, such as cellular proliferation and differentiation, embryogenesis, immunity and metabolism [1]. An active natural retinoid, all-*trans* retinoic acid (ATRA), is effective in differentiation therapy for acute promyelocytic leukemia (APL) [2]. APL is a subtype of acute myeloid leukemia, which is characterized by a specific chromosomal abnormality t(15,17) associated with a genetic rearrangement between retinoic acid receptor α (RARα) (gene symbol, *RARA*) and the promyelocytic leukemia gene *PML* [2]. RARα plays a role in granulocyte differentiation of hematopoietic cells and the abnormal chimeric receptor PML-RARα has been implicated in APL pathogenesis by blocking the myeloid differentiation program and enhancing self-renewal of leukemic cells [3,4]. Pharmacological doses of ATRA induce differentiation of APL cells into granulocytes through degradation of PML-RARα and recovery of physiological RARα signaling [3,4].

Retinoids, including ATRA, 9-*cis* retinoic acid (9cRA) and synthetic RAR ligands, exhibit anti-tumor effects not only on APL but also on other malignancies, such as breast cancer, lung cancer, and head and neck cancer [5]. With regard to leukemia, ATRA was first reported to induce the differentiation of human myeloid leukemia HL60 cells towards the granulocytic lineage [6,7]. Importantly, HL60 cells are derived from non-APL leukemia without t(15,17) [8], and ATRA can also induce differentiation of leukemia cells from non-APL myeloid leukemia patients [9]. Retinoids in combination with other differentiation inducers, such as 1α,25-dihydroxyvitamin D_3 (1,25(OH)$_2$D$_3$) and dibutyryl cAMP, synergistically induce differentiation of leukemia cells [10–13]. However, the underlying mechanisms of retinoid-induced differentiation of leukemia cells remain poorly understood and retinoids have not been utilized in the treatment of myeloid leukemia other than APL.

The active form of vitamin D_3, 1,25(OH)$_2$D$_3$, regulates calcium and bone homeostasis, immunity, and cellular growth and differentiation through direct binding to the vitamin D receptor

(VDR), and has been demonstrated to inhibit the proliferation and to induce the differentiation of various types of malignant cells, including breast, prostate and colon cancers as well as myeloid leukemia cells [14,15]. The administration of $1,25(OH)_2D_3$ and its analog has therapeutic effects in a mouse model of myeloid leukemia [16]. While ATRA induces granulocytic differentiation [6,7], $1,25(OH)_2D_3$ induces the differentiation of HL60 cells and other myeloid leukemia cells towards the monocyte and macrophage lineage [17,18]. Interestingly, ATRA induces monocytic differentiation of monoblastic leukemia U937 and THP-1 cells [13,19]. Combined treatment with $1,25(OH)_2D_3$ and retinoids induces the differentiation of HL60 cells and human monoblastic leukemia cells, such as THP-1 cells, to monocyte/macrophage-lineage cells more effectively than $1,25(OH)_2D_3$ alone [10,12,20]. Although $1,25(OH)_2D_3$ has been shown to exert its biological effects on cellular proliferation and differentiation by genomic and/or non-genomic pathways [21], the detailed mechanisms remain unclear. Macrophages have been classified into two cell types, classically activated M1 macrophages and alternatively activated M2 macrophages [22,23]. While M1 macrophages produce proinflammatory cytokines and enhance microbicidal and tumoricidal immunity, M2 macrophages are involved in wound healing and immune regulation. Although retinoids and $1,25(OH)_2D_3$ play functional roles in monocytes and macrophages [4,24], the macrophage cell type resulting from $1,25(OH)_2D_3$ and/or retinoid differentiation of myeloid leukemia cells has not been further characterized. In this study, we examined the effects of $1,25(OH)_2D_3$ in combination with retinoids on differentiation of myeloid leukemia cells and found that $1,25(OH)_2D_3$ in combination with 9cRA and ATRA induce the differentiation of myeloid leukemia cells to macrophages with M2-like phenotype.

Materials and Methods

Compounds

$1,25(OH)_2D_3$, ATRA and 9cRA were purchased from Wako Pure Chemical Industries (Osaka, Japan). Am80 (4-[(5,6,7,8-tetrahydro-5,5,8,8-tetramethyl-2-naphthalenyl)carbamoyl]benzoic acid) [25] and HX630 (4-[2,3-(2,5-dimethyl-2,5-hexano)dibenzo[b,f][1,4]-thiazepin-11-yl]benzoic acid) [26] were kindly provided by Dr. Koichi Shudo of Research Foundation ITSUU Laboratory (Tokyo, Japan).

Cell culture, cell growth, nitroblue tetrazolium (NBT) reduction, and interleukin-10 (IL-10) production

Human myeloid leukemia HL60 and THP-1 cells (RIKEN Cell Bank, Tsukuba, Japan) were maintained in RPMI1640 medium containing 10% fetal bovine serum, 100 unit/ml penicillin, and 100 μg/ml streptomycin in a humidified atmosphere containing 5% CO_2. Suspensions of cells (10^5 cells/ml) were cultured with or without test compounds at pharmacological concentrations (30−100 nM) according to our preliminary experiments and the previous reports [10–12,27]. Cell numbers were counted in a Z1S Coulter Counter (Beckman Coulter, Fullerton, CA). Cell morphology was examined in cell smears stained with May-Grünwald-Giemsa. NBT reduction was assayed colorimetrically and NBT-reducing activity data were normalized to the cell numbers [28]. IL-10 levels in culture media were determined with the Human IL-10 ELISA MAX Standard kit (BioLegend, San Diego, CA).

Flow cytometry

Expression of cell surface antigens, CD14, CD11b and CD163, were determined with immunofluorescence staining and flow cytometry [29]. FITC mouse anti-human CD14, PE mouse anti-human CD11b, PE mouse anti-human CD163, and isotype control antibodies were purchased from Becton, Dickinson and Company (Franklin Lakes, NJ). The stained cells were assayed with a flow cytometer (BD FACSCalibur; Becton, Dickinson and Company) and analyzed with the BD CellQuest software (Becton, Dickinson and Company).

Reverse transcription and real-time quantitative polymerase chain reaction

Total RNAs from samples were prepared by the acid guanidine thiocyanate-phenol/chloroform method [30]. cDNAs were synthesized using the ImProm-II Reverse Transcription system (Promega Corporation, Madison, WI). Intron-spanning primers were as follows: CD163 (GenBank accession no. NM_004244), 5′-ACT GCA AGA ACT GGC AAT GG-3′ and 5′-CCA TGC TTC ACT TCA ACA CG-3′; ARG1 (GenBank accession no. NM_000045), 5′-TCC AAG GTC TGT GGG AAA AG-3′ and 5′-ATT GCC AAA CTG TGG TCT CC-3′; IL10 (GenBank accession no. NM_000572), 5′-CCA AGA CCC AGA CAT CAA GG-3′ and 5′-GGC CTT GCT CTT GTT TTC AC-3′; IL12B (GenBank accession no. NM_002187), 5′-ATT GAG GTC ATG GTG GAT GC-3′ and 5′-TTC TTG GGT GGG TCA GGT TT-3′; TGFB1 (GenBank accession no. NM_000660), 5′-CAA CAA TTC CTG GCG ATA CCT C-3′ and 5′-AAA GCC CTC AAT TTC CCC TC-3′; TNF (GenBank accession no. NM_000594), 5′-TGC TTG TTC CTC AGC CTC TT-3′ and 5′-TGA GGT ACA GGC CCT CTG AT-3′; IL6 (GenBank accession no. NM_000600), 5′-AAA GAG GCA CTG GCA GAA AA-3′ and 5′-AAA GCT GCG CAG AAT GAG AT-3′; NOS2 (GenBank accession no. NM_000625), 5′-TAC CCC TCC AGA TGA GCT TC-3′ and 5′-TCT CCT TTG TTA CCG CTT CC-3′. Other primer sequences have been reported previously [28]. The mRNA values were normalized to the amount of β-actin mRNA.

Statistical analysis

All values are shown as mean ± S.D. We performed one-way ANOVA followed by Tukey's multiple comparisons or two-way ANOVA to assess significant differences using Prism 6 (Graphpad Software, La Jolla, CA).

Results

Induction of differentiation of human myeloid leukemia cells by retinoids plus $1,25(OH)_2D_3$

We examined the effects of 9cRA and ATRA in the absence or presence of $1,25(OH)_2D_3$ on NBT-reducing activity, a marker of myeloid differentiation, in monoblastic leukemia THP-1 cells and promyelocytic leukemia HL60 cells. 9cRA (100 nM) increased NBT-reducing activity in THP-1 and HL60 cells, while ATRA (100 nM) was not effective (Fig. 1A), consistent with the previous reports showing that 9cRA is more potent than ATRA in inducing differentiation of leukemia cells [20,31,32]. In combination with $1,25(OH)_2D_3$, 9cRA and ATRA effectively increased NBT-reducing activity in these cells (Fig. 1A). Am80 (also called tamibarotene) is a potent synthetic RAR agonist that is used in the treatment of recurrent APL in Japan [33,34]. HX630 is an RXR selective agonist derived from LE135, an RAR antagonist [26]. HX630 does not exhibit RAR antagonistic activity but enhances the differentiation-inducing activity of Am80 in HL60 cells [33]. We also examined the effects of Am80 and HX630 in the absence or presence of $1,25(OH)_2D_3$. Although Am80 and HX630 at 100 nM were not effective, the combination of

A

NBT reduction

THP-1 cells

HL60 cells

B   THP-1 cells   HL60 cells

C

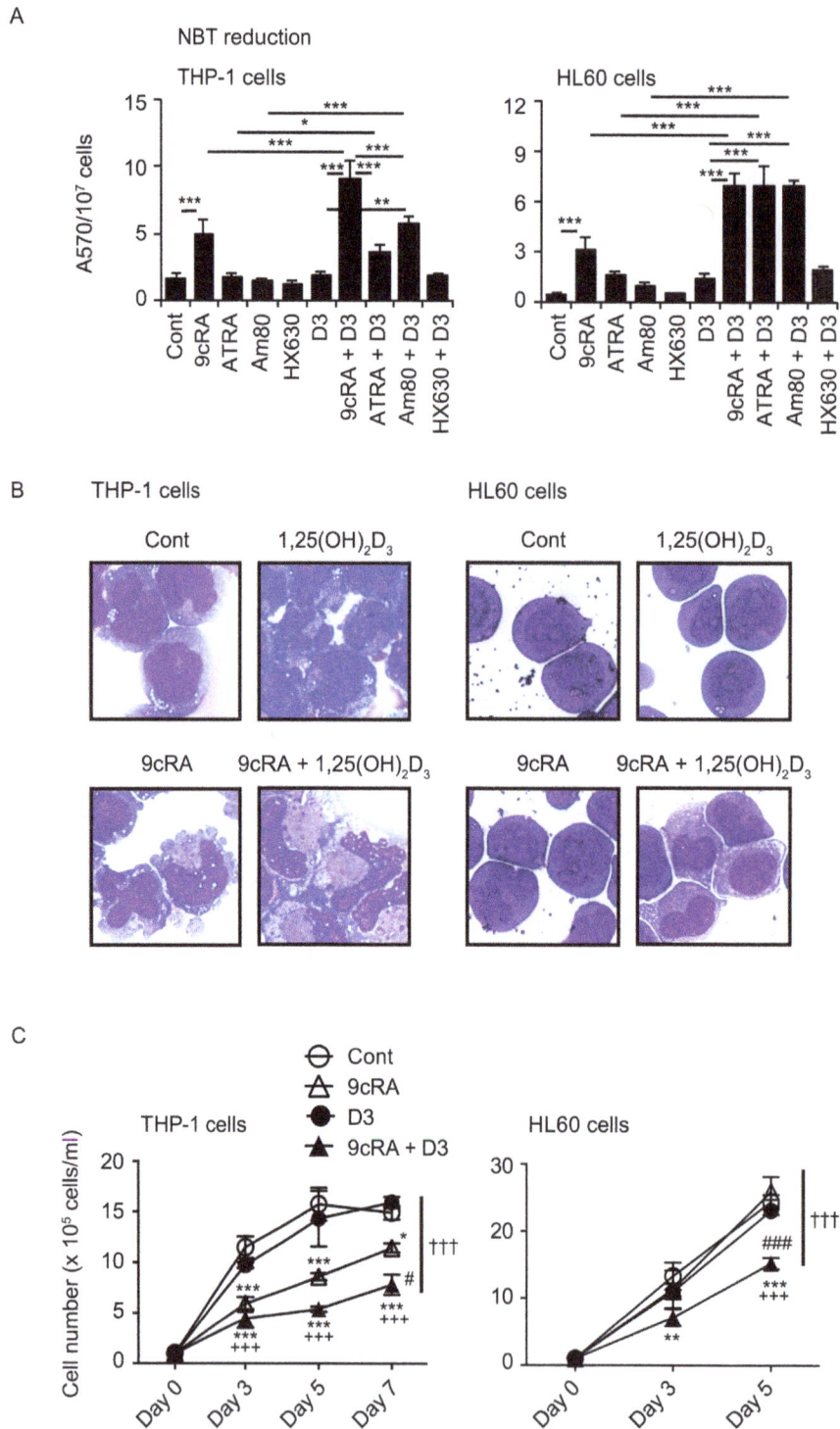

Figure 1. Induction of differentiation of THP-1 and HL60 cells by combined treatment with retinoid and 1,25(OH)₂D₃. (A) NBT-reducing activities. Cells were treated with vehicle control (Cont), 100 nM 9cRA, ATRA, Am80 or HX630 in the absence or presence of 100 nM 1,25(OH)$_2$D$_3$ (D3) for 5 days. *, $p<0.05$; **, $p<0.01$; ***, $p<0.001$ (one-way ANOVA followed by Tukey's multiple comparisons). (B) Morphological changes of THP-1 and HL60 cells treated with 9cRA and/or 1,25(OH)$_2$D$_3$. Cells were treated with vehicle control (Cont), 100 nM 9cRA and/or 100 nM 1,25(OH)$_2$D$_3$ for 5 days and the cell smears were stained with May-Grünwald-Giemsa. (C) Cell proliferations. Cells (1×10^5/ml) were cultured with vehicle control (Cont), 100 nM 9cRA and/or 100 nm 1,25(OH)$_2$D$_3$ (D3), and cell numbers were counted at indicated days. *, $p<0.05$; **, $p<0.01$; ***, $p<0.001$ vs Cont; ###, $p<0.001$ vs 9cRA; +++, $p<0.001$ vs D3 (one-way ANOVA followed by Tukey's multiple comparisons). †††, $p<0.001$ (two-way ANOVA).

$1,25(OH)_2D_3$ with Am80 but not HX630 significantly increased NBT-reducing activity in THP-1 and HL60 cells (Fig. 1A).

THP-1 cells and HL60 cells were treated with $1,25(OH)_2D_3$ and/or 9cRA and the morphological features were examined. While untreated THP-1 cells had a basophilic cytoplasm and large nuclei with several nucleoli, cells treated with 9cRA (100 nM) had grayish, enlarged cytoplasm and slightly lobulated nuclei (Fig. 1B). Although $1,25(OH)_2D_3$ (100 nM) treatment did not induce an apparent morphological change, the combination of 9cRA and $1,25(OH)_2D_3$ enlarged the grayish cytoplasm area more effectively than 9cRA alone. Untreated HL60 cells have promyelocytic features, although they are not derived from APL having t(15;17) [8]. While HL60 treated with $1,25(OH)_2D_3$ (100 nM) had slightly less basophilic cytoplasm and decreased nuclear-cytoplasmic ratio, 9cRA (100 nM) induced differentiation of HL60 cells into myelocytic cells having slightly lobulated nuclei and a decreased nuclear-cytoplasmic ratio (Fig. 1B). Combined treatment with 9cRA and $1,25(OH)_2D_3$ enhanced the monocytic features of HL60 cells with enlarged grayish cytoplasm and a further decrease in the nuclear-cytoplasmic ratio. These findings are consistent with the previous reports showing monocytic differentiation of myeloid leukemia cells by $1,25(OH)_2D_3$ plus 9cRA or ATRA [32;35]. 9cRA (100 nM) suppressed the proliferation of THP-1 cells, and although $1,25(OH)_2D_3$ (100 nM) was not effective, combined treatment with $1,25(OH)_2D_3$ enhanced the anti-proliferative effect of 9cRA (Fig. 1C). While treatment with 9cRA (100 nM) or $1,25(OH)_2D_3$ (100 nM) alone was not effective, the combined treatment with 9cRA and $1,25(OH)_2D_3$ effectively suppressed HL60 proliferation (Fig. 1C).

We next examined the effects of combined treatment with retinoids and $1,25(OH)_2D_3$ on expression of surface antigens, CD14 and CD11b, additional markers of myelomonocytic differentiation. $1,25(OH)_2D_3$ at 100 nM slightly increased CD14 expression in THP-1 cells (Fig. 2A). 9cRA at 100 nM increased CD14 expression and the combination of 9cRA and $1,25(OH)_2D_3$ increased CD14 expression more strongly than single use of these compounds. Interestingly, although ATRA and Am80 were not effective, these retinoids enhanced CD14 expression in combination with $1,25(OH)_2D_3$. HX630 did not increase CD14 expression in the absence or presence of $1,25(OH)_2D_3$. $1,25(OH)_2D_3$ also slightly increased CD11b expression in THP-1 cells (Fig. 2B). 9cRA, ATRA and Am80 at 30 nM increased CD11b expression, and effectively enhanced CD11b expression induced by $1,25(OH)_2D_3$. HX630 did not increase CD11b expression in the absence or presence of $1,25(OH)_2D_3$. Transcriptional induction of CD14, a VDR target gene [36], is also associated with myeloid differentiation [28]. Retinoid treatment did not increase CD14 mRNA levels in THP-1 and HL60 cells (Fig. 2C). Interestingly, while the effect of $1,25(OH)_2D_3$ (100 nM) alone was not significant, combinations of $1,25(OH)_2D_3$ with 9cRA, ATRA and Am80 effectively increased CD14 mRNA expression in these cells. The combination of HX630 and $1,25(OH)_2D_3$ was not effective in CD14 mRNA induction. Thus, when combined with $1,25(OH)_2D_3$, a RAR/RXR agonist (9cRA) and RAR agonists (ATRA and Am80), but not a RXR agonist (HX630), effectively induce differentiation of myeloid leukemia THP-1 and HL60 cells.

Induction of M2 macrophage markers in human myeloid leukemia cells by retinoids plus $1,25(OH)_2D_3$

As shown in Figure 1B and the previous reports [10;20;32], combined treatment with retinoid and $1,25(OH)_2D_3$ induces differentiation of myeloid leukemia cells into the monocytic lineage rather than the granulocytic lineage. We examined whether leukemia cells treated with retinoid plus $1,25(OH)_2D_3$ exhibit M1 or M2 macrophage phenotypes. Expression of the CD163, ARG1, IL10 and TGFB1 marker genes is associated with M2 macrophage activation, whereas IL12B, TNF, IL6 and NOS2 expression is increased in M1 macrophages [23]. Treatment of THP-1 cells with 9cRA, ATRA or $1,25(OH)_2D_3$ alone did not induce CD163 mRNA expression, but the combination of 9cRA and $1,25(OH)_2D_3$ effectively increased CD163 mRNA levels (Fig. 3A). ATRA plus $1,25(OH)_2D_3$ also increased CD163 expression but less effectively than 9cRA plus $1,25(OH)_2D_3$. Although CD163 mRNA expression was not detected in HL60 cells treated with 9cRA or ATRA alone, 9cRA plus $1,25(OH)_2D_3$ and ATRA plus $1,25(OH)_2D_3$ tended to increase CD163 mRNA levels. 9cRA plus $1,25(OH)_2D_3$ also effectively increased ARG1 mRNA expression in THP-1 cells, while ATRA plus $1,25(OH)_2D_3$ tended to increase its expression, an effect that did not reach statistical significance (Fig. 3B). Interestingly, combination of ATRA and $1,25(OH)_2D_3$ effectively increased ARG1 mRNA levels in HL60 cells, while the combined effect of 9cRA and $1,25(OH)_2D_3$ did not reach statistical significance. IL10 mRNA expression was also elevated in THP-1 cells treated with 9cRA plus $1,25(OH)_2D_3$ and, to a lesser extent, ATRA plus $1,25(OH)_2D_3$ (Fig. 3C). Although treatment of HL60 cells with $1,25(OH)_2D_3$ decreased IL10 mRNA levels, the combination of $1,25(OH)_2D_3$ with 9cRA or ATRA increased them to control levels. Combination of $1,25(OH)_2D_3$ with 9cRA or ATRA did not increase IL12B mRNA levels in THP-1 and HL60 cells (Fig. 3D). IL12B mRNA levels in THP-1 cells treated with 9cRA were decreased by combined treatment with $1,25(OH)_2D_3$. Addition of 9cRA increased TGFB1 mRNA levels in THP-1 cells treated with $1,25(OH)_2D_3$ (Fig. 3E). 9cRA increased TNF mRNA expression in THP-1 cells but combined treatment with $1,25(OH)_2D_3$ decreased its expression. IL6 mRNA expression was increased by the combination of 9cRA and $1,25(OH)_2D_3$. 9cRA and/or $1,25(OH)_2D_3$ induced no significant change in NOS2 mRNA expression. Thus, the combination of retinoid and $1,25(OH)_2D_3$ increases expression of genes associated with M2 macrophages.

We further examined expression of CD163 as a cell surface marker of M2 macrophages in THP-1 cells. Figure 4A shows representative flow cytometric analysis of THP-1 cells treated with or without 9cRA and $1,25(OH)_2D_3$ using anti-CD14 and anti-CD163 antibodies. 9cRA but not $1,25(OH)_2D_3$ increased CD163 mean fluorescence intensity in THP-1 cells, and the combination of 9cRA and $1,25(OH)_2D_3$ effectively enhanced the intensity values (Fig. 4B). 9cRA increased and $1,25(OH)_2D_3$ slightly decreased surface CD14 mean fluorescence intensity, but 9cRA plus $1,25(OH)_2D_3$ also strongly increased the CD14 intensity (Fig. 4B). 9cRA treatment increased the percentage of both CD163+/CD14+ cells and CD163−/CD14+ cells (Fig. 4B). Combination of $1,25(OH)_2D_3$ with 9CRA increased the percentage of CD163+/CD14+ cells but not of CD163−/CD14+ cells. These findings are consistent with induction of the M2 macrophage phenotype in THP-1 cells by 9cRA plus $1,25(OH)_2D_3$.

The combination of 9cRA and 1,25(OH)2D3 induces IL-10 protein secretion in THP-1 and HL60 cells

Finally, we examined IL-10 protein levels in conditioned media of THP-1 and HL60 cells treated with 9cRA and/or $1,25(OH)_2D_3$. IL-10 protein levels from THP-1 cells treated with 9cRA and $1,25(OH)_2D_3$ alone were below detection limits, but the combination of these compounds effectively induced IL-10 protein secretion from these cells (Fig. 5). While IL-10 protein was detected in the culture media of untreated HL60 cells, 9cRA increased and $1,25(OH)_2D_3$ decreased the protein level. 9cRA plus $1,25(OH)_2D_3$ effectively increased the IL-10 protein levels in

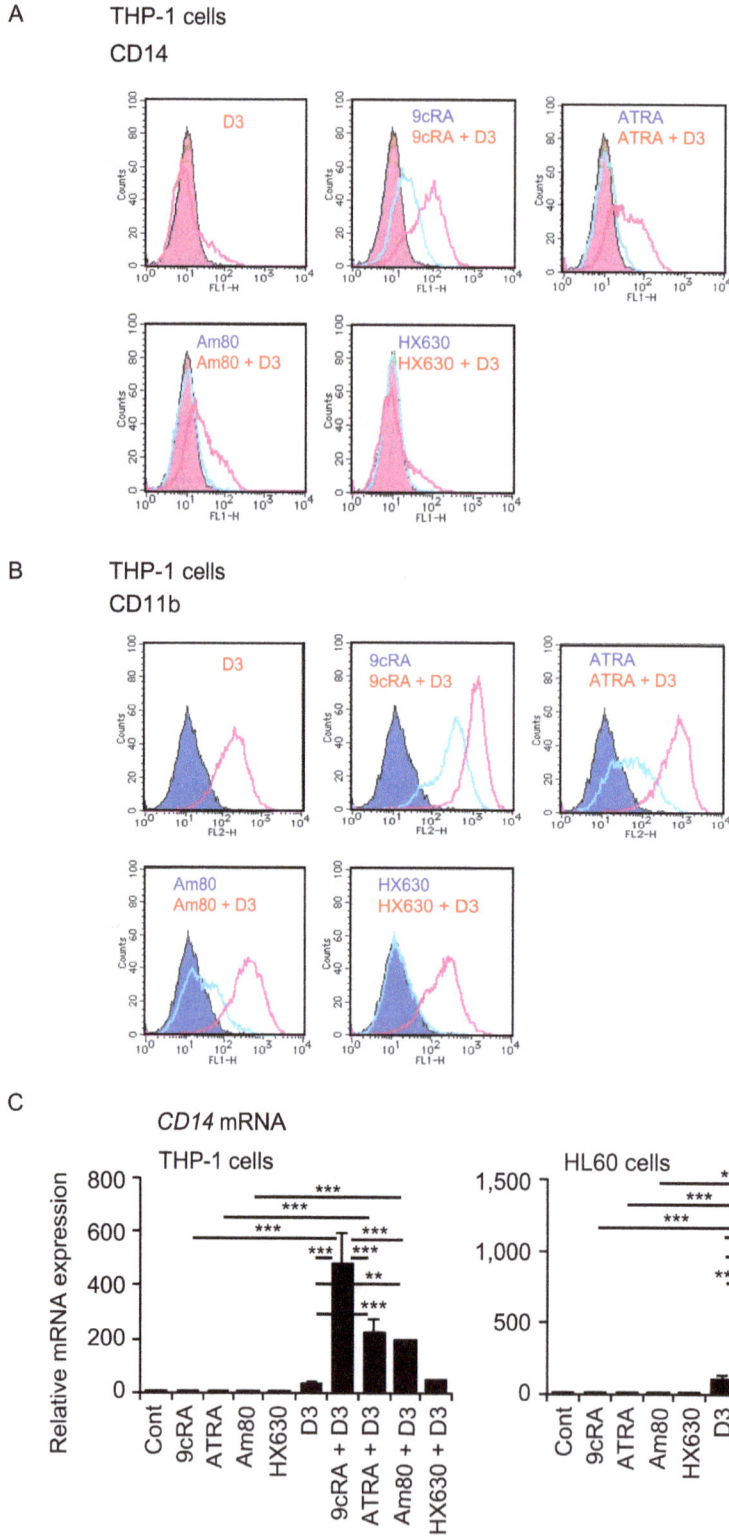

Figure 2. Effects of combined treatment with retinoid and 1,25(OH)₂D₃ on cell surface CD14 and CD11b expression and *CD14* mRNA expression. Representative histograms of CD14 expression (A) and CD11b expression (B) in THP-1 cells. Cells were treated with vehicle control (Cont), 100 nM 9cRA, ATRA, Am80 or HX630 in the absence or presence of 100 nM 1,25(OH)₂D₃ (D3) for 96 hours. Filled curves, vehicle control. Similar results were obtained from repeated experiments. (C) *CD14* mRNA levels in THP-1 and HL60 cells. Cells were treated with vehicle control (Cont), 30 nM 9cRA, ATRA, Am80 or HX630 in the absence or presence of 100 nM 1,25(OH)₂D₃ (D3) for 72 hours. **, $p<0.01$; ***, $p<0.001$ (one-way ANOVA followed by Tukey's multiple comparisons).

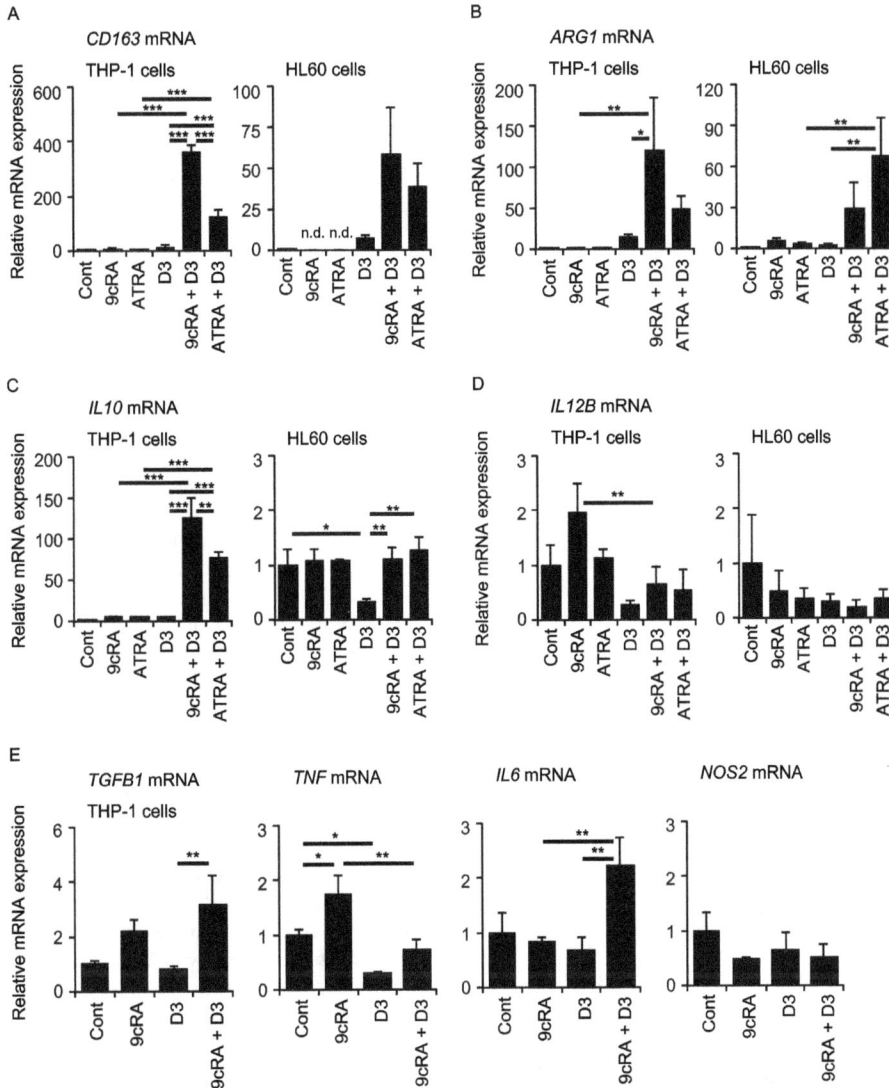

Figure 3. Expression of marker genes of M1 and M2 macrophages. mRNA levels of the M2 markers *CD163* (A), *ARG1* (B), *IL10* (C), and the M1 marker *IL12B* (D) in THP-1 and HL60 cells. (E) mRNA levels of the M2 marker *TGFB1*, the M1 markers *TNF*, *IL6*, and *NOS2* in THP-1 cells. Cells were treated with vehicle control (Cont), 30 nM 9cRA, or ATRA in the absence or presence of 100 nM 1,25(OH)$_2$D$_3$ (D3) for 72 hours. *, $p < 0.05$; **, $p < 0.01$; ***, $p < 0.001$ (one-way ANOVA followed by Tukey's multiple comparisons). n.d., not detected.

media. Thus, combined treatment of leukemia cells with 9cRA and 1,25(OH)$_2$D$_3$ induces IL-10 protein secretion as well as increased expression of M2 macrophage markers.

Discussion

In this study, we found that combined treatment with retinoid and 1,25(OH)$_2$D$_3$ induces the differentiation of human myeloid leukemia THP-1 and HL60 cells into the monocytic lineage with a M2 macrophage phenotype. ATRA induces granulocytic differentiation of promyelocytic leukemia HL60 cells but monocytic differentiation of monoblastic U937 and THP-1 cells [6,7,13,19]. Combination of ATRA or 9cRA with 1,25(OH)$_2$D$_3$ effectively induces monocyte/macrophage phenotypes, such as phagocytic activity, monocyte-specific esterase, lysozyme secretion, and *CSF1R* expression, in HL60 and U937 cells [10,32,37]. We observed a monocytic morphology and increased CD14 expression in HL60 and THP-1 cells treated with 9cRA plus

1,25(OH)$_2$D$_3$ (Figs. 1 and 2). ATRA plus 1,25(OH)$_2$D$_3$ also induces differentiation of promyelocytic AML-193 cells into cells that display both a typical neutrophilic morphology and monocyte-specific properties, such as CD14 expression and monocyte-specific esterase, a hybrid granulomonocytic phenotype [35]. RAR signaling plays an important role in hematopoiesis and RARα is involved in neutrophil development [4]. RAR and RXR signaling pathways have been reported to regulate monocyte/macrophage function [4]. However, it remains to be determined how retinoid signaling enhances monocytic differentiation induced by 1,25(OH)$_2$D$_3$ in myeloid leukemia cells.

Among retinoids, 9cRA, ATRA and Am80, but not HX630, in combination with 1,25(OH)$_2$D$_3$ exhibit effective differentiation-inducing activity in these cells (Figs. 1 and 2). 1,25(OH)$_2$D$_3$ acts as a ligand for the nuclear receptor VDR, which forms a heterodimer with RXR [38], and the VDR−RXR heterodimer is not permissive to RXR ligand activation [39]. RAR selective ligands exhibit stronger synergistic effects with 1,25(OH)$_2$D$_3$ than RXR

A

B

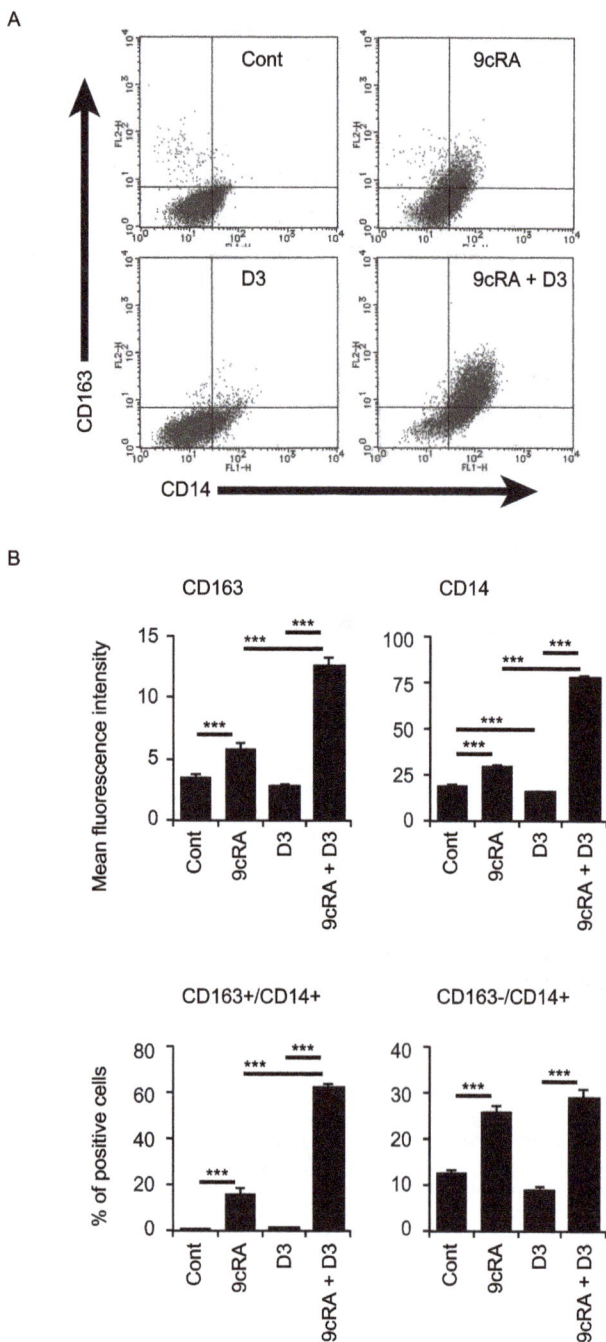

Figure 4. Cell surface expression of CD163 in THP-1 cells. (A) Representative histograms of CD14 and CD163 expression. (B) Quantification of mean fluorescence intensity of CD163 and CD14 expression. (C) Quantification of percentages of CD163+/CD14+ cells and CD163−/CD14+ cells. Cells were treated with vehicle control (Cont), 100 nM 9cRA and/or 100 nM 1,25(OH)$_2$D$_3$ (D3) for 96 hours. **, $p < 0.01$; ***, $p < 0.001$ (one-way ANOVA followed by Tukey's multiple comparisons).

selective ligands in inhibiting proliferation and inducing differentiation of monoblastic U937 cells [27]. Combined effects of retinoid and 1,25(OH)$_2$D$_3$ on differentiation of myelomonocytic leukemia cells are likely mediated by VDR and RAR activation. RXR also forms heterodimers with RAR and other nuclear receptors, including peroxisome proliferator-activated receptor

(PPAR) and liver X receptor (LXR) [38]. The RAR−RXR heterodimer is activated by RXR ligand only in the presence of RAR ligand, a feature known as conditional permissivity [39]. 9cRA exhibits differentiation-inducing activity more effectively than ATRA in the absence or presence of 1,25(OH)$_2$D$_3$ (Figs. 1 and 2), in agreement with previous reports [20,31,32]. Since 9cRA acts as a ligand for both RAR and RXR [40], synergistic activation may be due to binding to both RAR and RXR in the RAR−RXR heterodimer. In addition, RXR ligands can activate permissive heterodimers, such as PPAR−RXR and LXR−RXR [38]. PPARγ ligand and LXR ligand have been reported to induce differentiation of myeloid leukemia cells [41,42]. RXR ligand activation of these permissive heterodimers may also contribute to the effect of 9cRA. However, the pure RXR ligand HX630 alone and in combination with 1,25(OH)$_2$D$_3$ was not effective in inducing differentiation of THP-1 and HL60 cells, while the combination of 1,25(OH)$_2$D$_3$ with the RAR selective agonist Am80 induced the differentiation of these cells (Figs. 1 and 2). These findings suggest that cooperation between VDR signaling and RAR signaling, not RXR signaling, plays a role in the differentiation of myeloid leukemia cells. VDR activation changes expression of many genes, including those involved in cellular proliferation, differentiation and apoptosis [21]. 1,25(OH)$_2$D$_3$ treatment can modulate intracellular kinase pathways via a non-genomic mechanism, and it remains unknown whether the non-genomic actions are mediated through VDR or other proteins [21]. Although both genomic and non-genomic effects of 1,25(OH)$_2$D$_3$ have been shown to play roles in differentiation induction of leukemia cells, the detailed mechanisms remain to be elucidated. RAR signaling may modulate the vitamin D signaling pathway or regulate other differentiation mechanisms. Further studies are needed to elucidate molecular mechanisms involving VDR, RAR and RXR signaling pathways in the induced differentiation of leukemia cells.

Combined treatment with 9cRA and 1,25(OH)$_2$D$_3$ increased mRNA expression of *CD163*, *ARG1*, *IL10*, and *TGFB1* genes (Fig. 3), surface expression of CD163 proteins (Fig. 4) and IL-10 secretion in THP-1 cells (Fig. 5). This combination also increased *CD163*, *ARG1* and *IL10* mRNA levels (Fig. 3) and IL-10 secretion in HL60 cells (Fig. 5). This phenotype has been characterized as M2 macrophages, although the classification of human macrophages remains controversial [23]. 9cRA plus 1,25(OH)$_2$D$_3$ did not increase expression of the M1 macrophage gene *IL12B* in THP-1 and HL60 cells (Fig. 3). Although *TNF* mRNA levels were not increased, *IL6* mRNA expression was effectively induced by the combination of 9cRA and 1,25(OH)$_2$D$_3$ in THP-1 cells. ATRA plus 1,25(OH)$_2$D$_3$ has been reported to induce mRNA and protein levels of tumor necrosis factor (TNF) and IL-6 in U937 cells [43] and to increase expression of inducible nitric oxide synthase (encoded by *NOS2*) and nitric acid production in U937 cells [44], while we observed no significant change in *NOS2* mRNA expression in THP-1 and HL60 cells after treatment with ATRA or 9cRA in combination with 1,25(OH)$_2$D$_3$ (Fig. 3, and data not shown). Tumor necrosis factor (TNF) and IL-6 are cytokines produced from M1 macrophages and *NOS2* expression is a M1 macrophage marker [22,23,45]. Macrophages with a mixed phenotype expressing both M1 and M2 markers have been identified [46]. Thus, differentiated leukemia cells by 9cRA plus 1,25(OH)$_2$D$_3$ are macrophage-like cells expressing primarily M2 markers with some M1 markers. Further analysis is required to reveal their functional characteristics.

The RAR signaling pathways play an important role in hematopoiesis and granulocytic differentiation [4,47]. With regard

IL-10 protein

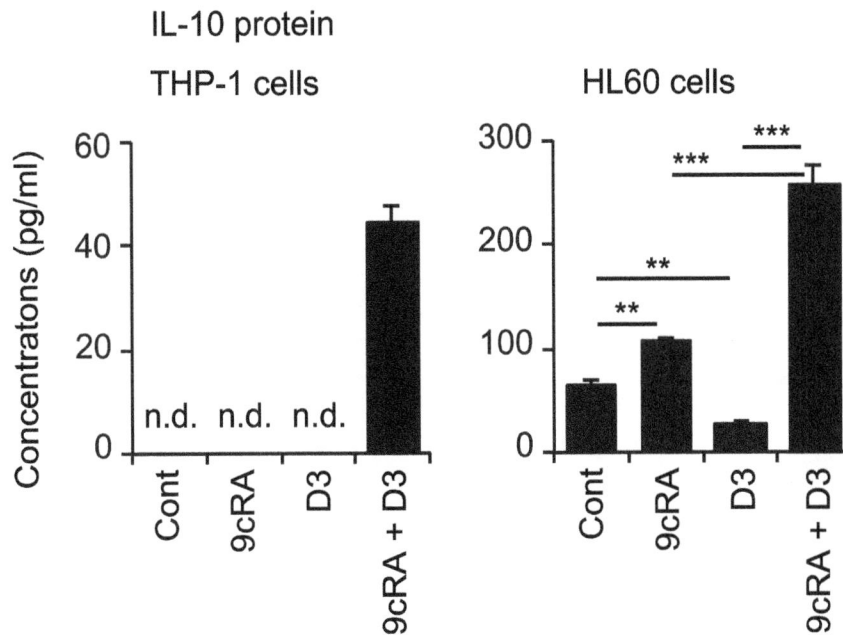

Figure 5. Secreted IL-10 production in THP-1 and HL60 cells. Cells were treated with vehicle control (Cont), 30 nM 9cRA and/or 100 nM 1,25(OH)$_2$D$_3$ (D3) for 72 hours and secreted IL-10 levels in media were measured. **, $p < 0.01$; ***, $p < 0.001$ (one-way ANOVA followed by Tukey's multiple comparisons). n.d., not detected.

to macrophages, ATRA inhibits TNF production in mouse peritoneal macrophages activated by lipopolysaccharide and interferon γ [48]. ATRA also reduces the synthesis of IL-12 and TNF and enhances IL-10 production in lipopolysaccharide-stimulated human macrophages [49]. Although VDR is dispensable for normal myelopoiesis [50], the vitamin D signaling pathway is involved in the regulation of macrophage/monocyte function [4]. 1,25(OH)$_2$D$_3$ suppresses activation of mouse macrophages by interferon γ [51], and enhances the immunoglobulin- and complement-dependent phagocytosis activity of human blood monocytes [52]. Thus, both ATRA and 1,25(OH)$_2$D$_3$ induce the macrophage/monocyte function common to M2 macrophages. Combined effects of retinoid and 1,25(OH)$_2$D$_3$ on physiological monocyte/macrophage function remain to be elucidated.

In contrast to 9cRA treatment, 1,25(OH)$_2$D$_3$ reduced *IL10* mRNA levels and IL-10 production in HL60 cells (Figs. 3 and 5). These findings agree with previous reports that show that 1,25(OH)$_2$D$_3$ suppresses *IL10* expression through VDR recruitment to the *IL10* promoter in monocytes [53,54]. Interestingly, 1,25(OH)$_2$D$_3$ enhances *IL10* expression of activated human B lymphocytes by recruiting VDR to the *IL10* promoter [55]. The combination of 9cRA with 1,25(OH)$_2$D$_3$ effectively induced IL-10 transcription and secretion in THP-1 and HL60 cells (Figs. 3 and 5). Thus, VDR activation induces or suppresses *IL10* expression in a manner dependent on cellular conditions. Treatment with 9cRA plus 1,25(OH)$_2$D$_3$ increased *CD163* mRNA levels and surface

CD163 expression (Figs. 3 and 4). CD163 mediates IL-10 secretion in human monocytes [56]. IL-10 plays an important role in immune regulation by macrophages [46,57]. Our findings may provide an insight into mechanisms of IL-10 induction.

In conclusion, our results indicate that combined treatment with retinoid and 1,25(OH)$_2$D$_3$ induces differentiation of human myeloid leukemia THP-1 and HL60 cells into macrophage-like cells expressing M2 markers. Further study of human leukemia cell differentiation has the potential to extend differentiation-inducing therapy to the treatment of non-APL myeloid leukemia and to expand the understanding of human macrophage function.

Acknowledgments

The authors thank Dr. Shinya Suzu of Center for AIDS Research, Kumamoto University, Dr. Takayoshi Suganami and Dr. Yoshihiro Ogawa of Tokyo Medical and Dental University for helpful comments, members of the Makishima laboratory for technical assistance and helpful comments, and Dr. Andrew I. Shulman for editorial assistance.

Author Contributions

Conceived and designed the experiments: HT Y. Hatta MM. Performed the experiments: HT NI Y. Hatta HU MN. Analyzed the data: HT Y. Hatta Y. Hasegawa MM. Contributed reagents/materials/analysis tools: NI. Contributed to the writing of the manuscript: HT Y. Hatta MM JT MT.

References

1. Al Tanoury Z, Piskunov A, Rochette-Egly C (2013) Vitamin A and retinoid signaling: genomic and non-genomic effects. J Lipid Res 54: 1761–1775.
2. Wang ZY, Chen Z (2008) Acute promyelocytic leukemia: from highly fatal to highly curable. Blood 111: 2505–2515.
3. de Thé H, Chen Z (2010) Acute promyelocytic leukaemia: novel insights into the mechanisms of cure. Nat Rev Cancer 10: 775–783.
4. Nagy L, Szanto A, Szatmari I, Szeles L (2012) Nuclear hormone receptors enable macrophages and dendritic cells to sense their lipid environment and shape their immune response. Physiol Rev 92: 739–789.
5. Connolly RM, Nguyen NK, Sukumar S (2013) Molecular pathways: current role and future directions of the retinoic acid pathway in cancer prevention and treatment. Clin Cancer Res 19: 1651–1659.

6. Honma Y, Takenaga K, Kasukabe T, Hozumi M (1980) Induction of differentiation of cultured human promyelocytic leukemia cells by retinoids. Biochem Biophys Res Commun 95: 507–512.

7. Breitman TR, Selonick SE, Collins SJ (1980) Induction of differentiation of the human promyelocytic leukemia cell line (HL-60) by retinoic acid. Proc Natl Acad Sci USA 77: 2936–2940.

8. Dalton WJ, Ahearn M, McCredie K, Freireich E, Stass S, et al. (1988) HL-60 cell line was derived from a patient with FAB-M2 and not FAB-M3. Blood 71: 242–247.

9. Honma Y, Fujita Y, Kasukabe T, Hozumi M, Sampi K, et al. (1983) Induction of differentiation of human acute non-lymphocytic leukemia cells in primary culture by inducers of differentiation of human myeloid leukemia cell line HL-60. Eur J Cancer Clin Oncol 19: 251–261.

10. Brown G, Bunce CM, Rowlands DC, Williams GR (1994) All-trans retinoic acid and 1α,25-dihydroxyvitamin D₃ co-operate to promote differentiation of the human promyeloid leukemia cell line HL60 to monocytes. Leukemia 8: 806–815.

11. Taimi M, Chateau MT, Cabane S, Marti J (1991) Synergistic effect of retinoic acid and 1,25-dihydroxyvitamin D₃ on the differentiation of the human monocytic cell line U937. Leuk Res 15: 1145–1152.

12. Makishima M, Kanatani Y, Yamamoto-Yamaguchi Y, Honma Y (1996) Enhancement of activity of 1α,25-dihydroxyvitamin D₃ for growth inhibition and differentiation induction of human myelomonocytic leukemia cells by tretinoin tocoferil, an α-tocopherol ester of all-trans retinoic acid. Blood 87: 3384–3394.

13. Olsson IL, Breitman TR (1982) Induction of differentiation of the human histiocytic lymphoma cell line U-937 by retinoic acid and cyclic adenosine 3':5'-monophosphate-inducing agents. Cancer Res 42: 3924–3927.

14. Nagpal S, Na S, Rathnachalam R (2005) Noncalcemic actions of vitamin D receptor ligands. Endocr Rev 26: 662–687.

15. Haussler MR, Whitfield GK, Kaneko I, Haussler CA, Hsieh D, et al. (2013) Molecular mechanisms of vitamin D action. Calcif Tissue Int 92: 77–98.

16. Honma Y, Hozumi M, Abe E, Konno K, Fukushima M, et al. (1983) 1α,25-Dihydroxyvitamin D₃ and 1α-hydroxyvitamin D₃ prolong survival time of mice inoculated with myeloid leukemia cells. Proc Natl Acad Sci USA 80: 201–204.

17. Abe E, Miyaura C, Sakagami H, Takeda M, Konno K, et al. (1981) Differentiation of mouse myeloid leukemia cells induced by 1α,25-dihydroxyvitamin D₃. Proc Natl Acad Sci USA 78: 4990–4994.

18. Mangelsdorf DJ, Koeffler HP, Donaldson CA, Pike JW, Haussler MR (1984) 1,25-Dihydroxyvitamin D₃-induced differentiation in a human promyelocytic leukemia cell line (HL-60): receptor-mediated maturation to macrophage-like cells. J Cell Biol 98: 391–398.

19. Mehta K, Lopez-Berestein G (1986) Expression of tissue transglutaminase in cultured monocytic leukemia (THP-1) cells during differentiation. Cancer Res 46: 1388–1394.

20. Defacque H, Sevilla C, Piquemal D, Rochette-Egly C, Marti J, et al. (1997) Potentiation of VD-induced monocytic leukemia cell differentiation by retinoids involves both RAR and RXR signaling pathways. Leukemia 11: 221–227.

21. Okamoto R, Koeffler HP (2011) Hematological malignancy. In: Feldman D, Pike JW, Adams JS, editors. Vitamin D. 3 ed. Waltham: Academic Press. 1731–1750.

22. Mosser DM, Edwards JP (2008) Exploring the full spectrum of macrophage activation. Nat Rev Immunol 8: 958–969.

23. Murray PJ, Allen JE, Biswas SK, Fisher EA, Gilroy DW, et al. (2014) Macrophage activation and polarization: nomenclature and experimental guidelines. Immunity 41: 14–20.

24. Hewison M (2012) Vitamin D and immune function: an overview. Proc Nutr Soc 71: 50–61.

25. Kagechika H, Kawachi E, Hashimoto Y, Himi T, Shudo K (1988) Retinobenzoic acids. 1. Structure-activity relationships of aromatic amides with retinoidal activity. J Med Chem 31: 2182–2192.

26. Umemiya H, Fukasawa H, Ebisawa M, Eyrolles L, Kawachi E, et al. (1997) Regulation of retinoidal actions by diazepinylbenzoic acids. Retinoid synergists which activate the RXR-RAR heterodimers. J Med Chem 40: 4222–4234.

27. Makishima M, Shudo K, Honma Y (1999) Greater synergism of retinoic acid receptor (RAR) agonists with vitamin D₃ than that of retinoid X receptor (RXR) agonists with regard to growth inhibition and differentiation induction in monoblastic leukemia cells. Biochem Pharmacol 57: 521–529.

28. Amano Y, Cho Y, Matsunawa M, Komiyama K, Makishima M (2009) Increased nuclear expression and transactivation of vitamin D receptor by the cardiotonic steroid bufalin in human myeloid leukemia cells. J Steroid Biochem Mol Biol 114: 144–151.

29. Iriyama N, Yuan B, Hatta Y, Horikoshi A, Yoshino Y, et al. (2012) Granulocyte colony-stimulating factor potentiates differentiation induction by all-trans retinoic acid and arsenic trioxide and enhances arsenic uptake in the acute promyelocytic leukemia cell line HT93A. Oncol Rep 28: 1875–1882.

30. Tavangar K, Hoffman AR, Kraemer FB (1990) A micromethod for the isolation of total RNA from adipose tissue. Anal Biochem 186: 60–63.

31. Sakashita A, Kizaki M, Pakkala S, Schiller G, Tsuruoka N, et al. (1993) 9-cis-retinoic acid: effects on normal and leukemic hematopoiesis in vitro. Blood 81: 1009–1016.

32. Nakajima H, Kizaki M, Ueno H, Muto A, Takayama N, et al. (1996) All-trans and 9-cis retinoic acid enhance 1,25-dihydroxyvitamin D₃-induced monocytic differentiation of U937 cells. Leuk Res 20: 665–676.

33. Kagechika H (2002) Novel synthetic retinoids and separation of the pleiotropic retinoidal activities. Curr Med Chem 9: 591–608.

34. Tobita T, Takeshita A, Kitamura K, Ohnishi K, Yanagi M, et al. (1997) Treatment with a new synthetic retinoid, Am80, of acute promyelocytic leukemia relapsed from complete remission induced by all-trans retinoic acid. Blood 90: 967–973.

35. Masciulli R, Testa U, Barberi T, Samoggia P, Tritarelli E, et al. (1995) Combined vitamin D₃/retinoic acid induction of human promyelocytic cell lines: enhanced phagocytic cell maturation and hybrid granulomonocytic phenotype. Cell Growth Differ 6: 493–503.

36. Carlberg C, Seuter S, de Mello VDF, Schwab U, Voutilainen S, et al. (2013) Primary vitamin D target genes allow a categorization of possible benefits of vitamin D₃ supplementation. PLoS ONE 8: e71042.

37. Bunce CM, Wallington LA, Harrison P, Williams GR, Brown G (1995) Treatment of HL60 cells with various combinations of retinoids and 1α,25 dihydroxyvitamin D₃ results in differentiation towards neutrophils or monocytes or a failure to differentiate and apoptosis. Leukemia 9: 410–418.

38. Evans RM, Mangelsdorf DJ (2014) Nuclear receptors, RXR, and the big bang. Cell 157: 255–266.

39. Shulman AI, Larson C, Mangelsdorf DJ, Ranganathan R (2004) Structural determinants of allosteric ligand activation in RXR heterodimers. Cell 116: 417–429.

40. Allenby G, Bocquel MT, Saunders M, Kazmer S, Speck J, et al. (1993) Retinoic acid receptors and retinoid X receptors: interactions with endogenous retinoic acids. Proc Natl Acad Sci USA 90: 30–34.

41. Tsao T, Kornblau S, Safe S, Watt JC, Ruvolo V, et al. (2010) Role of peroxisome proliferator-activated receptor-γ and its coactivator DRIP205 in cellular responses to CDDO (RTA-401) in acute myelogenous leukemia. Cancer Res 70: 4949–4960.

42. Sanchez PV, Glantz ST, Scotland S, Kasner MT, Carroll M (2014) Induced differentiation of acute myeloid leukemia cells by activation of retinoid X and liver X receptors. Leukemia 28: 749–760.

43. Taimi M, Defacque H, Commes T, Favero J, Caron E, et al. (1993) Effect of retinoic acid and vitamin D on the expression of interleukin-1β, tumour necrosis factor-α and interleukin-6 in the human monocytic cell line U937. Immunology 79: 229–235.

44. Dugas N, Mossalayi MD, Calenda A, Leotard A, Becherel P, et al. (1996) Role of nitric oxide in the anti-tumoral effect of retinoic acid and 1,25-dihydroxyvitamin D₃ on human promonocytic leukemic cells. Blood 88: 3528–3534.

45. Mantovani A, Sica A, Sozzani S, Allavena P, Vecchi A, et al. (2004) The chemokine system in diverse forms of macrophage activation and polarization. Trends Immunol 25: 677–686.

46. Noy R, Pollard JW (2014) Tumor-associated macrophages: from mechanisms to therapy. Immunity 41: 49–61.

47. Chanda B, Ditadi A, Iscove NN, Keller G (2013) Retinoic acid signaling is essential for embryonic hematopoietic stem cell development. Cell 155: 215–227.

48. Mehta K, McQueen T, Tucker S, Pandita R, Aggarwal BB (1994) Inhibition by all-trans-retinoic acid of tumor necrosis factor and nitric oxide production by peritoneal macrophages. J Leukoc Biol 55: 336–342.

49. Wang X, Allen C, Ballow M (2007) Retinoic acid enhances the production of IL-10 while reducing the synthesis of IL-12 and TNF-α from LPS-stimulated monocytes/macrophages. J Clin Immunol 27: 193–200.

50. O'Kelly J, Hisatake J, Hisatake Y, Bishop J, Norman A, et al. (2002) Normal myelopoiesis but abnormal T lymphocyte responses in vitamin D receptor knockout mice. J Clin Invest 109: 1091–1099.

51. Helming L, Bose J, Ehrchen J, Schiebe S, Frahm T, et al. (2005) 1α,25-Dihydroxyvitamin D₃ is a potent suppressor of interferon gamma-mediated macrophage activation. Blood 106: 4351–4358.

52. Xu H, Soruri A, Gieseler RK, Peters JH (1993) 1,25-Dihydroxyvitamin D3 exerts opposing effects to IL-4 on MHC class-II antigen expression, accessory activity, and phagocytosis of human monocytes. Scand J Immunol 38: 535–540.

53. Matilainen JM, Husso T, Toropainen S, Seuter S, Turunen MP, et al. (2010) Primary effect of 1α,25(OH)₂D₃ on IL-10 expression in monocytes is short-term down-regulation. Biochim Biophys Acta 1803: 1276–1286.

54. Matilainen JM, Rasanen A, Gynther P, Vaisanen S (2010) The genes encoding cytokines IL-2, IL-10 and IL-12B are primary 1α,25(OH)₂D₃ target genes. J Steroid Biochem Mol Biol 121: 142–145.

55. Heine G, Niesner U, Chang HD, Steinmeyer A, Zugel U, et al. (2008) 1,25-dihydroxyvitamin D₃ promotes IL-10 production in human B cells. Eur J Immunol 38: 2210–2218.

56. Philippidis P, Mason JC, Evans BJ, Nadra I, Taylor KM, et al. (2004) Hemoglobin scavenger receptor CD163 mediates interleukin-10 release and heme oxygenase-1 synthesis: antiinflammatory monocyte-macrophage responses in vitro, in resolving skin blisters in vivo, and after cardiopulmonary bypass surgery. Circ Res 94: 119–126.

57. Ng TH, Britton GJ, Hill EV, Verhagen J, Burton BR, et al. (2013) Regulation of adaptive immunity; the role of interleukin-10. Front Immunol 4: 129.

9

Prognostic Significance of Neutrophil Lymphocyte Ratio in Patients with Gastric Cancer

Xi Zhang[2⁹], Wei Zhang[1⁹], Li-jin Feng[1]*

1 Department of Pathology, Shanghai Tenth People's Hospital, Tongji University, School of Medicine, Shanghai, China, 2 Department of Medical Oncology, Shanghai Tenth People's Hospital, Tongji University, School of Medicine, Shanghai, China

Abstract

Background: Several studies have shown that neutrophil lymphocyte ratio (NLR) may be associated with the prognosis of gastric cancer (GC), but the results are controversial.

Methods: This study was performed to evaluate the prognostic implications of neutrophil lymphocyte ratio of GC in all available studies. We surveyed 2 medical databases, PubMed and EMBASE, to identifyall relevant studies. Data were collected from studies comparing overall survival (OS), disease-free survival (DFS) and progression-free survival (PFS) in patients with GC.

Results: Ten studies (n = 2,952) evaluated the role of NLR as a predictor of outcome were involved for this meta-analysis (10 for OS, 3 for DFS, and 2 for PFS). Overall and disease-free survival were significantly better in patients with low NLR value and the pooled HRs was significant at 1.83 ([95% CI], 1.62–2.07) and 1.58 ([95% CI], 1.12–2.21), respectively. For progression-free survival, the pooled hazard ratio of NLR was significant at 1.54 ([95% CI], 1.22–1.95). No evidence of significant heterogeneity or publication bias for OS and DFS was seen in any of the included studies.

Conclusion: This meta-analysis indicated that elevated NLR may be associated with a worse prognosis for patients with GC.

Editor: Masaru Katoh, National Cancer Center, Japan

Funding: The authors have no support or funding to report.

Competing Interests: The authors have declared that no competing interests exist.

* Email: fenglijinmd@163.com

⑨ These authors contributed equally to this work.

Introduction

Despite the incidence of gastric cancer is decreasing, it remains one of the most frequent causes of cancer-related death worldwide [1]. The incidence of gastric cancer varies widely in different regions and is particularly common in East Asia [2]. In china, where gastric cancer is endemic, more patients are diagnosed in middle or late stage, which is reflected by poor overall survival rates. Although there have been great improvements in diagnostic and treatment technologies, most of the gastric patients still have either regional or distant metastatic disease with the 5-year overall survival less than 10% [3]. Therefore, it is important to identify prognostic factors for these patients in order to select patients for tailor treatment. Up to now, the prognosis significance of lymph node status [4], depth of tumor invasion [5] and macroscopic tumor size [6] are well known in GC. In addition, elevations of serum tumor markers can also be an independent predictor of adverse prognosis [7]. However, none of these have been demonstrated to be sufficiently effective for clinical use. More recently, established systemic inflammation-based prognostic scores have been explored extensively, such as NLR and serum C-reactive protein (CRP). CRP is an acute-phase response protein, which has been proven to be an independent prognostic factor for

survival in malignancy [8]. However, CRP is not routinely measured in many hospitals, and CRP level displays nonspecific change after treatment [9]. NLR can be suggested as the balance between pro-tumor inflammatory status and anti-tumor immune status. Patients with elevated NLR have a relative lymphocytopenia and neutrophil leukocytosis in favor of protumor inflammatory response, which gained its prognostic value in patients with colorectal cancer [10], lung cancer [11], pancreatic ductal adenoma [12], etc. Elevated level of NLR in GC patients may predict poorer clinical outcome [13], while some authors did not agree with the former results [14]. The aim of this study was to comprehensively and quantitatively summarize the global results to evaluate its prognostic value for patients with GC.

Methods

Search strategy and eligibility criteria

This meta-analysis was executed in accordance with the Preferred Reporting Items for Systematic Reviews and Meta-Analyses (PRISMA) guidelines [15]. A systematic literature search of relevant studies was conducted in PubMed and EMBASE up to June 2014. We used the following search terms without restrictions: "NLR", "neutrophil to lymphocyte ratio", "neutro-

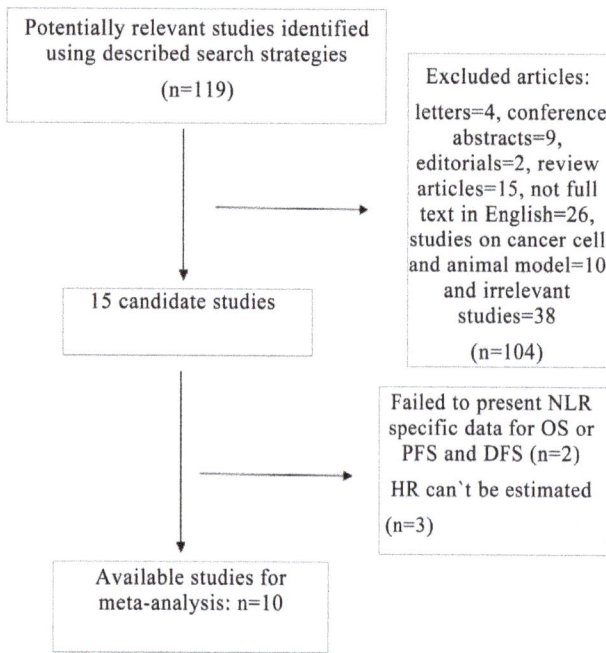

Figure 1. Flow chart of the meta-analysis.

phil lymphocyte ratio", "prognosis" and "gastric cancer" or "GC". Moreover, reference lists of retrieved articles were also reviewed to identify any studies that were not identified from the preliminary literature searches. Studies were included if they met the following criteria: (1) patients with gastric cancer in the studies were histopathologically confirmed (2) neutrophil-lymphocyte ratio values were reported (3) they evaluated the corelation between neutrophil lymphocyte ratio and the survival outcome of GC and (4) if studies' hazard ratios (HRs) were not directly repored, estimation of the HR could be reconstruct by other data. Articles were excluded from the meta-analysis based on the following criteria: (1) letters, conference abstracts, editorials, review articles, not full text in English, studies on cancer cell and animal model and irrelevant studies (2) studies had overlapping or duplicate data (3) studies failed to present the cut-off value for elevated NLR.

Quality Assessment

The quality of studies was assessed according to Newcastl-Ottawa Quality Assessment Scale (NOS) [16] by two reviewers (Xi Z and Wei Z). This scale includes three aspects of evaluation: selection, comparability, and outcome between the case group and control group. Studies that scored ≥6 were assigned as high-quality studies. Any disagreement was resolved by discussion.

Data extraction

Two investigators independently evaluated and extracted the data. All studies were double-checked by both and disagreements were resolved by consensus. The extracted data elements of this review included the following: (1) publication details, including first author's last name, publication year, and origin of the studied population (2) characteristics of the studied population, including sample size, age, and stage of disease and (3) HR of NLR for OS, DFS and PFS as well as their 95% CIs and p values and (4) follow-up time (5) cut-off values for elevated HR. If data for HR was not available, we extracted the total numbers of observed deaths and

Table 1. Main characteristics of all the studies included in the meta-analysis.

First author, date(ref.)	Study region	No (M/F, n)	Treatment (predominant)	Follow-up(M) (median and range)	Age(ys) (median and range)	NO. of Distal metastasis	Survival Analysis	Cutoff Value(<CV/≥CV)	HR	Summary results	Clinical stage	(III+IV)/All (n%)	Outcome
Lee et al.(2013)	Korea	174(114/60)	chemotherapy	14.9(1-47.9)	18-79	104	prospective	3.0(112/62)	R	positive	I-IV	145/174(83.3%)	OS
Wang et al.(2012)	China	324(225/99)	surgery	39.9(23.8-57.4)	NR	0	retrospective	5.0(313/11)	R	negative	III	324/324(100%)	OS/DFS
Jeong et al.(2012)	Korea	104(69/35)	chemotherapy	11.9(10.2-11.9)	52.5(28-82)	104	retrospective	3.0(49/55)	R	positive	IV	104/104(100%)	OS
Jung et al.(2011)	Korea	293(193/100)	surgery	38.2(4.2-65.5)	63(21-96)	120	retrospective	2.0(138/155)	R	positive	III-IV	293/293(100%)	OS/DFS
Shimada et al.(2010)	Japan	1028(709/319)	surgery	23(12-84)	65(26-89)	27	retrospective	4.0(127/901)	R	positive	I-IV	312/1028(30.3%)	OS
Jin et al.(2013)	China	46(36/10)	Chemotherapy	NR	60(37-77)	6	prospective	2.5(26/20)	E	negative	I-IV	34/46(73.9%)	OS/PFS
Aurello et al.(2014)	Italy	102(62/40)	surgery	40.8(8-107)	69±10.6	0	retrospective	5.0(74/28)	R	negative	I-IV	53/102(51.9%)	OS/DFS
Cho et al.(2014)	Japan	268(175/93)	chemotherapy	11.3(2.4-57.8)	55.4±12.48	187	retrospective	3.0(130/138)	R	positive	IV	268/268(100%)	OS/PFS
Jiang et al.(2014)	China	377(253/124)	surgery	42(1-103)	64±11.7	0	prospective	1.44(68/309)	R	positive	I-III	236/377(62.5%)	OS
Dirican et al.(2013)	Turkey	236(162/74)	multiple therapy	NR	58(30-86)	105	retrospective	3.8(147/89)	R	positive	I-IV	210/236(88.9%)	OS

OS: overall survival; DFS: Disease-free survival; PFS: progression-free survival; NR: not reported; R: reported; E: estimated; HR: hazard ratio; CV: cutoff value; Assessment Scale; All: all patients.

Prognostic Significance of Neutrophil Lymphocyte Ratio in Patients with Gastric Cancer

Table 2. Quality Assessment of included studies based on the Newcastle-Ottawa Scales.

Study	How representative was the exposed Cohort	Selection of non-exposed cohort	Ascertainment of exposure	Demonstration that outcome of interest was not present at start of study	Of cohorts on basis of design or analysis	Assessment of outcome	Follow up Long enough for outcomes to occur	Adequacy of cohort follow-up
Lee et al.(2013)	Somewhat representative of GC patients	Drawn from the same community as exposed cohort	Written self-report	Yes	Study controls for multiple covariate	confirmation of the outcome by reference to secure records	Yes	No description
Wang et al.(2012)	Somewhat representative of GC patients	Drawn from the same community as exposed cohort	From structured interview	Yes	Study controls for multiple covariate	confirmation of the outcome by reference to secure records	Yes	No description
Jeong et al.(2012)	Somewhat representative of GC patients	Drawn from the same community as exposed cohort	Secure record	Yes	Study controls for multiple covariate	confirmation of the outcome by reference to secure records	Yes	Complete follow-up
Jung et al.(2011)	Somewhat representative of GC patients	Drawn from the same community as exposed cohort	Secure record	Yes	Study controls for multiple covariate	confirmation of the outcome by reference to secure records	Yes	No description
Shimada et al.(2010)	Representative of GC patients	Drawn from the same community as exposed cohort	From structured interview	Yes	Study controls for multiple covariate	confirmation of the outcome by reference to secure records	Yes	No description
Jin et al.(2013)	Somewhat representative of GC patients	Drawn from the same community as exposed cohort	Secure record	Yes	Study controls for multiple covariate	confirmation of the outcome by reference to secure records	No	No description
Aurello et al.(2014)	Representative of GC patients	Drawn from the same community as exposed cohort	From structured interview	Yes	Study controls for multiple covariate	confirmation of the outcome by reference to secure records	Yes	Complete follow-up
Cho et al.(2014)	Somewhat representative of GC patients	Drawn from the same community as exposed cohort	Secure record	Yes	Study controls for multiple covariate	confirmation of the outcome by reference to secure records	Yes	No description
Jiang et al.(2014)	Somewhat representative of GC patients	Drawn from the same community as exposed cohort	Secure record	Yes	Study controls for multiple covariate	confirmation of the outcome by reference to secure records	Yes	No description
Dirican et al.(2013)	Somewhat representative of GC patients	Drawn from the same community as exposed cohort	Secure record	Yes	Study controls for multiple covariate	confirmation of the outcome by reference to secure records	No	No description

Study ID	HR (95% CI)	% Weight
OS		
Lee (2013)	2.24 (2.09, 3.63)	19.37
Dirican (2013)	2.74 (1.90, 3.70)	13.28
Wang (2012)	1.87 (0.90, 3.87)	2.78
Shimada (2010)	1.85 (1.24, 2.75)	9.25
Jung (2011)	1.46 (1.03, 2.07)	12.25
Jeong (2012)	1.65 (1.03, 2.64)	6.66
Jiang (2014)	1.60 (1.04, 2.43)	8.24
Aurello (2014)	1.15 (0.69, 3.28)	2.43
Cho (2014)	1.57 (1.23, 2.01)	24.42
Jin (2013)	1.92 (0.67, 5.51)	1.33
Subtotal (I-squared = 29.8%, p = 0.171)	1.83 (1.62, 2.07)	100.00
DFS		
Aurello (2014)	0.95 (0.35, 2.56)	11.48
Wang (2012)	1.76 (0.88, 3.51)	23.80
Jung (2011)	1.65 (1.09, 2.52)	64.72
Subtotal (I-squared = 0.0%, p = 0.565)	1.58 (1.12, 2.21)	100.00
PFS		
Jin (2013)	2.33 (1.07, 5.07)	9.16
Cho (2014)	1.48 (1.15, 1.89)	90.84
Subtotal (I-squared = 16.0%, p = 0.275)	1.54 (1.22, 1.95)	100.00

.181   1   5.51

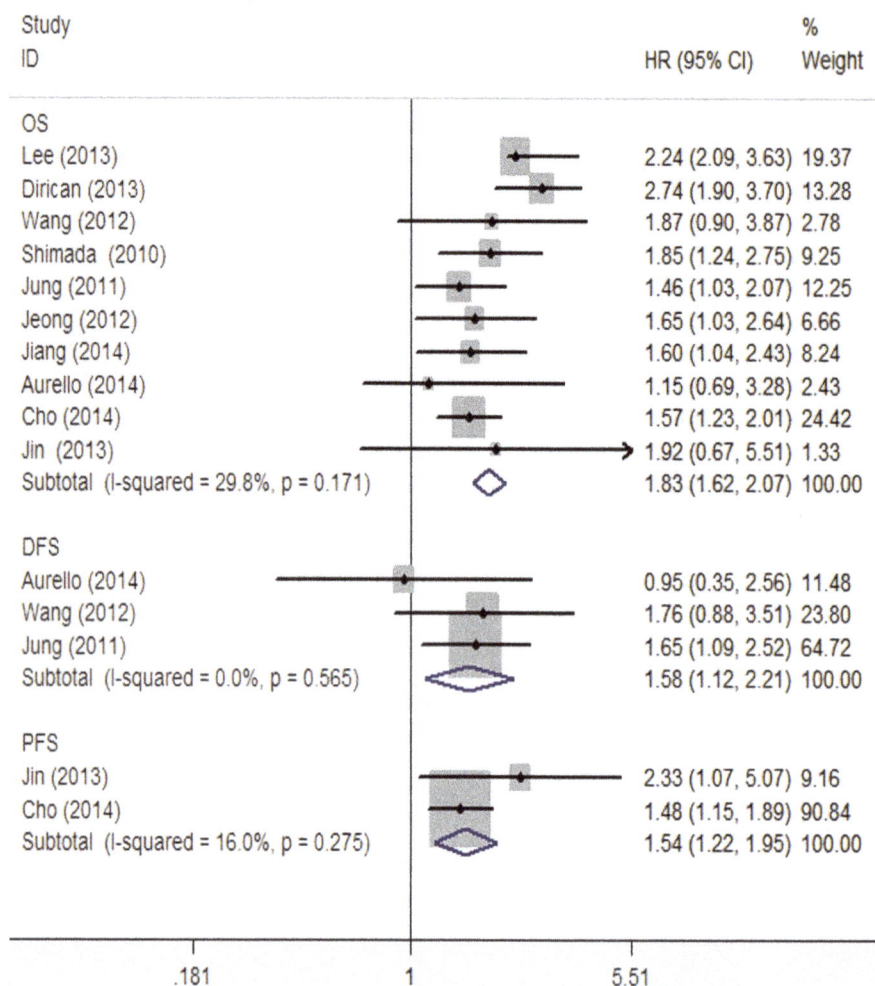

Figure 2. Forest plots of studies evaluating hazard ratios (HR) with 95% confidence interval (95% CI) for high NLR levels as compared with low levels. Survival data are reported as overall survival, disease-free survival and progression-free survival.

the numbers of patients in each group to calculate HR. Data were extracted from the graphical survival plots when data were only available as Kaplan-Meier curves [17]. If several estimates were reported in the same article, we chose the most powerful one (multivariate analysis was superior to univariate analysis).

Statistical Analysis

HRs and their 95% CIs from each study were used to calculate pooled HRs. The heterogeneity of the combined HRs was performed using Cochran's Q test and Higgins' I-squared statistics. A P value <0.05 was considered significant. We used the random effects model (Der Simonian and Laird method) if heterogeneity was observed (P<0.05). The fixed effects model was applied in the absence of between-study heterogeneity (P≥0.05) [18]. Publication bias of literature was evaluated using Begg's funnel plot and the Egger's linear regression test and a p<0.05 was considered significant. Statistical analyses were carried out using the statistical software Stata (version 12.0).

Results

Literature search

A flow diagram of our literature search is shown in Figure 1. We identified 15 potentially relevant articles concerning NLR and prognosis of gastric cancer. Three studies were excluded as HR can't be calculated by the described method [19–21] and 2 studies were excluded as failed to present NLR specific data for OS or DFS and PFS [22–23]. A total of 10 articles [13–14,24–31] that met the inclusion and exclusion criteria were retrieved. Of these reports selected for further evaluation, 10 investigated the prognostic role of NLR for OS, 3 for DFS and 2 for PFS, respectively.

Study Characteristics

The characteristics of the included studies were summarized in Table 1. We collected the data from 10 studies, which involved a total of 2,952 patients from the Korea, China, Japan, Italy and Turkey. Treatment methods for nine studies were surgery and chemotherapy. Patients of one study were treated by multiple-therapy. Four studies enrolled less than 200 patients and six studies

Table 3. Summary of the subgroup meta analysis results for OS.

Subgroup	N	Random-effects model HR(95%)CI	Fixed-effects model HR(95%)CI	Heterogeneity	
				I²(%)	P Value
Treatment method					
Surgery	5	1.59(1.30–1.95)	1.59(1.30–1.95)	0	0.808
Chemotherapy	4	1.82(1.48–2.23)	1.82(1.53–2.15)	21	0.284
Sample size					
Sample size <200	4	1.94(1.52–2.47)	1.97(1.58–2.46)	7.3	0.357
Sample size ≥ 200	6	1.79(1.46–2.20)	1.77(1.54–2.05)	44.4	0.11
Cut-off value					
Cut-off value>3	4	2.01(1.44–2.80)	2.14(1.70–2.70)	42.7	0.157
Cut-off value≦3	6	1.72(1.49–1.99)	1.72(1.49–1.99)	2.9	0.398
Geographic region					
Eastern countries	8	1.74(1.53–1.99)	1.74(1.53–1.99)	0	0.625
Western countries	2	1.80(0.65–4.97)	2.46(1.80–3.38)	74.5	0.048
TNM stage					
(III+IV)/All = 100%	4	1.57(1.31–1.87)	1.57(1.31–1.87)	0	0.936
(III+IV)/All<100%	6	2.03(1.65–2.21)	2.09(1.77–2.47)	28.7	0.220

HR: hazard ratio; CI: confidence interval; All: all patients.

had more than 200 patients. The risk of bias in included studies was outlined based on the Newcastle-Ottawa Quality Assessment Scales. (Table 2) HR and 95%CI were reported directly in 9 of the enrolled cohorts. Jung et al presented separate cut-off value with cut-off value = 3.0 for OS and cut-off value = 2.0 for DFS. In the study by Jin, HR and its 95% CIs before treatment was calculated from Kaplan-Meier curves.

Outcome from eligible studies

In the 10 studies evaluating OS, there was no significant heterogeneity between studies for categorized NLR (I-squared = 29.8%; p = 0.171). The fixed-effect model was applied to calculate the pooled HR, and its 95% CI. The pooled HR of 1.83 (95%CI: 1.62–2.07) indicated that patients with elevated NLR have shorter OS (Figure 2).

Subgroup analyses was conducted for OS. Subgroup analyses by treatment methods showed that elevated NLR predicted poor prognosis in patients treated with both surgery and chemotherapy [(HR = 1.59, 95%CI: (1.30–1.95); HR = 1.82, 95%CI:(1.53–2.15)]. Stratification by sample size, we found the pooled HRs was 1.77, 95%CI: (1.54–2.05) for studies with more than 200 cases and 1.97, 95%CI: (1.58–2.46) for studies with less than 200 cases. The results revealed that high NLR remained to be a worse prognostic marker regardless of sample size. Stratification by cut-off value≤3.0 and cut-off value>3.0, it was found that the pooled HRs was still a poor predictor for GC [HR = 1.72, 95%CI: (1.49–1.99)] for cut-off value≤3.0 and [HR = 2.14, 95%CI: (1.70–2.70)] for cut-off value>3.0. In the subgroup analyses by geographic region, we found that elevated NLR was still a poor predictor for eastern patients [HR = 1.74, 95%CI: (1.53–1.99)] but not for western patients [HR = 1.80, 95%CI: (0.65–4.97)]. When per-

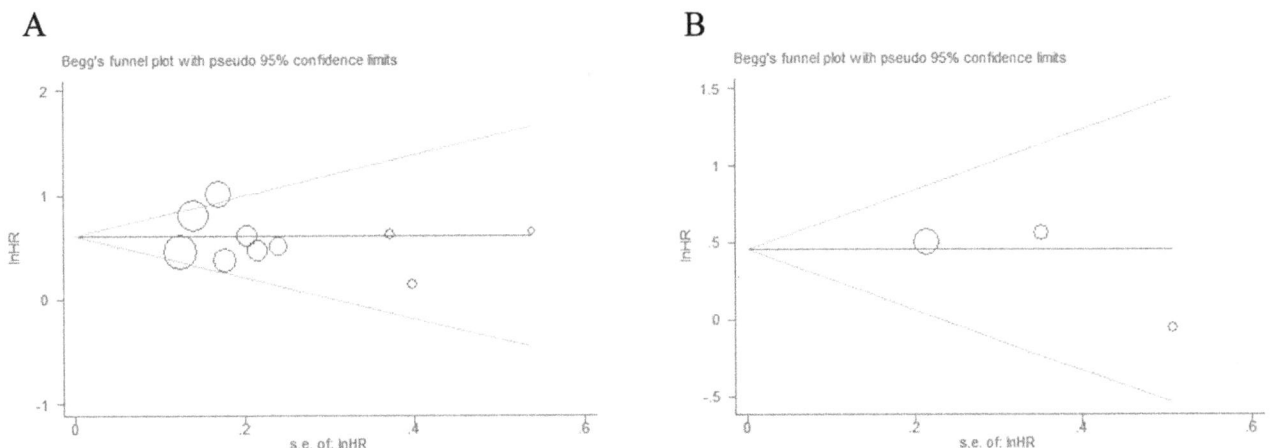

Figure 3. Funnel plots of studies included in the meta-analyses: A) overall survival, B) disease-free survival.

forming subgroup analyses stratified by TNM stage, we found that increased NLR was a negative predictor in patients with stage III or IV[HR = 1.57,95%CI: (1.31–1.87)]and patients with stage I–IV[HR = 2.09,95%CI: (1.77–2.47)], however, NLR might be a more important prognostic factor for early TNM stage patients with the higher pooled HRs (Table 3).

Meta-regression was also conducted to explore the potential source of heterogeneity. The results showed that TNM stage (p = 0.049) may contribute to the source of inter-study heterogeneity.

For DFS and PFS, there were three studies reporting the data of NLR for DFS and two studies reporting the data of NLR for PFS in GC patients. The P values between-study heterogeneity for DFS and PFS were (I-squared = 0%; p = 0.565) and (I-squared = 16%; p = 0.275), respectively. As for the ability to evaluate DFS, the combined HR of 1.58 (95%CI: 1.12–2.21) showed that the high NLR had significant relationship with DFS in GC (Figure 2). As illustrated in Figure 2, elevated NLR predicted poor prognosis for PFS whose pooled HR was significant at 1.54 (95%CI: 1.22–1.95).

Publication Bias

We applied funnel plots and Egger's test to evaluate publication bias of the included studies. As shown in Figure 3, the funnel plot was symmetrical. There was no evidence for significant publication bias for OS and DFS, since their p values for Egger were more than 0.1.

Discussion

Our results from this meta-analysis including 10 studies with 2952 cases showed that elevated NLR was associated with OS, DFS and PFS. Subgroup analyses revealed that poor OS with high NLR could be found in patients treated with both surgery and chemotherapy. Elevated NLR was a significant prognostic marker to predict poor OS regardless of sample size and cut-off values. When subgroup was analyzed by geographic region, we found that elevated NLR was still a poor OS predictor for eastern patients but not for western patients. Moreover, when the prognostic significance of elevated NLR was evaluated by TNM stage, NLR might be a more crucial prognostic factor for early TNM stage patients.

Chronic inflammation is known to promote carcinogenesis contributing to the onset or progression of cancer [32]. Tumors can not only develop at the sites of inflammation, such as Helicobacter pylori infection is recognized as a causative agent for gastric cancer [33], but they can also trigger regional immune response and release inflammatory factors around the tumor which result in the formation of an inflammatory microenvironment. Inflammatory processes always accompany with progression of cancer, which can contribute to tumorigenesis by supplying cytokines, such as vascular endothelial growth factor (VEGF), interleukin-18 and matrix metalloproteinases [34–36] to the tumor microenvironment that promotes angiogenesis, and thus promotes tumor growth and metastasis.

In recent decades, a variety of predictors have been identified and applied for predicting GC outcomes. CEA, Her-2 are currently used in routine pathological assessment of GC. Ki-67, caspase-3 and p53 have also been reported associated with GC survival [37]. In addition, it is well known today that miRNAs have very important regulatory functions in cancer. Up to now, accumulating studies have investigated the diagnostic and prognostic values of miRNAs in GC. For example, Ueda T found that microRNAs are expressed differentially in gastric cancers and unique microRNAs are associated with progression and prognosis of GC [38]. However, the above-mentioned biomarkers should be examined in cancerous tissues. Thus it is impossible to monitor their levels continuously throughout disease progression. In contrast, NLR as an indicator of inflammation can be easily assayed in plasma or serum, which may be widely applied in the clinic.

NLR is known to possess prognostic value in cancer population. There are a number of possible mechanisms by which NLR is associated with worse outcome in patients with cancer. Firstly, the antitumor responses of natural killer cells and activated T cells may be suppressed by increased number of neutrophils around the tumor [39]. A high NLR reflects both a heightened neutrophil-dependent inflammatory response and a decreased lymphocyte mediated antitumor immune reaction, which may weaken the lymphocyte-mediated anti-tumor cellular immune response and contribute to aggressive tumor biology, cancer progression and poor prognosis. Secondly, circulating neutrophils contributes to tumor growth and progression by producing cytokines, such as tumor necrosis factor (TNF), IL-1, IL-6, and angiogenic factor vascular endothelial growth factor (VEGF) [40]. Thirdly, a reduced number of lymphocytes may weaken the lymphocyte-mediated anti-tumor cellular immune response. The neutrophil count alone may not reflect the prognostic information of a decreased lymphocyte mediated immune response, and a low lymphocyte count alone may not reflect the neutrophil driven tumor growth process. Hence, it is likely that the combined effects of neutrophilia and lymphocytopenia lead to a high NLR which may reflect the combined prognostic information of these two processes, and be a stronger predictor of outcome than either alone.

There are some limitations in this study. First, there is some heterogeneity of subjects for NLR in the OS group. Heterogeneity might be caused by characteristics of the patients, such as age, differentiation or disease stage, cut off values, treatment they might have received, the duration of follow-up, and adjustments for other cofactors. Moreover, our results are likely to be affected by the wide range of cutoff values for elevated NLR, which may affect the positive associations between NLR and GC prognosis. For example, cut-off scores of NLR were defined as 1.44, 2.5, 3.0, 4.0 or 5.0 by analyzing the ROC curve, median value or based on previous studies, however, subgroup analyses stratified by cut-off values showed that the NLRs prognostic value was not affected substantially. Second, the NLR is usually regarded as a prognostic marker in several diseases which are related to survival, such as cardiovascular diseases [41]. Thus, we cannot consider NLR as a "predictor" for survival unless the involved patients don't have other severe diseases related to NLR. Finally, only English studies were included in this analysis and small studies with null results tended not to be published, which may cause potential publication bias.

Conclusions

In conclusion, our meta-analysis, including a quantified synthesis of all published studies, showed that elevated NLR was a poor predictor for survival in patients with gastric cancer. The critical role of NLR in cancer prognosis may contribute to its clinical utility. Considering the limitations of the present meta-analysis, further research with large-scale and standard investigations should be conducted.

Supporting Information

Checklist S1 PRISMA checklist.

Acknowledgments

We would like to acknowledge Dr. Zhu-Qing Liu for statistical advice.

Author Contributions

Conceived and designed the experiments: XZ WZ LJF. Performed the experiments: XZ WZ LJF. Analyzed the data: XZ. Contributed reagents/materials/analysis tools: XZ. Wrote the paper: XZ.

References

1. Parkin DM, Bray F, Ferlay J, Pisani P (2005) Global cancer statistics. CA Cancer J Clin 55: 74–108.
2. Jemal A, Bray F, Center MM, Ferlay J, Ward E, et al. (2011) Global cancer statistics. CA Cancer J Clin 2011; 61: 69–90.
3. Wagner AD, Grothe W, Haerting J, Kleber G, Grothey A, et al. (2006) Chemotherapy in advanced gastric cancer: a systematic review and meta-analysis based on aggregate data. J Clin Oncol 24(18): 2903–2909.
4. Shiraishi N, Inomata M, Osawa N, Yasuda K, Adachi Y, et al. (2000) Early and late recurrence after gastrectomy for gastric carcinoma. Univariate and multivariate analyses. Cancer 89: 255–61.
5. Kim JP, Lee JH, Kim SJ, Yu HJ, Yang HK et al. (1998) Clinicopathologic characteristics and prognostic factors in 10783 patients with gastric cancer. Gastric Cancer 1: 125–33.
6. Aoyama T, Yoshikawa T, Watanabe T, Hayashi T, Ogata T, et al. (2011) Macroscopic tumor size as an independent prognostic factor for stage II/III gastric cancer patients who underwent D2 gastrectomy followed by adjuvant chemotherapy with S-1. Gastric Cancer 14(3): 274–8.
7. Mihmanli M, Dilege E, Demir U, Coskun H, Eroglu T, et al. (2004) The use of tumor markers as predictors of prognosis in gastric cancer. Hepatogastroenterology 51(59): 1544–7.
8. Han Y, Mao F, Wu Y, Fu X, Zhu X, et al. (2011) Prognostic role of C-reactive protein in breast cancer: a systematic review and meta-analysis. Int J Biol Markers 26(4): 209–15.
9. Cook EJ, Walsh SR, Farooq N, Alberts JC, Justin TA, et al. (2007) Post-operative neutrophil-lymphocyte ratio predicts complications following colorectal surgery. Int J Surg 5: 27–30.
10. Li MX, Liu XM, Zhang XF, Zhang JF, Wang WL, et al. (2014) Prognostic Role of Neutrophil-to-lymphocyte Ratio in Colorectal Cancer: A Systematic Review and Meta-Analysis. Int J Cancer 134(10): 2403–13.
11. Teramukai S, Kitano T, Kishida Y, Kawahara M, Kubota K, et al. (2009) Pretreatment neutrophil count as an independent prognostic factor in advanced non-small-cell lung cancer: an analysis of Japan Multinational Trial Organisation LC00-03. Eur J Cancer 45 (11): 1950–8.
12. Stotz M, Gerger A, Eisner F, Szkandera J, Loibner H, et al. (2013) Increased neutrophil-lymphocyte ratio is a poor prognostic factor in patients with primary operable as well as inoperable pancreatic cancer. Br J Cancer 23; 109 (2): 416–21.
13. Lee S, Oh SY, Kim SH, Lee JH, Kim MC, et al. (2013) Prognostic significance of neutrophil lymphocyte ratio and platelet lymphocyte ratio in advanced gastric cancer patients treated with FOLFOX chemotherapy. BMC Cancer 22; 13: 350.
14. Wang DS, Ren C, Qiu MZ, Luo HY, Wang ZQ, et al. (2012) Comparison of the prognostic value of various preoperative inflammation-based factors in patients with stage III gastric cancer. Tumour Biol 33(3): 749–56.
15. Moher D, Liberati A, Tetzlaff J, Altman DG (2009) Preferred reporting items for systematic reviews and meta-analyses: the PRISMA statement. BMJ 339: b2535.
16. Wells GA, Shea B, O'Connell D, J Peterson, V Welch, et al. (2011) The Newcastle-Ottawa Scale (NOS) for assessing the quality of nonrandomised studies in meta-analyses 2010. Available at: URL: http://www.ohri.ca/programs/clinical_epidemiology/oxford.asp. Accessed: 2011 January 10.
17. Parmar MKB, Torri V, Stewart L (1998) Extracting summary statistics to perform meta-analyses of the published literature for survival endpoints. Stat Med 17: 2815–34.
18. DerSimonian R, Laird N (1986) Meta-analysis in clinical trials. Control Clin Trials 7: 177–188.
19. Aliustaoglu M, Bilici A, Ustaalioglu BB, Konya V, Gucun M, et al. (2010) The effect of peripheral blood values on prognosis of patients with locally advanced gastric cancer before treatment. Med Oncol 27(4): 1060–5.
20. Lee DY, Hong SW, Chang YG, Lee WY, Lee B (2013) Clinical Significance of Preoperative Inflammatory Parameters in Gastric Cancer Patients. J Gastric Cancer 13(2): 111–6.
21. Nakayama Y, Gotohda N, Shibasaki H, Nomura S, Kinoshita T, et al. (2014) Usefulness of the neutrophil/lymphocyte ratio measured preoperatively as a predictor of peritoneal metastasis in patients with advanced gastric cancer. Surg Today 16. Epub ahead of print.
22. Dutta S, Crumley AB, Fullarton GM, Horgan PG, McMillan DC (2012) Comparison of the prognostic value of tumour and patient related factors in patients undergoing potentially curative resection of gastric cancer. Am J Surg 204(3): 294–9.
23. Aizawa M, Gotohda N, Takahashi S, Konishi M, Kinoshita T (2011) Predictive Value of Baseline Neutrophil/Lymphocyte Ratio for T4 Disease in Wall-Penetrating Gastric Cancer. World J Surg 35(12): 2717–22.
24. Dirican A, Ekinci N, Avci A, Akyol M, Alacacioglu A, et al. (2013) The effects of hematological parameters and tumor-infiltrating lymphocytes on prognosis in patients with gastric cancer. Cancer Biomarkers 13(1): 11–20.
25. Jeong JH, Lim SM, Yun JY, Rhee GW, Lim JY, et al. (2012) Comparison of two inflammation-based prognostic scores in patients with unresectable advanced gastric cancer. Oncology 83(5): 292–9.
26. Jin H, Zhang G, Liu X, Liu X, Chen C, et al. (2013) Blood neutrophil-lymphocyte ratio predicts survival for stages III-IV gastric cancer treated with neoadjuvant chemotherapy. World J Surg Oncol 24; 11: 112.
27. Jung MR, Park YK, Jeong O, Seon JW, Ryu SY, et al. (2011) Elevated preoperative neutrophil to lymphocyte ratio predicts poor survival following resection in late stage gastric cancer. J Surg Oncol 104(5): 504–10.
28. Shimada H, Takiguchi N, Kainuma O, Soda H, Ikeda A, et al. (2010) High preoperative neutrophil-lymphocyte ratio predicts poor survival in patients with gastric cancer. Gastric Cancer 13(3): 170–6.
29. Aurello P, Tierno SM, Berardi G, Tomassini F, Magistri P, et al. (2014) Value of Preoperative Inflammation-Based Prognostic Scores in Predicting Overall Survival and Disease-Free Survival in Patients with Gastric Cancer. Ann Surg Oncol 21(6): 1998–2004.
30. Cho IR, Park JC, Park CH, Jo JH, Lee HJ, et al. (2014) Pre-treatment neutrophil to lymphocyte ratio as a prognostic marker to predict chemotherapeutic response and survival outcomes in metastatic advanced gastric cancer. Gastric Cancer. Jan 19. Epub ahead of print.
31. Jiang N, Deng JY, Liu Y, Ke B, Liu HG, et al. (2014) The role of preoperative neutrophil–lymphocyte and platelet–lymphocyte ratio in patients after radical resection for gastric cancer. Biomarkers, Jun 9: 1–8 Epub ahead of print.
32. Hanahan D, Weinberg RA (2011) Hallmarks of cancer: the next generation. Cell 144: 646–74.
33. Parsonnet J, Friedman GD, Vandersteen DP, Chang Y, Vogelman JH, et al. (1991) Helicobacter pylori infection and the risk of gastric carcinoma. N Engl J Med 17; 325(16): 1127–31.
34. Webb NJ, Myers CR, Watson CJ, Bottomley MJ, Brenchley PE (1998) Activated human neutrophils express vascular endothelial growth factor (VEGF). Cytokine 10(4): 254–7.
35. Jablonska E, Puzewska W, Grabowska Z, Jablonski J, Talarek L, et al. (2005) VEGF, IL-18 and NO production by neutrophils and their serum levels in patients with oral cavity cancer. Cytokine 30(3): 93–99.
36. Ardi VC, Kupriyanova TA, Deryugina EI, Quigley JP (2007) Human neutrophils uniquely release TIMP-free MMP-9 to provide a potent catalytic stimulator of angiogenesis. Proc Natl Acad Sci USA 104: 20262–20267.
37. Xiao LJ, Zhao S, Zhao EH, Zheng X, Gou WF, et al. (2013) Clinicopathological and prognostic significance of Ki-67, caspase-3 and p53 expression in gastric carcinomas. Oncol Lett 6(5): 1277–1284.
38. Ueda T, Volinia S, Okumura H, Shimizu M, Taccioli C, et al. (2010) Relation between microRNA expression and progression and prognosis of gastric cancer: a microRNA expression analysis. Lancet Oncol 11(2): 136–46.
39. Shau H, Kim A. (1988) Suppression of lymphokine-activated killer induction by neutrophils. J Immunol 141: 4395–4402.
40. An X, Ding PR, Li YH, Wang FH, Shi YX, et al. (2010) Elevated neutrophil to lymphocyte ratio predicts survival in advanced pancreatic cancer. Biomarkers 15: 516–22.
41. Tamhane UU, Aneja S, Montgomery D, Rogers EK, Eagle KA, et al. (2008) Association between admission neutrophil to lymphocyte ratio and outcomes in patients with acute coronary syndrome. Am J Cardiol 15; 102(6): 653–7.

10

Hematopoietic Stem/Progenitor Cell Sources to Generate Reticulocytes for *Plasmodium vivax* Culture

Florian Noulin[1]*, Javed Karim Manesia[2], Anna Rosanas-Urgell[1], Annette Erhart[1], Céline Borlon[1], Jan Van Den Abbeele[3], Umberto d'Alessandro[4], Catherine M. Verfaillie[2]

1 Unit of Malariology, Institute of Tropical Medicine, Antwerp, Belgium, 2 Department of development and regeneration, Stem Cell Institute, Leuven, Belgium, 3 Unit of Veterinary Protozoology, Institute of Tropical Medicine, Antwerp, Belgium, 4 Medical Research Council Unit, Fajara, The Gambia

Abstract

The predilection of *Plasmodium vivax* (*P. vivax*) for reticulocytes is a major obstacle for its establishment in a long-term culture system, as this requires a continuous supply of large quantities of reticulocytes, representing only 1–2% of circulating red blood cells. We here compared the production of reticulocytes using an established *in vitro* culture system from three different sources of hematopoietic stem/progenitor cells (HSPC), i.e. umbilical cord blood (UCB), bone marrow (BM) and adult peripheral blood (PB). Compared to CD34+-enriched populations of PB and BM, CD34+-enriched populations of UCB produced the highest amount of reticulocytes that could be invaded by *P. vivax*. In addition, when CD34+-enriched cells were first expanded, a further extensive increase in reticulocytes was seen for UCB, to a lesser degree BM but not PB. As invasion by *P. vivax* was significantly better in reticulocytes generated *in vitro*, we also suggest that *P. vivax* may have a preference for invading immature reticulocytes, which should be confirmed in future studies.

Editor: Ana Paula Arez, Instituto de Higiene e Medicina Tropical, Portugal

Funding: The funding was provided by ITM Secondary Research Funding (SOFI-B), http://www.itg.be/itgtool_v2/Projecten/Project.asp?PNr = 755023. The funders had no role in study design, data collection and analysis, decision to publish, or preparation of the manuscript.

Competing Interests: The authors have declared that no competing interests exist.

* Email: flo_noulin@hotmail.com

Introduction

Plasmodium vivax (*P. vivax*) is the most widespread malaria parasite outside sub-Saharan Africa, and accounts for 80 to 300 million of malaria cases per year [1]. The predilection of *P. vivax* for reticulocytes is a major obstacle for the establishment of a long-term *P. vivax* culture system [2,3]. As reticulocytes represent only 1–2% of the circulating red blood cells (RBCs) with a half-life of 2 days (including 1 day in the peripheral blood), collecting sufficient reticulocytes to maintain a *P. vivax* culture is a challenge [3].

It has been previously shown that reticulocytes can be obtained by concentrating adult peripheral blood (PB) or umbilical cord blood (UCB) using either a 70% percoll solution [4] or a plasma autologous ultra-centrifugation [5]. One study suggested that *P. vivax* could be maintained in culture for up to 85 days with reticulocytes concentrated from umbilical blood cord (UCB) [6]; however, parasites did not develop beyond one schizogony cycle and parasite densities were very low [7]. In addition, it is possible to culture hematopoietic stem/progenitor cells (HSPC)/CD34+ cells to induce erythroid differentiation and consequently produce reticulocytes *in vitro* [8]. Reticulocytes generated from CD34+ cells from both bone marrow (BM) and peripheral blood mononuclear cells (PBMC) have been previously used for culturing *P. vivax*; but the authors did not provide data regarding the efficiency of invasion and the development of the parasites *in vitro* [9].

In this report, we compared different sources of hematopoietic stem/progenitor cells (HPSC), namely UCB, BM and peripheral blood, for their capacity to produce reticulocytes that allow invasion by *P. vivax*.

Materials and Methods

HSPCs expansion and reticulocytes differentiation

CD34+ cell isolation. The differentiation of HSPC into reticulocytes was done according to a previously described protocol [10]. UCB was obtained from the Belgian Cord Blood Bank at the Gasthuisberg Hospital Leuven, BM samples were obtained from volunteer donors; and human peripheral blood from the Antwerp Red Cross. Mononuclear cells from peripheral blood (PBMC), UCB and BM were isolated on a Ficoll gradient (GE Healthcare), by 30 minutes centrifugation at 400 g. The mononuclear cells were collected and washed twice with PBS. CD34+ enriched HSPCs were isolated using Magnetic Assorting Cell Sorting (MACS, Biotenyl Biotech). HSPC cell purity after MACS selection was assessed by FACS analysis, using CD34 and CD45 antibodies (eBioscience).

Reticulocytes differentiation

CD34+-enriched cells were dispensed in a 6-well plate with IMDM medium (Gibco) supplemented with L-glutamine (4 M, Sigma), penicillin-streptomycin (1%, Invitrogen), folic acid (10 µg/mL, Sigma), inositol (40 µg/mL, Sigma), transferrin (120 µg/mL, Sigma), monothioglycerol (1.6 10^{-4} M, Sigma), insulin (10 mg/mL, Sigma) and 10% human plasma. During the first 8 days, the medium was supplemented with the following factors: hydrocor-

Table 1. Hematopoietic stem progenitor cells (HSPC) expansion and reticulocyte differentiation for three different sources HSPCs (6 independent experiments were carried out for each HSPC source).

HSPC sources	Mean proportion (%) of reticulocytes at D14 (± SD) (n = 6)	Cell number mean fold increase (± SD) (n = 3)	
		After 5 days of expansion	After 7 days of differentiation
UCB	18.3±1.3	11.5±2.3	33.5±2.4
BM	20.5±1.5	3.1±0.3	8.6±0.5
PBMC	32±6	1.3±0.2	3.4±0.2

Results show the mean proportions of reticulocytes observed at the peak of enucleation after 14 days of culture, as well as the increase in total cell number after 5 days of expansion and 7 days of differentiation (3 independent experiments). After 5 days of expansion, the number of cells was counted and divided by the initial number of plated MACS/CD34+ cells, while after 7 days of HSPC differentiation, the cell count was compared to the number of cells not previously expanded, results are expressed in mean fold increase (± SD).

tisone (HDS, 10^{-6} M, Sigma), interleukin-3 (IL-3, 5 ng/mL, R&D system), stem cell factor (SCF, 100 ng/mL, Bioke) and erythropoietin (EPO, 3 IU/mL, R&D system) and placed at 37°C in a 5% CO_2 incubator. The initial volume of medium was 4 mL and after 4 days, an extra 3 mL was added. After 8 days, the cells were centrifuged for 5 minutes at 300 g, fresh IMDM medium supplemented with EPO (3 IU/mL) was added, and the cells were transferred in a 25 cm² flask. On day 11, the medium was changed and complete medium was added without EPO. Afterwards, medium was refreshed every 3 days and 10% heat inactivated human serum was added to protect the viability of the cells.

For CD34+ cell expansion, CD34+ enriched cells were dispensed in a 6-well plate with 4 mL Serum-free expansion medium (SFEM, Sigma) with SCF (50 ng/mL), thrombopoietin (TPO, 50 ng/mL, R&D system), FMS-like tyrosine kinase 3 (FLT3, 50 ng/mL, R&D system) and IL-6 (50 ng/mL, R&D system) for 5 days at 37°C, and 5% CO_2. On day 5, the cells were counted, and transferred into a new 6-well plate to induce the reticulocyte differentiation (using the protocol described above).

Reticulocyte concentration

Reticulocytes were enriched from UCB or PB by loading on a 70% isotonic percoll cushion which was spun for 15 minutes at 400 g. After two washes with PBS, reticulocytes were counted as described below.

Reticulocyte count

Cells were spun at 300 g for 5 minutes and re-suspended in 50 µL of PBS; 50 µL of Cresyl blue (Roche) diluted 1:1000 was added and cells were incubated at room temperature for 30 minutes. After a cytospin centrifugation (3 minutes at 700 rpm), the cells were fixed with methanol, and stained for 10 minutes with Giemsa (Sigma). The slides were then examined by microscopy (immersion objective, 630× magnification), and reticulocytes were counted against a minimum of 500 RBCs and the density per 100 RBCs was computed. A reticulocyte was morphologically defined as an enucleated cell with at least 3 dots of cresyl blue RNA.

Plasmodium vivax invasion assays

Cryopreserved P. vivax isolates [11] from infected patients were provided by the Shoklo Malaria Research Unit (SMRU, Mae Sot, Thailand). The samples were thawed with NaCl solutions and cultured for 36 to 40 hours with McCoy's medium (Gibco) supplemented with glucose (2%) and 20% heat inactivated human serum. P. vivax mature forms were concentrated on a 45% percoll

after a 5 minutes treatment with 0.05% trypsin. After 15 minutes of centrifugation at 1600 g, cells above the 45% percoll were collected and washed twice before checking the quality of the concentration. If more than 90% of the cells contained parasites, they were mixed with our previously differentiated and cryopreserved reticulocytes (chosen to contain the same percentage of reticulocytes for all the conditions tested) in a 96-well plate and the initial parasite density was adjusted on a 1:6 ratio (final volume 100 µL, hematocrit 2–5%). Cells were checked at 24 hours postinvasion by doing a cytospin slide stained with Giemsa. The parasite densities were computed after examining a minimum of 500 RBCs.

Data analysis

Data were entered and analyzed with STATA12 (StataCorp, Texas). Reticulocytes were counted after 14 days of differentiation and the mean±SD calculated for each source of HSPC. The Kruskall-Wallis test was used to compare population means. Means and standard deviations were calculated to summarize HSPC expansion rates.

Ethics statement

P. vivax samples collection was approved by the ethics committees of the faculty of tropical medicine, Mahidol University, Bangkok, Thailand (number MUTM-2008-15) and the University of Oxford, Centre for Clinical Vaccinology and Tropical Medicine, United Kingdom (Ethics approval number: OXTREC 027-025). UCB were collected from the cord blood bank at the Gasthuisberg Hospital, Leuven, Belgium (Ethics approval number ML6620). Bone marrow samples were taken from voluntary donors at the Gasthuisberg hospital, Leuven, Belgium (Ethics approval number B322201112107). Adult peripheral blood samples were bought from the Antwerp Red Cross blood bank.

A written inform consent was signed by each donor.

Results

Reticulocyte production from BM, PB and UCB CD34+-enriched cell populations

Reticulocyte differentiation was successfully induced from magnetically sorted CD34+-enriched populations from UCB, PBMC and BM in three independent experiments (n = 3). The enrichment for CD34+ cells in the sorted populations was 55% (SD±6) for UCB, 35% (SD±8) for BM and 16% (SD±6), for PBMC (3 independent experiments) as determined by FACS. The peak of enucleation occurred after 14 days of differentiation,

D0 of expansion

D5 of expansion

UCB:

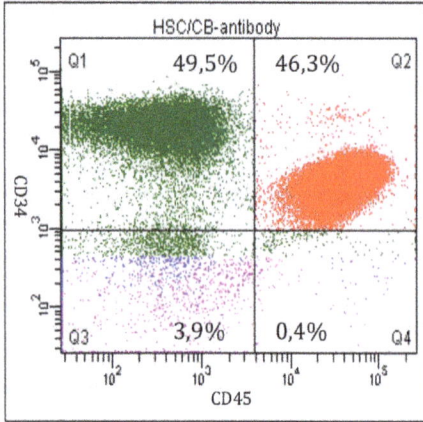 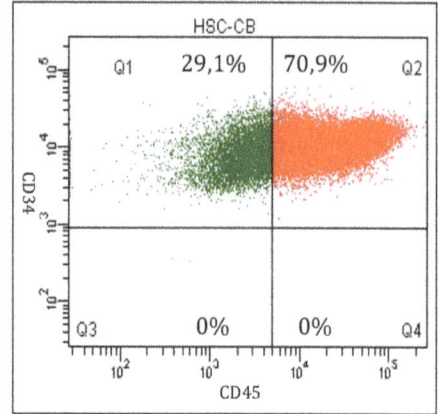

BM

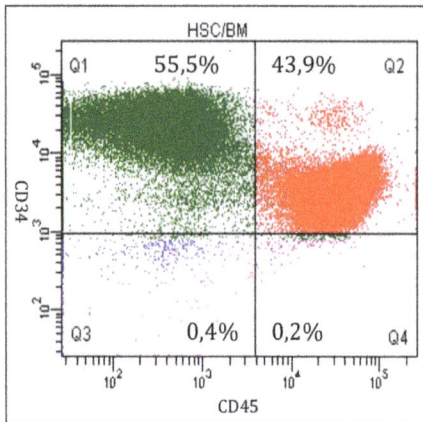 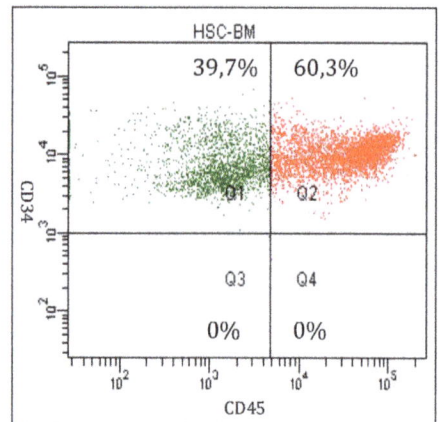

PBMC

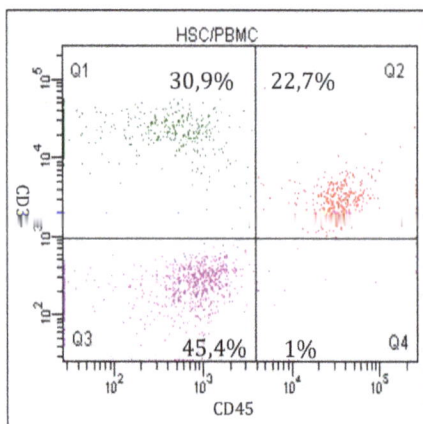 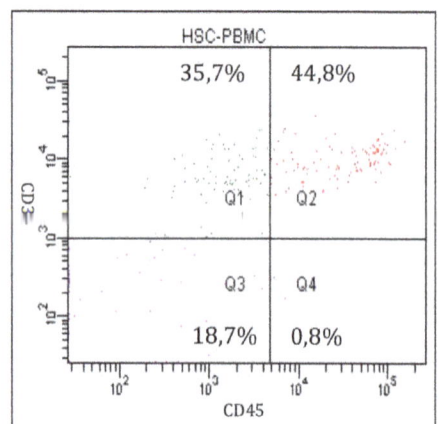

Figure 1. FACS analyses of the CD34$^+$/CD45$^+$ cells from UCB, PBMNC and BM, after isolation (Day 0) and following 5 days of expansion. The Q2 gate represents the population double positive for CD34 (APC) and CD45 (PE).

regardless of the source. The enucleation of erythroid cells from PBMC (mean = 32, SD±6) was significantly higher (p = 0.002) than that of UCB (18%, SD±1.3 and BM (21%, SD±1.5) (Table 1, 6 independent experiments).

Reticulocyte production from *ex vivo* expanded BM, PB and UCB CD34-enriched cell populations

We next tested if larger numbers of reticulocytes could be obtained from *ex vivo* expanded CD34$^+$-enriched cell populations. After 5 days of expansion in serum-free medium with TPO and SCF, the total cell populations increased >10-fold in cultures initiated with UCB/CD34$^+$-enriched cells, 3-fold for BM/CD34$^+$-enriched cells while for PBMC no expansion was observed (Table 1, 3 independent experiments). FACS analysis demonstrated an increase in the CD34$^+$/CD45$^+$ population between Day 0 and Day 5 for all three cell sources: from 55% to 70% (SD±2) for UCB, 35% to 55% (SD±5) for BM, and 16% to 29% (SD±16) for PBMC (n = 3 for CB and BM, n = 2 for PBMC)(Figure 1).

Following expansion, a similar number of cells (irrespective of the CD34$^+$ content or expansion) were cultured under reticulocyte differentiation conditions. After 7 days of erythroid differentiation, the total number of cells, previously subject to an expansion step, was 3 times higher compared to CD34$^+$ cells that were immediately induced to differentiate. After 14 days of differentiation, expanded cells expressed high levels of CD235a and CD71 receptors, regardless of cell source (respectively 87.4% for UCB, 81.7% for BM and 70.6% for PB; Figure 2). Compared to unexpanded cells, the proportion of reticulocytes obtained at day 14 from *in vitro* expanded CD34$^+$ cells was 5 to 10-fold higher.

P. vivax invasion

P. vivax parasites invaded reticulocytes derived from CD34$^+$ cells or directly obtained from enriched blood (PB or UCB;

Figure 3). The mean invasion rates for the different sources of HSPC sources were 3.05%, 3.05% and 3.15% respectively for UCB, BM and PB (n = 4). The means for UCB-concentrated reticulocytes (n = 4) and PB-concentrated reticulocytes (n = 3) were respectively 1.4% and 0.2%.

When using the same *P. vivax* isolate, the invasion rate between different HSPC sources did not differ for all of the 4 *P. vivax* isolates tested (Figure 4a); however, the invasion rate observed varied for each of the *P. vivax* isolates used. When we compared two different *P. vivax* isolates using the same HSPC-derived reticulocytes, the invasion rate varied significantly by isolate (Figure 4b; PV1 and PV2, p<0.001). After 3 days of culture, only few rings (parasite density <0.05%) could be observed and none survived longer than 72 hours, regardless of the HSPC source. Interestingly, the invasion rate of *P. vivax* in HSPC-derived reticulocytes appeared to be higher when compared with reticulocytes isolated directly from PB. For the same *P. vivax* isolate, the parasite density 24 hours post-invasion in UCB/HSPC-derived reticulocytes was up to 9-fold higher than in UCB-concentrated reticulocytes (1.8% *versus* 0.2%, respectively), and 18-fold higher than adult PB-concentrated reticulocytes (2.1% *versus* 0.1% respectively). Parasite densities were not significantly different between HSPC-derived reticulocytes (5%), UCB-concentrated reticulocytes (4.6% p = 0.056) and PB-concentrated reticulocytes (3.5% p = 0.06) when the reticulocyte percentage was 20% for HSPC-derived reticulocytes and respectively 60% and 70% for reticulocytes concentrated from PB and UCB.

Discussion

In this study, we compare for the first time different source of HSPC to generate reticulocytes suitable for *P. vivax* studies. We could demonstrate that compared with CD34$^+$-enriched populations from PB and BM, CD34$^+$-enriched populations from UCB

UCB   BM   PB

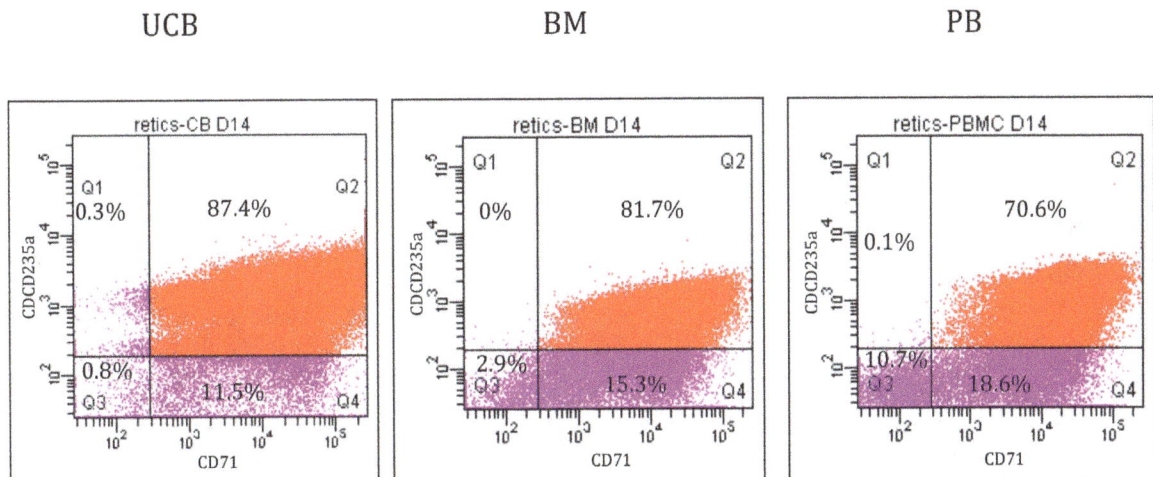

Figure 2. FACS analyses of the CD235a$^+$/CD71$^+$ cells from UCB, PBMNC and BM, after 5 days of expansion and 14 days of differentiation. The Q2 gate represents the population positive for CD235a (Per-CP-Cy5-5) and CD71 (PE).

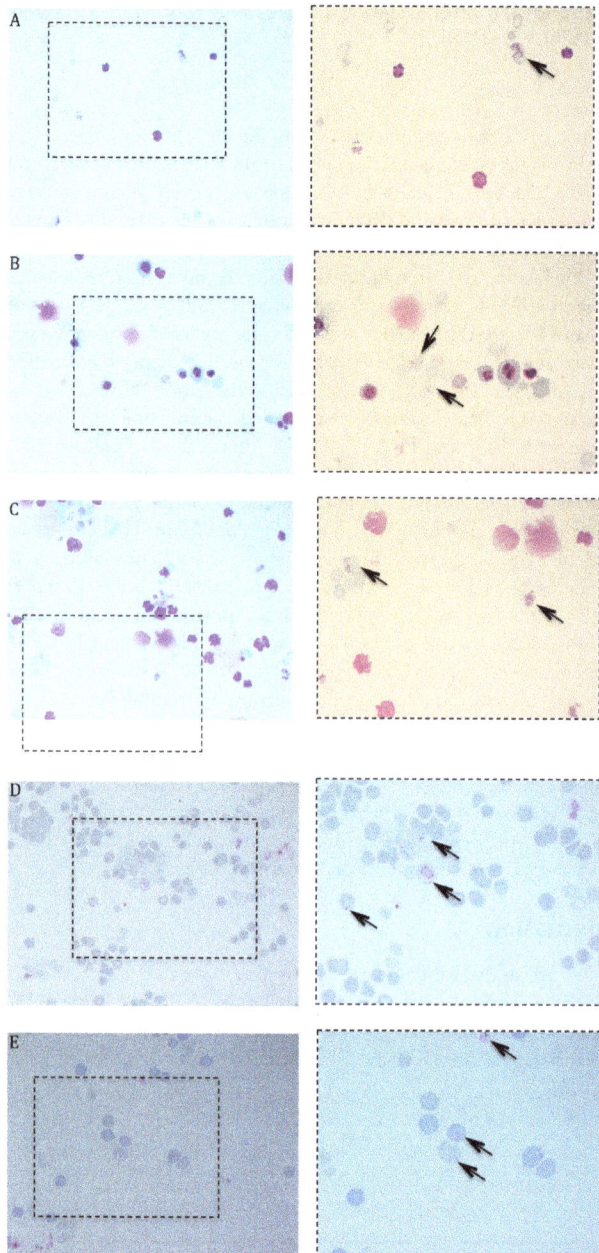

Figure 3. Cytopsin of the *P. vivax* culture 24 h post-invasion for different sources of reticulocytes. A) UCB/HSPC, B) BM/HSPC, C) PB/HSPC, D) reticulocytes-enriched UCB and E) reticulocytes-enriched PB. The left panels represent pictures with a 63× magnification and the corresponding right panels represent a 100× of the left picture square. *P. vivax* infected cells are under arrow.

produced the highest number of reticulocytes that can be invaded by *P. vivax*. Second, when CD34+-enriched cells were first expanded, a further extensive increase in reticulocytes was generated from UCB, to a lesser degree BM but not PB.

The number of reticulocytes derived from UCB CD34+ enriched cell populations could be substantially increased when the CD34+ cells were first expanded for 5 days. Noteworthy, in our experiments PB/HSPC cells showed a limited increase of the population after 5 days of expansion compared to UCB/HSPC and BM/HSPC. This is likely due to the low frequency of CD34+

cell in non-mobilized PBMC [12] and the more mature fate of HSPC in PB or BM compared to cells from UCB [13].

Reticulocytes derived from magnetically sorted CD34+ cells from either PBMC, BM or UCB could be invaded by *P. vivax* with similar efficiencies, while invasion was significantly influenced by the type of *P. vivax* isolate. Despite successful invasion, none of the produced reticulocyte population could support the full development and long-term culture of *P. vivax*. Reticulocytes generated in this study were more permissive for *P. vivax* invasion compared with the study published by Panichakul *et al* [6], who observed only 0.0015% of invasion, mainly due to a very low percentage of reticulocytes (0.5%); or Furuya *et al* [14] who used frozen erythroblast derived from UCB/HSPC (0.8% parasitemia). The 3.5% parasitemia rate observed in our study are in line with the invasion rate observed by Borlon *et al* (2.1%) [11] and Russell *et al* (3.7%) [4], both using reticulocyte-enriched UCB (percentage of reticulocytes greater than 50%).

Our observations might also suggest a preference of *P. vivax* for more immature reticulocytes as we observed a higher invasion rate of reticulocytes derived from any HSPC source compared to those concentrated from either UCB or PB. The higher invasion rate in HSPC derived reticulocytes concentrated from UCB compared to those from PB could be explained by the distribution of their reticulocytes populations. Indeed, Paterakis *et al* [15] classified reticulocytes according to their RNA content by FACS analysis and divided them into 3 categories, i.e. immature reticulocytes (high amount of RNA), median, and old reticulocytes (medium and low amount of RNA, respectively). They found that among the reticulocyte population, UCB contains more immature reticulocytes (13.6%) than adult peripheral blood (1%). Furthermore, HSPC-derived reticulocytes were collected at the peak of enucleation, i.e. when they were at an immature stage of development. This provides additional evidence for preference of *P. vivax* for immature reticulocytes and should be further investigated.

When reticulocyte-enriched blood from UCB and PB was used at 3-fold higher reticulocyte concentrations (70% and 60%, respectively), the invasion rates became similar to that obtained with HSPC-derived reticulocytes (20% for HSPC). This is in line with a recently published report by Martín-Jaular *et al* [16] wherein the authors observed a predominant invasion of CD71high-expression cells (CD71 being a marker of reticulocyte maturation, as their expression decrease while the reticulocyte maturate to the RBC stage) by *P. yoelii* (a mouse *Plasmodium* species also invading preferentially reticulocytes).

Our preliminary observations need further in-depth investigation to provide new insights into the invasion mechanisms of *P. vivax*, and more specifically on the critical stage-specific receptors. If confirmed, this hypothesis would justify the use of reticulocytes derived from HSPC instead of reticulocyte-enriched blood as target cells for the establishment of continuous *P. vivax* cultures.

In conclusion, our results demonstrate that it is possible to produce large amounts of immature reticulocytes that can be efficiently invaded by *P. vivax*. The ability to derive reticulocytes from UCB/HSPCs in in larger quantities than from PB or BM/HSPCs without loosing the permissiveness to *P. vivax* make this source of HSPC as more suitable and likely to develop into a standardized and continuous source of reticulocytes for the long-term culture of *P. vivax*.

The possibility to efficiently expand the CD34+ population to generate more reticulocytes coupled with the possibility to cryopreserve those HSPC-derived reticulocytes [7] opens also new perspectives to create stocks of reticulocytes to use as target cells for the establishment of an *in vitro* culture of *P. vivax*.

a) Parasite density for different sources of HSPC-derived reticulocytes with 1 *P. vivax* isolate.

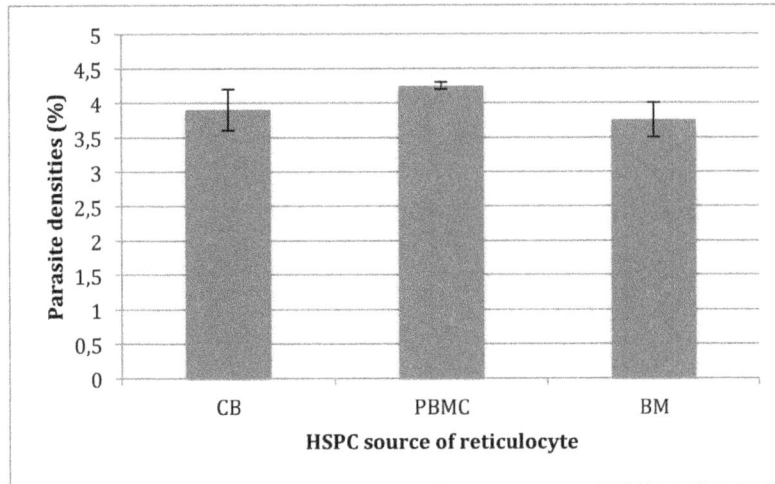

b) Parasite density for each source of reticulocytes with different *P. vivax* isolates.

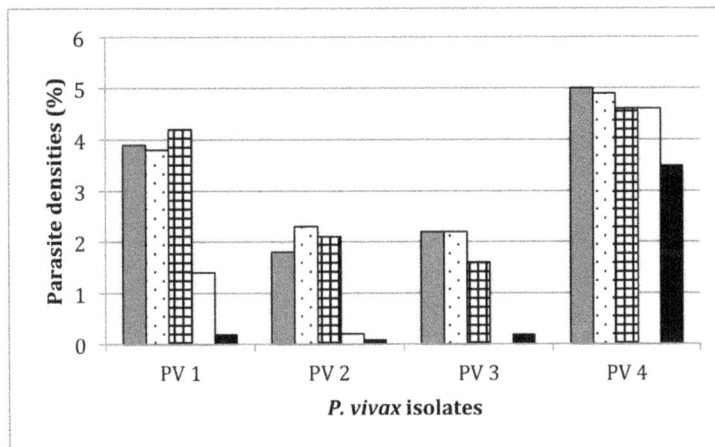

Figure 4. Parasite densities 24 hours post-invasion with *P. vivax*. The parasite density was counted for at least 500 red blood cells, dividing the number of infected enucleated cells by the total number of cells and multiplied by 100 (%). a) Parasite density for different sources of HSPC-derived reticulocytes with 1 *P. vivax* isolate. The mean and SD of 2 different batches of differentiated reticulocytes was calculated for each source of HSPC and tested for invasion with the same *P. vivax* isolate. b) Parasite density for each source of reticulocytes with different *P. vivax* isolates. Parasite densities (%) were counted by dividing the number of *P. vivax* ring-infected cells by the total number of counted RBCs and multiplying the result by 100. Different reticulocyte sources were tested: grey = UCB/HSPC-derived reticulocytes; dotted = BM/HSPC-derived reticulocytes; squared = PBMC/HSPC-derived reticulocytes; white = reticulocytes concentrated from UCB, black = reticulocytes concentrated from adult peripheral blood. PV1 and PV2 were tested with the same batches of HSPC-derived reticulocytes for the 3 different sources (UCB, BM and PBMC). For PV4, the proportion of reticulocytes was 20% for HSCP-derived reticulocytes and respectively 70% and 60% for reticulocytes concentrated from UCB adult peripheral blood.

Acknowledgments

We would like to thanks Prof. Michel Delforge for kindly providing us with the bone marrow samples and Thomas Vanwelden for isolation of bone marrow mononuclear cells. We also thank Prof François Nosten and his team (SMRU) for providing the *plasmodium vivax* isolates.

Author Contributions

Conceived and designed the experiments: FN JKM. Performed the experiments: FN. Analyzed the data: FN CMV AE. Contributed reagents/materials/analysis tools: ARU AE. Wrote the paper: FN JKM JVDA UDA AE CB ARU CMV.

References

1. Price RN, Tjitra E, Guerra CA, Yeung S, White NJ, et al. (2007) Vivax malaria: neglected and not benign. The American journal of tropical medicine and hygiene 77: 79–87.

2. Noulin F, Borlon C, Van Den Abbeele J, D'Alessandro U, Erhart A (2013) 1912–2012: a century of research on Plasmodium vivax in vitro culture. Trends in parasitology 29: 286–294.

3. Moreno-Perez DA, Ruiz JA, Patarroyo MA (2013) Reticulocytes: Plasmodium vivax target cells. Biology of the cell/under the auspices of the European Cell Biology Organization 105: 251–260.

4. Russell B, Suwanarusk R, Borlon C, Costa FT, Chu CS, et al. (2011) A reliable ex vivo invasion assay of human reticulocytes by Plasmodium vivax. Blood 118: e74–81.

5. Golenda CF, Li J, Rosenberg R (1997) Continuous in vitro propagation of the malaria parasite Plasmodium vivax. Proceedings of the National Academy of Sciences of the United States of America 94: 6786–6791.

6. Panichakul T, Sattabongkot J, Chotivanich K, Sirichaisinthop J, Cui L, et al. (2007) Production of erythropoietic cells in vitro for continuous culture of Plasmodium vivax. International journal for parasitology 37: 1551–1557.

7. Noulin F, Borlon C, van den Eede P, Boel L, Verfaillie CM, et al. (2012) Cryopreserved Reticulocytes Derived from Hematopoietic Stem Cells Can Be Invaded by Cryopreserved Plasmodium vivax Isolates. PloS one 7: e40798.

8. Douay L, Andreu G (2007) Ex vivo production of human red blood cells from hematopoietic stem cells: what is the future in transfusion? Transfusion medicine reviews 21: 91–100.

9. Fernandez-Becerra C, Lelievre J, Ferrer M, Anton N, Thomson R, et al. (2013) Red blood cells derived from peripheral blood and bone marrow CD34(+) human haematopoietic stem cells are permissive to Plasmodium parasites infection. Memorias do Instituto Oswaldo Cruz 108: 801–803.

10. Giarratana MC, Kobari L, Lapillonne H, Chalmers D, Kiger L, et al. (2005) Ex vivo generation of fully mature human red blood cells from hematopoietic stem cells. Nature biotechnology 23: 69–74.

11. Borlon C, Russell B, Sriprawat K, Suwanarusk R, Erhart A, et al. (2012) Cryopreserved Plasmodium vivax and cord blood reticulocytes can be used for invasion and short term culture. International journal for parasitology 42: 155–160.

12. Bender JG, Unverzagt K, Walker DE, Lee W, Smith S, et al. (1994) Phenotypic analysis and characterization of CD34+ cells from normal human bone marrow, cord blood, peripheral blood, and mobilized peripheral blood from patients undergoing autologous stem cell transplantation. Clinical immunology and immunopathology 70: 10–18.

13. Steidl U, Kronenwett R, Rohr UP, Fenk R, Kliszewski S, et al. (2002) Gene expression profiling identifies significant differences between the molecular phenotypes of bone marrow-derived and circulating human CD34+ hematopoietic stem cells. Blood 99: 2037–2044.

14. Furuya T, Sa JM, Chitnis CE, Wellems TE, Stedman TT (2014) Reticulocytes from cryopreserved erythroblasts support Plasmodium vivax infection in vitro. Parasitology international 63: 278–284.

15. Paterakis GS, Lykopoulou L, Papassotiriou J, Stamulakatou A, Kattamis C, et al. (1993) Flow-cytometric analysis of reticulocytes in normal cord blood. Acta haematologica 90: 182–185.

16. Martin-Jaular L, Elizalde-Torrent A, Thomson-Luque R, Ferrer M, Segovia JC, et al. (2013) Reticulocyte-prone malaria parasites predominantly invade CD71hi immature cells: implications for the development of an in vitro culture for Plasmodium vivax. Malaria journal 12: 434.

Defects in the Acquisition of Tumor-Killing Capability of CD8+ Cytotoxic T Cells in Streptozotocin-Induced Diabetic Mice

Shu-Ching Chen[1], Yu-Chia Su[2], Ya-Ting Lu[3], Patrick Chow-In Ko[4], Pei-Yu Chang[1], Hung-Ju Lin[3], Hong-Nerng Ho[5], Yo-Ping Lai[3]*

1 Department of Medical Research, National Taiwan University Hospital, Taipei, Taiwan, 2 National Laboratory Animal Center, National Applied Research Laboratories, Taipei, Taiwan, 3 Department of Internal Medicine, National Taiwan University Hospital, Taipei, Taiwan, 4 Department of Emergency Medicine, National Taiwan University Hospital, Taipei, Taiwan, 5 Department of Obstetrics and Gynecology, National Taiwan University, College of Medicine, Taipei, Taiwan

Abstract

Emerging evidences have shown that diabetes mellitus not only raises risk but also heightens mortality rate of cancer. It is not clear, however, whether antitumor CD8+ cytotoxic T lymphocyte (CTL) response is down-modulated in diabetic hosts. We investigated the impact of hyperglycemia on CTLs' acquisition of tumor-killing capability by utilizing streptozotocin-induced diabetic (STZ-diabetic) mice. Murine diabetes was induced by intraperitoneal injection of STZ (200 mg/kg) in C57BL/6 mice, 2C-T cell receptor (TCR) transgenic and P14-TCR transgenic mice. The study found that, despite harboring intact proliferative capacity measured with CFSE labeling and MTT assay, STZ-diabetic CD8+ CTLs displayed impaired effector functions. After stimulation, STZ-diabetic CD8+ CTLs produced less perforin and TNFα assessed by intracellular staining, as well as expressed less CD103 protein. Furthermore, adoptive transfer of STZ-diabetic P14 CD8+ effector cells showed an insufficient recruitment to the B16.gp33 melanoma and inadequate production of perforin, granzyme B and TNFα determined by immunohistochemistry in the tumor milieu. As a result, STZ-diabetic CD8+ effector cells were neither able to eliminate tumor nor to improve survival of tumor-bearing mice. Taken together, our data suggest that CD8+ CTLs are crippled to infiltrate into tumors and thus fail to acquire tumor-killing capability in STZ-diabetic hosts.

Editor: George Kassiotis, MRC National Institute for Medical Research, United Kingdom

Funding: The study was supported by grants from National Science Council (NSC 99-2314-B-002-081-MY3), National Taiwan University Hospital (NTUH. 98P22) and Liver Disease Prevention and Treatment Research Foundation. The funders had no role in study design, data collection and analysis, decision to publish, or preparation of the manuscript.

Competing Interests: The authors have declared that no competing interests exist.

* Email: yopinglai@ntu.edu.tw

Introduction

Diabetes and cancer are severe health concerns of worldwide significance. According to the estimation of World Health Organization, 347 million people worldwide have diabetes. In addition to severe complications caused by chronic hyperglycemia, epidemiological studies show that diabetic patients have higher risk of cancer [1–6], suggesting that diabetic patients carry impaired anti-tumor immunity.

CTL plays a cardinal role in anti-tumor defense. Upon activation, naïve CD8+ T cells are driven to clonal expansion and differentiation into the CTLs that exert cytokine production and tumor-lysis activity [7–10]. Glucose is essential fuel for T cell activation, proliferation, and acquisition of effector functions [11–15]. Chronic exposure to hyperglycemia may result in delayed response to antigen stimulation and failure to eliminate implanted ultraviolet-induced tumors [16–21]. The hypothesis is proposed that diabetes may cause defective CD8+ T cell responses that render diabetic hosts bearing poor tumor control. Nevertheless, two important questions remain unanswered. First, whether the diabetic condition hinders CD8+ T cell activation and differen-

tiation into functional effector cells remains undefined. Second, it remains elusive in what extent of CD8+ T cells that are hampered by acute hyperglycemia.

STZ is used to induce diabetes by damaging pancreatic β-cells, resulting in insulin deficiency and consequently hyperglycemia [22,23]. To investigate whether diabetes causes CD8+ T cell impairment, we used STZ-diabetic murine model to examine CD8+ T cell activation and differentiation both in vitro and in vivo. Furthermore, to evaluate anti-tumor immunity of STZ-diabetic CD8+ T cells, the effector functions at early and late differentiation stages were checked in vitro. Finally, we used murine melanoma model to assess tumor-killing capability of STZ-diabetic CD8+ T cells by monitoring tumor size and mice survival.

Materials and Methods

Ethical statements

All animal procedures in this study were followed guideline of the Use of Laboratory Animals published by National Taiwan University (NTU) and approved by Institutional Animal Care and

Use Committee (IACUC) of College of Medicine and College of Public Health of NTU (Permit Number: 20100131). Mice were housed on a 12 h light–dark cycle, with the dark cycle occurring from 8:00 P.M. to 8:00 A.M in a specific pathogen-free environment of the animal center at NTU hospital. The mice enrolled in the study were monitored at least three times per week. All surgery was performed under sodium pentobarbital (30–90 mg/kg, intraperitoneal injection) anesthesia, and all efforts were made to minimize suffering. The humane endpoint criteria were set following IACUC guidelines, including the body weight

loss of no more than 20% of pre-procedural weight, tumor size reaching 20 mm in diameter. At the end of experiment, mice were sacrificed by euthanasia with carbon dioxide gas inhalation. The spleens and tumors were collected after sacrifice of the mice.

Mice

Male C57BL/6, B10.A, CD45.1, 2C and P14 TCR-transgenic mice at age of 6–8 weeks were obtained from animal center at NTU Hospital. The mice used in this study included more than

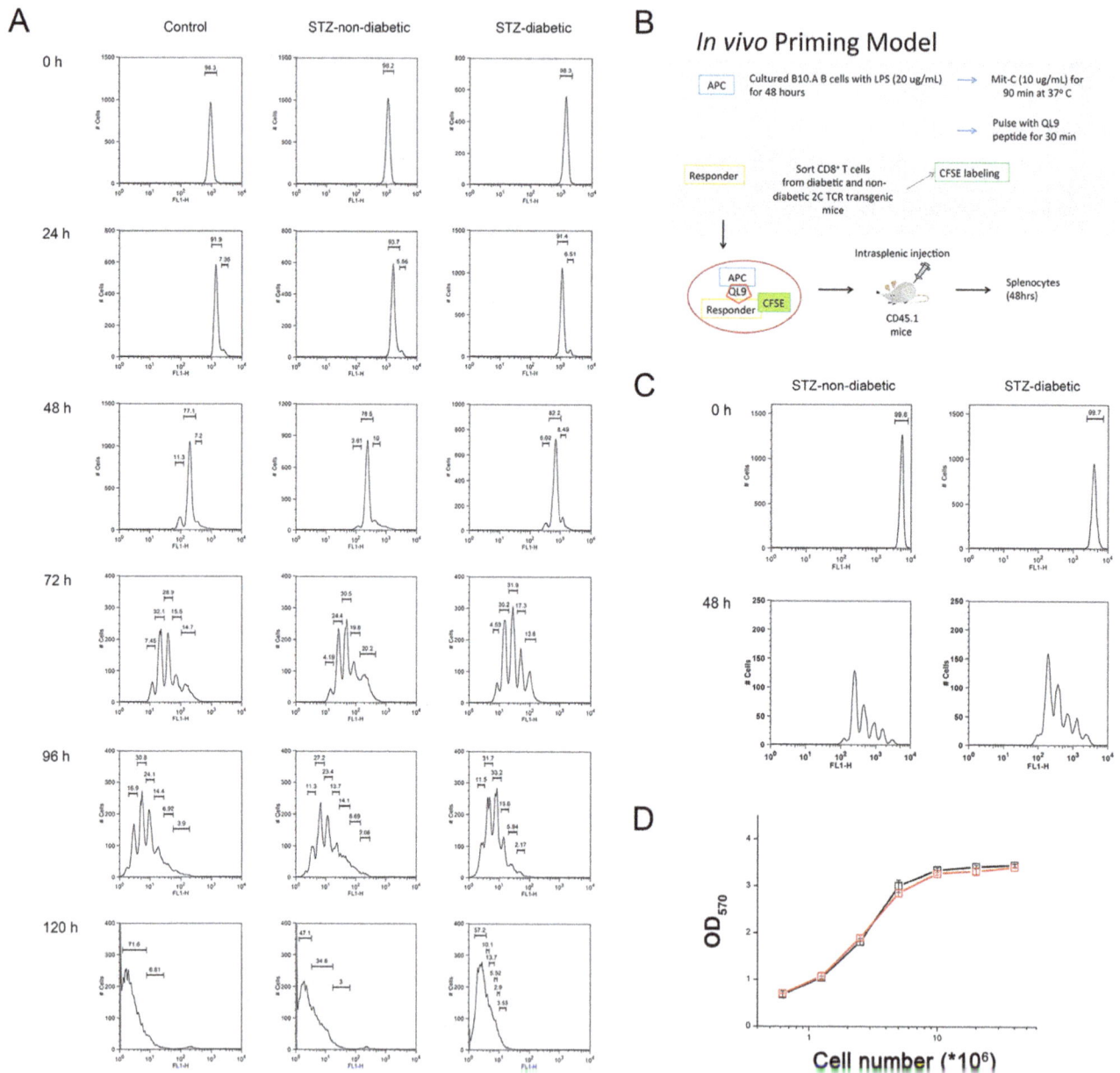

Figure 1. CD8+ T cell proliferation following stimulation. (A) CFSE-labeled STZ-diabetic, STZ-non-diabetic and control naïve CD8+ T cells from C57BL/6 mice were stimulated by anti-CD3/CD28 antibodies *in vitro* at the indicated time (24, 48, 72, 96 and 120 hours) and cell divisions were analyzed by flow cytometry. (B) *In vivo* CD8+ T cell priming model. (C) CFSE-labeled STZ-diabetic or STZ-non-diabetic 2C CD8+ T cells were co-administered with QL9-pulsed B10.A B blast cells into the spleen of healthy CD45.1 mice. Forty eight hours after priming, the splenocytes of CD45.1 mice were stained with PE anti-mouse CD45.2 antibody and cell divisions were analyzed by flow cytometry. (D) Five-day antigen-stimulated 2C CD8+ T cells from STZ-diabetic (red line) and STZ-non-diabetic (black line) mice were cultured in IL-2-containing medium for 24 hours, followed by MTT assay. Mit C, mitomycin C. APC, antigen-presenting cells. The data represent three independent experiments.

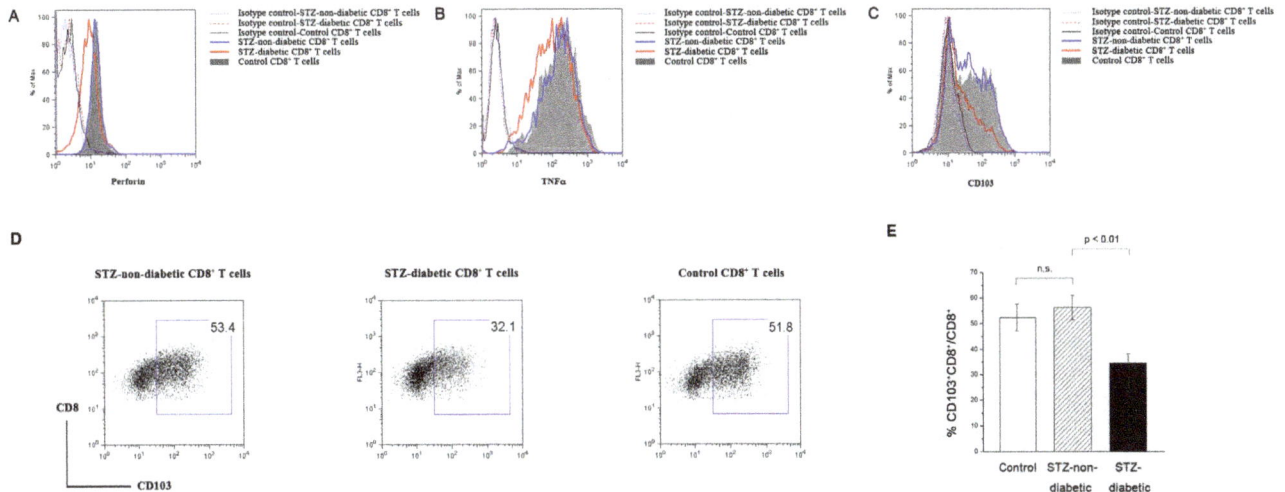

Figure 2. Effector functions of STZ-diabetic CD8$^+$ T cells. (A, B) Naïve CD8$^+$ T cells from STZ-diabetic (red line), STZ-non-diabetic (blue line) and control (gray-filled) C57BL/6 mice were stimulated by anti-CD3/CD28 antibodies *in vitro*. At 24 and 72 hours after stimulation, the production of perforin and TNFα was checked by intracellular staining and analyzed by flow cytometry. (C) At 120 hours of antigenic stimulation, 2C CD8$^+$ T cells from STZ-diabetic (red line) and STZ-non-diabetic (gray-filled) mice were harvested and surface CD103 expression was checked and analyzed by flow cytometry. Staining of isotype control for the three experimental groups was shown: STZ-non-diabetic (blue dot), STZ-diabetic (red dash) and control (black line) mice. (D) CD103-positive population was gated in 5 day-stimulated 2C CD8$^+$ T cells from STZ-non-diabetic, STZ-diabetic and control mice. (E) CD103-positive percentage in 5 day-stimulated 2C CD8$^+$ T cells was analyzed from the three experimental groups. Data are representative of three independent experiments with three to five mice per time point.

eight mice in each group and all experiments were repeated for at least three independent times.

Antibodies and reagents

Anti-mouse CD3 (clone 145-2C11) and anti-CD28 (clone 37.51) antibodies were prepared in our laboratory. DMEM, penicillin and streptomycin from GIBCO Inc. (Grand Island, NY, USA); fetal bovine serum (FBS) from HyClone Inc. (Logan, UT, USA); anti-mouse antibodies including FITC anti-CD3, -IFNγ and -granzyme B, PE anti-CD4, -CD19 and -perforin, PE-Cy5 anti-CD8 and APC anti-CD45.2 antibodies from eBioscience (San Diego, CA, USA); PE anti-TNFα and -CD103 antibodies from BioLegend (San Diego, CA, USA); STZ, Mitomycin C, LPS, MTT, phorbol myristic acid (PMA), Ionomycin and Brefeldin A from Sigma (St. Louis, MO, USA); CFSE from Molecular Probes (Eugene, OR, USA); QL9 (QLSPFPFDL) and KM9 (KAVTN-FATM) peptides from AnaSpec, Inc. (San Jose, CA, USA) were purchased.

Diabetes development

Diabetes was induced by intraperitoneal injection of STZ (200 mg/kg) into male mice as described previously [22,23]. Blood glucose and weight were measured before and after STZ administration. Blood glucose level above 400 mg/dL was defined as diabetes.

Cell preparation and culture conditions

Naïve (CD62L^{hi}CD44^{lo}) CD8$^+$ T cells were obtained from spleens of mice by positive isolation of CD8$^+$ T cells [24], and further by sorting on FACSAria (BD Bioscience, San Jose, CA, USA) through service provided by Flow Cytometric Analyzing and Sorting Core Facility (First Core Laboratory, NTU, College of Medicine). Cells culture was set up in DMEM containing 10% FBS and 5×10^{-5} M 2-Mercaptoethanol. To activate CD8$^+$ T cells, the naïve cells were stimulated by anti-CD3/CD28

antibodies for the indicated time. For activating 2C TCR-transgenic (2C) CD8$^+$ T cells, the cells were stimulated by mitomycin C-treated [25] LPS-stimulated B10.A B blasts [26] and QL9 peptide. Cells were grown in 5% CO_2 humidified air at 37°C. For *in vivo* priming, naïve 2C CD8$^+$ T cells mixed with QL9-pulsed B10.A B blast cells were injected into the spleens of CD45.1 mice.

Cell proliferation assays

CFSE (carboxyfluorescein succinimidyl ester) labeling. CFSE (5 mM) was added to the cells (10×10^6 cells/mL) according to the manufacturer's instructions.

MTT (3-[4,5-dimethylthiazol-2-yl]-2,5-diphenyltetrazolium bromide) assay. Cells were incubated with MTT (1 mg/mL) for 4 hours. The formazan was solubilized by dimethyl sulfoxide and colorimetric absorbance was quantified by measuring optical density (OD) at 570 nm by a spectrophotometer (Tecan Group Ltd., Mannedorf, Switzerland).

Intracellular cytokine staining

After 6-hour culture with PMA (10 ng/mL)/Ionomycine (1 μg/mL) and 4-hour culture with Brefeldin A (10 μg/mL), the cells were fixed and permeabilized with cytofix-cytoperm kit (BD Biosciences) and stained with specific antibodies according to the manufacturer's instructions.

B16.gp33 melanoma model with adoptive transfer of P14 CD8$^+$ effector cells

B16.gp33 cells derived from B16 melanoma cells and genetically modified to express gene encoding amino acid 33–41 of glycoprotein from lymphocytic choriomeningitis virus (LCMV) were kindly provided by Dr. Hanspeter Pircher [27] and cultured in DMEM supplemented with 10% FBS and 200 μg/mL G418. Following subcutaneous inoculation of B16.gp33 cells (1×10^6 cells/mouse), the tumor diameter and survival of mice

A

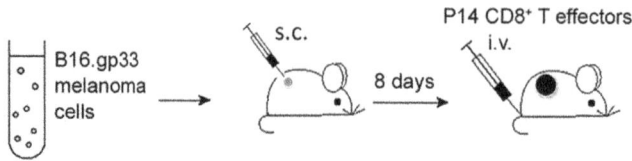

Model of B16.gp33 melanoma with
adoptive transfer of P14 CD8+ T effector cells

B

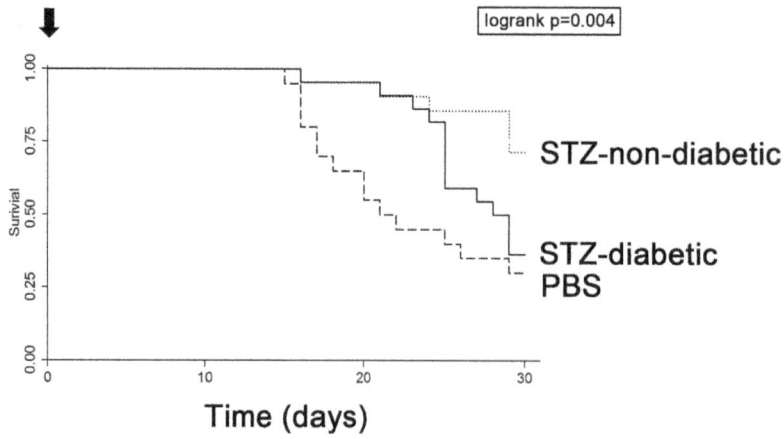

C

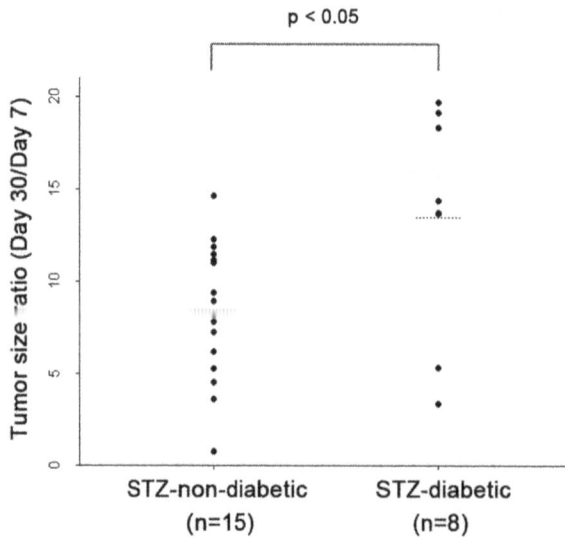

Figure 3. Impaired anti-tumor immunity of STZ-diabetic CTLs. (A) Murine model of B16.gp33 melanoma with adoptive transfer of P14 CD8$^+$ T effector cells. (B) After adoptive transfer of STZ-diabetic (n = 22) or STZ-non-diabetic (n = 21) P14 CD8$^+$ T effector cells into B16.gp33 melanoma-bearing C57BL/6 mice, the survival time of the mice was recorded. Tumor-bearing mice with PBS but not T cells injection were considered as the controls (n = 20). (C) Tumor size of the mice that survived on day 30 after tumor inoculation. The increased fold of tumor size was calculated as tumor size at day 30 divided by that at day 7.

were recorded. P14 CTLs specific for LCMV gp33 in the context of H-2D^b were generated by activating the P14 naïve CD8$^+$ T cells with mitomycin C-treated LPS-activated syngeneic B cell blasts and KM9 peptide, followed by harvest and cultured in recombinant human IL-2 (100 IU/mL)-containing medium as previously described [28]. The P14 CTLs in 1 X PBS (1×10^7 cells/0.15 mL/mouse) were injected intravenously into the mice that had B16.gp33 tumor inoculation for 8 days.

Detection of TNFα granzyme B and perforin in tumor-infiltrating lymphocytes

At 16 hours after transfer of P14 CTLs, the tumors were processed for cryosections and subjected to immunohistochemical staining by 2 μg/mL of FITC anti-granzyme B, PE anti-TNFα, PE anti-perforin and APC anti-CD45.2 antibodies.

Statistical analysis

Experiments were performed independently for at least three times. The percentage of CD103$^+$ cells in CD8$^+$ T cells between three groups was analyzed by unpaired Student's t-test. The difference of relative distribution of immune cells and increased fold of tumor size between two groups was analyzed by Student's t-test. The survival difference between two groups was analyzed by logrank test. The general linear model was fitted for the unbalanced data to assess the difference of CD 45.2$^+$ cell infiltration between two groups. Statistical significance was set at a p value of less than 0.05.

Results

STZ-diabetic mice and relative distribution of CD8$^+$ T cells in peripheral lymphoid tissues

C57BL/6 male mice at the age of 6–8 weeks were administered with STZ intraperitoneally. Twenty days after STZ injection, blood glucose level was significantly increased (>400 mg/dL vs. non-diabetic control: 142.9 ± 16.5 mg/dL, $p < 0.05$) and weight was significantly decreased (18.5 ± 1.7 g vs. 25.4 ± 1.7 g, $p < 0.05$) in STZ-diabetic mice (n = 22) compared to non-diabetic control mice (n = 15). The splenocytes of STZ-diabetic and C57BL/6 control mice were immune-phenotyped and analyzed by flow cytometry to study the relative distribution of CD8$^+$ T cells in peripheral lymphoid tissues in diabetic condition, showing no significant difference between STZ-diabetic and control mice. To investigate whether the numbers of naïve CD62L^{hi}CD44^{lo}CD8$^+$ T cells were changed in STZ-diabetic mice, the expression of CD62L and CD44 proteins in CD3$^+$CD8$^+$ T cells were further inspected. It showed that naïve CD8$^+$ T cells still remained a significant population in the spleen of STZ-diabetic mice (data not shown).

Proliferation of STZ-diabetic CD8$^+$ T cells after activation

To investigate STZ-diabetic CD8$^+$ T cell activation, CFSE-labeled naïve CD8$^+$ T cells from STZ-diabetic and control C57BL/6 mice were stimulated by anti-CD3/CD28 antibodies *in vitro*, respectively, and harvested at indicated time for analyzing cell proliferation. It showed that, as control cells, STZ-diabetic CD8$^+$ T cells had high proliferative capability (Figure 1A). To

further study diabetic CD8$^+$ T cell activation by specific antigenic peptide, the cell proliferation following *in vivo* priming was assessed (Figure 1B). It revealed that after priming for 48 hours, more than 50% of both STZ-diabetic and STZ-non-diabetic 2C CD8$^+$ T cells had 3–4 cell divisions (Figure 1C), indicating that STZ-diabetic CD8$^+$ T cells still attain proliferative capability upon stimulation *in vivo*. To further study the proliferative capability in late activated stage, 5-day stimulated 2C CD8$^+$ T cells were cultured in IL-2-containing medium for 24 hours and cell proliferation was analyzed, revealing no significant difference between STZ-diabetic and STZ-non-diabetic groups (Figure 1D). Taken together, the results indicated that as non-diabetic cells, the STZ-diabetic CD8$^+$ T cells possess proliferative potential.

Effector function of STZ-diabetic CD8$^+$ T cells

The anti-CD3/CD28-stimulated CD8$^+$ T cells from STZ-diabetic and non-diabetic control C57BL/6 mice were harvested at indicated time for checking the effector function. Significant production of IL-2, IFNγ and Granzyme B was observed in all groups (data not shown). However, STZ-diabetic CD8$^+$ T cells produced less perforin and TNFα at 24–72 hours after stimulation (Figures 2A and 2B), indicating an impaired effector function at early differentiation stage. Besides, expression of CD103protein was significantly lower in STZ-diabetic 2C CD8$^+$ T cells on day 5 following stimulation (Figure 2C). Of note, fewer CD103$^+$ cells were present in STZ-diabetic CD8$^+$ T cell population (Figures 2D and 2E), implying accumulation deficit of diabetic CTLs in tumor and thereby compromising anti-tumor immunity.

Anti-tumor immunity of STZ-induced diabetic CD8$^+$ T cells

To investigate tumor-killing capability of STZ-diabetic CD8$^+$ T cells *in vivo*, B16-gp33 melanoma cells were subcutaneously inoculated, followed by adoptive transfer of the tumor-specific P14 CD8$^+$ effector cells intravenously (Figure 3A). All the mice developed tumor and 70% of the PBS control group (14/20) died of tumor burden whereas, only 29% of the mice with adoptive transfer of STZ-non-diabetic P14 CD8$^+$ effector cells died (6/21) during the experimental observation period. It showed that adoptive transfer of STZ-non-diabetic P14 CD8$^+$ effector cells caused a prolonged survival from 36% (8/22 mice of STZ-diabetic group) to 71% (15/21 mice of STZ-non-diabetic group) of tumor-bearing mice on 30 days after tumor inoculation (Figure 3B, $p < 0.01$). By contrast, transfer of the STZ-diabetic P14 CD8$^+$ effector cells did not show beneficial effect on survival (8/22 mice of STZ-diabetic group vs. 6/20 mice of PBS injection group). Furthermore, smaller tumor size was revealed in STZ-non-diabetic P14 CD8$^+$ effector cells-treated group (Figure 3C, $p < 0.05$). Taken together, STZ-diabetic CD8$^+$ T cells are defective in tumor eradication *in vivo*. To elucidate the tumor-infiltrating efficacy of tumor-specific T cells, the tumor was removed and intra-tumor CD45.2$^+$ cells was analyzed by immunohistochemical staining at 16 hours after adoptive transfer of P14 CD8$^+$ effector cells (CD45.2$^+$) into tumor-bearing CD45.1 mice, (Figure 4A). Significantly fewer CD45.2$^+$ cells were found in the tumor of mice receiving STZ-diabetic P14 CD8$^+$ effector cells than STZ-non-diabetic group (Figure 4B), STZ-diabetic: 24.8, 95% confidence

A

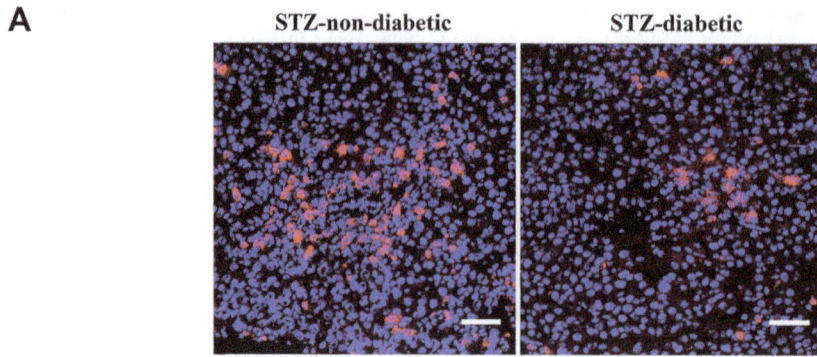

B

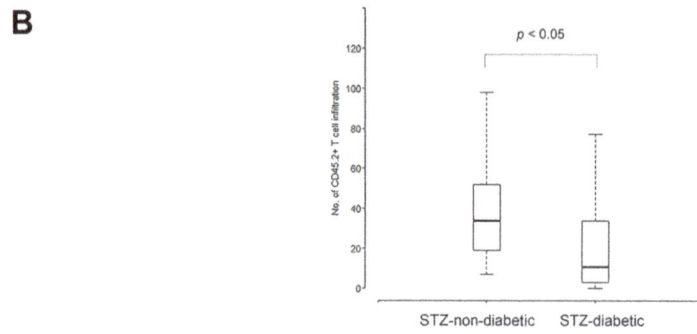

C

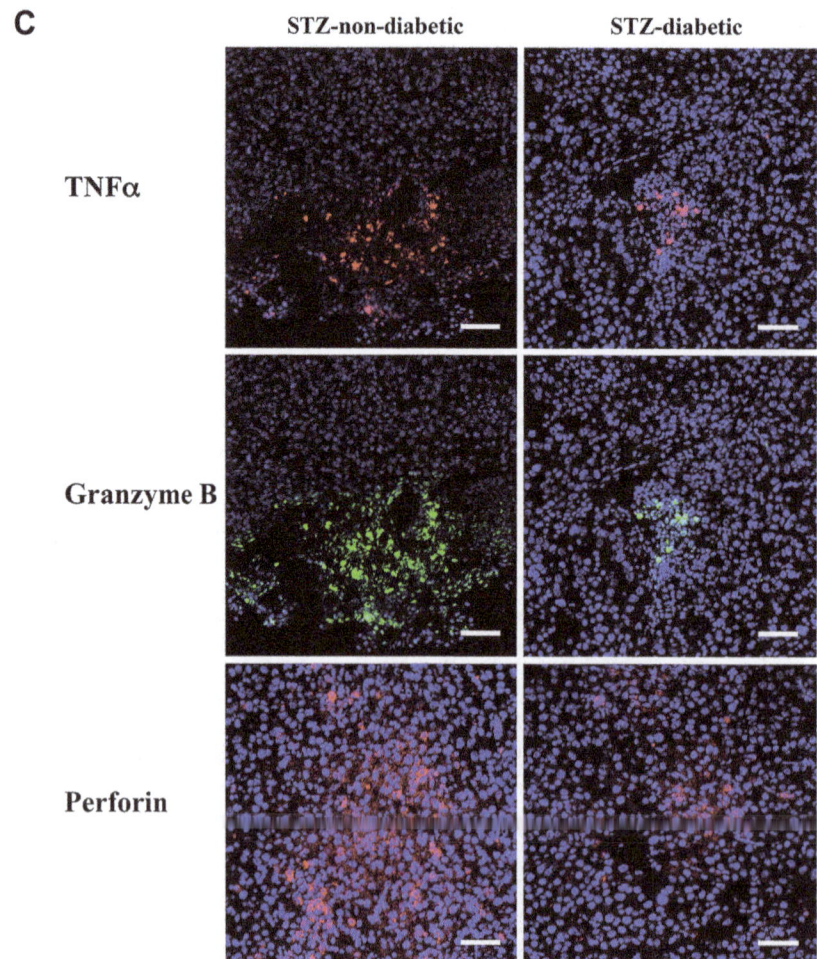

Figure 4. Infiltration and cytotoxicity of STZ-diabetic CTLs in tumor. (A, B) Assessment of the tumor-specific CTL infiltration in the tumor. Sixteen hours after adoptive transfer of STZ-diabetic or STZ-non-diabetic P14 CD8$^+$ T effector cells into tumor-bearing CD45.1 mice, the tumors were processed for cryosections and stained by APC anti-mouse CD45.2 antibody and Hoechst 33342. (C) The production of TNFα, granzyme B and perforin by STZ-diabetic or STZ-non-diabetic P14 CTLs was monitored by immunostaining the tumors with specific antibodies and Hoechst 33342, and were visualized by a Zeiss LSM 510 confocal microscope. Scale bar: 50 µm.

interval (CI), 14.8–34.8; STZ-non-diabetic: 43.7, 95% CI, 34.4–52.9; $p<0.01$. the difference: 18.9, 95% CI, 5.3–32.5; $p<0.01$). Moreover, there were significantly fewer perforin-, granzyme B- and TNFα-producing cells in the tumor of mice receiving STZ-diabetic P14 CD8$^+$ effector cells than STZ-non-diabetic group (Figure 4C). Therefore, STZ-diabetic P14 T cells had impaired effector function and were ineffective against tumor burden *in vivo*.

Discussion

Diabetic patients have an increased incidence of cancers [1–6], suggesting that diabetes hampers anti-tumor CTL function. Considerable evidence has accumulated supporting the importance of abundant tumor-infiltrating CTLs for better outcomes in various types of cancers [29–31]. Therefore, appropriate intra-tumor migration of CTLs is a prerequisite for antitumor surveillance. Our data showed that adoptive transfer of STZ-diabetic CD8$^+$ effector cells resulted in fewer tumor-infiltrating T cells as well as less production of perforin, Granzyme B and TNFα *in situ*. It is plausible that, in addition to defective cytotoxicity, the intra-tumor migration of STZ-diabetic CTLs is impeded.

Recent reports have shown that TNFα can promote influx of tumor-reactive T cells by remodeling intra-tumor vessels [32–34], and thereby exerts a local immunomodulatory function in tumor microenvironment. Our study showed that the less production of intra-tumor TNFα in STZ-diabetic CD8$^+$ T cells-treated mice may lead to insufficient infiltration of tumor-reactive CTLs. Furthermore, anti-tumor defense requires recognition of tumor antigens by CTLs' TCRs and strengthening CTL/tumor cell contacts by LFA-1-ICAM-1 and/or CD103-E-cadherin interaction [35–39]. This firm adhesion constructed by CD103-E-cadherin interaction is crucial for CTLs to kill tumor cells especially when tumors do not express ICAM-1 [37,39]. It ensures tumor killing by promoting the maturation of immunological synapse and polarized release of cytokine and lytic granules. Thus,

significantly less expression of CD103 protein on STZ-diabetic CTLs revealed in our study may cripple CTLs' intratumor migration and firm retention in tumors, leading to insufficient cytokine production and cytotoxicity toward tumor cells.

The findings from the current study strongly suggest that the effect of diabetes on CD8$^+$ T cell function should be reconsidered more precisely. Overall, these results provide values for identifying STZ-induced diabetes may hamper the CTL function as a result of impaired cell differentiation. The enfeebled CTLs with inadequate CD103 expression show ineffective tumor infiltration and insufficient production of the cytotoxic mediators. The elucidation of how effector functions of STZ-diabetic CD8$^+$ T cells are impeded will optimize strategies for advancing tumor-killing capability and inducing protective antitumor immunity in diabetic hosts.

Supporting Information

Checklist S1   The Arrive Guidelines Checklist for Animal Research reports *in vivo* experiments of this study.

Acknowledgments

We thank Dr. Chung-Jiuan Jeng for critical review of the manuscript. We are grateful for Yu-Ching Lin for excellent technical assistance. We appreciate the service provided by the Flow Cytometric Analyzing and Sorting Core Facility of the First Core Laboratory, College of Medicine, National Taiwan University.

Author Contributions

Conceived and designed the experiments: SCC YPL. Performed the experiments: SCC YCS YTL PYC. Analyzed the data: SCC YCS YTL PYC HJL. Contributed reagents/materials/analysis tools: PCIK HNH. Wrote the paper: SCC YPL.

References

1. Giovannucci E, Harlan DM, Archer MC, Bergenstal RM, Gapstur SM, et al. (2010) Diabetes and cancer: a consensus report. Diabetes Care 33: 1674–1685.
2. Stattin P, Bjor O, Ferrari P, Lukanova A, Lenner P, et al. (2007) Prospective study of hyperglycemia and cancer risk. Diabetes Care 30: 561–567.
3. Connolly GC, Safadjou S, Chen R, Nduaguba A, Dunne R, et al. (2012) Diabetes mellitus is associated with the presence of metastatic spread at disease presentation in hepatocellular carcinoma. Cancer Invest 30: 698–702.
4. Chen HF, Liu MD, Chen P, Chen LH, Chang YH, et al. (2013) Risks of Breast and Endometrial Cancer in Women with Diabetes: A Population-Based Cohort Study. PLoS One 8: e67420.
5. Williams JC, Walsh DA, Jackson JF (1984) Colon carcinoma and diabetes mellitus. Cancer 54: 3070–3071.
6. La Vecchia C, D'Avanzo B, Negri E, Franceschi S (1991) History of selected diseases and the risk of colorectal cancer. Eur J Cancer 27: 582–586.
7. Kaech SM, Hemby S, Kersh E, Ahmed R (2002) Molecular and functional profiling of memory CD8 T cell differentiation. Cell 111: 837–851.
8. Lyman MA, Aung S, Biggs JA, Sherman LA (2004) A spontaneously arising pancreatic tumor does not promote the differentiation of naive CD8+ T lymphocytes into effector CTL. J Immunol 172: 6558–6567.
9. Klebanoff CA, Gattinoni L, Torabi-Parizi P, Kerstann K, Cardones AR, et al. (2005) Central memory self/tumor-reactive CD8+ T cells confer superior antitumor immunity compared with effector memory T cells. Proc Natl Acad Sci U S A 102: 9571–9576.
10. Milstein O, Hagin D, Lask A, Reich-Zeliger S, Shezen E, et al. (2011) CTLs respond with activation and granule secretion when serving as targets for T-cell recognition. Blood 117: 1042–1052.
11. Maciver NJ, Jacobs SR, Wieman HL, Wofford JA, Coloff JL, et al. (2008) Glucose metabolism in lymphocytes is a regulated process with significant effects on immune cell function and survival. J Leukoc Biol 84: 949–957.
12. Bental M, Deutsch C (1993) Metabolic changes in activated T cells: an NMR study of human peripheral blood lymphocytes. Magn Reson Med 29: 317–326.
13. Jacobs SR, Herman CE, Maciver NJ, Wofford JA, Wieman HL, et al. (2008) Glucose uptake is limiting in T cell activation and requires CD28-mediated Akt-dependent and independent pathways. J Immunol 180: 4476–4486.
14. MacIver NJ, Michalek RD, Rathmell JC (2013) Metabolic regulation of T lymphocytes. Annu Rev Immunol 31: 259–283.
15. Fox CJ, Hammerman PS, Thompson CB (2005) Fuel feeds function: energy metabolism and the T-cell response. Nat Rev Immunol 5: 844–852.
16. Stentz FB, Kitabchi AE (2003) Activated T lymphocytes in Type 2 diabetes: implications from in vitro studies. Curr Drug Targets 4: 493–503.
17. De Maria R, Todaro M, Stassi G, Di Blasi F, Giordano M, et al. (1994) Defective T cell receptor/CD3 complex signaling in human type I diabetes. Eur J Immunol 24: 999–1002.
18. Delespesse G, Duchateau J, Bastenie PA, Lauvaux JP, Collet H, et al. (1974) Cell-mediated immunity in diabetes mellitus. Clin Exp Immunol 18: 461–467.
19. Eibl N, Spatz M, Fischer GF, Mayr WR, Samstag A, et al. (2002) Impaired primary immune response in type-1 diabetes: results from a controlled vaccination study. Clin Immunol 103: 249–259.

20. Mahmoud AA, Rodman HM, Mandel MA, Warren KS (1976) Induced and spontaneous diabetes mellitus and suppression of cell-mediated immunologic responses. Granuloma formation, delayed dermal reactivity and allograft rejection. J Clin Invest 57: 362–367.

21. Diepersloot RJ, Bouter KP, Beyer WE, Hoekstra JB, Masurel N (1987) Humoral immune response and delayed type hypersensitivity to influenza vaccine in patients with diabetes mellitus. Diabetologia 30: 397–401.

22. Rakieten N, Rakieten ML, Nadkarni MV (1963) Studies on the diabetogenic action of streptozotocin (NSC-37917). Cancer Chemother Rep 29: 91–98.

23. Junod A, Lambert AE, Stauffacher W, Renold AE (1969) Diabetogenic action of streptozotocin: relationship of dose to metabolic response. J Clin Invest 48: 2129–2139.

24. Lai YP, Lin CC, Liao WJ, Tang CY, Chen SC (2009) CD4+ T cell-derived IL-2 signals during early priming advances primary CD8+ T cell responses. PLoS One 4: e7766.

25. Janeway CA Jr, Ron J, Katz ME (1987) The B cell is the initiating antigen-presenting cell in peripheral lymph nodes. J Immunol 138: 1051–1055.

26. Kakiuchi T, Chesnut RW, Grey HM (1983) B cells as antigen-presenting cells: the requirement for B cell activation. J Immunol 131: 109–114.

27. Prevost-Blondel A, Zimmermann C, Stemmer C, Kulmburg P, Rosenthal FM, et al. (1998) Tumor-infiltrating lymphocytes exhibiting high ex vivo cytolytic activity fail to prevent murine melanoma tumor growth in vivo. J Immunol 161: 2187–2194.

28. Castellino F, Huang AY, Altan-Bonnet G, Stoll S, Scheinecker C, et al. (2006) Chemokines enhance immunity by guiding naive CD8+ T cells to sites of CD4+ T cell-dendritic cell interaction. Nature 440: 890–895.

29. Fridman WH, Pages F, Sautes-Fridman C, Galon J (2012) The immune contexture in human tumours: impact on clinical outcome. Nat Rev Cancer 12: 298–306.

30. Naito Y, Saito K, Shiiba K, Ohuchi A, Saigenji K, et al. (1998) CD8+ T cells infiltrated within cancer cell nests as a prognostic factor in human colorectal cancer. Cancer Res 58: 3491–3494.

31. Mahmoud SM, Paish EC, Powe DG, Macmillan RD, Grainge MJ, et al. (2011) Tumor-infiltrating CD8+ lymphocytes predict clinical outcome in breast cancer. J Clin Oncol 29: 1949–1955.

32. Johansson A, Hamzah J, Payne CJ, Ganss R (2012) Tumor-targeted TNFalpha stabilizes tumor vessels and enhances active immunotherapy. Proc Natl Acad Sci U S A 109: 7841–7846.

33. Ganss R, Ryschich E, Klar E, Arnold B, Hammerling GJ (2002) Combination of T-cell therapy and trigger of inflammation induces remodeling of the vasculature and tumor eradication. Cancer Res 62: 1462–1470.

34. Johansson A, Hamzah J, Ganss R (2012) Intratumoral TNFAlpha improves immunotherapy. Oncoimmunology 1: 1395–1397.

35. Anikeeva N, Somersalo K, Sims TN, Thomas VK, Dustin ML, et al. (2005) Distinct role of lymphocyte function-associated antigen-1 in mediating effective cytolytic activity by cytotoxic T lymphocytes. Proc Natl Acad Sci U S A 102: 6437–6442.

36. Springer TA, Dustin ML (2012) Integrin inside-out signaling and the immunological synapse. Curr Opin Cell Biol 24: 107–115.

37. Le Floc'h A, Jalil A, Vergnon I, Le Maux Chansac B, Lazar V, et al. (2007) Alpha E beta 7 integrin interaction with E-cadherin promotes antitumor CTL activity by triggering lytic granule polarization and exocytosis. J Exp Med 204: 559–570.

38. Franciszkiewicz K, Le Floc'h A, Jalil A, Vigant F, Robert T, et al. (2009) Intratumoral induction of CD103 triggers tumor-specific CTL function and CCR5-dependent T-cell retention. Cancer Res 69: 6249–6255.

39. Franciszkiewicz K, Le Floc'h A, Boutet M, Vergnon I, Schmitt A, et al. (2013) CD103 or LFA-1 engagement at the immune synapse between cytotoxic T cells and tumor cells promotes maturation and regulates T-cell effector functions. Cancer Res 73: 617–628.

12

Vancomycin Dosing in Neutropenic Patients

Michiel B. Haeseker[1,2]*, Sander Croes[3], Cees Neef[3], Cathrien A. Bruggeman[1,2], Leo M. L. Stolk[3], Annelies Verbon[1,4]

1 Department of Medical Microbiology, Maastricht University Medical Center, Maastricht, the Netherlands, 2 Care and Public Health Research Institute (CAPHRI), Maastricht, the Netherlands, 3 Department of Clinical Pharmacy and Toxicology, Maastricht University Medical Center, Maastricht, the Netherlands, 4 Department of Internal Medicine, Erasmus Medical Center, Rotterdam, the Netherlands

Abstract

Background: To compare vancomycin pharmacokinetic parameters in patients with and without neutropenia.

Methods: Patients $\geq$18 years admitted on general wards were included. Routinely vancomycin trough and peak plasma concentrations were measured with a fluorescence polarization immunoassay. Pharmacokinetic parameters of individual patients were determined with maximum a posterior Bayesian estimation (MW Pharm 3.60). Neutropenia was defined as neutrophils $<0.5\times10^9$ cells/L.

Principal Findings: A total of 171 patients were included. Patients with neutropenia (n = 56) had higher clearance of vancomycin (CLva), 67 ($\pm$26) mL/min, compared to patients without neutropenia (n = 115), CLva 50 ($\pm$22) mL/min (p< 0.001). No significant difference was found in serum creatinine and vancomycin volume of distribution. Neutropenia was positively associated with CLva, independently of relevant co-variables (B: 12.122, 95%CI: 1.095 to 23.149, p = 0.031). On average patients with neutropenia needed 33% higher doses of vancomycin to attain adequate exposure, i.e. AUC$_{24}$$\geq$ 400 mg$\times$h/L. Furthermore, 15 initially neutropenic patients in our study group received vancomycin for a second administration period. Ten patients received the second administration period during another neutropenic period and 5 patients during a non-neutropenic phase. All 5 patients with vancomycin during both neutropenic and non-neutropenic phase had higher CLva (91 ($\pm$26) mL/min) during the neutropenic period and lower CLva (45 ($\pm$10) mL/min) during the non-neutropenic phase (p = 0.009).

Conclusion: This study shows that most patients with neutropenia have augmented CLva. In a small group of patients that received vancomycin during two episodes, the augmented CLva seems to be reversible in the non-neutropenic period. Our data indicate that it is important to increase the daily dose with one third in patients with neutropenia (from 15 mg/kg twice daily to 13 mg/kg three times daily). Frequent performance of therapeutic drug monitoring in patients with neutropenia may prevent both therapy failure due to low AUCs and overcomes toxicity due to high vancomycin trough concentrations during recovery from neutropenia.

Editor: Jonghan Kim, Northeastern University, United States of America

Funding: The authors have no funding or support to report.

Competing Interests: The authors have declared that no competing interests exist.

* Email: m.haeseker@mumc.nl

Introduction

Mortality from infections after cytostatic conditioning regimens in hematologic neutropenic patients requiring hematopoietic cell transplantation is high [1]. Bacterial infections are common during neutropenic phases and antibiotics, such as vancomycin, are often required [2]. In a recent surveillance study, Gram positive organisms are the most common cause of bacteremia in hematology patients, i.e. coagulase negative staphylococci (36%), followed by, Streptococci (11%), *S. aureus* (8%) and Enterococci (4%) [3]. Antibiotics should be started within 1 hour in patients with severe sepsis. However, adequate dosing of vancomycin can be difficult. Augmented clearance has been increasingly described in critically ill patients at the Intensive Care Unit (ICU) [4–6]. Changes in volume of distribution (Vd), changes in renal function and severe hypoalbuminemia are often present, influencing

vancomycin plasma concentrations. Augmented clearance of vancomycin leads to lower vancomycin plasma concentrations, decreased 24-hour area under the curve (AUC$_{24}$) and leads to diminished clinical outcome [6]. Augmented clearance of vancomycin in patients with hematological malignancies has been reported, but the augmented clearance was not associated with population specific covariables [7]. In another study low teicoplanin trough concentrations in neutropenic patients were reported, suggesting augmented clearance of teicoplanin in neutropenic patients [8]. In addition, elevated clearance of piperacillin and ceftazidime has also been noticed in patients with febrile neutropenia [9,10]. The mechanism of augmented clearance of antibiotics is not completely understood and is poorly investigated in patients with hematologic malignancies or in patients with neutropenia. The aim of this study is to compare vancomycin pharmacokinetic parameters in patients with and without neutropenia at non-ICUs in a University Hospital.

Methods

Materials and Methods

Study group. In this observational study patients were prospectively followed. Patients older than 18 years treated with vancomycin intravenously (iv) and hospitalized at the Maastricht University Medical Center (MUMC), a 715 bed university hospital, were included from May 2011 until July 2013. Patients were excluded when admitted at the ICU or when insufficient data was collected. Vancomycin was started at the discretion of the attending physician, either empirically or as therapy for bacteria susceptible to vancomycin. Dose individualization was applied since an initial loading dose of 15 mg/kg was followed by dose adjustment based on therapeutic drug monitoring (TDM) and renal function. Demographic and clinical data, such as age, gender, weight, temperature, co-medication, length of hospital stay, time of administration of vancomycin and laboratory parameters, such as, serum creatinine (Jaffé method), and leucocytes were retrieved from the electronic patient file (SAP, the Netherlands). Neutropenia was defined as $<0.5 \times 10^9$ cells/L. Creatinine clearance (CLcr) was calculated with the Cockcroft and Gault formula [(140 - age in years) × weight in kg]/[serum creatinine in μmol × factor] using total bodyweight [11].

Ethics statement. This study was conducted according to the principles expressed in the Declaration of Helsinki. This study was registered at the Dutch Trial Register (NTR 1725). The Medical Ethical Committee of the Maastricht University Medical Center (MEC 08-4-063) approved this study and waived the necessity to obtain informed consent from participants because of the observational design. Electronic health records were anonymized prior to use.

Measurement of vancomycin. Vancomycin plasma concentrations were measured as standard clinical care with a fluorescence polarization immune assay using of Cobas Integra 800 system (Roche Diagnostics). The calibration curve ranged from 2.0 to 80 mg/L. The accuracy and coefficients of variation (CV) of the controls (6.9, 17.7 and 31.0 mg/L) were within 90%–110% and $<3.3\%$, respectively. Patients with at least two plasma samples available, drawn in such a manner to ensure calculations of vancomycin clearance (CLva) were included. Blood samples were collected at least one hour after the end of infusion and trough levels were obtained just before the next dose.

PK-analysis. Pharmacokinetic parameters (CLva, Vd) of vancomycin in individual patients were calculated with maximum a posterior (MAP) Bayesian estimation computer program (MW/Pharm 3.60, Mediware, the Netherlands). Bayesian priors from a two compartment open pharmacokinetic model based on previous studies, were applied: V1 0.21 ± 0.04 L/kg, k_{elm} 0.0143 ± 0.0029 h^{-1}, $k_{elr} = k_{slope} \times CLcr$ (mL/min), 0.00327 ± 0.00109 h^{-1}/mL/min, k_{12} 1.12 ± 0.28 h^{-1}, and k_{21} 0.48 ± 0.12 h^{-1} [12,13], where V1 is volume of distribution central compartment (L/kg); k_{elm}, metabolic elimination rate constant (h^{-1}); k_{slope}, renal elimination rate constant (h^{-1}/mL/min); k_{elr}, renal elimination rate constant (h^{-1}); k_{12} (h^{-1}), rate constant from the 1st to the 2nd compartment; and k_{21}(h^{-1}), vice versa. The elimination rate constant $k_{el} = k_{elm} + k_{elr} = k_{elm} + (k_{slope} \times CLcr)$ [14]. With MAP Bayesian estimation all patient characteristics and measured vancomycin concentrations are fitted on an existing population model. With at least two concentrations per patient individual pharmacokinetic parameters can be adequately derived with MAP Bayesian estimation [15,16]. With these individual pharmacokinetic parameters, dosing simulations were made to adjust the dose individually; this MAP Bayesian

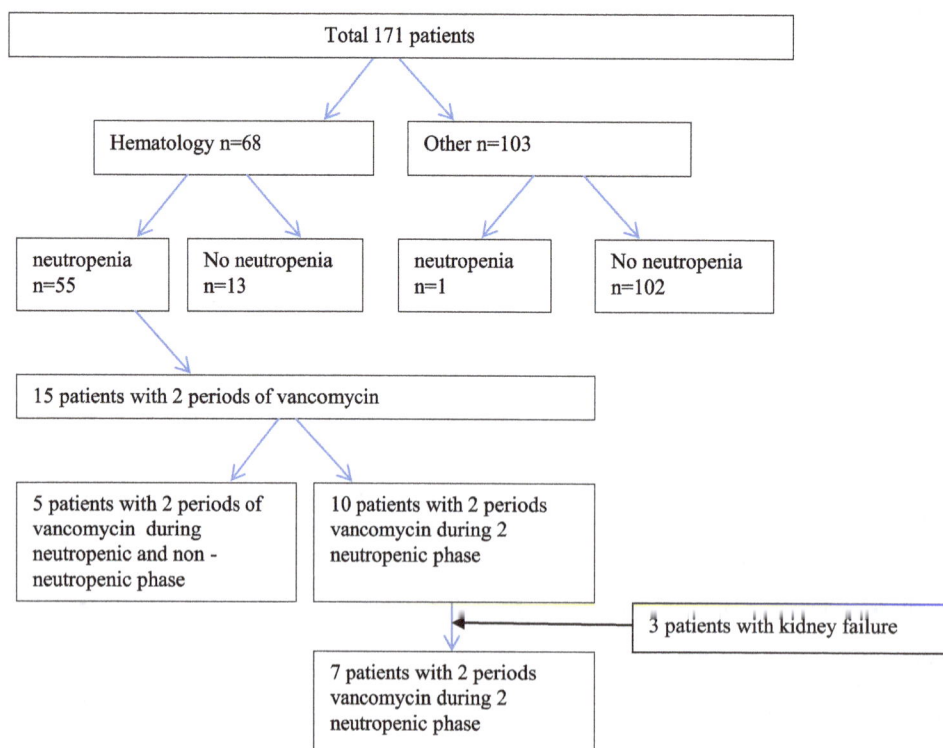

Figure 1. Flow of the 171 included patients with regard to hematology, neutropenia and two vancomycin administration periods.

Table 1. Mean (±SD) for Age, CLcr, CLva, Vd, Dose 24 h and AUC of patients with and without neutropenia in all patients (A) and in patients with haematological malignancy (B).

A] All patients (n = 171)								
Neutro-penia	N	Age year	CLcr mL/min	Creatinine μmol/L	CLva mL/min	Vd L	Dose 24 h mg	AUC mg*24 h/L
No	115	61(±14)	107(±78)	95(±67)	50(±22)	56(±29)	1521(±727)	499(±102)
Yes	56	55(±13)	113(±57)	80(±31)	67(±26)	62(±32)	2017(±719)	507(±87)
p		0.01	0.142	0.873	<0.001	0.304	<0.001	0.259
B] Patients with haematological malignancy (n = 68)								
Neutro-penia	N	Age Year	CLcr mL/min	Creatinine μmol/L	CLva mL/min	Vd L	Dose 24 h mg	AUC mg ×24 h/L
No	13	57(±11)	111(±58)	96(±59)	53(±16)	59(±18)	1604(±646)	502(±102)
Yes	55	55(±14)	114(±57)	79(±29)	68(±26)	62(±32)	2040(±705)	509(±87)
p		0.839	0.714	0.779	0.024	0.691	0.028	0.697

CLva: vancomycin clearance.
CLcr: creatinine clearance calculated from serum creatinine with Cockcroft and Gault [11].
Vd: volume of distribution.
AUC: 24 hour area under the curve.

estimation is a standard procedure in institutes which provide TDM service.

The AUC_{24} in steady-state was calculated with the formula: 24-hour dose/CLva.

Analysis of patients with and without neutropenia. Pharmacokinetic, clinical and demographic parameters were compared in patients with and without neutropenia in all patients and in patients with hematological malignancies. Furthermore, pharmacokinetic parameters of two vancomycin administration periods within the same patients were compared. Both patients with two vancomycin administrations during two different neutropenia periods and patients with two vancomycin administrations during one neutropenia period and one period without neutropenia were compared.

Statistical analysis. Normal distribution was evaluated for metric variables by means of the Shapiro-Wilk test and presented as mean (±SD). If not, median and ranges were given. Categorical variables are presented as frequencies and percentages. Metric and categorical variables were evaluated between patients with and without neutropenia using the Student t-test or non-parametric test (Kruskal Wallis), respectively.

First, the influence of co-variables on CLva was determined in univariable (Pearson) analysis. Subsequently, only the significant co-variables in the univariable analyses were included in the multivariable analysis, after checking the assumptions. The Enter method was used in the multivariable linear regression. CLcr is estimated with the C&G formula which includes serum creatinine, age, weight and gender [11]. To avoid multicollinearity, serum creatinine, age, weight and gender were left out of the multivariable model. Data analysis was done with IBM SPSS-pc version 20.0. A p-value of <0.05 was considered to be statistically significant.

Results

Study group

The mean age was 59 (±14) years and 61% were male. Patients were admitted on different general wards; hematology ward (40%, 68/171), surgery ward (19%, 32/171), internal ward (11%, 19/171), neurosurgery ward (11%, 18/171), orthopedic ward (10%, 17/171), cardiac (9%, 15/171) and eye ward (1%, 2/171). The majority of patients had sepsis (46%, 79/171), implant infection (16%, 27/171) or abdominal infection (15%, 25/171). A total of 171 patients with a mean (±SD) of 6 (±3) vancomycin plasma concentrations were included.

Pharmacokinetics analysis

The mean dose (±SD) of vancomycin per 24 hours was 1683 (±759) mg, with a mean Vd of 58 (±30) L and AUC_{24} of 502 (±97) mg×h/L. The mean (±SD) trough concentration in steady state (SS) was 13 (±4) mg/L, CmeanSS was 21 (±4) mg/L, peak concentration in SS was 49 (±14) mg/L, CLva was 56 (±25) mL/min and serum creatinine was 89 (±68) μmol/L.

Analysis of patients with and without neutropenia

Sixty eight patients had a hematological malignancy and 56 patients were neutropenic, Figure 1. Neutropenic patients (n = 56) had higher CLva, 67 (±26) mL/min, compared to non-neutropenic patients (n = 115), CLva 50 (±22) mL/min (p< 0.001). No significant difference in serum creatinine and Vd was found, Table 1 and Figure 2. Forty eight percent (27/56) of the neutropenic patients had CLva >70 mL/min, compared to 21% (24/115) without neutropenia. Of the 68 patients with a hematological malignancy, 55 patients were neutropenic and 13

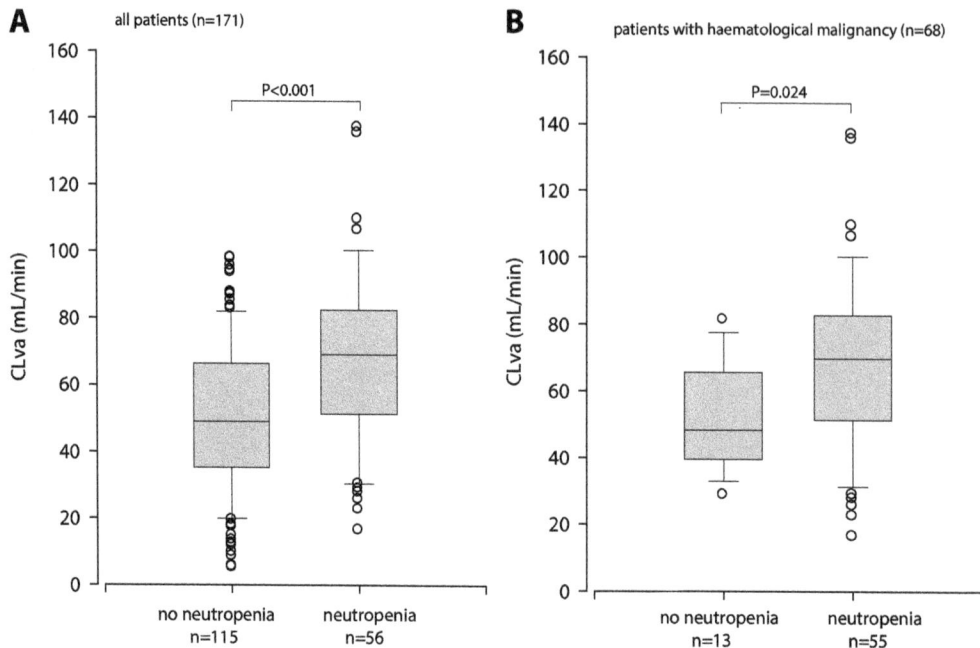

Figure 2. Boxplot for vancomycin clearance (CLva) in patients with and without neutropenia in all patients (A) and in patients with haematological malignancy (B). Lower and higher boundary of the box indicates 25th and 75th percentile, respectively, the line within the box marks the median, the whiskers above and below the box indicate the 90th and 10th percentiles and the open circles indicate outside the 90th and 10th percentiles.

were not neutropenic. Within the hematologic malignancy patients, neutropenic patients had higher CLva, than non-neutropenic patients, Table 1 and Figure 2. Physicians used TDM and adjusted vancomycin dosing as shown by the mean dose of vancomycin in patients with neutropenia of 2017 ($\pm$720) mg compared to 1521 ($\pm$727) mg in patients without neutropenia, p<0.001. On average, among patients with neutropenia the daily vancomycin dose was 33% (500 mg/day) higher to achieve the same AUC_{24} (Table 1). Patients with sepsis (n = 79) had higher CLva and were younger than patients without sepsis (n = 92). Vd and CLcr were not different, Table 2. Neutropenic patients with sepsis (n = 47) seemed to have slightly higher CLva of 69 ($\pm$27) mL/min than neutropenic patients without sepsis (n = 9) CLva 60 ($\pm$22) mL/min, p = 0.269. Both neutropenic patients with sepsis and without sepsis had higher CLva than non-neutropenic patients.

Of the 171 patients, 15 neutropenic patients received a second period of vancomycin, of which 5 patients received vancomycin during both an neutropenic and non neutropenic period. Ten patients received two vancomycin episodes during neutropenic periods. However, 3 patients developed kidney failure and were taken out. Leaving 7 patients with two vancomycin periods during neutropenia, Figure 1. Therefore, the data of 7 patients with two neutropenic periods and 5 patients with both a neutropenic and non-neutropenic period could be compared. The median (range) of time between the two vancomycin administrations was 30 (20–108) days for these 7 patients and 21 (14–136) days for the 5 patients with both a neutropenic and non-neutropenic period. For the 7 patients with vancomycin administrations in two neutropenic periods, the CLva remained similar: 77 ($\pm$30) to 70 ($\pm$23) mL/min (p = 0.748), as did the serum creatinine 68 ($\pm$13) to 66 ($\pm$11) µmol/L (p = 0.701) and CLcr 120 ($\pm$41) to 117 ($\pm$35) mL/min (p = 0.848). The 5 patients with vancomycin administrations in both a neutropenic and non-neutropenic period had a statistically

significantly higher CLva, 91 ($\pm$26) mL/min, during the neutropenic phase compared to CLva, 45 ($\pm$10) mL/min during the non-neutropenic phase (p = 0.009). Serum creatinine, 65 ($\pm$10) and 69 ($\pm$11) µmol/L (p = 0.462) and CLcr, 141 ($\pm$70) and 113 ($\pm$48) mL/min during the neutropenic and non-neutropenic periods, respectively, were not significantly different (p = 0.402), Figure 3 and neither was the Vd was 74 ($\pm$24) L during neutropenic and 51 ($\pm$10) L during non-neutropenic phase (p = 0.175).

CLcr, neutropenia, hematologic malignancy and sepsis were correlated with CLva in the univariable analysis, Table 3. In the multivariable analysis, CLva was positively associated with CLcr (B: 0.205, 95%CI: 0.164–0.245, p<0.001) and neutropenia (B: 12.122, 95%CI: 1.095 to 23.149, p = 0.031), Table 3.

Discussion

Our study shows that higher doses of vancomycin are needed during neutropenic periods to achieve vancomycin target AUC_{24} and target trough concentrations. The augmented clearance of vancomycin in neutropenic patients seems reversible. Augmented clearance of vancomycin cannot be predicted with the estimated CLcr, as serum creatinine and estimated CLcr in our analysis are not significantly different in neutropenic and non-neutropenic patients. Moreover, the estimated CLcr is not reliable above 125 µmol/L and shows a poor agreement with measured CLcr in urine in critically ill patients displaying augmented clearance of creatinine [17,18]. Our Bayesian calculated CLva is in line with the population estimated CLva in patients with hematological malignancies in the simulations by Buelga *et al.* [7]. However, our routine patient care observations demonstrate that augmented clearance is associated with neutropenia rather than hematological malignancy and sepsis. In the multivariable analysis neutropenia (yes/no) was positively associated with CLva, independently of the

Table 2. Mean (±SD) for Age, CLcr, CLva, Vd, Creatinine for patients with sepsis and without sepsis.

	N	Age years	CLva mL/min	Vd L	CLcr mL/min	Creatinine µmol/L
Sepsis	79	56 (±13)	60 (±27)	57 (±26)	108 (±56)	84 (±38)
No sepsis	92	61 (±14)	52 (±23)	58 (±33)	110 (±83)	96 (±71)
p		0.017	0.048	0.639	0.535	0.894

CLva: vancomycin clearance.
CLcr: creatinine clearance calculated from serum creatinine with Cockcroft and Gault [11].
Vd: volume of distribution.

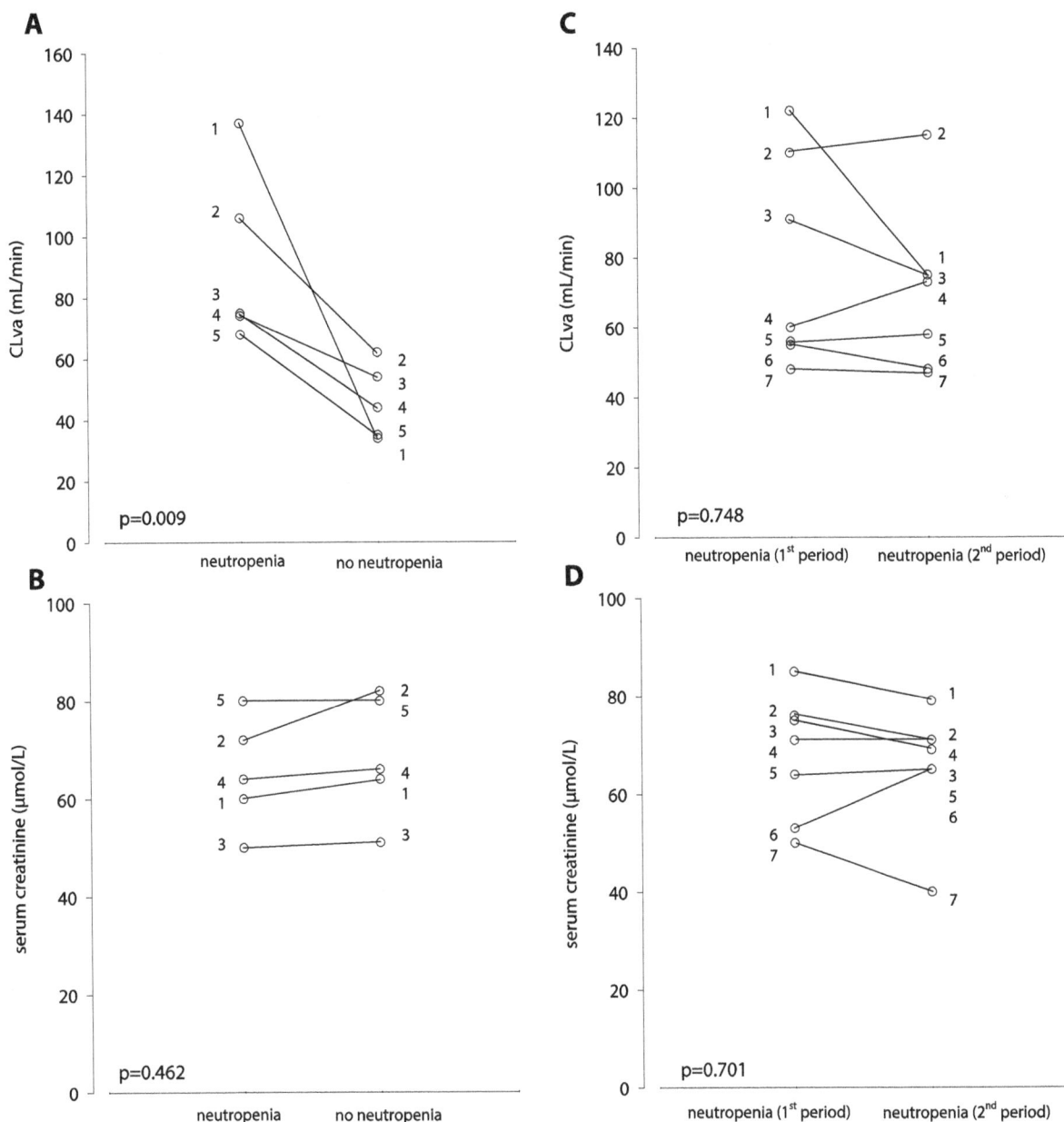

Figure 3. A. Vancomycin clearance (CLva) and B. serum creatinine of 5 patients (number 1–5) during both a neutropenic and a non-neutropenic phase and C. CLva and D. serum creatinine of 7 patients (number 1–7) during two neutropenic phases.

Table 3. Univariable and multivariable correlation coefficients between CLva and predictors used in this study.

	Univariable[a]		Multivariable[b]			
	R	P-value	B	95% confidence interval for B		p-value
				Lower bound	Upper bound	
CLcr	0.599	<0.001	0.205	0.164	0.245	<0.001
Neutropenia	0.322	<0.001	12.122	1.095	23.149	0.031
Hematologic malignancy	0.300	<0.001	3.582	−8.404	15.569	0.556
Sepsis	0.170	0.027	0.427	−7.236	8.090	0.913
Vd	0.008	0.915	-	-	-	-

CLva: vancomycin clearance.
CLcr: creatinine clearance.
Vd: volume of distribution.
[a]Pearson correlation was performed as the univariable analysis.
[b]Only co-variates that were significantly correlated with CLva in the univariable analysis (P<0.05) were included in the multivariable analysis.

other co-variables. Although, our group of patients that received a second administration of vancomycin is small, the augmented clearance of vancomycin seems to be temporarily and reversible, as the CLva returned to normal during the non-neutropenic phase. The mechanism of augmented clearance is not completely clarified; most likely more than one factor is involved in developing augmented clearance. Young age, increased blood flow to the kidneys, genetic factors and other medication has been proposed to influence the CLva [5,6]. Neutropenia might be added to this list. Most likely augmented clearance also influences other renally cleared antibiotics [9,10]. Therefore, TDM of these antibiotics or/ and at least one 24-hour creatinine measurement in urine to determine the most accurate CLcr at the ICU is recommended [5,19,20]. Our data suggest that this recommendation may be extended to neutropenic patients.

Our study has a couple of limitations. Firstly, our study is a real-life observational study and we assumed the TDM protocol was strictly followed by clinicians, especially the timing of peak concentrations. Secondly, our group of patients with a second vancomycin administration was rather small to prove the demonstrated tendency of reversibility of elevated CLva, at the moment when patients are recovering from neutropenia. Further research is needed to fully understand the complex pharmacokinetics of vancomycin and other antibiotics in patients with

neutropenia. A prospective study may elucidate which other factors are involved in augmented CLva, but such a study would need a multicenter design and inclusion of many patients. Until, we fully understand augmented clearance, we suggest to increase the initial daily dose of vancomycin with 33% (13 mg/kg three times daily) in patients with neutropenia and to perform TDM after the first vancomycin dose in patients to prevent low plasma concentrations of vancomycin and consequently reduced efficacy. When patients are recovering from neutropenia, TDM is again necessary to adjust the vancomycin dose to prevent toxicity due to high vancomycin exposure.

Acknowledgments

The authors acknowledge the support provided by department of Pharmacy laboratory and the excellent statistical advice of Casper den Heijer.

Author Contributions

Conceived and designed the experiments: AV LMLS CAB CN. Performed the experiments: MBH SC LMLS. Analyzed the data: MBH SC LMLS AV. Contributed reagents/materials/analysis tools: MBH SC LMLS CN. Wrote the paper: MBH SC LMLS CN CAB AV.

References

1. Scott BL, Park JY, Deeg HJ, Marr KA, Boeckh M, et al. (2008) Pretransplant neutropenia is associated with poor-risk cytogenetic features and increased infection-related mortality in patients with myelodysplastic syndromes. Biol Blood Marrow Transplant 14: 799–806.

2. Sepkowitz KA (2002) Antibiotic prophylaxis in patients receiving hematopoietic stem cell transplant. Bone Marrow Transplant 29: 367–371.

3. Schelenz S, Nwaka D, Hunter PR (2013) Longitudinal surveillance of bacteraemia in haematology and oncology patients at a UK cancer centre and the impact of ciprofloxacin use on antimicrobial resistance. J Antimicrob Chemother 68: 1431–1438.

4. Revilla N, Martin-Suarez A, Perez MP, Gonzalez FM, Fernandez de Gatta Mdel M (2010) Vancomycin dosing assessment in intensive care unit patients based on a population pharmacokinetic/pharmacodynamic simulation. Br J Clin Pharmacol 70: 201–212.

5. Udy AA, Roberts JA, Boots RJ, Paterson DL, Lipman J (2010) Augmented renal clearance: implications for antibacterial dosing in the critically ill. Clin Pharmacokinet 49: 1–16.

6. Claus BO, Hoste EA, Colpaert K, Robays H, Decruyenaere J, et al. (2013) Augmented renal clearance is a common finding with worse clinical outcome in critically ill patients receiving antimicrobial therapy. J Crit Care 28: 695–700.

7. Buelga DS, del Mar Fernandez de Gatta M, Herrera EV, Dominguez-Gil A, Garcia MJ (2005) Population pharmacokinetic analysis of vancomycin in

patients with hematological malignancies. Antimicrob Agents Chemother 49: 4934–4941.

8. Pea F, Viale P, Candoni A, Pavan F, Pagani L, et al. (2004) Teicoplanin in patients with acute leukaemia and febrile neutropenia: a special population benefiting from higher dosages. Clin Pharmacokinet 43: 405–415.

9. Pea F, Viale P, Damiani D, Pavan F, Cristini F, et al. (2005) Ceftazidime in acute myeloid leukemia patients with febrile neutropenia: helpfulness of continuous intravenous infusion in maximizing pharmacodynamic exposure. Antimicrob Agents Chemother 49: 3550–3553.

10. Sime FB, Roberts MS, Warner MS, Hahn U, Robertson TA, et al. (2014) Altered pharmacokinetics of piperacillin in febrile neutropenic patients with haematological malignancy. Antimicrob Agents Chemother.

11. Cockcroft DW, Gault MH (1976) Prediction of creatinine clearance from serum creatinine. Nephron 16: 31 41.

12. Pryka RD, Rodvold KA, Garrison M, Rotschafer JC (1989) Individualizing vancomycin dosage regimens: one- versus two-compartment Bayesian models. Ther Drug Monit 11: 450–454.

13. Rodvold KA, Pryka RD, Garrison M, Rotschafer JC (1989) Evaluation of a two-compartment Bayesian forecasting program for predicting vancomycin concentrations. Ther Drug Monit 11: 269–275.

14. Manual MP. Available: http://www.mwpharm.nl/downloads/documentation/UK-315-VOL3.PD.

15. van der Meer AF, Marcus MA, Touw DJ, Proost JH, Neef C (2011) Optimal sampling strategy development methodology using maximum a posteriori Bayesian estimation. Ther Drug Monit 33: 133–146.

16. Proost JH, Meijer DK (1992) MW/Pharm, an integrated software package for drug dosage regimen calculation and therapeutic drug monitoring. Comput Biol Med 22: 155–163.

17. Grootaert V, Willems L, Debaveye Y, Meyfroidt G, Spriet I (2012) Augmented renal clearance in the critically ill: how to assess kidney function. Ann Pharmacother 46: 952–959.

18. Hoste EA, Damen J, Vanholder RC, Lameire NH, Delanghe JR, et al. (2005) Assessment of renal function in recently admitted critically ill patients with normal serum creatinine. Nephrol Dial Transplant 20: 747–753.

19. Udy AA, Putt MT, Shanmugathasan S, Roberts JA, Lipman J (2010) Augmented renal clearance in the Intensive Care Unit: an illustrative case series. Int J Antimicrob Agents 35: 606–608.

20. Troger U, Drust A, Martens-Lobenhoffer J, Tanev I, Braun-Dullaeus RC, et al. (2012) Decreased meropenem levels in Intensive Care Unit patients with augmented renal clearance: benefit of therapeutic drug monitoring. Int J Antimicrob Agents 40: 370–372.

13

High Levels of Soluble Ctla-4 Are Present in Anti-Mitochondrial Antibody Positive, but Not in Antibody Negative Patients with Primary Biliary Cirrhosis

Daniele Saverino[1]*, Giampaola Pesce[2], Princey Antola[2], Brunetta Porcelli[3], Ignazio Brusca[4], Danilo Villalta[5], Marilina Tampoia[6], Renato Tozzoli[7], Elio Tonutti[8], Maria Grazia Alessio[9], Marcello Bagnasco[2], Nicola Bizzaro[10]

1 Department of Experimental Medicine – Section of Human Anatomy, University of Genova, Genova, Italy, 2 Autoimmunity Unit, Department of Internal Medicine, University of Genova, Genova, Italy, 3 Department of Internal Medicine, University of Siena, Siena, Italy, 4 Department of Clinical Pathology, Buccheri La Ferla Hospital, Palermo, Italy, 5 Allergology and Clinical Immunology, S. Maria degli Angeli Hospital, Pordenone, Italy, 6 Laboratory of Clinical Pathology, University Hospital, Bari, Italy, 7 Clinical Pathology, Department of Laboratory Medicine, S. Maria degli Angeli Hospital, Pordenone, Italy, 8 Immunopathology and Allergology Unit, S. Maria della Misericordia Hospital, Udine, Italy, 9 Department of Laboratory Medicine, Biochemistry Laboratory, Riuniti Hospital, Bergamo, Italy, 10 Laboratory of Clinical Pathology, San Antonio Hospital, Tolmezzo, Udine, Italy

Abstract

Primary biliary cirrhosis (PBC) is a chronic autoimmune cholestatic liver disease frequently characterized by anti-mitochondrial autoantibodies (AMA). A minority of patients are AMA-negative. Cytotoxic-T-Lymphocyte-Antigen-4 (CTLA-4) is a surface molecule expressed on activated T-cells delivering a critical negative immunoregulatory signal. A soluble form of CTLA-4 (sCTLA-4) has been detected at high concentrations in several autoimmune diseases, and its possible functional meaning has been suggested. We aimed to evaluate sCTLA-4 concentration in sera of patients with PBC and to correlate it to immunological abnormalities associated with the disease. Blood samples were collected from 82 PBC-patients diagnosed according to international criteria (44 AMA-positive/MIT3-positive and 38 AMA-negative-MIT3-negative), and 65 controls. sCTLA-4 levels were evaluated by ELISA and Western blot. Increased sCTLA-4 concentrations were found in all AMA-positive PBC-patients, but in none of the AMA-negative ones, nor in normal controls or in controls with unrelated liver diseases. sCTLA-4 presence was associated with autoantibodies against MIT3, but not with nuclear autoantibodies (sp100, gp210). This is the first study to demonstrate that levels of sCTLA-4 are elevated in sera of PBC patients. However, they are clearly restricted to patients with AMA positivity, suggesting an immunological difference with respect to AMA-negative ones.

Editor: Aftab A. Ansari, Emory University School of Medicine, United States of America

Funding: This work was funded by University of Genova, Italy (PRA2012). The funders had no role in study design, data collection and analysis, decision to publish, or preparation of the manuscript.

Competing Interests: The authors have declared that no competing interests exist.

* Email: daniele.saverino@unige.it

Introduction

Primary biliary cirrhosis (PBC) is a chronic cholestatic liver autoimmune disease characterized by slow progressive immune-mediated destruction of the small- and medium-sized bile ducts, leading to liver fibrosis, cirrhosis, eventually requiring transplantation [1–6]. The prevalence of PBC ranges from 30 to 400 per million. PBC preferentially affects middle-aged women (m:f ratio 9 to 1), sharing this characteristic with other autoimmune diseases [7]. Progression of PBC is usually slow-paced, but symptoms of portal hypertension and hepatic decompensation (jaundice, ascites, or variceal bleeding) may develop several years after the initial diagnosis [1,2,4,8,9]. The aetiology of PBC is unknown; however, it is believed that genetic susceptibility, and environmental factors are involved in concert [10]. Studies in animal models suggest that specific infectious and environmental triggers can induce PBC-specific pathological features, probably by the mechanism of molecular mimicry [10–14]. This would occur in the setting of T

regulatory impairment, particularly in susceptible individuals [15,16].

The autoimmune pathogenesis of PBC is supported by a large amount of experimental and clinical data, such as the presence of autoreactive T cells, and serum autoantibodies characteristic of the disease [17–19]. High-titer serum AMA positivity is pathognomonic for PBC, and is present in 90–95% of patients [8,17–19]. Patients lacking detectable AMA but presenting signs and symptoms of PBC should be considered as having "AMA-negative PBC". AMA are specific to the lipolylated domains within components of the 2-oxoacid dehydrogenase family of enzymes, particularly the E2 component of the pyruvate dehydrogenase complex (PDC-E2) [17–19]. In addition to AMA, PBC-specific anti-nuclear autoantibodies (ANA) including the "multiple nuclear dot" and "nuclear membrane/rim" patterns are present in approximately 30% of patients [17–19]. The "multiple nuclear dot" pattern corresponds to autoantibodies against sp100, sp140, promyelocytic leukaemia nuclear body proteins, and small ubiquitin-like modifiers [20]. The "nuclear envelope/rim" pattern corresponds to reactivity specific for gp210 and nucleoporin p62 [21]. Up to 30% of PBC patients have both patterns, which demonstrate significant disease specificity. PBC-specific ANA may be present in AMA-negative PBC patients, in asymptomatic individuals and in family members of PBC patients [17–19].

Whether AMA-negative PBC and AMA-positive PBC are the same or two immunologically different diseases is debated. The use of more sensitive techniques other than immunofluorescence, such as ELISA and immunoblotting, has revealed that a number of patients who were classified as AMA-negative by immunofluorescence assay, display a positivity for AMA related autoantigens. This would suggest that the different expression of AMA refers to a single autoimmune disorder and that the AMA-negative PBC cohort results from analytical limits. Nevertheless, a small proportion of PBC patients that are definitely AMA-negative, whatever the detection method employed, does exist. [19].

In general, the activity of T cells is controlled by several activatory and inhibitory co-receptors. Among various inhibitory pathways, Cytotoxic-T-Lymphocyte-Antigen-4 (CTLA-4), a member of the immunoglobulin superfamily, plays a key role in restraining T-cell responses during antigenic stimulation. CTLA-4 is homologous to the activating coreceptor CD28, but its affinity for CD80 and CD86 molecules is much higher than that of CD28. Thus, it can efficiently compete with CD28 for its ligands and maintain homeostasis during T-cell responsiveness [22–24]. CTLA-4 has steady-state messenger RNA (mRNA) levels for two known isoforms: a full-length isoform (flCTLA-4) encoded by exon 1 (leader peptide), exon 2 (ligand-binding domain), exon 3 (transmembrane domain) and exon 4 (cytoplasmic tail) and a soluble form (sCTLA-4), which lacks exon 3. sCTLA-4, originating from alternative splicing, results in the loss of a cysteine residue and is found in the serum as a soluble monomeric protein [24–26]. The presence of high concentrations of sCTLA-4 was observed in sera of patients with autoimmune thyroid diseases [26,27], as well as in patients with other autoimmune diseases, such as type-1 diabetes, diffuse cutaneous systemic sclerosis [28], systemic lupus erythematosus [29] and myasthenia gravis [30,31].

As for other diseases of autoimmune origin, polymorphisms of *CTLA-4* (particularly, CTLA-4+49G>A polymorphism) could play a role on susceptibility to PBC [32].

Although our understanding of the role of the *CTLA-4* gene and its protein products is incomplete, we analysed the presence of sCTLA-4 in sera from PBC patients, under the hypothesis that its levels could be related to the immunological abnormalities associated with the disease. Furthermore, we separately studied a consistent group of clinically and histologically diagnosed PBC patients selected on the basis of AMA negativity, and compared the results obtained with those of AMA-positive patients. The results showed relevant differences between the two groups.

Materials and Methods

Patients

Blood samples were collected from PBC patients from different regions of Italy, following the ethical guidelines of the most recent Declaration of Helsinki (Edinburg 2000) and all patients enrolled in this study provided written informed consent. The Ethics Committee of Azienda Ospedaliero-Universitaria di Udine, Italy, approved the research. Ninety % of them were female with a median age of 61 years (range 37–89).

The diagnosis of PBC was formulated by experienced gastroenterologists from 2006 to 2008. For each patient at least two out of three internationally accepted criteria were fulfilled, i.e., presence of serum AMA, increased enzymes indicating cholestasis

(i.e., alkaline phosphatase) for longer than 6 months, and compatible or diagnostic liver histology [8,17–19]. All AMA-negative patients (see below) fulfilled the latter two criteria. All sera were collected at diagnosis before starting any kind of specific medication.

The study population was composed by two distinct groups of PBC sera. The first included 44 AMA-positive PBC sera from consecutively diagnosed patients. As a second group, 46 sera were randomly selected from a previously described cohort of 100 AMA-negative PBC cases [19]. Among them, 8 were excluded on the basis of positivity for MIT3 (see below): thus, 38 "true" AMA-negative patients were eventually included.

An overlap syndrome with systemic sclerosis was observed in only 2 out of the total pool of PBC patients studied.

Sera from 20 patients with hepatitis B virus infection and 45 blood donor volunteers (17 and 36 women, aged 32–64 and 30–61 years, respectively) were included as controls. Sera were stored frozen until the use and freezing and thawing was avoided.

Methods

Serum samples were first assayed for AMA and ANA by IIF on sections of rat kidney, stomach and liver, and on HEp2 cells, respectively (test kits from EUROIMMUN, Lübeck, Germany, and INOVA Diagnostics, San Diego, CA, USA) and by an ELISA screening test (PBC Screen, INOVA Diagnostics, and EURO-IMMUN) using three coating antigens: recombinant pMIT3 and purified gp210 and sp100 with anti-IgG and anti-IgA dual conjugate. The manufacturer's cut-off was established at 25 units. Samples were considered as negative (≤20.0 units), equivocal (20.1–24.9 units), or positive (≥25.0 units). A negative result indicated the absence of antibodies to MIT3, gp210, or sp100. A positive result indicated the presence of antibodies to one or more of the antigens included in the PBC Screen assay. Subsequently, sera from patients with PBC were tested on the individual MIT3, gp210 and sp100 IgG Quanta Lite ELISAs (INOVA Diagnostics) [19].

sCTLA-4 measurement

A specific ELISA method was used for measuring serum sCTLA-4 levels (Bender Med System, Prodotti Gianni SpA, Milano, Italy), according to the manufacturer's protocol. Each sample was diluted 1:10 in assay buffer provided by the manufacturer and tested in triplicate. Deviation between triplicates was <10% for any reported value. The lowest sensitivity threshold was 0.1 ng/ml.

The analytical response was linear approximately between 0.162 and 1.200 of absorbance values (corresponding to 0.1–50 ng/ml) as assessed by serial dilution test using a strongly positive serum (data not shown). For samples with sCTLA-4 concentration higher than 50 ng/ml, the ELISA tests were repeated using a greater dilution factor (1:100) [27].

Western blotting was used to confirm the presence of sCTLA-4 by testing four different samples (three positive and one negative by ELISA). Proteins were separated by loading 200 μl of sera on 10–20% gradient PAGE in a discontinuous buffer system on a Mini-Protean system (Bio-Rad, Segrate, Milano, Italy). The separated components were electroblotted onto polyvinylidene difluoride membranes. The blots were washed with 0.15 M NaCl, 0.05 M Tris (TBS), pH 7.5, with 0.3% Tween 20 and reacted with a 1:100 dilution of the anti-CTLA-4 mAb (clone 14D3, IgG2a, eBiosciences, San Diego, CA) for 1 hour at room temperature, washed, and then reacted with reporter antibody (HRP-conjugated anti-mouse IgG) for 1 hour. The blots were then developed by the use of a commercially available chemiluminescence detection

Table 1. Biochemical, serological and histological features in AMA-positive and in AMA-negative PBC patients (values are expressed as median and range).

	AMA-positive (n = 44)	AMA-negative (n = 38)	P value
Women (*n*)	38	33	n.s.
Age (*years*)	38–82	37–82	n.s.
PBC screen (*units*)	152.44 (78–200)	39.46 (2–119)	<0.0001
gp210 (*units*)	4 (1–11)	2 (1–33)	<0.0001
sp100 (*units*)	4 (2–16)	3 (1–179)	0.0064
ALP (*UI/l*)	289 (147–2675)	302 (138–2943)	n.s.
gammaGT (*U/l*)	156 (37–1335)	140 (39–1822)	n.s.
ALT (*UI/l*)	61 (37–240)	40 (32–555)	n.s.
Total bilirubin (*mg/dl*)	1.7 (0.8–2.91)	0.8 (0.3–41.4)	n.s.
Direct bilirubin (*mg/dl*)	0.9 (0.3–1.6)	0.2 (0.1–4.7)	n.s.
Albumin (*g/l*)	4.4 (3–5.8)	4 (2.9–5.1)	0.0751
Histological Scheuer stage	III (I–IV)	II (I–IV)	n.s.
I	11 patients	10 patients	
II	6 patients	18 patients	
III	16 patients	1 patient	
IV	11 patients	4 patients	
sCTLA-4 (*ng/ml*)	14.3 (0.9–81.8)	1 (0.1–15.1)	<0.0001
	Hepatitis B virus infection (n = 20)	**Healthy donors** (n = 45)	**P value**
Women (*n*)	17	36	n.s.
Age (*years*)	32–64	30–61	n.s.

kit (BMB, Indianapolis, IN) according to the manufacturer's instructions.

Statistical analysis

Statistical analysis was performed using the Mann–Whitney U-test for comparison of sCTLA-4 levels among AMA-positive and AMA-negative patients. Spearman regression analysis was used to evaluate the correlation between sCTLA-4 and other parameters (such as PBC Screen, MIT3, gp210, sp100, alkaline phosphatase (ALP), gamma–glutamyl transpeptidase (gammaGT), alanine aminotransferase (ALT), total and direct bilirubin, albumine, and Scheuer stage). A P value less than 0.05 was considered statistically significant. All analyses were performed by using the GraphPad Prism4 software 4.0 (GraphPad Software Inc., La Jolla, CA).

Results

Serological characteristics of PBC patients

All IIF AMA-positive PBC sera (44/44) tested positive at the PBC Screen assay. When single antigens were used, all sera recognized MIT3, whereas none recognized gp210 alone, nor sp100 alone.

Among IIF AMA-negative PBC sera, 25/38 tested positive at the PBC Screen assay. When single antigens were used, none of 38 sera recognized MIT3 alone, 2/38 recognized gp210 only, and 8/38 sp100. Finally, no serum reacted against two different antigens.

As expected, the difference of PBC screen, gp210 and sp100 between the two groups of AMA-IIF positive and AMA IIF-negative PBC patients was statistically significant, p<0.05 (Table 1). In fact, our previous data confirm the hypothesis that a substantial part of IIF AMA-negative (a so called "probable") PBC cases manifest disease-specific autoantibodies when tested using newly available tools [19].

As shown in Table 1, increased enzyme values (i.e., ALP, ALT, and gammaGT) indicating cholestasis and stage determination did not reveal a statistical difference between the two groups of patients, though the majority of AMA-positive PBC patients were in stage 3 (characterized by fibrous scaring bridging portal tracts with occasional foci of bile duct loss), whereas AMA-negative were in stage 2 (showing portal enlargement with bile ductular reaction and inflammatory cell infiltration).

Finally, none of the control sera showed elevation of ALP or positivity for AMA.

sCTLA-4 is present in sera from PBC patients and its level is related to AMA

We assessed the presence of the soluble form of CTLA-4 in sera from PBC patients and controls by using a sensitive ELISA. sCTLA-4 levels were markedly raised in virtually all of AMA-positive PBC patients at diagnosis and significantly higher compared to AMA-negative PBC patients and controls (p< 0.001) (Fig. 1A). Only 6 out 45 healthy subjects and none of the 20 hepatitis B virus-infected patients had detectable sCTLA-4. No correlation was found between sCTLA-4 levels and age or presence of symptoms.

We confirmed the presence of sCTLA-4 by Western-blot testing three different samples that were positive by ELISA. As shown in Fig. 1B, a characteristic band of approximately 23 kDa is apparent, which is consistent with previous reports [26,27]. For comparison, a serum undetectable amount of sCTLA-4 is shown.

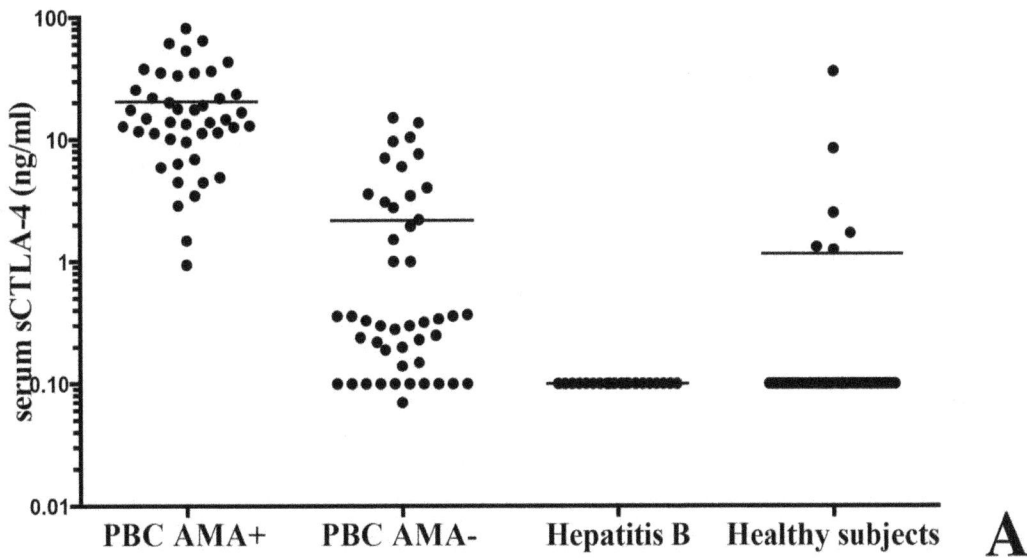

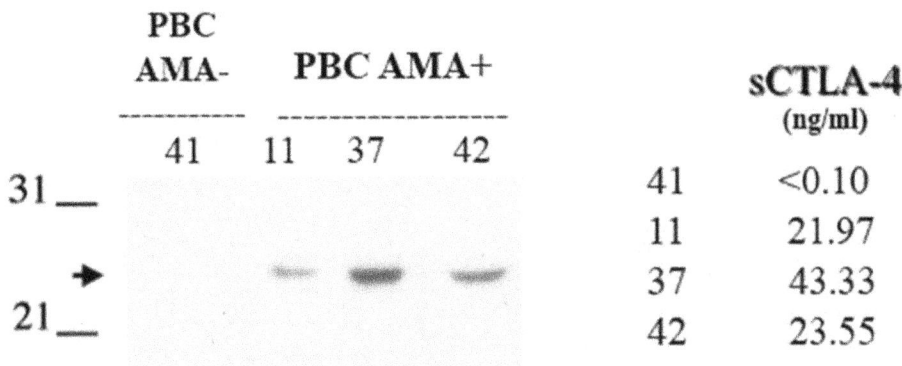

Figure 1. A sCTLA-4 is found in serum of PBC AMA-positive patients. Panel A, The concentration of sCTLA-4 was evaluated by ELISA on sera collected from AMA-positive PBC patients, AMA-negative PBC patients, and hepatitis B-infected patients and healthy donors as controls. Results are expressed as nanogram per milliliter. Each sample was diluted 1:10 and tested in triplicate. Samples showing values higher then the detection limit of the test (50 ng/ml) were diluted appropriately and tested again. Deviation between triplicates was <10% for any reported value. Panel B, Immunoprecipitation of sCTLA-4 was performed on sera from a representative group of AMA-positive PBC patients. In addition, a serum undetectable sCTLA-4 dosing (below the sensibility of the text) was shown. Arrow marks 23 kDa species.

Correlation among sCTLA-4 and classical PBC clinical and functional parameters

As observed above, the levels of sCTLA-4 strongly correlated with AMA-positivity. For this reason we compared serum sCTLA-4 levels to other specific autoantibodies characteristically present in PBC patients. Otherwise, all the other clinical/functional parameters analysed failed to show any significant correlation with serum sCTLA-4 levels. Similarly, no correlation was found between sCTLA-4 levels and sp100 or gp210 positivity. As far as sp100 is concerned, out of 8 sp100-positive sera, 4 had undetectable, and 4 had detectable sCTLA-4.

In addition, we divided AMA-positive and AMA-negative PBC patients in two subgroups based on low (i.e. 0.1–10 ng/ml), and high sCTLA-4 concentration (i.e. >10.1 ng/ml) (Fig. 2). Of interest, MIT3 was the only marker showing a significant positive correlation with sCTLA-4, both comparing low and high sCTLA-4 levels (p<0.0001). A significant difference between AMA-

positive and AMA-negative with low sCTLA-4 levels for PBC screen and sp100 was apparent (p<0.0001 and p=0.0174, respectively). All the other clinical/functional parameters analysed failed to show any significant correlation with serum sCTLA-4 levels.

Of interest, when we stratified all PBC patients as low (i.e. 0.1–10 ng/ml), and high sCTLA-4 concentration (i.e. >10.1 ng/ml), we could observe a positive correlation between sCTLA-4 and the PBC screen test, IIF-AMA results, MIT3, and gp210 presence (Table 2). Otherwise, all the other clinical/functional parameters analysed failed to show any significant correlation with serum sCTLA-4 levels.

Discussion

Increased serum levels of sCTLA-4 have been demonstrated in several autoimmune diseases [31]. The results of the present study

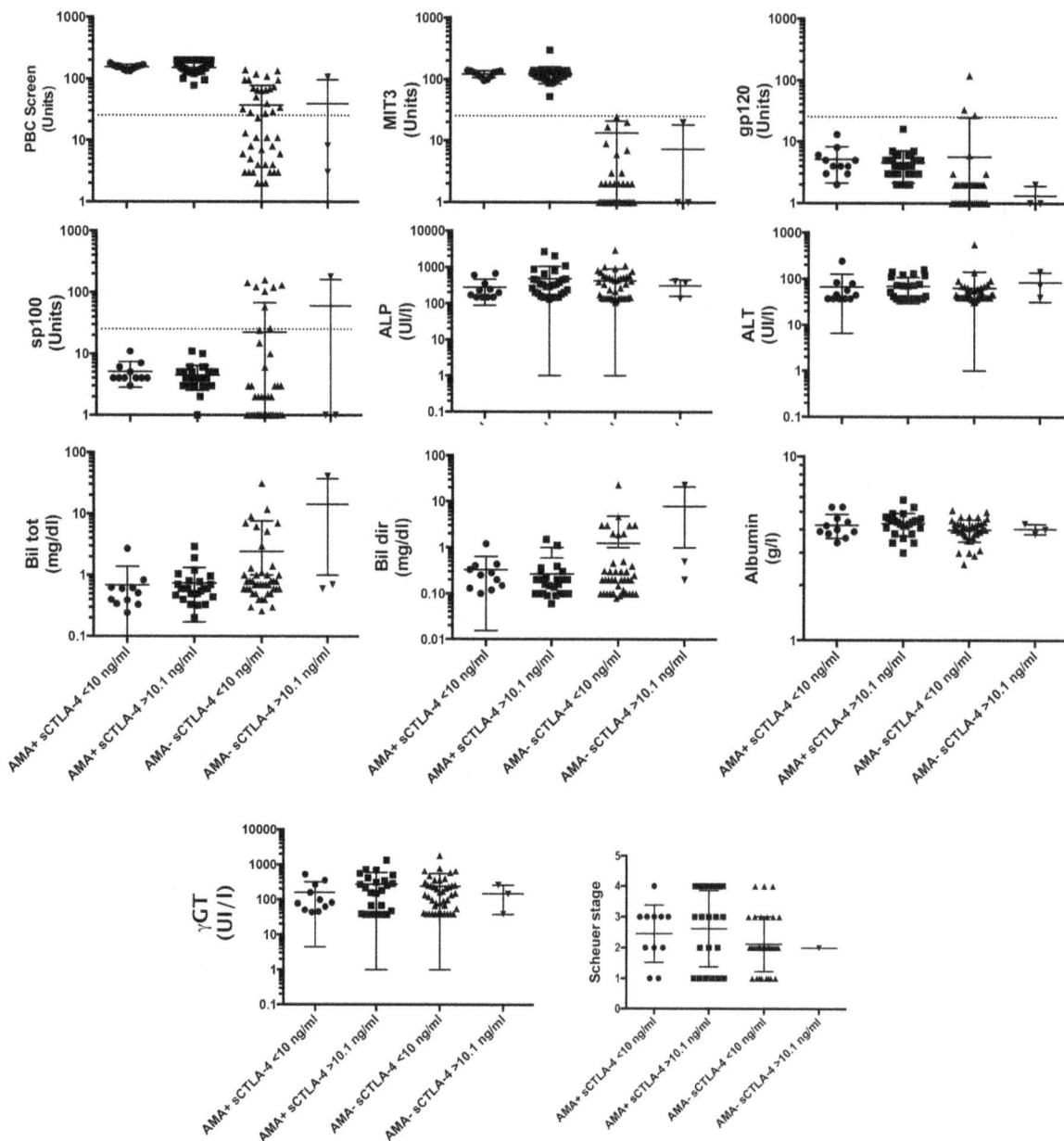

Figure 2. Correlation of sCTLA-4 amounts and cholestatic liver biochemistry, histology, and serum anti-mitochondrial autoantibodies. The AMA-positive and AMA-negative patients were divided in two subgroups in base of the sCTLA-4 values (low 0.1–10 ng/ml, and high >10.1 ng/ml). MIT3 was the only marker of PBC showing a significant positive correlation with the amount of sera sCTLA-4, both comparing low and high sCTLA-4 levels. In addition, a difference between AMA-positive and AMA-negative with low sCTLA-4 levels for PBC screen and sp100 was apparent. Dotted lines indicate the cut off value (25 Units), respectively for PBC screen, MIT3, gp210, and sp100.

showed for the first time that high levels of the soluble form of CTLA-4 are detectable in sera from patients with PBC displaying positivity for AMA. This did not occur in control subjects with viral (HBV) hepatitis, nor in normal individuals. The presence of sCTLA-4 was confirmed by Western blot, which allowed the demonstration of the caracteristic 23-kDa band in ELISA positive sera only. Although it was not possible to performe absorption experiments with specific monoclonal antibodies, we think this finding strongly support the specificity of our data.

Preliminary experiments (comparing 44 AMA-positive vs. 16 AMA-negative patients) demonstrated the presence of sCTLA-4 only in the sera of the first group of patients (data not shown) [32].

In order to better evidentiate this difference, we increased the number of AMA-negative patients included in this study: only patents who were negative for MIT3 the most relevant fine specificity responsible for AMA IIF reactivity, were considered. Interestingly, in this selected group of AMA-negative patients with histologically proven PBC, serum sCTLA-4 was almost invariably undetectable, as in control subjects. At variance, no relationship was found between sCTLA-4 concentration and positivity for other PBC-related autoantibodies directed against nuclear antigens, such as sp100 and gp210.

Altogether, these findings may prompt two types of considerations.

Table 2. Biochemical, serological and histological parameters from PBC patients (values are expressed as median and range) according to sCTLA-4 levels (low 0.1–10 ng/ml, and high >10.1 ng/ml).

	sCTLA-4 low (n = 28)	sCTLA-4 high (n = 55)	P value
Women (n)	24	50	n.s.
Age (years)	37–82	38–82	n.s.
PBC screen (units)	69 (2–178)	144.5 (3–200)	p<0.0001
AMA+ (n)	11	52	p<0.0001
MIT3 (units)	5 (1–139)	118.5 (1–300)	p<0.0001
gp210 (units)	2 (1–33)	4 (1–16)	p = 0.0007
sp100 (units)	4 (1–159)	4 (1–179)	n.s.
ALP (UI/l)	128 (55–2943)	339.5 (144–2675)	p = 0.0011
gammaGT (U/l)	67 (39–1822)	166.5 (37–1335)	n.s.
ALT (UI/l)	42 (32–555)	51 (37–159)	n.s.
Total bilirubin (mg/dl)	0.63 (0.3–11.7)	0.8 (0.5–41.4)	n.s.
Direct bilirubin (mg/dl)	0.15 (0.1–4.7)	0.2 (0.3–1.8)	n.s.
Albumin (g/l)	4.1 (2.9–5.3)	4.3 (3–5.8)	n.s.
Histological Scheuer stage	II (I–IV)	III (I–IV)	n.s.
I	8 patients	13 patients	
II	12 patients	13 patients	
III	7 patients	17 patients	
IV	2 patients	12 patients	

First of all, they are reminiscent of similar observations reported by a number of research groups, including our own, in other autoimmune diseases (both systemic and organ-specific) [26–31,33,34], and in other immunological or haematological disorders, such as IgE-mediated reaction to hymenoptera venom [35], or acute lymphoblastic leukemia (ALL) in paediatric patients [36]. In some of these conditions, sCTLA-4 concentrations appeared to be somehow correlated with disease activity or outcome (e.g. severity of histological lesion, and gluten exposure in patients with celiac disease) [34]. In addition, in a different model disease, a correlation was observed among CD1d expression and higher levels of sCTLA-4 in B-ALL patients, suggesting a possible role of this soluble molecule as a marker of progression to malignancy, or as a marker of severity of this neoplastic disease [36]. Moreover, in vitro experiments proved that the soluble form of CTLA-4 present in autoimmune sera is functionally active, namely, it is able to bind its physiological ligands and to interfere with cell-to-cell interaction crucial for the costimulation process (which in turn is crucial for mounting an efficient, as well as pathological immune response) [27, 31, 32 34–36]. The nature of such interference seems to depend upon the activation state of T-cells. Specifically, sCTLA-4 in vitro appeared to favor the expansion and cytokine production of chronically activated T-cells by blocking the triggering and negative signaling of their membrane CTLA-4, whereas sCTLA-4 interaction with naïve, membrane CTLA-4-negative T-cells had the opposite effect [27,31,32,34–37]. Thus, the presence of sCTLA-4 was suggested to be a relevant mechanism of perpetuation of immunological injury, possibly somehow related to disease outcome. That this is not simply a nonspecific inflammatory phenomenon is suggested by the lack of sCTLA-4 rise in controls with infectious diseases. Of note, the possible role of sCTLA-4 in modulating tissue damage was also suggested in a murine model [38].

The second relevant consideration rised by the findings of the present study is the apparent relationship of sCTLA-4 with AMA reactivity. As AMA-negative PBC patients are rare, we selected a consistent group of such patients and compared their sCTLA-4 levels with a comparable AMA-positive group of patients. It is debated whether AMA-negative PBC patients represent or not a distinct subset of PBC: they account for 2 to 5% of total PBC patients [19] and it has been suggested that the relatively low sensitivity of IIF method for AMA is at least in part responsible for AMA negativity. Nevertheless, the limits of sensitivity of IIF explain only in part AMA-negative PBC. In fact, in our series we selected a relatively large group of AMA-negative/MIT3-negative patients. In addition, the comparison of functional data and histology seems to suggest that AMA-negative patients have a milder disease than AMA-positive ones. In fact, the distribution of patients according to the Scheuer stage shows a higher damage in AMA-positive (with the majority of III and IV stage) versus the AMA-negative ones (with the majority of I and II stage). The striking difference in sCTLA-4 serum concentrations in relationship to AMA presence does support the concept that a major immunological difference exist between the two groups of patients. In fact, some literature data underline the possible pathogenetic role of anti-mitochondrial reactivity per se via molecular mimicry [11–13,17–19], and a meta-analysis on the role of CTLA-4 SNP (+ 49A/G) as a predisposing factor in PBC suggests, though circumstantially, a link with AMA positivity [34].

However, several points have to be clarified. There is some doubt about the molecular heterogeneity of sCTLA-4 and the relationship between the ability to produce sCTLA-4 and the CTLA-4 polymorphisms observed in some autoimmune diseases. In particular, no correlation has been recently found between three recurrent single nucleotide mutations, CT60 (rs3087243), + 49 A/G (rs231775) and −318 (rs5742909) and sCTLA-4 production [38]. As mentioned above, a role of other related genes is likely, although no data are available to date. Finally, there is still a debate about the spliced/shaded nature of the soluble variant of CTLA-4 [27,34,36,39]. Moreover, the relationship between *CTLA-4* polymorphism(s) described associated with autoimmune diseases (including PBC) [33] and the ability to produce the spliced soluble form of the molecule has been not yet elucidated.

Conclusion

In conclusion, we have shown that serum sCTLA-4 values were elevated only in AMA (MIT3)-positive and not in AMA (MIT3)-negative PBC patients. Thus, some immunological difference of AMA-positive patients with respect to AMA-negative ones seems to exist. Data on sCTLA-4 in asymptomatic AMA-positive individuals could help to elucidate its possible role in the natural history of the disease.

Author Contributions

Conceived and designed the experiments: DS GP MB NB. Performed the experiments: PA DS. Analyzed the data: DS GP MB NB. Contributed reagents/materials/analysis tools: BP IB DV MT RT ET MGA NB. Wrote the paper: DS MB NB.

References

1. Gershwin ME, Selmi C, Worman HJ, et al. (2005) Risk factors and comorbidities in primary biliary cirrhosis: a controlled interview-based study of 1032 patients. Hepatology 42: 1194–202.
2. Selmi C, Zuin M, Gershwin ME (2008) The unfinished business of primary biliary cirrhosis. J Hepatology 49: 451–60.
3. Hudson M, Rojas-Villarraga A, Coral-Alvarado P, López-Guzmán S, Mantilla RD, et al. (2008) Polyautoimmunity and familial autoimmunity in systemic sclerosis. J Autoimmun 31: 156–9.
4. Kumagi T, Onji M (2008) Presentation and diagnosis of primary biliary cirrhosis in the 21st century. Clinical Liver Disease 12: 243–59.
5. Hohenester S, Oude-Elferink RP, Beuers U (2009) Primary biliary cirrhosis. Semininars Immunopathol 31: 283–307.
6. Milkiewicz P (2008) Liver transplantation in primary biliary cirrhosis. Clin Liver Dis 12: 461–472.
7. Gleicher N, Barad DH (2007) Gender as risk factor for autoimmune diseases. J Autoimmun 28: 1–6.
8. Kaplan MM, Gershwin ME (2005) Primary biliary cirrhosis. New England Journal of Medicine 353: 1261–73.
9. Pares A, Caballeria L, Rodes J (2006) Excellent long-term survival in patients with primary biliary cirrhosis and biochemical response to ursodeoxycholic Acid. Gastroenterol 130: 715–720.
10. Invernizzi P, Selmi C, Gershwin ME (2010) Update on primary biliary cirrhosis. Dig Liver Disease 42: 401–418.
11. Bogdanos D, Pusl T, Rust C, Vergani D, Beuers U. (2008) Primary biliary cirrhosis following Lactobacillus vaccination for recurrent vaginitis. J Hepatol 49: 466–473.
12. Smyk D, Cholongitas E, Kriese S, Rigopoulou EI, Bogdanos DP (2011) Primary biliary cirrhosis: family stories. Autoimmune Dis 2011: 189585.
13. Hirschfield GM, Gershwin ME (2011) Primary biliary cirrhosis: one disease with many faces. The Israel Medical Association Journal 13: 55–59.
14. Smyk DS, Mytilinaiou MG, Milkiewicz P, Rigopoulou EI, Invernizzi P, et al. (2012) Towards systemic sclerosis and away from primary biliary cirrhosis: the case of PTPN22. Autoimmun Highligths 3: 1–9.
15. Bernuzzi F, Fenoglio D, Battaglia F, Fravega M, Gershwin ME, et al. (2010) Phenotypical and functional alterations of CD8 regulatory T cells in primary biliary cirrhosis. J Autoimmun 35: 176–180.
16. Longhi MS, Ma Y, Bogdanos DP, Cheeseman P, Mieli-Vergani G, et al. (2004) Impairment of CD4(+)CD25(+) regulatory T-cells in autoimmune liver disease. J Hepatol 41: 31–37.
17. Liu H, Norman GL, Shums Z, Worman HJ, Krawitt EL, et al Invernizzi P (2010) PBC screen: an IgG/IgA dual isotype ELISA detecting multiple mitochondrial and nuclear autoantibodies specific for primary biliary cirrhosis. J Autoimmun 35: 436–442.
18. Bogdanos DP, Komorowski L (2011) Disease-specific autoantibodies in primary biliary cirrhosis. Clinica Chimica Acta 412: 502–512.
19. Bizzaro N, Covini G, Rosina F, Muratori P, Tonutti E, et al. (2012) Overcoming a "probable" diagnosis in antimitochondrial antibody negative primary biliary cirrhosis: study of 100 sera and review of the literature. Clin Reviews Allergy Immunol 42: 288–297.
20. Duarte-Rey C, Bogdanos D, Yang CY, Roberts K, Leung PS, et al. (2012) Primary biliary cirrhosis and the nuclear pore complex. Autoimmun Rev 11: 898–902.
21. Courvalin JC, Worman HJ (1977) Nuclear envelope protein autoantibodies in primary biliary cirrhosis. Seminar Liver Dis 17: 79–90.

22. Harper K, Balzano C, Rouvier E, Mattéi MG, Luciani MF, et al. (1991) CTLA-4 and CD28 activated lymphocyte molecules are closely related in both mouse and human as to sequence message expression gene structure and chromosomal location. J Immunol 147: 1037–1044.
23. Karandikar NJ, Vanderlugt CL, Walunas TL, Miller SD, Bluestone JA. (1996) CTLA-4: a negative regulator of autoimmune disease. J Exp Med 184: 783–788.
24. Salomon B, Bluestone JA (2001) Complexities of CD28/B7: CTLA-4 costimulatory pathways in autoimmunity and transplantation. Annual Rev Immunol 19: 225–252.
25. Magistrelli G, Jeannin P, Herbault N, Benoit De Coignac A, Gauchat JF, et al. (1999) A soluble form of CTLA-4 generated by alternative splicing is expressed by nonstimulated human T cells. Eur J Immunol 29: 3596–3602.
26. Oaks MK, Hallett KM (2000) A soluble form of CTLA-4 in patients with autoimmune thyroid disease. J Immunol 164: 5015–5018.
27. Saverino D, Brizzolara R, Simone R, Chiappori A, Milintenda-Floriani F, et al. (2007) Soluble CTLA-4 in autoimmune thyroid diseases: Relationship with clinical status and possible role in the immune response dysregulation. Clin Immunol 123: 190–198.
28. Sato S, Fujimoto M, Hasegawa M, Komura K, Yanaba K, et al. (2004) Serum soluble CTLA-4 levels are increased in diffuse cutaneous systemic sclerosis. Rheumatol 43: 1261–126.
29. Wong CK, Lit LC, Tam LS, Li EK, Lam CW. (2005) Aberrant production of soluble costimulatory molecules CTLA-4. CD28. CD80 and CD86 in patients with systemic lupus erythematosus. Rheumatol 44: 989–994.
30. Wang XB, Kakoulidou M, Giscombe R, Qiu Q, Huang D, et al. (2002) Abnormal expression of CTLA-4 by T cells from patients with myasthenia gravis: effect of an AT-rich gene sequence. J Neuroimmunol 130: 224–232.
31. Saverino D, Simone R, Bagnasco M, Pesce G (2010) The soluble CTLA-4 receptor and its role in autoimmune diseases: an update. Autoimmun Highlights 1: 73–81.
32. Simone R, Pesce G, Antola G, Rumbullaku M, Bagnasco M, et al. (2014) The Soluble Form of CTLA-4 from Serum of Patients with Autoimmune Diseases Regulates T-Cell Responses, BioMed Res Int: 215763.
33. Chen RR, Han ZY, Li JG, Shi YQ, Zhou XM, et al. (2011) Cytotoxic T-lymphocyte antigen 4 gene +49A/G polymorphism significantly associated with susceptibility to primary biliary cirrhosis: a meta-analysis. J Dig Dis 12: 428–435.
34. Simone R, Brizzolara R, Chiappori A, Milintenda-Floriani F, Natale C, et al. (2009) A functional soluble form of CTLA-4 is present in the serum of celiac patients and correlates with mucosal injury. Int Immunol 21: 1037–1045.
35. Riccio AM, Saverino D, Pesce G, Rogkakou A, Severino M, et al. (2012) Effects of different up-dosing regimens for hymenoptera venom immunotherapy on serum CTLA-4 and IL-10. PLoS One 7: e37980.
36. Simone R, Tenca C, Fais F, Luciani M, De Rossi G, et al. (2012) A Soluble Form of CTLA-4 Is Present in Paediatric Patients with Acute Lymphoblastic Leukaemia and Correlates with CD1d(+) Expression. PLoS One 7: e44654.
37. Cutolo M, Nadler SG (2013) Advances in CTLA-4-Ig-mediated modulation of inflammatory cell and immune response activation in rheumatoid arthritis. Autoimmun Rev 12: 758–767.
38. Dhirapong A, Yang GX, Nadler S, Zhang W, Tsuneyama K, et al. (2012) Therapeutic effect of cytotoxic T lymphocyte antigen 4/immunoglobulin on a murine model of primary biliary cirrhosis. Hepatology 57: 708–715.
39. Berry A, Tector M, Oaks MK (2008) Lack of association between sCTLA-4 levels in human plasma and common CTLA-4 polymorphisms. J Neg Res Biomed 7: 8.

Differential Antigen Expression Profile Predicts Immunoreactive Subset of Advanced Ovarian Cancers

Kevin H. Eng[1]*, Takemasa Tsuji[2]

1 Department of Biostatistics and Bioinformatics, Roswell Park Cancer Institute, Buffalo, NY, United States of America, **2** Center for Immunotherapy, Roswell Park Cancer Institute, Buffalo, NY, United States of America

Abstract

The presence and composition of lymphocytes characterizing an immune response has been connected to prognosis in advanced ovarian cancer. Our aim is to establish novel associations between prognosis and the expression of immune-related genes through a focused screen utilizing publicly available high-throughput assays. We consider transcriptome profiles from $n = 1137$ advanced ovarian cancer patients observed in four separate studies divided into discovery/validation sets ($n = 503/n = 634$). We focus on a subset of lymphocyte markers, antigen presentation and processing genes, T cell receptor associated co-stimulatory/repressor genes and cancer testis (CT) antigens. We modeled differential expression and co-expression using these subsets and tested for association with overall survival. Fifteen of 64 immune-related genes are associated with survival of which 5 are reproduced in the validation set. The expression of these genes defines an immunoreactive (IR) subgroup of patients with a favorable prognosis. Phenotypic characterization of the immune compartment signal includes upregulation of markers of CD8$^+$ T-cell activation in these patients. Using multivariate model building, we find that the expression of 6 CT antigens can predict IR status in the discovery and validation sets. These analyses confirm that a genomic approach can reproducibly detect lymphocyte signals in tumor tissue suggesting a novel way to study the tumor microenvironment. Our search has identified new candidate prognostic markers associated with immune components and uncovered preliminary evidence of prognostic subgroups associated with different immune mechanisms.

Editor: Rolf Müller, Philipps University, Germany

Funding: CA016056 www.cancer.gov National Cancer Institute core grant to Roswell Park Cancer Institute. Roswell Park Alliance Foundation www.roswellpark.org/giving award to KHE. The funders had no role in study design, data collection and analysis, decision to publish, or preparation of the manuscript.

Competing Interests: The authors have declared that no competing interests exist.

* Email: kevin.eng@roswellpark.org

Introduction

Recent, high-throughput gene expression profiling studies in ovarian cancer have identified a theme of differentially regulated immune signaling molecules related to prognosis [1,2]. The finding is consistent with mounting evidence that ovarian cancers are strongly immunogenic: spontaneous humoral and cellular immune reactions develop in response to disease [3], form characteristic epitopes [4], and are subject to complex up- and down-regulation by immune processes [5,6]. The degree of tumor infiltration by host immune cells has been associated with good prognosis [7] as well as the balance of lymphocyte subtypes.

Subtypes of lymphocytes have diverse functions related to antigen recognition and immune suppression [8] and are thought to indicate a dynamic and evolving response to cancer [9]. For example, an increase in CD8$^+$ T cells was found to be associated with good prognosis, but a rise in regulatory T cells was found to counteract this benefit [10]. Thus, studying components of the ovarian tumor microenvironment [11] is a critical angle for identifying prognostic associations [12].

However, few array-based expression studies have sampled both the host's reaction as well as the tumor. Most large observational studies [1,2,13,14] considered only tumor tissue because their goal was prognostic modeling; immune associations were made *post hoc* based only on enrichment inferred from a small number of significant immune genes. Other array-based studies that focused on immune characterization were small and observational (n = 38) [15] or case control (n = 25, n = 25) [16]. These studies showed positive associations between lymphocyte-specific markers and prognosis implying that the sampled tissue contained some microenvironment signal.

Recent work in expression arrays is able to computationally separate tumor, stromal and immune components of these complex tissues. For example, the ESTIMATE algorithm [17] uses 141 genes to estimate the fraction of expression signal attributable to the immune compartment. While this approach is useful for eliminating the noise due to impure samples, this study noted that the immune signals did seem to carry mild association with clinical outcomes. Based on the presence and potential prognostic value of immune markers, we conjecture that the apparent associations can be traced to residual lymphocyte RNA and that further analysis of these markers can be attributed to signal from the microenvironment. As such, we might simply model markers that we suspect are highly likely to be immune-specific *a priori*.

We rely on two large cohorts of public data organized into a discovery set and a validation set: 503 biobanked high-grade serous ovarian cancer samples from the Cancer Genome Atlas (TCGA) [2] form a focused training and exploration set and a more clinically-representative mix of 634 samples from 3 Gene Expression Omnibus (GEO) studies [1,13,14] form the validation set. The clinical features of the data are described in their original papers, but briefly, all of the patients in these studies have advanced, primary ovarian cancer (a small number of primary peritoneal and fallopian tube in the validation set) and received adjuvant platinum and taxane treatments following surgery.

We study first the specificity of immune-related genes to lymphocyte tissues and then explore univariate prognostic associations. Using clustering algorithms, we identify a subset of cancer cases with high adaptive immunity signals and we show that this subset can be predicted by the tumor expression of cancer-testis antigens. Taken together, these results imply that significant prognostic value remains untapped in the tumor microenvironment.

Methods

Clinical and Gene Expression Data

TCGA is a biorepository study of $n=503$ high-grade serous ovarian cancers from multiple centers in the United States and is described extensively in the original article [2]. Relevant to our analysis, this study strictly included ovarian primaries and papillary serous histologies. Samples were originally assessed as Stage III-IV and Grade 2,3 (later re-staged by a TCGA pathologist) and the patient received adjuvant platinum and taxane based chemotherapy. We adopt the view that these cases reflect a biased but homogenous clinical presentation more likely to yield a consistent biological mechanism.

Three clinical datasets were downloaded from the NCBI GEO database and are described below. Table 1 is a summary of clinically relevant differences between the studies.

GEO:GSE9891 is an Australian observational study [14] of $n=285$ mostly serous (227) ovarian cancer including some peritoneal (34) and fallopian (5) primaries. Conditioning on patients receiving platinum/taxol and removing the LMP samples,

we analyze $n=240$ samples. For reproducibility purposes, we work with normalized data from GEO.

GEO:GSE32062 is a Japanese observational study [1] of $n=270$ samples including 10 control samples, 193 recurrences, 121 deaths yielding $n=260$ samples to analyze. An adjuvant platinum/taxol regimen was recorded for all patients.

GEO:GSE3149 is an observational study [13] of $n=134$ arrays after combining redundant ones. Significant work has been have been published on the difficulties in the original analysis of this data [18]; we have implemented the recommended similarity checks and averaged arrays when they appear to come from the same patient. This analysis begins with the GEO banked data and should be immune to data conversion problems.

A biological dataset, NCI-60 cell line data were taken from GEO:GSE5846 [19] where all of the cell lines were measured under untreated conditions. As positive controls, ovary cell lines, IGROV-1, OVCAR-3, OVCAR-4, OVCAR-5, OVCAR-8, SK-OV-3 and NCI/ADR-RES; should express no immune markers. For negative controls, we also study leukemia lines CCRF-CEM, HL-60(TB), MOLT-4, RPMI-8226, SR, and K-562.

Candidate Immune-related and Cancer-Testis Antigen Genes

Candidate genes were selected from KEGG:Antigen processing and presentation (hsa04612) focusing on surface receptors and genes involved in plasma membrane transport. Surface markers and co-regulatory molecules of the T-cell receptor signaling pathway (hsa04660) were added, excluding the internal signaling mechanisms (for example: phospholipases, secondary messengers, and the kinase cascades) as these are non-specific and related to other signaling pathways. Cancer-testis antigen genes were defined based on overlap with the CT Database [20]. The full gene list is provided in Tables S1 and S4.

All genes were aligned using official gene names mapped using the provided GEO platform annotation (i.e., an associated GPL file) and R package hthgu133a.db-2.8.0 [21]. Expression values were scaled and centered for comparability across genes. Note that the highly variable parts of the T-cell receptor (TCA, TCB) cannot be measured on the hybridization-based oligonucleotide arrays.

Table 1. Descriptive statistics for data sets used in this study.

Study	Discovery	Validation		
	TCGA [2]	Australian [14]	Japanese [1]	US [13]
n	503	240	260	134
GEO Array Type	GPL570*	GPL570	GPL6480	GPL96
GEO identifier	NA	GSE9891	GSE32062	GSE3149
Age (Range)	59.7 (30–89)	60.2 (23–80)	NA	NA
Stage (% III, IV)	92%	5%	100%	NA
Grade (% 3,4)	87%	61%	50%	NA
Residual Disease (% None)	23%	27%	40%	NA
Neoadjuvant (% Yes)	0%	7%	0%	NA
Median Months OS	44 (40–48)	44 (38–57)	60 (50–80)	74 (35–98)
Median Months PFS	18 (15–19)	15 (14–18)	19 (18–23)	NA

* TCGA uses 3 array types. Only the Affymetrix array was used for completeness.

Computational Methods

Univariate associations were performed with proportional hazards regression. No time truncation, to reduce the effect of long survivors, was performed. Significance was cut at $p < 0.05$ and was adjusted for multiple testing unless otherwise noted. The reported FDR calculation is based on the expected number of false positives assuming all tests are null.

Clustering analysis in the TCGA data is based on complete hierarchical clustering under Euclidean distance. Subgroups were picked by splitting the tree at 4 leaves based on visual inspection and a within/between group sum of squares criterion. Cluster centers were used to seed a k-means clustering algorithm in the validation data and the p-value is reported for a study-stratified 4-group log-rank test.

The volcano plot uses literature-based surface markers and co-regulators based on a simple t-test. Highlighted genes were significant above the Bonferroni $p < 0.001$ mark and had biologically extreme fold change values.

Partial correlations were computed using the class averages for genes assigned to CD4, CD8, CD3, MHCI and MHCII-based sets. The GeneNet algorithm [22] using FDR < 0.05 and hard thresholding at absolute correlation 0.15 was used to infer Gaussian graphical models.

To infer the missing nodes in the GGM, a hidden node must satisfy three properties. Using MHCII - X - CD8 as an example: MHCII and CD8 must be conditionally independent given Gene X ($p > 0.05$); MHCII and Gene X must be conditionally dependent given all other genes (Bonferroni $p < 0.05$); CD8 and Gene X must be conditionally dependent given other genes (Bonferroni $p < 0.05$). Each of these can be reduced to a p-value statement using standard linear model theory and added variable analysis.

Predictions from a multivariate logistic regression model were categorized into immunoreactive class calls based on thresholding the predicted value from the model. This threshold was chosen using the sensitivity/specificity intersection point across all validation datasets.

All statistical analysis was performed in the R statistical programming language.

Results

Expression of genes specific to lymphocytes is measurable in tumor samples

We observed that selected lymphocyte specific markers are present in measurable quantities in sampled tumor tissue from our discovery set. The distribution of average expression (Figure 1A) shows the typical multimodal pattern in expression arrays: the lower peak reflects the background noise for genes that are not expressed in the sample and the higher peak represents signal. The lymphocyte marker CD45 is in the signal peak and is relatively highly expressed (Table S2). We conjecture that a measurable portion of the cells in each sample contain lymphocyte RNA which would represent the tumor microenvironment.

Comparison with the GeneAtlas tissues [23] confirms that the nominal action of these expression array probes is lymphocyte-specific. We considered probe expression in ovarian NCI-60 cell lines [19] to exclude the possibility that genes are normally expressed in tumor tissue (Table S2). Considering the mean quantile of expression versus other probes, surface markers CD64, CD1D, CD14, CD33, CD8A, CD16b, CD45 maintain a low level in cell lines versus microdissected tumor (all lower than the 35th quantile, $p < 0.05$). The near absence of IL6, IL12, IFNB1, and IFNG (between the 2nd and 25th quantile) suggests that the ability

to measure cytokine signaling is lost in this in vitro system; notably, the IL12 receptor is measurable, so surface markers do appear. The exception to this pattern is that CD4 is over-expressed (51st and 61st quantiles in tumor and cell line samples respectively).

This establishes that a reproducible immune signal can be measured in sampled tumor tissue and we proceed assuming that these markers form a representative cross-section of tumor and immune system interaction.

Reproducible associations between candidate genes and overall survival

Of the 64 candidate genes, 15 have univariate associations (score test p-value < 0.05) with overall survival (OS) following surgery and primary chemotherapy in the TCGA study (Table S1). A further 5 of these can be validated in the withheld independent studies ($FDR = 0.032$).

The validated set can be organized by function: major histocompatibility complex (MHC) I genes, HLA-F, and HLA-G; an MHCII gene, HLA-DOB; the MHCI associated transporter, TAP1; and the co-receptor complex subunit, CD3D (TCR-δ). Increasing expression of each of these transcripts is associated with better survival (Table 2). T-cell related genes are highly correlated, which likely accounts for an indirect but positive association between the suppressor HLA-DOB and survival (Univariate HR = 0.74, 95% CI: 0.65–0.85, $p < 0.0001$). We will examine the multivariate expression of these genes next.

Using a hierarchical clustering algorithm, the discovery set patients can be divided into four groups (Figure 1B) associated with OS (p = 1.2e-05). Represented in the heatmap in Figure 1C, the simultaneous expression of all five genes (colored purple) confers the most benefit. The simultaneous expression of all five genes is consistent with T cell activation, so we deem the high expressing subgroup an immunoreactive (IR) subset.

The degree of expression is not associated with variation in poor prognosis: the low expression of all genes (orange) does no worse than a heterogenous pattern of high and medium expression (yellow) or uniformly medium expression (green subgroup). This suggests that the deficient expression of any one gene is sufficient to lead to poor prognosis.

We assign validation patients to their most similar discovery set subgroup by k-means clustering. In the second heatmap (Figure 1D), the patients (columns) are ordered by hierarchical clustering within the validation data set. So, the clustered subgroups are strengthened by the observation that the class labels are preserved in the validation set.

In the discovery data, the survival benefit for the high expressers (n = 55, 10%) is a median of 70.9 months (95% CI: 58.1–98.0) versus 41.4 (36.9–45, p = 3.5e-05) OS; the median progression free survival (PFS) benefit is significant (p = 3.1e-04) at 30.4 (18.2–91.3) months versus 16.4 (14.7–18). This subgroup accounts for 5% of the deaths observed in the dataset and 7% of the recurrent cases. This benefit is weakly reproduced in the validation data: (p = 0.0335) with a difference of 64.0 months versus 51 months median OS. The PFS difference was not significant in the validation set.

Association with immunoreactive subgroup and immune markers

The TCGA analysis confirmed a set of genetic subsets [2] identified in a previous study [14]. Our high expression subgroup (purple, n = 55) is associated with their IR subgroup (38/55, 69%) (p < 0.0001) (Table 3). The orange subgroup (n = 39) is mostly proliferative (31/37, 84%). Both of these associations hold in the

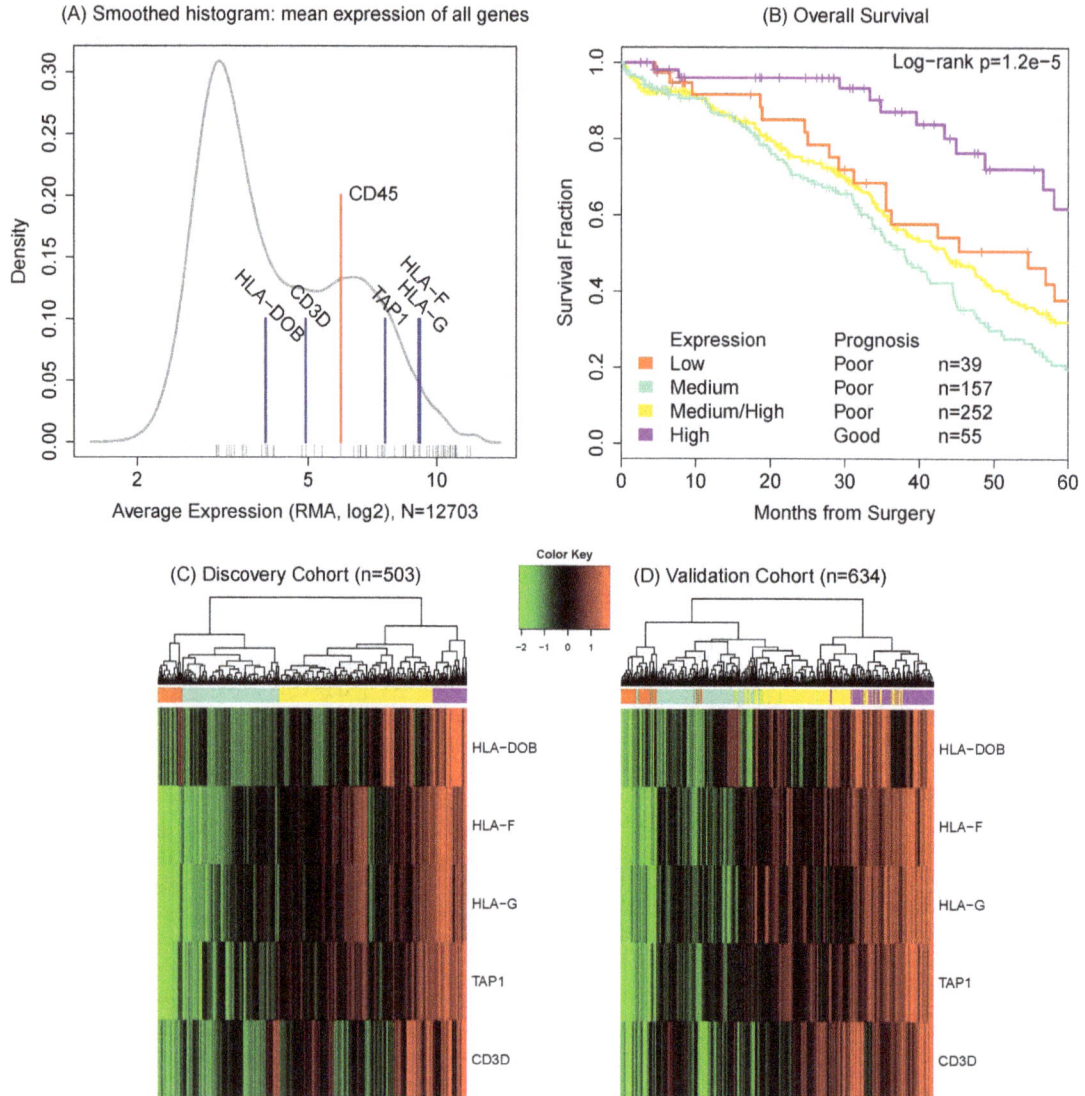

Figure 1. Mean relative expression of the selected genes confirms that they are all expressed in the samples (A). Black ticks indicate the mean expression of immune-related genes. CD45 is highlighted as a lymphocyte specific marker indicating the presence of lymphocytes. Subgroup-based survival estimates (B) are shown for the TCGA data based on hierarchical clustering of relative expression of selected T-cell genes (C and D). The four color bar on the left identifies the subgroups. The purple subset (n = 55, 11%) represents a significant survival benefit associated with the expression of all five genes.

Table 2. Validated immune genes related to overall survival and their correlation structure.

| Gene Name | HR (95% CI) | p-value | Correlation | | | |
			HLA-G	HLA-DOB	TAP1	CD3D
HLA-F	0.89 (0.79–1.00)	0.0429	0.95	0.51	0.84	0.60
HLA-G	0.88 (0.79–0.99)	0.0282		0.48	0.81	0.54
HLA-DOB	0.74 (0.65–0.85)	<0.0001			0.57	0.41
TAP1	0.88 (0.79–0.98)	0.0238				0.58
CD3D	0.85 (0.75–0.96)	0.0087				

Table 3. Association between derived subgroups and previously identified TCGA subgroups in discovery and validation sets.

Class	Purple	Yellow	Aqua	Orange
n	55	252	157	39
Overall Survival				p = 1.2e-05
median months	71	43	38	55
Progression-Free Survival				p = 6.7e-04
median months	30	18	15	17
Age				p = 6.2e-03
Mean Years	58	57	61	63
Stage				p = 2.8e-05
I/II	7	13	3	1
III/IV	48	239	154	38
Debulking Status				p = 3.2e-03
Optimal	17	51	21	13
Suboptimal	29	170	124	25
Platinum Status				p = n/s
Resistant	7	42	34	7
Sensitive	20	103	59	14
TCGA Class				p < 2.2e-16
Immunoreactive	38	59	7	0
Other	12	184	141	37
TCGA Class (Validation set)				p = 6.4e-11
Immunoreactive	35	27	8	0
Other	15	52	58	29

The colors are consistent with Figure 1. Note that only one study in the validation set had predicted TCGA classes and totals may not sum to 503 due to missing data.

validation data with TCGA subtypes. Altogether, this suggests that the hierarchical clustering derived subgroup is meaningful and that it nuances the TCGA subtypes as the latter were found to have no significant survival associations. Note that our study focuses on the IR subset and we make no attempt to model the other TCGA subtypes.

We examined the differential expression of standard immunology markers in the good prognosis subgroup. Figure 2 plots the change in expression across prognosis subgroups versus the

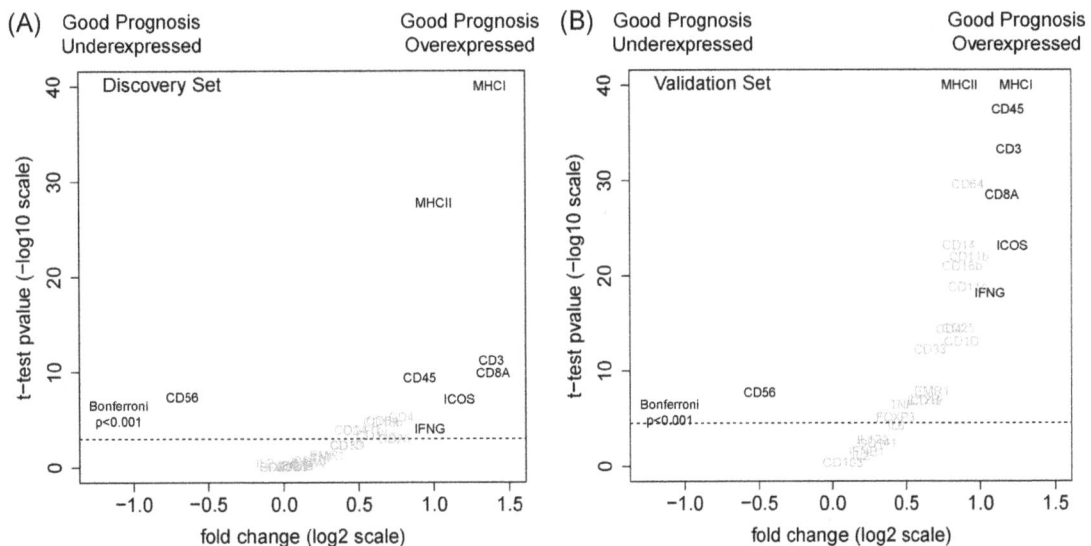

Figure 2. Differential expression of immunological markers in discovery (n = 503) and validation (n = 634) sets. Markers with strong biological and statistical significance (t-test Bonferroni p < 0.001) are chosen in the discovery set and highlighted in both plots.

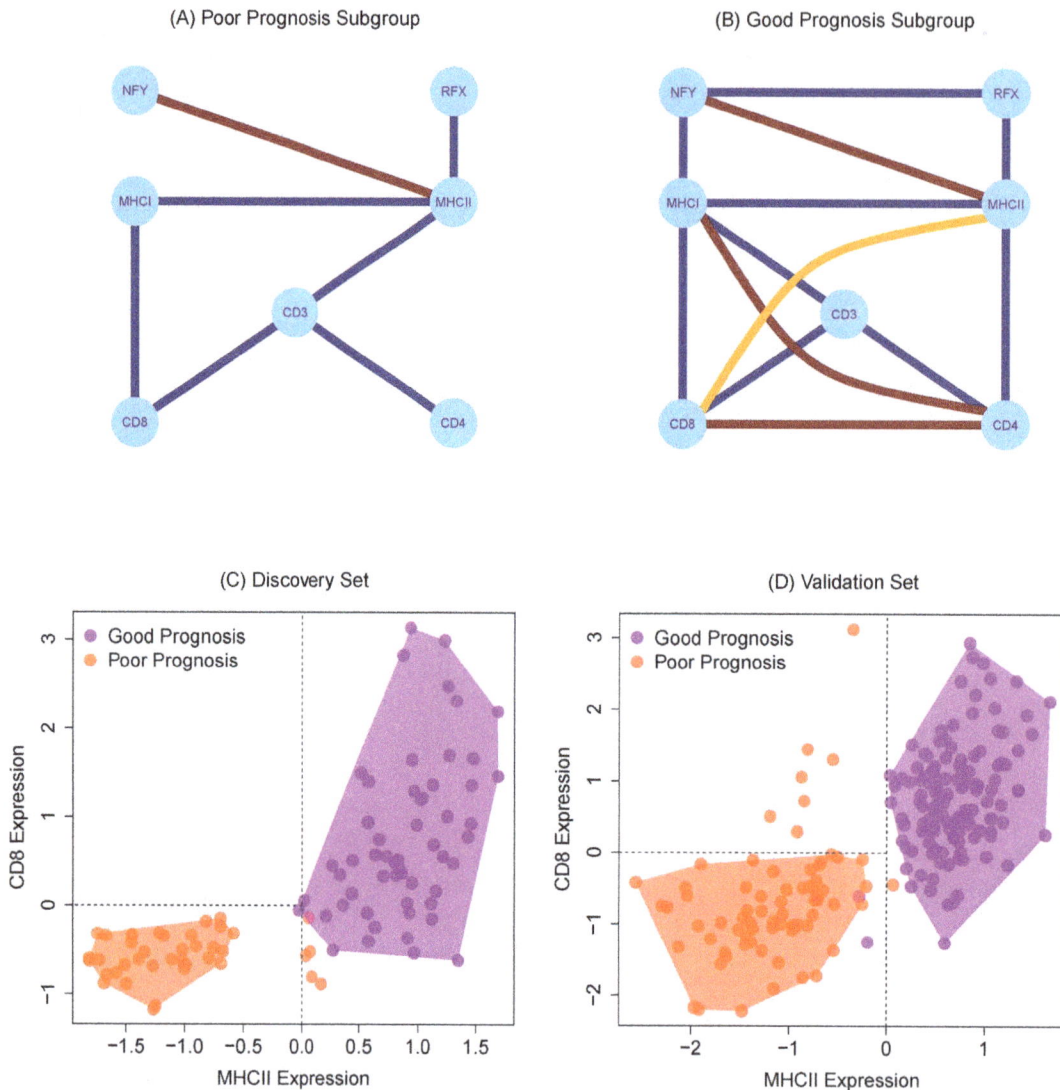

Figure 3. Partial correlation graphs indicating conditional relationships between genes in poor prognosis (n = 39)(A) and good prognosis (n = 55)(B) subgroups. Blue edges are positive associations and red are inhibitory associations. The highlighted orange edge can be removed by considering an independent set of genes. CD8 and MHCII array expression separate good and poor prognosis subgroups in discovery (C) and validation (D) data sets. MHCII expression is positively prognostic but appears in CD8 expressing samples. Shading is added for emphasis.

statistical evidence in both datasets. These markers imply an inflammatory response mediated by the recruitment of CD45[+] cells: CD8[+] cells and antigen-presenting cells (APC). No change in CD4 expression suggests that there is likely to be an latent background presence of CD4[+] T-cells and that the different action is attributable to activation (represented by differential *ICOS* expression). Absent are the NK cells (CD56[+]) reinforcing the idea that the process is part of adaptive immunity.

We conjecture that these observations are consistent with an immunoediting concept. The good prognosis group represents equilibrium where a prevalence of APCs and activated CD4[+] cells recruit CD8[+] T-cells to maintain adaptive immunity.

Prognostic co-expression suggests T-cell activation

To infer functional interactions between immune-related genes, we performed a co-expression analysis which summarizes correlation in the IR subgroup and the poor prognosis subgroups graphically. Edges in these Gaussian graphical models (GGMs)

represent statistical dependence between immune components (Figure 3A, 3B); positive dependence implies that both components are present and are likely to be interacting while negative edges imply mutually exclusive function or repression.

As in the differential expression analysis, CD4 and MHCII are correlated in the IR subgroup and not in the poor prognosis subgroups. Consistent with its reported function, RFX family (*RFX5, RFXANK, RFXAP*) of transcription factors' expression increases concordantly with the rise in MHCII expression [24]. In the IR subgroup, two edges imply anti-correlation between CD4 and MHCI which implies mutually exclusive function, and correlation between CD8 and MHCII (Figure 3C, 3D) which appears contrary to the specificity of MHC classes.

To explain this effect, we searched for missing genes whose inclusion in the graph would remove these edges. A missing link between CD8 and MHCII is *GZMA* a protease reflecting the activity of cytolytic T-cells. Between CD4 and MHCI we infer that CCR5, a cytokine receptor related to the activation of the T-cells,

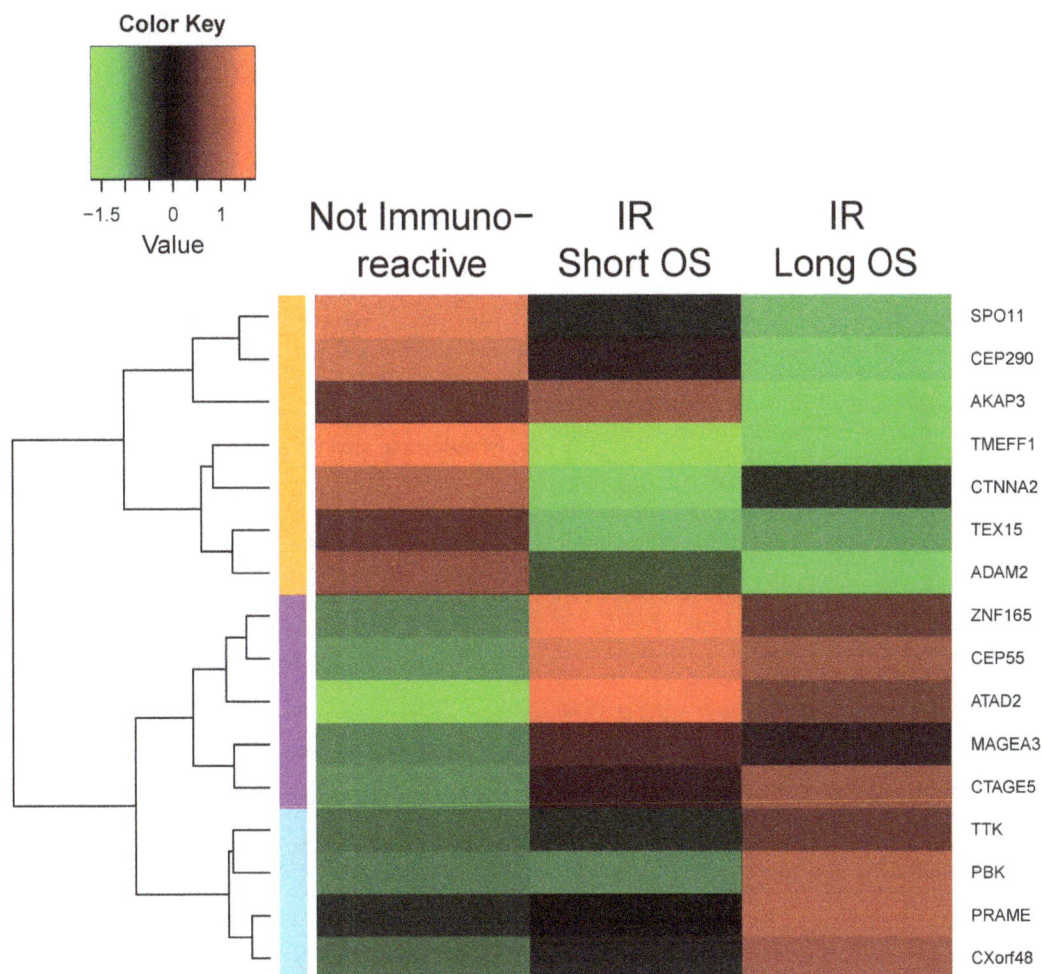

Figure 4. Cancer testis antigens associated with prognosis or immunoreactive (IR) subgroup can be divided into three classes: non-IR (orange), IR (purple) and immune stimulatory (cyan).

is missing. The common observation is that transcript associations likely need to be considered alongside measures of T-cell activation. The relevance of these genes is supported by the statistical significance of the transcriptome-wide search (adjusted $p < .05$) and the specificity of the selected genes' expression in lymphocyte tissues.

Focusing on CD8 and MHCII expression, we note that the good prognosis group can be defined by high MHCII expression where CD8 expression varies; CD8 expression is restricted when MHCII expression is low. Therefore, we hypothesize that MHC class II-mediated activation of CD4$^+$ T-cells are required for infiltration by CD8$^+$ T-cells that provide protection.

Immunoreactivity predicted by cancer-testis antigen profiles

We investigated the association of the IR subgroup with the cancer testis (CT) family of antigens [20]. These genes are frequently over-expressed in cancer cells and induce spontaneous immune responses, which make them a primary target for immunotherapy [25]. In particular, CT antigen expression is believed to influence the IR subset by regulating T-cell responses in the ovarian tumor microenvironment. The discovery set arrays measured 98 CT antigens (Table S4) of which 3 were associated

with the IR subset (Bonferroni $p < 0.05$): *CEP290*, *CTNNA2*, *TMEFF1*.

Because membership in the IR class is binary, we used logistic regression to model the multivariate set of antigens associated with IR status. Table S3 is the regression table for a model fit using BIC-based stepwise selection. Here, *CEP290*, *CTNNA2*, *TMEFF1*, and *TEX15* expression decreases the likelihood that a patient is in the IR class. Antigens *ZNF164* and *MAGEA3* increase the chance. Other than *CTNNA2*, which is twice as important as *MAGEA3*, the other genes have about the same effect. In the independent data, predictions from this model are strongly associated with the k-means derived associations (HR = 3.96, 95% CI: 2.59–6.14, p = 1.47e-11) tuned for equal sensitivity and specificity (0.66) given a moderate prevalence (140/634, 20.5%).

We further stratified patients in IR subgroup into good and poor prognosis based on OS to 33.5 months (overall study population median OS). A set of 16 antigens includes the union of the 3 IR subset genes and antigens associated with the difference in survival. Figure 4 is a heatmap comprising the mean expression of the 16 genes organized into three classes. The first class (orange) is expressed in non-IR cases and may reflect the activity of immunosuppressive elements. The second set (purple) is expressed in IR cancers but is unrelated to prognosis. The third (cyan) is expressed strongly in IR cases with good prognosis and may indicated immune stimulatory effects. A viable hypothesis might be to see if T cells responding to the second set of antigens (*ZNF165, CEP55, ATAD2, MAGEZ3, CTAGE5*) have regulatory phenotypes.

Discussion

We have analyzed the expression of 64 T-cell co-receptor and antigen presentation/processing genes in advanced serous ovarian cancer using a standard univariate screen and an analysis of their co-expression. These analyses define a subset of ovarian cancer cases with prognostically meaningful expression associated with T-cell activation and a previously defined immunoreactive subgroup [2]. In contrast to previous work [17,26], the subgroup can be identified reproducibly with just 5 genes versus over a hundred. This efficiency comes from our initial immunologic perspective. We reduce significantly the extraneous genes, but trade the ability to make a pan-ovarian cancer genetic characterization. As a result, we make no claim about or attempt to model non-immunologic signals.

We now have a small set of markers and antigens that may make translational and biomarker work more feasible for immunotherapy. With respect to the use of CT antigens, we have found a set which predicts non-immunogenic cancers (putatively, ones with low T-cell activation) and a set that might be targeted for blockade type immunotherapy. Both biological studies to verify regulatory activity of T cells in these cases and retrospective clinical studies may be the next investigative step. We speculate that the set of IR specific CT antigens stimulate immune responses (e.g., recruiting activated T cells), but are insufficiently immunogenic to induce tumor eradicating immune reaction. Alternatively, this group may prompt mixed effects: inducing immune responses while promoting tumor progression.

Inferentially, we have adopted a discovery/validation framework that allows us to make preliminary confirmations and to avoid over-interpreting high-dimensional artifacts. The data are limited by the nature of expression data from tumor samples; we rely on the conjecture that even after microdissection, assayed samples retain a portion of lymphocyte genetic material. Because this effect appears independently in multiple studies, these observations may be applicable to assays using this platform and are less likely to be subject to batch effect bias. Additionally, this work motivates the investigation of a structured way to analyze residual stromal signal from the tumor samples and therefore infer genetic interaction in the tumor microenvironment.

Supporting Information

Table S1 Univariate associations between genes and overall survival measured by score test p-value.

Table S2 Tissue specific quantiles of expression of lymphocyte specific markers. Low quantiles imply relatively low or no expression.

Table S3 Regression table for multivariate logistic regression model using antigen expression to predict immunoreactive class status.

Table S4 List of identified cancer testis (CT) antigens.

Acknowledgments

The results published here are in whole or part based upon data generated by The Cancer Genome Atlas pilot project established by the NCI and NHGRI. Information about TCGA and the investigators and institutions who constitute the TCGA research network can be found at http://cancergenome.nih.gov/.

Author Contributions

Conceived and designed the experiments: KHE TT. Performed the experiments: KHE. Analyzed the data: KHE TT. Contributed reagents/materials/analysis tools: KHE. Wrote the paper: KHE TT.

References

1. Yoshihara K, Tsunoda T, Shigemizu D, Fujiwara H, Hatae M, et al. (2012) High-risk ovarian cancer based on 126-gene expression signature is uniquely characterized by downregulation of antigen presentation pathway. Clinical Cancer Research 18: 1374–1385.
2. The Cancer Genome Atlas Research Network (2011) Integrated genomic analyses of ovarian carcinoma. Nature 474: 609–615.
3. Gnjatic S, Ritter E, Büchler MW, Giese NA, Brors B, et al. (2010) Seromic profiling of ovarian and pancreatic cancer. Proceedings of the National Academy of Sciences 107: 5088–5093.
4. Matsuzaki J, Gnjatic S, Mhawech-Fauceglia P, Beck A, Miller A, et al. (2010) Tumor-infiltrating NY-ESO-1-specific CD8+ t cells are negatively regulated by LAG-3 and PD-1 in human ovarian cancer. Proceedings of the National Academy of Sciences 107: 7875–7880.
5. Curiel TJ, Coukos G, Zou L, Alvarez X, Cheng P, et al. (2004) Specific recruitment of regulatory T cells in ovarian carcinoma fosters immune privilege and predicts reduced survival. Nature Medicine 10: 942–949.
6. Qian F, Gnjatic S, Jager E, Santiago D, Jungbluth A, et al. (2004) Th1/Th2 CD4+ T cell responses against NY-ESO-1 in HLA-DPB1*0401/0402 patients with epithelial ovarian cancer. Cancer Immunology 4: 12.
7. Zhang L, Conejo-Garcia JR, Katsaros D, Gimotty PA, Massobrio M, et al. (2003) Intratumoral T cells, recurrence, and survival in epithelial ovarian cancer. New England Journal of Medicine 348: 203–213.
8. Preston CC, Goode EL, Hartmann LC, Kalli KR, Knutson KL (2011) Immunity and immune suppression in human ovarian cancer. Immunotherapy 3: 539–556.
9. Dunn GP, Old LJ, Schreiber RD (2004) The immunobiology of cancer immunosurveillance and immunoediting. Immunity 21: 137–148.
10. Sato E, Olson SH, Ahn J, Bundy B, Nishikawa H, et al. (2005) Intraepithelial CD8+ tumor-infiltrating lymphocytes and a high cd8+/regulatory t cell ratio are associated with favorable prognosis in ovarian cancer. Proceedings of the National Academy of Sciences 102: 18538–18543.
11. Matsuzaki J, Qian F, Luescher I, Lele S, Ritter G, et al. (2008) Recognition of naturally processed and ovarian cancer reactive CD8+ t cell epitopes within a promiscuous HLA class II T-helper region of NY-ESO-1. Cancer Immunology Immunotherapy 57: 1185–1195.
12. Vaughan S, Coward JI, Bast RC, Berchuck A, Berek JS, et al. (2011) Rethinking ovarian cancer: recommendations for improving outcomes. Nature Reviews Cancer 11: 719–725.
13. Dressman HK, Berchuck A, Chan G, Zhai J, Bild A, et al. (2007) An integrated genomic-based approach to individualized treatment of patients with advanced-stage ovarian cancer. Journal of Clinical Oncology 25: 517–525.
14. Tothill RW, Tinker AV, George J, Brown R, Fox SB, et al. (2008) Novel molecular subtypes of serous and endometrioid ovarian cancer linked to clinical outcome. Clinical Cancer Research 14: 5198–5208.
15. Callahan MJ, Nagymanyoki Z, Bonome T, Johnson ME, Litkouhi B, et al. (2008) Increased hla-dmb expression in the tumor epithelium is associated with increased ctl infiltration and improved prognosis in advanced-stage serous ovarian cancer. Clinical Cancer Research 14: 7667–7673.
16. Leffers N, Fehrmann R, Gooden M, Schulze U, Ten Hoor K, et al. (2010) Identification of genes and pathways associated with cytotoxic T lymphocyte infiltration of serous ovarian cancer. British Journal of Cancer 103: 685–692.
17. Yoshihara K, Shahmoradgoli M, Martinez E, Vegesna R, Kim H, et al. (2013) Inferring tumour purity and stromal and immune cell admixture from expression data. Nature communications 4.
18. Baggerly KA, Coombes KR, Neeley ES (2008) Run batch effects potentially compromise the usefulness of genomic signatures for ovarian cancer. Journal of Clinical Oncology 26: 1186–1187.
19. Lee JK, Havaleshko DM, Cho H, Weinstein JN, Kaldjian EP, et al. (2007) A strategy for predicting the chemosensitivity of human cancers and its application to drug discovery. Proceedings of the National Academy of Sciences 104: 13086–13091.

20. Almeida LG, Sakabe NJ, Silva MCC, Mundstein AS, Cohen T, et al. (2009) CTdatabase: a knowledge-base of high-throughput and curated data on cancer-testis antigens. Nucleic Acids Research 37: D816–D819.

21. Carlson M (2014) hthgu133a.db: Affymetrix HT Human Genome U133 Array Plate Set annotation data (chip hthgu133a). R package version 2.8.0.

22. Schaefer J, Opgen-Rhein R, Strimmer K (2013) GeneNet: Modeling and Inferring Gene Networks. URL http://CRAN.R-project.org/package=GeneNet. R package version 1.2.8.

23. Su AI, Wiltshire T, Batalov S, Lapp H, Ching KA, et al. (2004) A gene atlas of the mouse and human protein-encoding transcriptomes. Proceedings of the National Academy of Sciences 101: 6062–6067.

24. Emery P, Durand B, Mach B, Reith W (1996) RFX proteins, a novel family of DNA binding proteins conserved in the eukaryotic kingdom. Nucleic Acids Research 24: 803–807.

25. Simpson AJ, Caballero OL, Jungbluth A, Chen YT, Old LJ (2005) Cancer/testis antigens, gametogenesis and cancer. Nature Reviews Cancer 5: 615–625.

26. Verhaak RG, Tamayo P, Yang JY, Hubbard D, Zhang H, et al. (2013) Prognostically relevant gene signatures of high-grade serous ovarian carcinoma. The Journal of clinical investigation 123: 517–525.

Assessment of CD4+ T Cell Responses to Glutamic Acid Decarboxylase 65 Using DQ8 Tetramers Reveals a Pathogenic Role of GAD65 121–140 and GAD65 250–266 in T1D Development

I-Ting Chow[1], Junbao Yang[1], Theresa J. Gates[1], Eddie A. James[1], Duy T. Mai[1], Carla Greenbaum[1], William W. Kwok[1,2]*

1 Benaroya Research Institute at Virginia Mason, Seattle, WA, United States of America, 2 Department of Medicine, University of Washington, Seattle, WA, United States of America

Abstract

Susceptibility to type 1 diabetes (T1D) is strongly associated with MHC class II molecules, particularly HLA-DQ8 (DQ8: DQA1*03:01/DQB1*03:02). Monitoring T1D-specific T cell responses to DQ8-restricted epitopes may be key to understanding the immunopathology of the disease. In this study, we examined DQ8-restricted T cell responses to glutamic acid decarboxylase 65 (GAD65) using DQ8 tetramers. We demonstrated that $GAD65_{121-140}$ and $GAD65_{250-266}$ elicited responses from DQ8+ subjects. Circulating CD4+ T cells specific for these epitopes were detected significantly more often in T1D patients than in healthy individuals after in vitro expansion. T cell clones specific for $GAD65_{121-140}$ and $GAD65_{250-266}$ carried a Th1-dominant phenotype, with some of the $GAD65_{121-140}$-specific T cell clones producing IL-17. $GAD65_{250-266}$-specific CD4+ T cells could also be detected by direct ex vivo staining. Analysis of unmanipulated peripheral blood mononuclear cells (PBMCs) revealed that $GAD65_{250-266}$-specific T cells could be found in both healthy and diabetic individuals but the frequencies of specific T cells were higher in subjects with type 1 diabetes. Taken together, our results suggest a proinflammatory role for T cells specific for DQ8-restricted $GAD65_{121-140}$ and $GAD65_{250-266}$ epitopes and implicate their possible contribution to the progression of T1D.

Editor: Matthias G. von Herrath, La Jolla Institute for Allergy and Immunology, United States of America

Funding: This work was supported by JDRF center funding for Translational Research at BRI and DP3 DK097653 grant from National Institutes of Health. The funders had no role in study design, data collection and analysis, decision to publish, or preparation of the manuscript.

Competing Interests: The authors have declared that no competing interests exist.

* Email: bkwok@benaroyaresearch.org

Introduction

Type 1 diabetes (T1D) results from destruction of the insulin-producing beta cells of the pancreas. A number of genes have been implicated in T1D development, but genes within the HLA class II region confer most of the disease risk [1]; in particular, it is estimated that 90% of T1D subjects have either an HLA-DQ8 or DQ2 allele [2]. Subjects with the DRB1*04:01 (DR0401)-DQ8 haplotype have an odds ratio of 8.4 for T1D [3], and the predisposing effect of this haplotype is supported by meta-analysis of data sets from different geographic regions [4]. In accordance with the importance of MHC class II molecules in antigen presentation, DQ8-restricted CD4+ T cells are likely to have an essential and pathogenic role in the progression of T1D.

A special feature of DQ8 is the absence of an aspartic acid residue at position 57 of the beta chain [5]. Lack of this Asp residue at beta 57 leads to reduced affinity for antigenic peptides, giving rise to diabetic pathology as a result of ineffective tolerance induction in the thymus [6,7]. Identification and characterization of DQ8-restricted self-epitopes may be key to comprehending

DQ8-mediated autoimmunity. A number of DQ8-restricted self-epitopes have been identified using DQ8 transgenic mice (for a recent review see [8]). Some of the reported peptides also elicit responses in HLA-DQ8+ individuals. However, monitoring of specific CD4+ T cells during the progression of diabetes, especially direct assessment of responses in the periphery, has been hampered by low frequencies of effector cells [9] and heterogeneity of the disease.

Autoantibodies against insulin (IA), glutamic acid decarboxylase 65 (GAD65), islet tyrosine phosphatase (IA-2), and zinc transporter 8 (ZnT8) have been used as predictive markers for T1D [10–13]. The appearance of autoantibodies is clear indication of beta cell autoimmunity and the combined measurement of insulin, GAD65, IA-2, and ZnT8 autoantibodies raise the detection rate to 98% at disease onset [12]. Despite their predictive value, some people with autoantibodies never develop diabetes [14]. In addition, the presence of autoantibodies does not necessarily indicate insulitis, the histopathologic hallmark of T1D that is mainly mediated by T-lymphocytes [15,16]. Therefore, identification of T cell biomarkers correlated with pathogenesis of T1D, together with the presence of autoantibodies, will facilitate disease prediction and prevention.

In this study, we investigated DQ8-restricted CD4+ T cell responses to GAD65. Responses of CD4+ T lymphocytes from T1D subjects to GAD65$_{121-140}$ and GAD65$_{250-266}$ were visualized using DQ8 tetramers after in vitro expansion of antigen-specific cells with the relevant peptides. In vitro responses and intracellular cytokine staining suggested a strong association of GAD65$_{121-140}$ and GAD65$_{250-266}$ to the disease. Direct ex vivo staining of peripheral blood mononuclear cells (PBMCs) for GAD65$_{250-266}$ revealed higher frequencies of CD4+ and CD4+CD45RO+ T cells in the T1D group. Collectively, our work indicates that T cells specific for GAD65$_{121-140}$ and GAD65$_{250-266}$ may contribute to the pathogenesis of T1D, and suggests GAD65$_{250-266}$-specific T cells as a potential biomarker for T1D.

Results

CD4+ T cell responses to GAD65$_{121-140}$ and GAD65$_{250-266}$ are detected more often in subjects with type 1 diabetes after in vitro expansion

Seven peptides derived from GAD65 were selected in this study to evaluate their relevance to the progression of autoimmune diabetes. All seven peptides are immunogenic in DQ8 transgenic mice [17–19], but DQ8-restricted responses in human subjects were not well demonstrated. Among the seven peptides, GAD65$_{121-140}$, GAD65$_{206-220}$, GAD65$_{250-266}$ bound to DQ8 with strong affinities (Table 1). The IC$_{50}$ values of GAD65$_{121-140}$, GAD65$_{206-220}$, and GAD65$_{250-266}$ were comparable to that of influenza A/Puerto Rico/8/34 Matrix Protein M1 (H1MP$_{185-204}$) epitope.

The three strong DQ8 binders were used to stimulate CD4+ T cells from DQ8+ T1D subjects. After two-week stimulation, GAD65$_{121-140}$ and GAD65$_{250-266}$ elicited CD4+ T cell responses in multiple subjects. Examples of positive tetramer staining for the two epitopes that elicited responses are shown in Fig. 1. Responses to GAD65$_{206-220}$ were negative in five T1D subjects examined and were not further investigated. The association of GAD65$_{121-140}$ and GAD65$_{250-266}$ with T1D was next examined by comparing the prevalence of specific CD4+ T cell responses in T1D patients and healthy controls. GAD65$_{121-140}$- and GAD65$_{250-266}$-specific CD4+ T cell responses were detected more often in T1D subjects than controls (GAD65$_{121-140}$: 6/10 T1D and 0/9 controls ($p = 0.0108$); GAD65$_{250-266}$: 9/17 T1D and 1/11 controls (Table 2, $p = 0.0407$); p value evaluated by two-tailed Fisher's exact tests), demonstrating a clear association of DQ8-restricted GAD65 T cell responses with disease.

DQ8-restricted self-epitopes elicit pathogenic responses

Self-peptides can modulate autoimmunity by induction of pathogenic (Th1/Th17) or suppressive (Th2/Treg) responses. To examine functional properties of DQ8-restricted self epitopes, GAD65$_{121-140}$- and GAD65$_{250-266}$-specific CD4+ T cells were cloned from in vitro expanded cultures of multiple subjects with type 1 diabetes. Representative tetramer staining for a GAD65$_{121-140}$ and a GAD65$_{250-266}$ clone is shown in Fig. 2A. These DQ8 tetramer-sorted clones were antigen-specific and the responses could be blocked by anti-DQ (SPVL3) antibodies (Fig. 2B). The GAD65-specific cells were assayed for cytokine production by intracellular cytokine staining (ICS) (Fig. S1A). All GAD65$_{250-266}$-specific clones produced Th1-type cytokine IFN-γ (Fig. 2C). One GAD65$_{250-266}$-specific clone also produced IL-4, but production of IFN-γ was still dominant in these cells (Fig. S1B). IL-17 was not detected in GAD65$_{250-266}$ cells. The ICS data were in agreement with the cytokine ELISA results as IFN-γ was the main cytokine secreted from GAD65$_{250-266}$ clones after peptide specific stimulation (Fig. 2D). Conversely, the cytokine profile for the four GAD65$_{121-140}$-specific T clones was more diversified. Two GAD65$_{121-140}$-specific clones isolated from different patients produced IL-17 (Fig. 2C). One of the IL-17-producing cells exhibited a Th1/Th17 double positive phenotype by co-expressing IFN-γ. Production of IL-17 was not a result of in vitro priming of naïve cells, as cells isolated from the memory population (CD45RA-CD4+) maintained the Th17-like phenotype (data not shown). The two IL-17-negative GAD65$_{121-140}$-specific clones were positive for IFN-γ, IL-4, and IL-10. However, these two clones might have distinct functionality as suggested by the ratio of IFN-γ to IL-4 producing cells (Fig. S1B) and the cytokine ELISA results (Fig. 2D). Although multiple clones isolated from one donor might be the same T cell captured at different stages of differentiation, our T cell clone data from different patients suggest that DQ8-restricted GAD65-specific epitopes could induce proinflammatory responses in T1D subjects.

Higher frequencies of GAD65$_{250-266}$-specific T cells are observed in subjects with type 1 diabetes

In vitro responses can be affected by numbers and activity of monocytes and lymphocytes in the blood samples. To confirm the disease association of DQ8/GAD65-specific cells in an unmanipulated state, ex vivo tetramer staining was performed for DQ8-specific T cells in DQ8+ patients and DQ8+ controls (average age for patients: 28.8, and for controls: 34.6, $p = 0.2809$). Direct ex vivo analysis was able to detect GAD65$_{250-266}$-specific CD4+ T cells in DQ8+ subjects, but not for GAD65$_{121-140}$-specific cells

Table 1. List of DQ8-restricted GAD65 peptides used in this study.

Peptide	IC$_{50}$ (µM)	Sequence
GAD65 121–140	1.6	YVVKS**FDRSTKVID**FHYPNE
GAD65 176–190	>50	PRY**FNQLSTGLD**MVG
GAD65 206–220	1.5	TYEI**APVFVLLE**YVT
GAD65 250–266	2.3	AMMI**ARFKMFPE**VKEKG
GAD65 427–441	>50	FQQDKH**YDLSYDTGD**
GAD65 461–475	>50	AKG**TTGFEAHVD**KCL
GAD65 508–521	>50	YIPPS**LRTLEDNEE**

*IC$_{50}$ value for the control H1MP$_{185-204}$ peptide was 1.4 µM.
*Predicted binding registers are indicated in boldface.

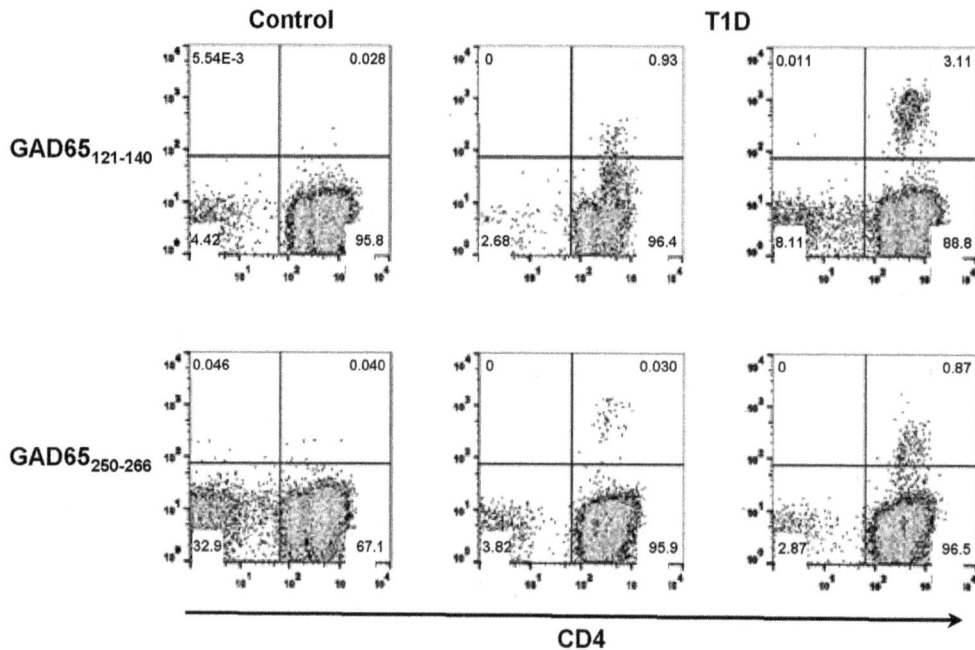

Figure 1. Detection of DQ8-specific self-reactive T cells in T1D patients. CD4+ T cells from T1D patients were stimulated with self-peptides derived from GAD65. The cells were cultured for two weeks and stained with PE-tetramers. CD4+ T cell responses to GAD65$_{121-140}$ and GAD65$_{250-266}$ were detected in multiple subjects. Representative tetramer staining of DQ8-specific self-reactive T cells was shown. Left column: negative staining from a healthy control. Middle and right columns: positive staining from two different T1D patients. Subjects were considered tetramer-positive if a distinct population that was more than three-fold above background in the same experiment was labeled.

(Fig. S2A and S2B). The unsuccessful detection might be due to low avidity or low frequencies of T cells specific for DQ8/GAD65$_{121-140}$. A representative ex vivo staining for DQ8/GAD65$_{250-266}$ from one T1D and one healthy subject is shown in Fig. 3A. The ex vivo staining for DQ8/GAD65$_{250-266}$ is specific as these cells can be co-stained by DQ8/GAD65$_{250-266}$ tetramers labeled with two different fluorochromes (PE or APC) (Fig. 3B).

Results of the ex vivo experiments are summarized in Table 3. The average frequencies of GAD65$_{250-266}$-specific cells and GAD65$_{250-266}$-specific CD45RO+ cells were found to be higher in the T1D group compared to the healthy control (Fig. 3C). There was no correlation between frequencies of GAD65$_{250-266}$-specific CD45RO+ cells and disease duration ($r^2 = 0.0218$).

Discussion

DQ8 possesses a predisposing non-aspartic acid residue at beta 57 and confers the highest risk to T1D. Substantial efforts have been made to identify DQ8-restricted responses which can closely monitor the progression of diabetes in human. However, detection of disease-related reactions from the rare islet-specific T cell populations is extremely challenging. In this study, we demonstrated DQ8 tetramers as a tool to study islet-specific T cell reactivity and identified two disease-associated peptides, GAD65$_{121-140}$ and GAD65$_{250-266}$ (Table 2, Fig. 2). In addition, T cells specific for GAD65$_{250-266}$ possessed several attributes that render these cells a potential biomarker for T1D. GAD65$_{250-266}$-

Table 2. Prevalence of GAD65-specific T cells in T1D and healthy subjects.

	Responses			
	+	-	Total	P
GAD65 121–140				
T1D	6	4	10	0.0108
Control	0	9	9	
Total	6	13	19	
GAD65 250–266				
T1D	9	8	17	0.0407
Control	1	10	11	
Total	10	18	28	

Not all peptides were tested on each subject.
Statistical analysis was performed using two-tailed Fisher's exact tests.

A

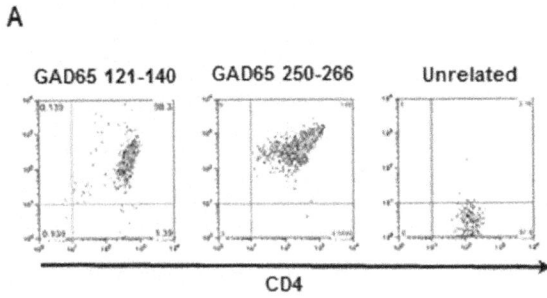

B

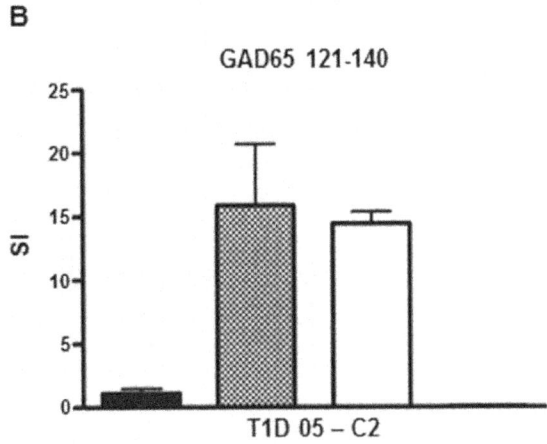

C

	Clone	IFN-γ	IL-10	IL-4	IL-17
GAD65 250-266	T1D 01 – C1	+	-	-	-
	– C2	+	-	-	-
	– C3	+	-	-	-
	– C4	+	-	-	-
	– C5	+	-	-	-
	– C6	+	+	+	-
	– C7	+	-	-	-
	T1D 02 – C1	+	-	-	-
	T1D 03 – C1	+	-	-	-
	– C2	+	-	-	-
	T1D 04 – C1	+	-	-	-
GAD65 121-140	T1D 05 – C1	+	-	-	+
	– C2	+	+	+	-
	– C3	+	+	+	-
	T1D 06 – C4	-	-	+	+

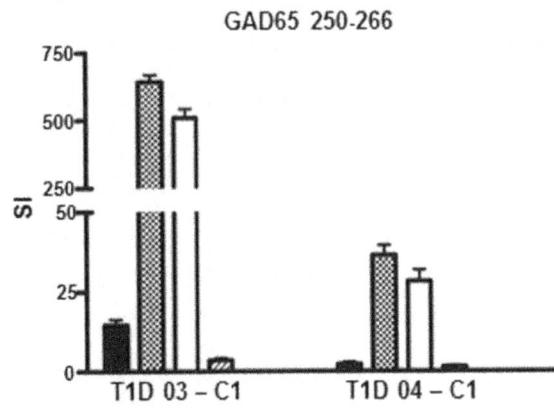

■ 1 μg/ml peptide

▨ 10 μg/ml peptide

□ 10 μg/ml peptide + anti-DR (L243)

▨ 10 μg/ml peptide + anti-DQ (SPVL3)

D

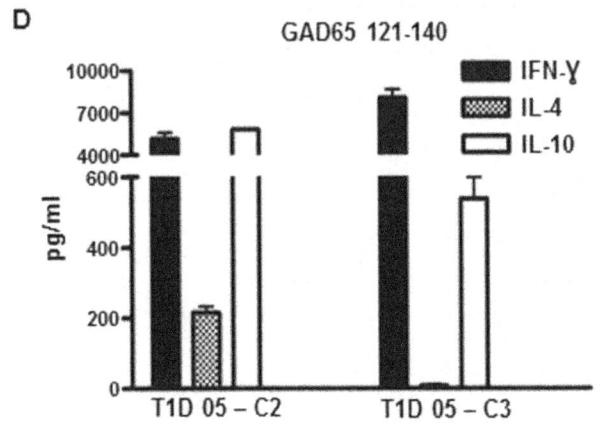

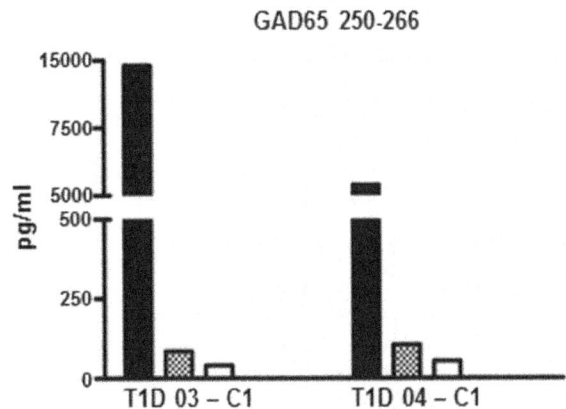

Figure 2. Functional analysis of DQ8-specific self-reactive T cells. T cell clones isolated by DQ8 tetramers were assayed for specificity and functionality. (**A**) Tetramer staining for GAD65$_{121-140}$-specific (clone T1D05-C2), GAD65$_{250-266}$-specific (clone T1D04-C1) and unrelated T cell clones. (**B**) Representative proliferation results of one GAD65$_{121-140}$- and two GAD65$_{250-266}$-specific T cell clones using APCs from a DR0401/DQ8 homozygous individual. Cells were stimulated with specific or irrelevant control peptide in the absence or presence of 20 μg/ml of L243 (HLA-DR blocking antibody) or SPVL3 (HLA-DQ blocking antibody). SI: stimulation index; cpm of specific peptide divided by cpm of irrelevant peptide. (**C**) Summary of cytokine-positive clones (for definition see Materials and methods) for GAD65$_{121-140}$ and GAD65$_{250-266}$. T cell clones were stimulated with 50 ng/mL phorbol 12-myristate 13-acetate and 1 μg/mL ionomycin in the presence of 10 μg/mL Brefeldin A in 1 mL of T cell medium for 4 hours at 37°C. Cells were fixed, permeabilized, stained with antibodies for IFN-γ, IL-10, IL-4, and IL-17, and analyzed on a LSRII multicolor flow cytometer. (**D**) Secretion of IFN-γ, IL-4, and IL-10 from two GAD65$_{121-140}$-specific and two GAD65$_{250-266}$-specific T cell clones. Clones were stimulated in the presence of 10 μg/ml of specific peptide with DQ8 antigen presenting cells.

specific cells exhibited robust responses upon peptide stimulation (Fig. 1), and could be detected directly in unmanipulated PBMCs (Fig. 3A). Most importantly, differences between patients and healthy subjects in frequencies of CD4+ and CD4+CD45RO+ cells specific for GAD65$_{250-266}$ could readily be seen by ex vivo analysis (Fig. 3C). Monitoring of GAD65$_{250-266}$-specific T cells can potentially provide new insights into the etiology and treatment of the disease, although further longitudinal studies to link specific responses to the beta cell function are essential to confirm its suitability as a biomarker.

Schneider et al. suggest that self-reactive T effector cells are less resistant to peripheral regulation in T1D patients [20]. The current GAD65$_{121-140}$- and GAD65$_{250-266}$-reactive T cell data support this model as responses to both peptides were more prevalent in T1D patients compared to controls (Fig. 1). Higher numbers of total antigen specific cells and CD4+CD45RO+ cells for GAD65$_{250-266}$ (Fig. 3C) were also found in the periphery of subjects with T1D by ex vivo tetramer staining. Other studies show that DRB1*04:01 (DR0401)-restricted GAD65-reactive T cells of certain specificities are preferentially activated in T1D patients while other specificities are not [21–24]. The discrepancy in GAD65 responses to peripheral regulation might reflect that self-reactive T cells for different specificities are subjected to various degree of regulation. Further study in examining whether discrepancy in regulation of DR0401 and DQ8 restricted responses will be of interest. Previous studies show some islet-reactive T cells exhibit protective phenotype in healthy subjects [25,26]. The presence of multiple effector properties for GAD65$_{121-140}$ (Fig. 2C, Fig. 2D, and Fig. S1B) implies the potential of GAD65$_{121-140}$-specific cells to modulate the immune balance between tolerance and autoimmunity. Future studies to compare the dynamics of T cell responses for each HLA haplotype during disease development will help to shed more insight into the immunopathology of T1D.

The presence of self-reactive T cells in healthy individuals highlights the importance of peripheral regulation as a checkpoint in the progression of T1D. The higher frequencies of GAD65$_{250-266}$-specific total and memory CD4+ T cells in subjects with type 1 diabetes (Fig. 3C) suggest that quantity and phenotypic changes for self-reactive T cells might be an indicator for loss of tolerance. DQ8 tetramers can therefore be a useful tool for the identification of disease-related self-reactive T cells as reliable biomarkers. Monitoring of these cells could assist with early-detection of risk or progression to T1D. In conclusion, DQ8-restricted CD4+ T cells specific for GAD65$_{121-140}$ and GAD65$_{250-266}$ were detected in multiple T1D subjects. GAD65$_{121-140}$- and GAD65$_{250-266}$-reactive T cells were more prevalent in T1D patients. Further evaluation of T cell responses for beta cell autoantigens should facilitate our understanding of the role of autoreactive DQ8 T cells in type 1 diabetes and selection of autoreactive DQ8 T cells as T1D biomarkers.

Materials and Methods

Subjects

The studies were approved by the Institutional Review Board of Benaroya Research Institute (BRI, Seattle, WA). All DQ8+ subjects were volunteers of Caucasian descent and were recruited with written consent from participating individuals or their guardians. HLA typing was conducted by BRI sequencing and genotyping core facilities. Samples from DQ8-positive T1D (n = 33, age from 9 to 56, days of disease duration from 281 to 7507) or DQ8-positive individuals without T1D or other autoimmune disease (healthy controls, n = 23, age from 18 to 56) were obtained under the auspices of the BRI JDRF Center for Translational Research at Benaroya Research Institute and Seattle Children's.

DQ8 protein and tetramers

Recombinant DQ8 protein was produced as previously described [27]. Briefly, soluble DQ8 was purified from insect cell culture supernatants by affinity chromatography and dialyzed against citric/phosphate storage buffer, pH 5.4. For the preparation of HLA class II tetramers, DQ8 protein was in vivo biotinylated in Drosophila S2 cells [28] prior to harvest and dialyzed into citric/phosphate buffer. The biotinylated monomer was loaded with 0.2 mg/ml of peptide by incubating at 37°C for 72 h in the presence of 0.2 mg/ml n-Dodecyl-β-maltoside and 1 mM Pefabloc SC (Sigma–Aldrich, St. Louis, MO). Peptide loaded monomers were subsequently conjugated into tetramers using R-PE streptavidin (Biosource International, Camarillo, CA) at a molar ratio of 8:1.

Peptides

Peptides derived from GAD65 (Table 1) were synthesized by Mimotopes (Clayton, Australia). The biotinylated reference peptide GAD65$_{250-266}$ (AMMIARFKMFPEVKEKG) was synthesized by Genscript with one 6-aminohexanoic acid spacer added between the N-terminal biotin label and the remainder of the peptide sequence.

Peptide binding competition

GAD65$_{250-266}$ is a good binder for DQ8 [29] and was used as the index peptide in the competition study. Various concentrations of each test peptide were incubated in competition with 0.04 μM biotinylated GAD65$_{250-266}$ peptide in wells coated with DQ8 protein. After washing, the remaining biotin-GAD65$_{250-266}$ peptide was labeled using europium-conjugated streptavidin (Perkin Elmer) and quantified using a Victor2 D time resolved fluorometer (Perkin Elmer). Peptide binding curves were simulated by non-linear regression with Prism software (Version 5, GraphPad Software Inc.) using a sigmoidal dose–response curve. IC$_{50}$ binding values were calculated from the resulting curves as

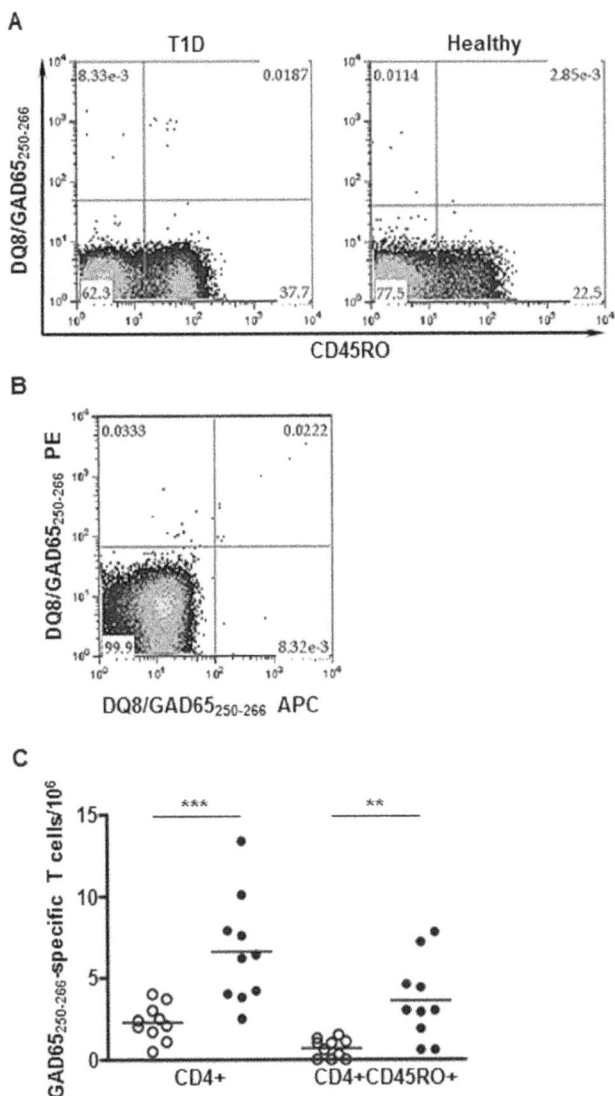

Figure 3. Direct ex vivo analysis of GAD65-specific T cells.
Unmanipulated PBMCs were stained with DQ8/GAD65$_{250-266}$ PE-tetramer. Antigen-specific CD4+ T cells were enriched, stained with antibodies against surface markers of interest, and analyzed on a Calibur multi-color flow cytometer. (**A**) Representative ex vivo analysis of the surface memory marker CD45RO for GAD65$_{250-266}$. The frequency of GAD65$_{250-266}$-specific CD45RO+CD4+ T cells was 4.4 per million CD4+ T cells for the T1D patient (left panel) and 0.6 per million for the healthy subject (right panel). (**B**) Ex vivo co-staining of GAD65$_{250-266}$-specific cells with DQ8/GAD65$_{250-266}$ PE- and DQ8/GAD65$_{250-266}$ APC-tetramers. Cells were stained with PE-labeled DQ8/GAD65$_{250-266}$ tetramers first. After enrichment, tetramer-positive cells were stained again with APC-labeled DQ8/GAD65$_{250-266}$ tetramers at 37°C for 1 h. (**C**) Cumulative total CD4+ and CD45RO+CD4+ T cell frequencies for GAD65$_{250-266}$ in controls (open circles, n = 10) and T1D patients (closed circles, n = 10). *** P<0.001, ** P<0.01, as evaluated by Mann-Whitney U-test.

the peptide concentration needed for 50% inhibition of reference peptide binding.

Self-reactive T cell identification

PBMCs were prepared from the blood of T1D or healthy DQ8 subjects by Ficoll underlay. CD4+ T cells were isolated using the Miltenyi CD4+ T cell isolation kit, plated in 48-well plates with

APCs, and stimulated with 20 µg/ml peptides from the selected peptide set. The cells were cultured for two weeks in the presence of T cell medium (RPMI-1640 (Gibso) +10% pooled human serum +1% penicillin-streptomycin) and IL-2 (Hemagen Diagnostics, Inc.) at 37°C, stained with PE-tetramers and antibodies of interest, and analyzed by flow cytometry. 20000 total events were collected for each staining. Lymphoid cells were gated based on forward and side scatter profile. The negative threshold for gating for Fig. 1 was set based on the staining of samples with empty tetramers. Our criterion for positivity was distinct staining that labeled a compact tetramer positive CD4+ population, and was more than three-fold above background (cells from an unstimulated well) in the same experiment.

Ex vivo analysis of self-reactive T cells

Ex vivo tetramer staining was performed as previously described [30]. Briefly, 30 million PBMCs in culture medium at a concentration of 150 million/mL were incubated with 50 nM dasatinib (LC Laboratories, dissolved in DMSO) for 10 min at 37°C. The cells were next stained with 20 µg/mL phycoerythrin (PE)–labeled tetramers at room temperature for 120 minutes, followed by antibody staining for 20 minutes at 4°C with CD4 APC (clone RPA-T4, eBioscience), CD45RO FITC (clone UCHC1, eBioscience), and a combination of CD14 PerCP (clone MφP9, BD PharMingen) and CD19 PerCP (clone SJ25C1, BD PharMingen) to exclude B cells and monocytes from the analysis. Cells were washed twice with FACS running buffer (0.5% BSA and 2mM EDTA in PBS) and incubated with anti-PE magnetic beads (Miltenyi Biotec, Bergisch Gladbach, Germany) at 4°C for another 20 minutes. The cells were washed again and enriched with a Miltenyi MS magnetic column. Samples were labeled with ViaProbe (BD Biosciences) and analyzed on a BD FACS Calibur flow cytometer. Frequencies were calculated by dividing the number of tetramer positive cells in the bound fraction by the number of total CD4+ T cells in the sample.

Statistical analysis

Statistical analysis was performed with Prism software (Version 5.03, GraphPad Software Inc.). The Mann-Whitney U-test was used to preform two group comparisons of T cell frequency. Fisher's exact test was used to compare the prevalence of T cell responses in T1D and healthy subjects.

T cell clone isolation

T cell clones were generated by staining cultured T cells with tetramers, sorting gated tetramer-positive CD4+ cells using a FACS Aria (at single-cell purity, applying a singlet gate to the lymphocyte population) and expanding in a 96-well plate in the presence of 1.0×10^5 irradiated PBMCs and 2 µg/ml phytohemagglutinin (Remel Inc. Lenexa, KS). After expansion of each T cell clone to a single 48 well, clones were stained again with tetramer and also stimulated in parallel with the corresponding peptides (10 µg/mL), adding HLA-DQ-matched irradiated PBMCs as antigen presenting cell and measuring thymidine uptake to verify epitope specificity.

Intracellular cytokine staining

Autoreactive-T cell clones isolated from T1D patients were resuspended in 200 µl of T cell medium (RPMI-1640 (Gibco) + 10% pooled human serum +1% penicillin-streptomycin), and stimulated with 50 ng/mL phorbol 12-myristate 13-acetate and 1 µg/mL ionomycin in the presence of 10 µg/mL Brefeldin A for 4 hours at 37°C. After incubation cells were stained with surface

Table 3. Summary of ex vivo results for GAD65$_{250-266}$.

T1D

Age	Duration (Days)	Frequency per 10^6 cells		% Memory	IAA	GADA	IA-2A	ZnT8A
		CD4+	CD4+CD45RO+					
14	1632	2.5	0.6	24.0	-	-	-	-
14	2439	3.8	0.6	15.8	+	-	-	+
17	1190	13.4	7.8	58.2	N/A	-	+	N/A
24	1379	6.2	2.9	46.8	+	+	+	+
25	292	7.9	3.0	38.0	-	+	+	+
25	1247	7.6	4.6	60.5	+	+	-	+
30	6564	4.2	1.9	45.2	-	-	+	+
41	1094	4.0	3.0	75.0	-	+	-	-
42	281	6.4	4.4	68.8	-	+	+	+
56	7507	10.1	7.2	71.0	+	+	-	-

Healthy

Age	Frequency per 10^6 cells		% Memory	IAA	GADA	IA-2A	ZnT8A
	CD4+	CD4+CD45RO+					
21	3.7	1.5	40.5	-	-	-	-
29	2.5	1.3	52.0	-	-	-	-
29	2.1	0.0	0.0	-	+	-	-
33	2.0	1.0	50.0	-	-	-	-
33	3.0	0.6	20.0	-	-	-	-
33	2.4	0.0	0.0	-	-	-	-
35	1.7	1.1	64.7	-	-	-	-
35	4.0	1.0	25.0	-	-	-	-
42	1.1	0.0	0.0	-	-	-	-
56	0.5	0.3	60.0	-	-	-	-

N/A: not available.

antibodies including CD3 PE-Cy5 (clone HIT3a, BioLegend) and CD4 v500 (clone RPA-T4, BD Biosciences) as well as Fixable Viability Stain 450 (BD Horizon). Cells were then fixed and permeabilized as per the manufacturer's instructions (eBioscience). Cells were next stained with antibodies against IFN-γ AF700 (clone 4S.B3, BioLegend), IL-10 PE Cy7 (clone MQ1-17H12, BioLegend), IL-17A APC Cy7 (clone BL168, BioLegend), and IL-4 FITC (clone 8D4-8, eBioscience) for 20 minutes at 4°C. Cells were then washed in PBS and immediately analyzed by flow cytometry on a BD LSRII multi-color flow cytometer. Clones were considered cytokine positive if more than 10% of the cells produced that particular cytokine.

Supporting Information

Figure S1 Intracellular cytokine staining for DQ8-specific T cell clones. T cell clones specific for $GAD65_{121-140}$ and $GAD65_{250-266}$ were stimulated with 50 ng/mL phorbol 12-myristate 13-acetate and 1 mg/mL ionomycin in the presence of 10 mg/mL Brefeldin A in 1 mL of T cell medium for 4 hours at 37°C. Cells were fixed, permeabilized, stained with antibodies for IFN-γ, IL-10, IL-4, and IL-17, and analyzed on a LSRII multicolor flow cytometer. (**A**) Representative intracellular cytokine staining analysis for the $GAD65_{250-266}$ T cell clone T1D01-C6. Staining results (open histograms) were compared to cells incubated with nonspecific isotype matched IgG control antibodies (gray histograms). Numbers indicate the percentage of cytokine-producing cells. (**B**) The ratio of IFN-γ producing cells to IL-4 producing cells in IFN-γ $^+$ IL-4$^+$ clones for $GAD65_{121-140}$ and

$GAD65_{250-266}$. Each dot represents one IFN-γ $^+$IL-4$^+$ clone from Fig 2(C) (T1D05-C2 and T1D05-C3 for $GAD65_{121-140}$, and T1D01-C6 for $GAD65_{250-266}$, respectively).

Figure S2 Direct ex vivo flow cytometric analysis of DQ8/GAD65-specific T cells. (**A**) Gating strategy for Tetramer+ cells. Lymphoid cells were selected based on forward and side scatter profile. A dump channel was used to exclude monocytes (CD14+), B cells (CD19+), and dead cells (ViaProbe) from lymphocytes. Viable Tetramer+CD4+CD45RO+ T cells were gated based on the staining of unenriched cells, and the gating was applied to enriched populations. Numbers indicate the percentage of cells in the gated regions or each quadrant. (**B**) Representative ex vivo analysis of the surface memory marker CD45RO for $GAD65_{121-140}$-specific cells in a T1D subject. The frequency of these cells is below the threshold of detection.

Acknowledgments

We thank Dr Catherine Pihoker, Seattle Children's, and coordinators from BRI and Seattle Children's for help with subject recruitment. The administrative support of Diana Sorus is greatly appreciated.

Author Contributions

Conceived and designed the experiments: IC JY WWK. Performed the experiments: IC JY TJG EAJ DTM. Analyzed the data: IC. Contributed reagents/materials/analysis tools: IC. Wrote the paper: IC CG WWK.

References

1. Todd JA, Walker NM, Cooper JD, Smyth DJ, Downes K, et al. (2007) Robust associations of four new chromosome regions from genome-wide analyses of type 1 diabetes. Nat Genet 39: 857–864.

2. Ide A, Eisenbarth GS (2003) Genetic susceptibility in type 1 diabetes and its associated autoimmune disorders. Rev Endocr Metab Disord 4: 243–253.

3. Erlich H, Valdes AM, Noble J, Carlson JA, Varney M, et al. (2008) HLA DR-DQ haplotypes and genotypes and type 1 diabetes risk: analysis of the type 1 diabetes genetics consortium families. Diabetes 57: 1084–1092.

4. Thomson G, Valdes AM, Noble JA, Kockum I, Grote MN, et al. (2007) Relative predispositional effects of HLA class II DRB1-DQB1 haplotypes and genotypes on type 1 diabetes: a meta-analysis. Tissue Antigens 70: 110–127.

5. Todd JA, Bell JI, McDevitt HO (1987) HLA-DQ beta gene contributes to susceptibility and resistance to insulin-dependent diabetes mellitus. Nature 329: 599–604.

6. Corper AL, Stratmann T, Apostolopoulos V, Scott CA, Garcia KC, et al. (2000) A structural framework for deciphering the link between I-Ag7 and autoimmune diabetes. Science 288: 505–511.

7. Yoshida K, Corper AL, Herro R, Jabri B, Wilson IA, et al. (2010) The diabetogenic mouse MHC class II molecule I-Ag7 is endowed with a switch that modulates TCR affinity. J Clin Invest 120: 1578–1590.

8. Di Lorenzo TP, Peakman M, Roep BO (2007) Translational mini-review series on type 1 diabetes: Systematic analysis of T cell epitopes in autoimmune diabetes. Clin Exp Immunol 148: 1–16.

9. Oling V, Marttila J, Ilonen J, Kwok WW, Nepom G, et al. (2005) GAD65- and proinsulin-specific CD4+ T-cells detected by MHC class II tetramers in peripheral blood of type 1 diabetes patients and at-risk subjects. J Autoimmun 25: 235–243.

10. Achenbach P, Warncke K, Reiter J, Naserke HE, Williams AJ, et al. (2004) Stratification of type 1 diabetes risk on the basis of islet autoantibody characteristics. Diabetes 53: 384–392.

11. Bingley PJ (2010) Clinical applications of diabetes antibody testing. J Clin Endocrinol Metab 95: 25–33.

12. Wenzlau JM, Juhl K, Yu L, Moua O, Sarkar SA, et al. (2007) The cation efflux transporter ZnT8 (Slc30A8) is a major autoantigen in human type 1 diabetes. Proc Natl Acad Sci U S A 104: 17040–17045.

13. Achenbach P, Lampasona V, Landherr U, Koczwara K, Krause S, et al. (2009) Autoantibodies to zinc transporter 8 and SLC30A8 genotype stratify type 1 diabetes risk. Diabetologia 52: 1881–1888.

14. Narendran P, Estella E, Fourlanos S (2005) Immunology of type 1 diabetes. QJM 98: 547–556.

15. Willcox A, Richardson SJ, Bone AJ, Foulis AK, Morgan NG (2009) Analysis of islet inflammation in human type 1 diabetes. Clin Exp Immunol 155: 173–181.

16. Gianani R, Campbell-Thompson M, Sarkar SA, Wasserfall C, Pugliese A, et al. (2010) Dimorphic histopathology of long-standing childhood-onset diabetes. Diabetologia 53: 690–698.

17. Wen L, Wong FS, Burkly L, Altieri M, Mamalaki C, et al. (1998) Induction of insulitis by glutamic acid decarboxylase peptide-specific and HLA-DQ8-restricted CD4(+) T cells from human DQ transgenic mice. J Clin Invest 102: 947–957.

18. Herman AE, Tisch RM, Patel SD, Parry SL, Olson J, et al. (1999) Determination of glutamic acid decarboxylase 65 peptides presented by the type I diabetes-associated HLA-DQ8 class II molecule identifies an immunogenic peptide motif. J Immunol 163: 6275–6282.

19. Liu J, Purdy LE, Rabinovitch S, Jevnikar AM, Elliott JF (1999) Major DQ8-restricted T-cell epitopes for human GAD65 mapped using human CD4, DQA1*0301, DQB1*0302 transgenic IA(null) NOD mice. Diabetes 48: 469–477.

20. Schneider A, Rieck M, Sanda S, Pihoker C, Greenbaum C, et al. (2008) The effector T cells of diabetic subjects are resistant to regulation via CD4+ FOXP3+ regulatory T cells. J Immunol 181: 7350–7355.

21. Danke NA, Yang J, Greenbaum C, Kwok WW (2005) Comparative study of GAD65-specific CD4+ T cells in healthy and type 1 diabetic subjects. J Autoimmun 25: 303–311.

22. Yang J, James EA, Sanda S, Greenbaum C, Kwok WW (2013) CD4+ T cells recognize diverse epitopes within GAD65: implications for repertoire development and diabetes monitoring. Immunology 138: 269–279.

23. Monti P, Scirpoli M, Rigamonti A, Mayr A, Jaeger A, et al. (2007) Evidence for in vivo primed and expanded autoreactive T cells as a specific feature of patients with type 1 diabetes. J Immunol 179: 5785–5792.

24. Oling V, Reijonen H, Simell O, Knip M, Ilonen J (2012) Autoantigen-specific memory CD4+ T cells are prevalent early in progression to Type 1 diabetes. Cell Immunol 273: 133–139.

25. Arif S, Tree TI, Astill TP, Tremble JM, Bishop AJ, et al. (2004) Autoreactive T cell responses show proinflammatory polarization in diabetes but a regulatory phenotype in health. J Clin Invest 113: 451–463.

26. van Lummel M, Duinkerken G, van Veelen PA, de Ru A, Cordfunke R, et al. (2014) Posttranslational modification of HLA-DQ binding islet autoantigens in type 1 diabetes. Diabetes 63: 237–247.

27. Novak EJ, Liu AW, Gebe JA, Falk BA, Nepom GT, et al. (2001) Tetramer-guided epitope mapping: rapid identification and characterization of immunodominant CD4+ T cell epitopes from complex antigens. J Immunol 166: 6665–6670.

28. Yang J, Jaramillo A, Shi R, Kwok WW, Mohanakumar T (2004) In vivo biotinylation of the major histocompatibility complex (MHC) class II/peptide

complex by coexpression of BirA enzyme for the generation of MHC class II/
tetramers. Hum Immunol 65: 692–699.

29. Kwok WW, Domeier ML, Raymond FC, Byers P, Nepom GT (1996) Allele-
specific motifs characterize HLA-DQ interactions with a diabetes-associated
peptide derived from glutamic acid decarboxylase. J Immunol 156: 2171–2177.

30. Scriba TJ, Purbhoo M, Day CL, Robinson N, Fidler S, et al. (2005)
Ultrasensitive detection and phenotyping of CD4+ T cells with optimized
HLA class II tetramer staining. J Immunol 175: 6334–6343.

Increased CD112 Expression in Methylcholanthrene-Induced Tumors in CD155-Deficient Mice

Yoko Nagumo[1,2], Akiko Iguchi-Manaka[2,3], Yumi Yamashita-Kanemaru[2,4], Fumie Abe[2,4], Günter Bernhardt[6], Akira Shibuya[2,4,5*], Kazuko Shibuya[2*]

1 Faculty of Life and Environmental Sciences, University of Tsukuba, Tsukuba, Japan, 2 Department of Immunology, Faculty of Medicine, University of Tsukuba, Tsukuba, Japan, 3 Department of Breast and Endocrine Surgery, Faculty of Medicine, University of Tsukuba, Tsukuba, Japan, 4 Japan Science and Technology Agency, Core Research for Evolutional Science and Technology (CREST), University of Tsukuba, Tsukuba, Japan, 5 Life Science Center of Tsukuba Advanced Research Alliance (TARA), University of Tsukuba, Tsukuba, Japan, 6 Institute of Immunology, Hannover Medical School, Hannover, Germany

Abstract

Tumor recognition by immune effector cells is mediated by antigen receptors and a variety of adhesion and costimulatory molecules. The evidence accumulated since the identification of CD155 and CD112 as ligands for DNAM-1 in humans and mice has suggested that the interactions between DNAM-1 and its ligands play an important role in T cell– and natural killer (NK) cell–mediated recognition and lysis of tumor cells. We have previously demonstrated that methylcholanthrane (MCA) accelerates tumor development in DNAM-1–deficient mice, and the *Cd155* level on MCA-induced tumors is significantly higher in DNAM-1–deficient mice than in wild-type (WT) mice. By contrast, *Cd112* expression on the tumors is similar in WT and DNAM-1-deficient mice, suggesting that CD155 plays a major role as a DNAM-1 ligand in activation of T cells and NK cells for tumor immune surveillance. To address this hypothesis, we examined MCA-induced tumor development in CD155-deficient mice. Unexpectedly, we observed no significant difference in tumor development between WT and CD155-deficient mice. Instead, we found that *Cd112* expression was significantly higher in the MCA-induced tumors of CD155-deficient mice than in those of WT mice. We also observed higher expression of DNAM-1 and lower expression of an inhibitory receptor, TIGIT, on CD8[+] T cells in CD155-deficient mice. These results suggest that modulation of the expression of receptors and CD112 compensates for CD155 deficiency in immune surveillance against MCA-induced tumors.

Editor: Xue-feng Bai, Ohio State University, United States of America

Funding: This research was supported by a Grant-in-Aid from the Ministry of Education, Culture, Sports, Science and Technology of Japan (Grant Number 24249021 and 25114701 to AS and KS, respectively). The funders had no role in study design, data collection and analysis, decision to publish, or preparation of the manuscript.

Competing Interests: The authors have declared that no competing interests exist.

* Email: ashibuya@md.tsukuba.ac.jp (AS); kazukos@md.tsukuba.ac.jp (KS)

Introduction

Cancer immune surveillance to suppress tumor development is an important host protection process. Several immune effector cell types and secreted cytokines play a critical role in this process. Among them, cytotoxic T lymphocytes (CTL) and natural killer (NK) cells are major players in cell-mediated immunity against tumors [1,2]. Interaction of cell surface receptors on CTL and NK cells with their respective ligands expressed on tumors activates the CTL and NK cells [2,3], resulting in their secretion of cytokines and cytotoxicity against tumors [4,5].

The leukocyte adhesion molecule DNAX accessory molecule-1 (DNAM-1, also known as CD226) is a member of the immunoglobulin (Ig) superfamily and is constitutively expressed on most CD4[+] and CD8[+] T cells, NK cells, monocytes, and macrophages [6]. The poliovirus receptor (PVR) CD155 and another member of the same family, CD112 (PVR-related family 2 [PRR-2], also called nectin-2), are the ligands of DNAM-1 in humans and mice [7–9]. Interactions between DNAM-1 on NK cells and CD8[+] T cells and CD112 and CD155 on tumor cells augment cell-mediated cytotoxicity and cytokine production [7,8].

CD155 and CD112 are present on various types of epithelial and endothelial cells in many tissues [10,11]. A number of studies have demonstrated that CD155 and CD112 are overexpressed on certain hematopoietic and nonhematopoietic tumors [12–17], suggesting that DNAM-1 ligand expression might be induced by tumorigenesis and might stimulate CTL- and NK cell–mediated tumor immunity. Of note, CD155 and CD112 also bind TIGIT (T cell immunoreceptor with Ig and ITIM [immunoreceptor tyrosine-based inhibitory motif] domains), which is expressed on T cells and NK cells and mediates an inhibitory signal (either directly or indirectly) in these cells [18,19]. CD155 also binds an immunoreceptor, CD96 (also called T cell-activated increased late expression [TACTILE]), that is expressed on both activated T cells and NK cells [20–22]. Taken together, the available data suggest that CD155 might be a double-edged sword balancing tumor growth and elimination.

We have previously demonstrated that the chemical carcinogens methylcholanthrane (MCA) and 7,12-dimethylbenz[a]anthracene (DMBA) result in significantly greater development of fibrosarcoma and papilloma, respectively, in DNAM-1–deficient mice than in wild-type (WT) mice [23]. Interestingly, we found that although

Cd155 expression on MCA-induced fibrosarcomas was significantly higher in DNAM-1–deficient mice than in WT mice, *Cd112* expression was similar, suggesting that CD155, rather than CD112, is the tumor ligand involved in DNAM-1–mediated immune surveillance against MCA-induced fibrosarcoma. In the present study, we used CD155-deficient mice to examine the role of CD155 on MCA-induced fibrosarcomas in tumor immune surveillance.

Materials and Methods

Mice

C57BL/6N and BALB/c mice were purchased from CLEA (Tokyo, Japan). CD155-deficient C57BL/6N and BALB/c mice were described previously [24]; they were additionally backcrossed twice with C57BL/6N and BALB/c mice, respectively (a total of 12 generations). All mice were housed and bred under specific-pathogen-free conditions at the Animal Resource Center of the University of Tsukuba. Animal experiments were carried out in a humane manner after receiving approval from the Animal Experiment Committee of the University of Tsukuba (Approval No.: 10-237, 11-231, 12-231), and in accordance with Fundamental Guideline for Proper Conduct of Animal Experiment and Related Activities in Academic Research Institutions under the Jurisdiction of the Ministry of Education, Culture, Sports, Science and Technology, and Japanese Act on Welfare and Management of Animals (No.105).

Flow cytometry

CD4$^+$ T, CD8$^+$ T, and NK cells from *peripheral* blood were analyzed using an LSRFortessa flow cytometer (BD Biosciences, San Jose, CA). The anti-DNAM-1 monoclonal antibody (mAb) TX42 (rat IgG2a) was generated in our laboratory [13]. All other antibodies for flow cytometry analyses were purchased from BD Biosciences. CD8$^+$ T cells were purified by magnetic separation from spleen cells on a Mini-MACS system (Miltenyi Biotec, Bergisch Gladbach, Germany). Purified CD8$^+$ T cells were cultured in the presence of 20 ng/ml exogenous IL-2 (BD Biosciences) in a 24-well plate coated with 1 μg/ml of anti-CD3e mAb (BD Biosciences). The cells were harvested at various time points, and the cell surface molecules were analyzed by flow cytometry. Antibodies against TIGIT and CD96 were from eBioscience (San Diego, CA) and R&D Systems (Minneapolis, MN), respectively. Cell staining and flow cytometry were performed according to standard procedures. The CellQuest (BD Biosciences) and FlowJo (Tree Star, Inc., Ashland, OR) programs were used for data acquisition and analysis.

Tumor growth assay and survival of mice

Groups of 10–20 WT or CD155-deficient male mice (8–12 week-old) were injected subcutaneously (s.c.) in the back with 5 or 100 μg (as specified in the figure legends) MCA (Sigma-Aldrich, St. Louis, MO) dissolved in 0.1 ml corn oil (Sigma-Aldrich) after anesthetization (7:3 mixture of polyethylene glycol and isoflurane).

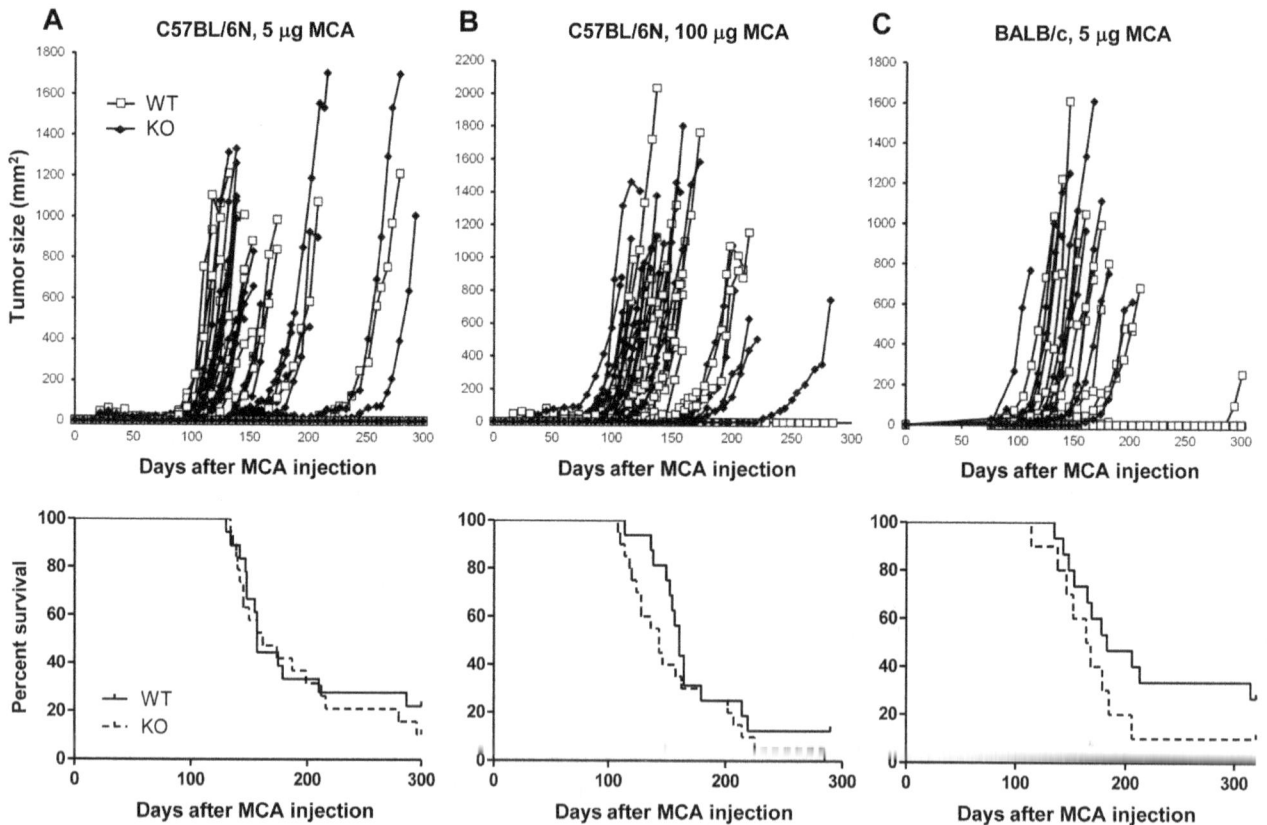

Figure 1. MCA-induced tumor development in WT and CD155-deficient mice. (A, B) WT (*n* = 18 and 16, respectively) or CD155-deficient (KO; *n* = 19 and 20, respectively) C57BL/6N mice were injected s.c. with 5 μg (A) or 100 μg (B) methylcholanthrane (MCA) on day 0. (C) WT (*n* = 15) or KO (*n* = 10) BALB/c mice were injected s.c. with 5 μg MCA on day 0. Tumor size in each mouse was measured once a week. Tumor size (top) and survival data (bottom) are shown.

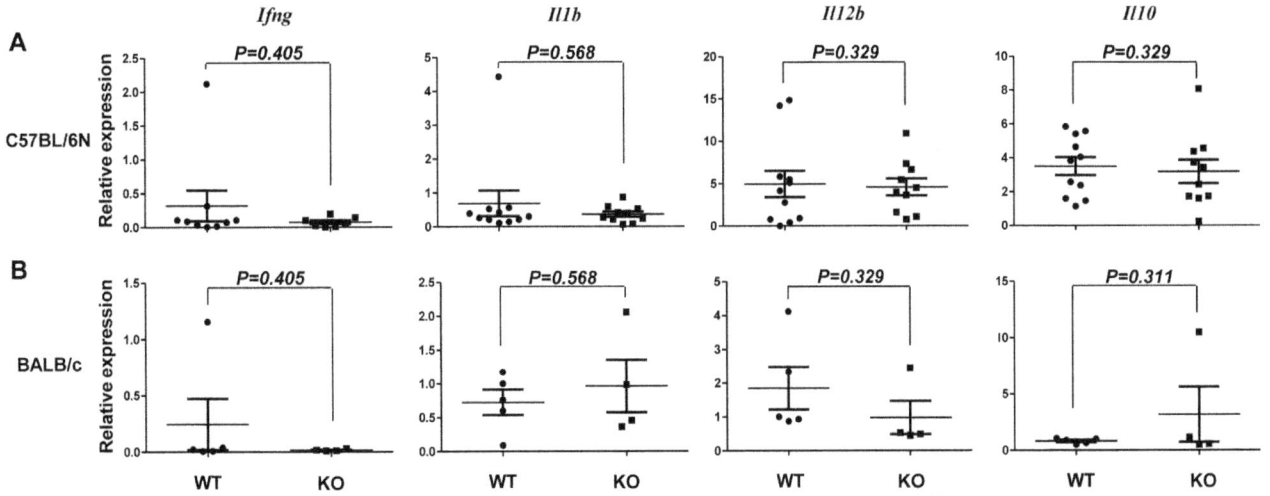

Figure 2. Relative cytokine mRNA levels in MCA-induced tumors. (A, B) Fibrosarcomas induced by 5 µg MCA in WT or CD155-deficient (KO) C57BL/6N (A) or BALB/c (B) mice were resected from each mouse and subjected to quantitative qRT-PCR for transcripts of the indicated cytokines. Horizontal bars represent means and error bars represent means ± SEM. P Values for Student's t test are shown.

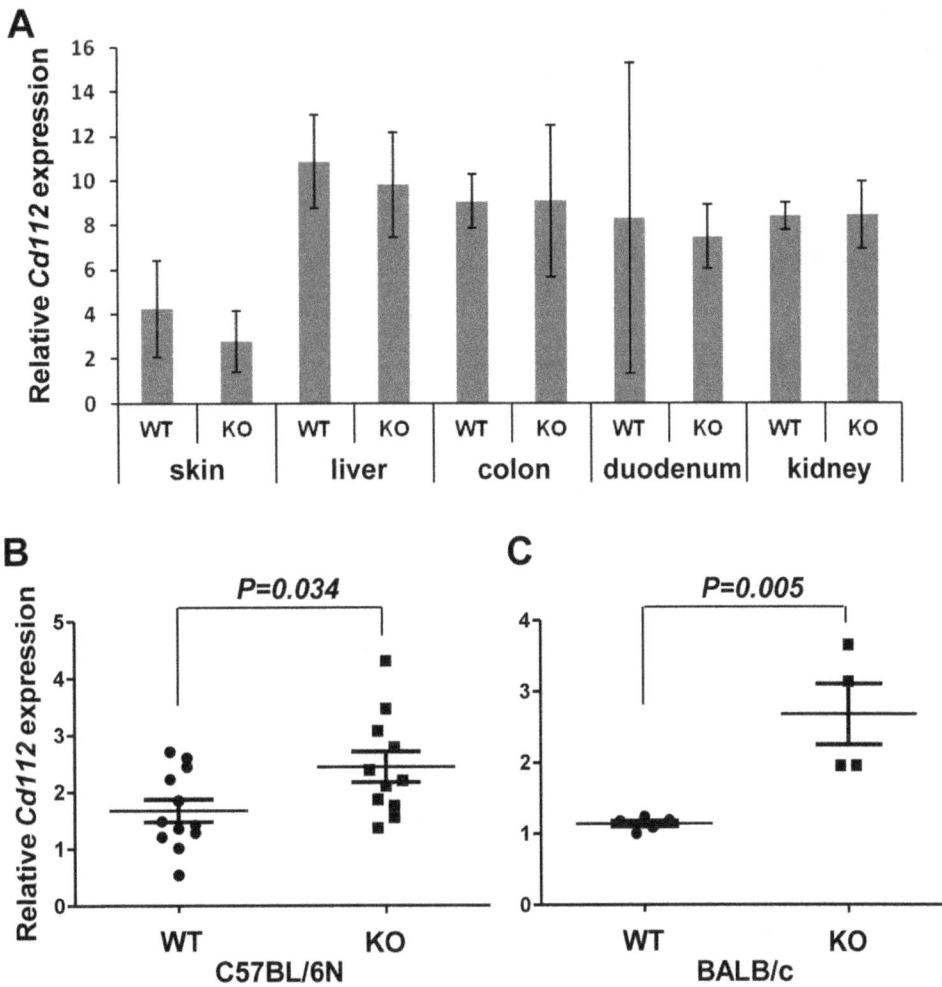

Figure 3. Relative *Cd112* mRNA levels in organs and MCA-induced tumors. (A) Tissues from WT (*n* = 3) or CD155-deficient (KO; *n* = 3) mice were subjected to quantitative qRT-PCR for *Cd112*. Error bars represent means ± SD. (B, C) Fibrosarcomas induced in WT or CD155-deficient C57BL/6N (B) or BALB/c (C) mice by 5 µg MCA were resected from each mouse and subjected to qRT-PCR for *Cd112*. Horizontal bars represent means and error bars represent means ± SEM. P Values for Student's t test are shown.

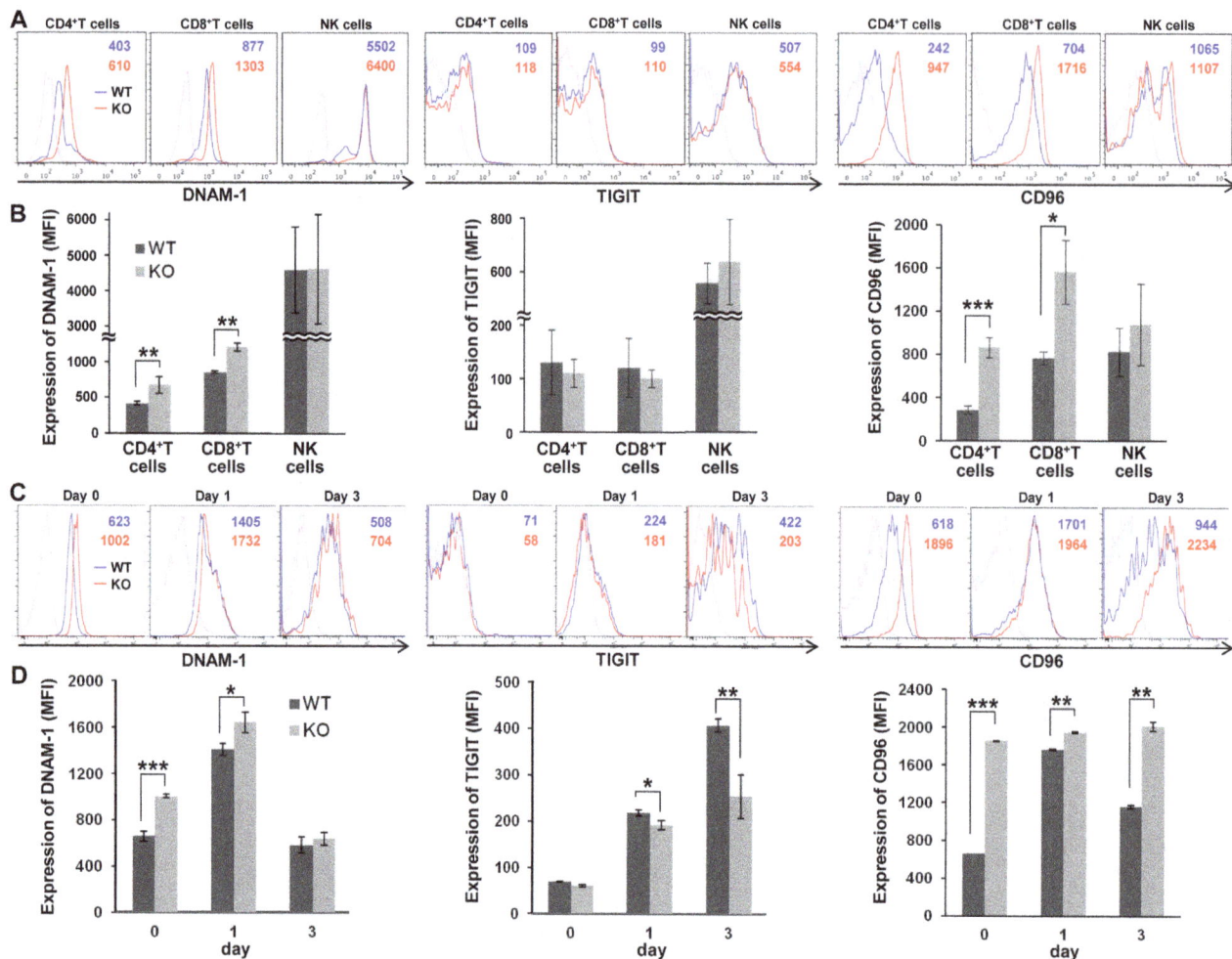

Figure 4. Expression of CD155 ligands on resting and activated T cells from WT and CD155-deficient mice. (A) Peripheral blood lymphocytes from WT ($n = 3$) or CD155-deficient (KO; $n = 3$) C57BL/6N mice were stained with anti-DNAM-1, anti-TIGIT, or anti-CD96 antibodies (WT; blue lines, KO; red lines) or control antibodies (WT; light blue lines, KO; pink lines), and analyzed by flow cytometry. The numbers (WT; in blue, KO; in red) indicate the mean fluorescence intensity (MFI) of DNAM-1, TIGIT, and CD96 staining. Representative data are shown. (B) MFI was used to analyze DNAM-1 expression on CD4$^+$ T, CD8$^+$ T, and NK cells as in (A). Error bars represent means ± SD. (C) CD8$^+$ T cells purified from spleen were activated with anti-CD3 antibody and IL-2 for the indicated number of days. Cells were stained and analyzed by flow cytometry, as described in (A). (D) The expression of DNAM-1, TIGIT, and CD96 on CD8$^+$ T cells is shown as MFI as in (C). *, $P < 0.05$; **, $P < 0.01$; ***, $P < 0.001$.

Mice were examined at least once a week for tumor size with a caliper square as previously described [13]. Mouse survival was closely monitored 3 times per week during the experimental period and the humane endpoint was applied for euthanization by excess anesthetization.

Quantitative real-time PCR (qRT-PCR)

Total RNA was extracted from fibrosarcomas and naive tissues with the Isogen reagent (Nippon Gene, Tokyo, Japan). For reverse transcription, we used 2 µg of total RNA and a High-Capacity cDNA Reverse Transcription Kit (Applied Biosystems, Carlsbad, CA) in a final volume of 20 µl. qRT-PCR was performed on a 7500 FAST Real-Time PCR System (Applied Biosystems) with Platinum SYBR Green qPCR SuperMix-UDG (Invitrogen, Grand Island, NY). The primers were as follows: *Ifng*, 5'-TCA-AGTGGCATAGATGTGGAAGAA-3' (forward) and 5'-TGGC-TCTGCAGGATTTTCATG-3' (reverse); *Il1b*, 5'-TGAAGCAG-CTATGGCAACTG-3' (forward) and 5'-CAGGTCAAAGGTT-TGGAAGC-3' (reverse); *Il12b*, 5'-GGAGACCCTGCCCATTG-AACT-3' (forward) and 5'-CAACGTTGCATCCTAGGATCG-3 (reverse); *Il10*, 5'-GCTGGACAACATACTGCTAACC-3' (forward) and 5'-ATTTCCGATAAGGCTTGGCAA-3' (reverse); *Cd112d*, 5'-CTCTGTGGATCGAATGGTCA-3' (forward) and 5'-GGCAGCGATAATACCTCCAA-3' (reverse); *Cd226*, 5'-T-CGCTCAGAGGCCATTACAG-3' (forward) and 5'-CCCTG-GGCTCTTTAAGTGGAA-3' (reverse); *Tigit*, 5'-CTGATACA-GGCTGCCTTCCT-3' (forward) and 5'-TGGGTCACTTCAG-CTGTGTC-3' (reverse); *Cd96*, 5'-TCCCCAATATGGCCTCT-AGTG-3' (forward) and 5'-GAGTGTAGTGTTCATCCCTT-CTG-3' (reverse). The level of the *β-actin* or *Cd2* transcripts were measured as internal controls. *β-actin*, 5'-GGCTGTATTCCC-CTCCATCG-3' (forward) and 5'-CCAGTTGGTAACAATGC-CATGT-3' (reverse); *Cd2*, 5'- TGGTAACTCATGTTCTTC-TGG-3' (forward) and 5'- GTAATGGTGTATGGCACAA-ATG-3' (reverse). PCR conditions were as follows: an initial denaturation step at 95°C for 10 min, followed by 40 cycles at

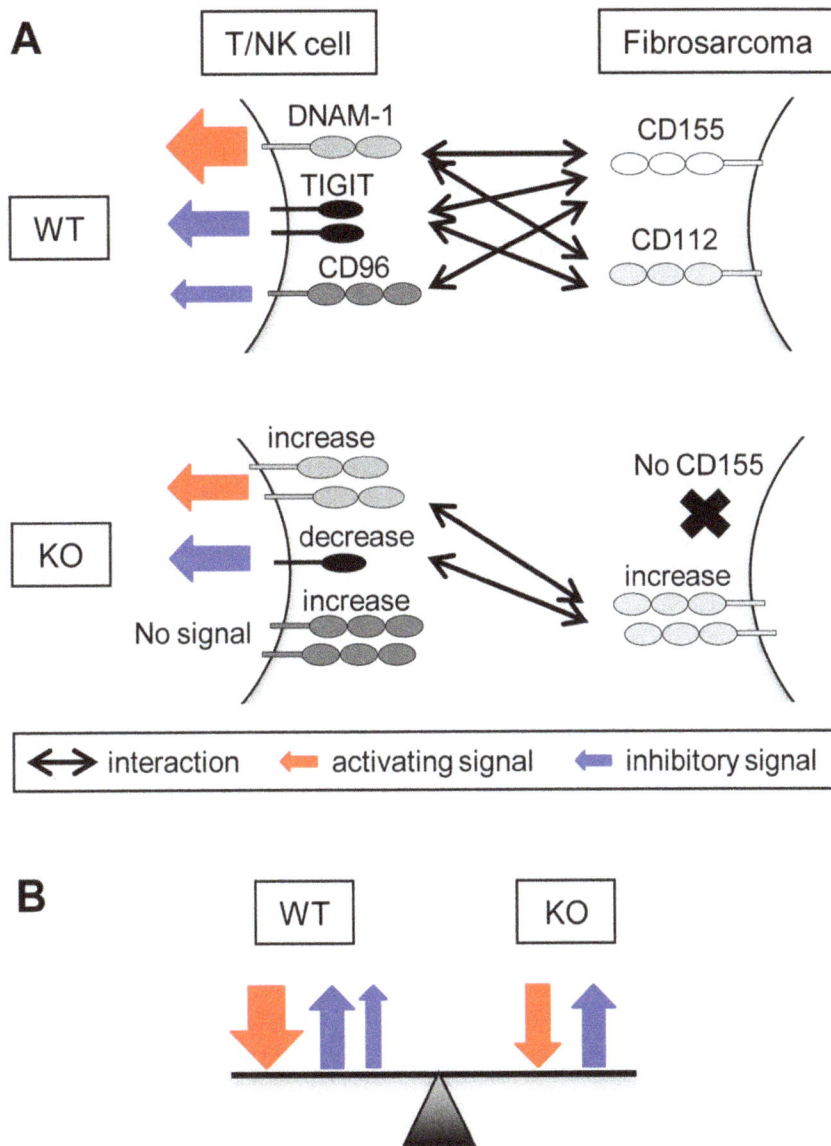

Figure 5. A hypothetical model for interactions between activating/inhibitory receptors DNAM-1, TIGIT and CD96 on T or NK cells and CD155/CD112 ligands expressed on MCA-induced fibrosarcoma in WT or CD155-deficient mice. (A) DNAM-1 and TIGIT bind to both of CD155 and CD112, while CD96 interacts with CD155 only. Each receptor-ligand interaction transduces either activating or inhibitory signal, as shown by the red or blue arrow, respectively. The modulation of the receptors and ligand expression on CD155-deficient (KO) fibrosarcoma are indicated. (B) The sums of the activating and inhibitory signals are similar between WT and KO.

95°C for 15 s and 60°C for 1 min. Data were analyzed by the $2^{-\Delta\Delta Ct}$ method. All values were determined in triplicate.

Statistics

The survival of mice was analyzed by the Kaplan–Meier survival method followed by the log-rank test. All other statistical analyses were performed using the unpaired Student's t test. $P < 0.05$ was considered statistically significant.

Results

MCA-induced tumor development is similar in WT and CD155-deficient mice

To examine the effect of CD155 on MCA-induced fibrosarcoma in tumor immune surveillance, WT and CD155-deficient mice in the C57BL/6N background were injected with MCA. Unexpectedly, both groups showed a similar course of fibrosarcoma development 80–250 days after MCA injection, and their survival rates were similar (**Fig. 1A, B**). Similar results were obtained for WT and CD155-deficient mice in the BALB/c background (**Fig. 1C**). These results suggest that, although DNAM-1 expressed on T cells and NK cells plays an important role in immune surveillance against MCA-induced fibrosarcoma, the counterpart of DNAM-1 on the fibrosarcoma may not be CD155 alone.

Expression of cytokine genes is similar in tumors from WT and CD155-deficient mice

Cytokines expressed in immune cells infiltrating tumor tissues are involved in tumor immune responses. Because there was no difference in MCA-induced tumor development between WT and CD155-deficient mice, we next investigated cytokine expression in tumor tissues from the two types of mice. qRT-PCR revealed that the levels of mRNA for the proinflammatory cytokines *Ifng, Il1b,* and *Il12b* and the anti-inflammatory cytokine *Il10* in fibrosarcomas induced by 5 μg MCA were similar in WT and CD155-deficient mice in both C57BL/6N and BALB/c backgrounds (**Fig. 2**). These results suggest that cytokine expression levels in immune cells infiltrating into tumors were similar in CD155-defficient mice and WT mice.

Cd112 expression is increased in MCA-induced fibrosarcoma in CD155-deficient mice

We next examined the expression of *Cd112* in MCA-induced fibrosarcoma in WT and CD155-defficient mice. In naïve C57BL/6N mice, *Cd112* expression was similar in several organs, including the skin, in WT and CD155-deficient mice (**Fig. 3A**). However, in MCA-induced fibrosarcoma, *Cd112* expression was significantly higher in CD155-deficient mice than in WT mice (**Fig. 3B**). Similar results were obtained for CD155-deficient mice in the BALB/c background (**Fig. 3C**). These results suggest that *Cd112* expression is upregulated in MCA-induced fibrosarcoma in CD155-deficient mice during the transformation.

DNAM-1 and CD96 expressions on resting T cells are increased in CD155-deficient mice

A previous report demonstrated that DNAM-1 expression on T cells was significantly higher in CD155-deficient mice than in WT mice [25]. Consistent with this, our flow cytometry analysis demonstrated significantly higher expression of DNAM-1 on peripheral blood CD4$^+$ and CD8$^+$ T cells (**Fig. 4A**). Fluorescence intensity analysis confirmed a significant increase in DNAM-1 expression on CD4$^+$ and CD8$^+$ T cells (**Fig. 4B**). At the same time, we also analyzed the expressions of TIGIT and CD96 on those cells and found that CD96 but not TIGIT expression on CD4$^+$ and CD8$^+$ T cells was also significantly higher in CD155-deficient mice than in WT mice. As to NK cells, however, we did not observe a difference of these molecules' expression between in WT and in CD155-deficient mice. TIGIT was markedly expressed on NK cells compared to CD4$^+$ and CD8$^+$ T cells, although there was no significant difference between WT and CD155-deficient mice.

Receptor modulation by CD8$^+$ T cell activation

As CD155 binds CD96, TIGIT, and DNAM-1, we examined the expression of these receptors on activated CD8$^+$ T cells. CD8$^+$ T cells from the spleens of WT and CD155-deficient mice were stimulated with anti-CD3 mAb in the presence of IL-2. DNAM-1 and CD96 expression was significantly higher on resting CD155-deficient CD8$^+$ T cells than on resting WT CD8$^+$ T cells, whereas TIGIT expression was not detected (**Fig. 4C, D**). Activated CD8$^+$ T cells increased expression of TIGIT on both WT and CD155-deficient CD8$^+$ T cells after stimulation. Upon stimulation, the levels of DNAM-1 and CD96 were still significantly higher on CD155-deficient than on WT CD8$^+$ T cells, whereas TIGIT expression was significantly lower on CD155-deficient CD8$^+$ T cells than on WT CD8$^+$ T cells (**Fig. 4C, D**).

To analyze the expressions of DNAM-1, TIGIT, and CD96 on tumor-resident immune cells, fibrosarcomas induced by 5 μg MCA in WT or CD155-deficient mice were resected and subjected to quantitative RT-PCR by using *Cd2* expression, which is specifically expressed on T cells and NK cells, but not on non-hematopoietic cells, for normalization. The average tumor size and time points of resection after MCA injection were

comparable between two groups. However, we did not observe different expression levels of those receptors in tumors between WT and CD155-deficient mice (**Fig. S1**).

Discussion

CD155 and CD112 are involved in tumor immune surveillance, because ectopic expression of CD155 or CD112 on tumors can induce cell-mediated cytotoxicity [13]. Although the binding affinities of DNAM-1 to CD155 and CD112 are similar [8], CD155 rather than CD112 appears to play a predominant role in DNAM-1-dependent NK cell triggering [7]. CD112, but not CD155, mediates not only heterophilic but also homophilic binding. This ability may adversely affect DNAM-1 binding to CD112, suggesting that DNAM-1 may prefer CD155 to CD112 as a physiological ligand [8,26].

Our previous study demonstrated that the development of MCA-induced fibrosarcoma and DMBA-induced papilloma was enhanced in DNAM-1-deficient mice, suggesting that DNAM-1 on T cells, NK cells, or both plays an important role in immune surveillance against DNAM-1 ligand–expressing tumors [23]. In this study, we used CD155-deficient mice to examine whether CD155 on MCA-induced fibrosarcoma plays a reciprocal role in tumor immunity. Unexpectedly, however, we found that MCA-induced tumors developed similarly in WT and CD155-deficient mice. We suggest several possible explanations of why the absence of CD155 on tumors did not affect tumor immunity (**Fig. 5**). First, *Cd112* expression in fibrosarcomas was significantly higher in CD155-deficient mice than in WT mice, suggesting that DNAM-1 interaction with CD112 compensated for the loss of the DNAM-1–CD155 interaction. CREB and c-Jun may regulate *Cd112* transcription [27] and are often activated in cancers [28,29]. The relative amounts of *Cd112* mRNA are higher in poorly differentiated gastric cancer than in normal gastric tissue [13]. Second, DNAM-1 expression was significantly upregulated on CD4$^+$ and CD8$^+$ T cells from CD155-deficient mice, consistent with a previous report [25]. DNAM-1 upregulation in CD8$^+$ T cells was independent of antigen-driven activation because it was already observed in resting T cells, but it was still upregulated after stimulation. We also found that, although TIGIT expression was upregulated after stimulation with anti-CD3 mAb in both WT and CD155-deficient CD8$^+$ T cells, it was significantly lower in CD155-deficient cells than in WT cells. TIGIT is an inhibitory receptor that binds to both CD155 and CD112 [18]. Thus, upregulated expression of the activating receptor DNAM-1 and downregulated expression of the inhibitory receptor TIGIT should be favorable for cytotoxicity mediated by T cells, NK-cells, or both against tumors with upregulated CD112, even if the affinity of CD112 for binding DNAM-1 or TIGIT is lower than that of CD155. CD96 expression was also significantly higher on CD155-deficient CD8$^+$ T cells than WT cells. Recent evidence indicates that CD96, which binds CD155 but not CD112, negatively regulates tumor immunity and cytokine secretion by NK cells [21]. Thus, the absence of CD155 on tumors would downregulate CD96-mediated NK cell inhibition, resulting in an increase in cytotoxicity against CD155-deficient tumors. It remains unclear how the expression of DNAM-1, TIGIT, CD96, and CD112 is modulated in CD155-deficient mice. A better understanding of the mechanisms that regulate the levels of these molecules may provide new insights into possible ways to improve cancer immunotherapy.

In contrast to the peripheral blood lymphocytes, we did not observe any different expression levels of DNAM-1, TIGIT, and CD96 in tumors after normalization by *Cd2* expression between

WT and CD155-deficient mice. It is unclear at present how these results can be explained. However, it is possible that, during tumor development for more than 100 days, immune cell activation might be modified. For example, myeloid-derived suppressor cells (MDSC) in tumors tissues suppress both innate and adaptive immunities by secretion of various cytokines [30], which might affect the expression of the cell surface molecules.

We have previously shown that abrogating DNAM-1 activity on CD8+ T cells results in development of milder graft-versus-host disease (GVHD) [31,32]. On the other hand, Seth et al. reported that the absence of CD155 aggravated acute GVHD, which is mainly caused by CD4$^+$ T cells [33]. Although there are differences in the experimental settings between the two GVHD models, these observations and the results of our current study indicate that phenotypes of CD155 and DNAM-1 deficiencies are not two sides of the same coin.

Supporting Information

Figure S1 Relative DNAM-1, TIGIT, and CD96 mRNA levels in MCA-induced tumors. Fibrosarcomas induced by 5 μg MCA in WT or CD155-deficient (KO) C57BL/6N mice were resected and subjected to quantitative RT-PCR for the expression of transcripts

of the indicated receptors as described in Materials and Methods. (A) Tumor size, days of resection after MCA injection, and relative expressions of the transcripts are shown. (B) Relative expressions of indicated receptors are shown. Horizontal bars represent means and error bars represent means ± SEM. P Values for Student's t test are shown.

Material S1 The ARRIVE Guidelines Checklist. We followed the ARRIVE (Animal Research: Reporting of *In Vivo* Experiments) guidelines and the ARRIVE Checklist is available as supporting information.

Acknowledgments

We thank S. Mitsuishi and Y. Nomura for secretarial assistance.

Author Contributions

Conceived and designed the experiments: YN AI-M AS KS. Performed the experiments: YN YY-K FA. Analyzed the data: YN AI-M YY-K FA GB AS KS. Contributed reagents/materials/analysis tools: YN YY-K FA GB. Contributed to the writing of the manuscript: YN AI-M AS KS.

References

1. Dunn GP, Old LJ, Schreiber RD (2004) The three Es of cancer immunoediting. Annu Rev Immunol 22: 329–360.
2. Swann JB, Smyth MJ (2007) Immune surveillance of tumors. J Clin Invest 117: 1137–1146.
3. Lanier LL (2005) NK cell recognition. Annu Rev Immunol 23: 225–274.
4. Dunn GP, Koebel CM, Schreiber RD (2006) Interferons, immunity and cancer immunoediting. Nat Rev Immunol 6: 836–848.
5. Springer TA (1990) Adhesion receptors of the immune system. Nature 346: 425–434.
6. Shibuya A, Campbell D, Hannum C, Yssel H, Franz-Bacon K, et al. (1996) DNAM-1, a novel adhesion molecule involved in the cytolytic function of T lymphocytes. Immunity 4: 573–581.
7. Bottino C, Castriconi R, Pende D, Rivera P, Nanni M, et al. (2003) Identification of PVR (CD155) and nectin-2 (CD112) as cell surface ligands for the human DNAM-1 (CD226) activating molecule. J Exp Med 198: 557–567.
8. Tahara-Hanaoka S, Shibuya K, Onoda Y, Zhang H, Yamazaki S, et al. (2004) Functional characterization of DNAM-1 (CD226) interaction with its ligands PVR (CD155) and nectin-2 (PRR-2/CD112). Int Immunol 16: 533–538.
9. Tahara-Hanaoka S, Miyamoto A, Hara A, Honda S, Shibuya K, et al. (2005) Identification and characterization of murine DNAM-1 (CD226) and its poliovirus receptor family ligands. Biochem Biophys Res Commun 329: 996–1000.
10. Lopez M, Aoubala M, Jordier F, Isnardon D, Gomez S, et al. (1998) The human poliovirus receptor related 2 is a new hematopoietic/endothelial homophilic adhesion molecule. Blood 92: 4602–4611.
11. Iwasaki A, Welker R, Mueller S, Linehan M, Nomoto A, et al. (2002) Immunofluorescence analysis of poliovirus receptor expression in Peyer's patches of humans, primates, and CD155 transgenic mice: Implications for poliovirus infection. J Infect Dis 186: 585–592.
12. Masson D, Jarry A, Baury B, Blanchardie P, Laboisse C, et al. (2001) Overexpression of the *CD155* gene in human colorectal carcinoma. Gut 49: 236–240.
13. Tahara-Hanaoka S, Shibuya K, Kai H, Miyamoto A, Morikawa Y, et al. (2006) Tumor rejection by the poliovirus receptor family ligands of the DNAM-1 (CD226) receptor. Blood 107: 1491–1496.
14. Carlsten M, Bjorkstrom NK, Norell H, Bryceson Y, van Hall T, et al. (2007) DNAX accessory molecule-1 mediated recognition of freshly isolated ovarian carcinoma by resting natural killer cells. Cancer Res 67: 1317–1325.
15. Castriconi R, Dondero A, Corrias MV, Lanino E, Pende D, et al. (2004) Natural killer cell-mediated killing of freshly isolated neuroblastoma cells: Critical role of DNAX accessory molecule-1–poliovirus receptor interaction. Cancer Res 64: 9180–9184.
16. Pende D, Spaggiari GM, Marcenaro S, Martini S, Rivera P, et al. (2005) Analysis of the receptor-ligand interactions in the natural killer-mediated lysis of freshly isolated myeloid or lymphoblastic leukemias: Evidence for the involvement of the poliovirus receptor (CD155) and nectin-2 (CD112). Blood 105: 2066–2073.
17. El-Sherbiny YM, Meade JL, Holmes TD, McGonagle D, Mackie SL, et al. (2007) The requirement for DNAM-1, NKG2D, and NKp46 in the natural killer cell-mediated killing of myeloma cells. Cancer Res 67: 8444–8449.
18. Yu X, Harden K, Gonzalez LC, Francesco M, Chiang E, et al. (2009) The surface protein TIGIT suppresses T cell activation by promoting the generation of mature immunoregulatory dendritic cells. Nat Immunol 10: 48–57.
19. Stanietsky N, Simic H, Arapovic J, Toporik A, Levy O, et al. (2009) The interaction of TIGIT with PVR and PVRL2 inhibits human NK cell cytotoxicity. Proc Natl Acad Sci U.S.A. 106: 17858–17863.
20. Wang PL, O'Farrell S, Clayberger C, Krensky AM (1992) Identification and molecular cloning of tactile. A novel human T cell activation antigen that is a member of the Ig gene superfamily. J Immunol 148: 2600–2608.
21. Chan CJ, Martinet L, Gilfillan S, Souza-Fonseca-Guimaraes F, Chow MT, et al. (2014) The receptors CD96 and CD226 oppose each other in the regulation of natural killer cell functions. Nat Immunol 15: 431–438.
22. Fuchs A, Cella M, Giurisato E, Shaw AS, Colonna M (2004) Cutting edge: CD96 (tactile) promotes NK cell-target cell adhesion by interacting with the poliovirus receptor (CD155). J Immunol 172: 3994–3998.
23. Iguchi-Manaka A, Kai H, Yamashita Y, Shibata K, Tahara-Hanaoka S, et al. (2008) Accelerated tumor growth in mice deficient in DNAM-1 receptor. J Exp Med 205: 2959–2964.
24. Maier MK, Seth S, Czeloth N, Qiu Q, Ravens I, et al. (2007) The adhesion receptor CD155 determines the magnitude of humoral immune responses against orally ingested antigens. Eur J Immunol 37: 2214–2225.
25. Seth S, Qiu Q, Danisch S, Maier MK, Braun A, et al. (2011) Intranodal interaction with dendritic cells dynamically regulates surface expression of the co-stimulatory receptor CD226 protein on murine T cells. J Biol Chem 286: 39153–39163.
26. Liu J, Qian X, Chen Z, Xu X, Gao F, et al. (2012) Crystal structure of cell adhesion molecule nectin-2/CD112 and its binding to immune receptor DNAM-1/CD226. J Immunol 188: 5511–5520.
27. Lui WY, Sze KL, Lee WM (2006) Nectin-2 expression in testicular cells is controlled via the functional cooperation between transcription factors of the Sp1, CREB, and AP-1 families. J Cell Physiol 207: 144–157.
28. Sakamoto KM, Frank DA (2009) CREB in the pathophysiology of cancer: Implications for targeting transcription factors for cancer therapy. Clin Cancer Res 15: 2583–2587.
29. Angel P, Hattori K, Smeal T, Karin M (1988) The jun proto-oncogene is positively autoregulated by its product, Jun/AP-1. Cell 55: 875–885.
30. Ostrand-Rosenberg S, Sinha P (2009) Myeloid-derived suppressor cells: linking inflammation and cancer. J Immunol 182: 4499–4506.
31. Nabekura T, Shibuya K, Shibuya A (2011) Reply to Seth, et al.: DNAX accessory molecule-1 (DNAM-1) plays an important role in alloreactive CD8+ T cells responsible for the exacerbation of acute graft-versus-host disease. Proc Natl Acad Sci U.S.A 108: E34.
32. Nabekura T, Shibuya K, Takenaka E, Kai H, Shibata K, et al. (2010) Critical role of DNAX accessory molecule-1 (DNAM-1) in the development of acute graft-versus-host disease in mice. Proc Natl Acad Sci U.S.A. 107: 18593–18598.
33. Seth S, Ravens I, Lee CW, Glage S, Bleich A, et al. (2011) Absence of CD155 aggravates acute graft-versus-host disease. Proc Natl Acad Sci U.S.A. 108: E32–E33.

Peripheral CD4+ T Cell Cytokine Responses Following Human Challenge and Re-Challenge with *Campylobacter jejuni*

Kelly A. Fimlaid[1,2]*, **Janet C. Lindow**[2], **David R. Tribble**[3], **Janice Y. Bunn**[4], **Alexander C. Maue**[5], **Beth D. Kirkpatrick**[1,2]

1 Department of Microbiology and Molecular Genetics, University of Vermont, Burlington, Vermont, 05405, United States of America, 2 University of Vermont College of Medicine, Vaccine Testing Center and Unit of Infectious Diseases, Burlington, Vermont, United States of America, 3 Infectious Disease Clinical Research Program, Uniformed Services University of the Health Sciences, Bethesda, Maryland, United States of America, 4 University of Vermont College of Mathematics, Burlington, Vermont, United States of America, 5 Naval Medical Research Center, Enteric Diseases Department, Silver Spring, Maryland, United States of America

Abstract

Campylobacter jejuni is a leading cause of human gastroenteritis worldwide; however, our understanding of the human immune response to *C. jejuni* infection is limited. A previous human challenge model has shown that *C. jejuni* elicits IFNγ production by peripheral blood mononuclear cells, a response associated with protection from clinical disease following re-infection. In this study, we investigate T lymphocyte profiles associated with campylobacteriosis using specimens from a new human challenge model in which *C. jejuni*-naïve subjects were challenged and re-challenged with *C. jejuni* CG8421. Multiparameter flow cytometry was used to investigate T lymphocytes as a source of cytokines, including IFNγ, and to identify cytokine patterns associated with either campylobacteriosis or protection from disease. Unexpectedly, all but one subject evaluated re-experienced campylobacteriosis after re-challenge. We show that CD4+ T cells make IFNγ and other pro-inflammatory cytokines in response to infection; however, multifunctional cytokine response patterns were not found. Cytokine production from peripheral CD4+ T cells was not enhanced following re-challenge, which may suggest deletion or tolerance. Evaluation of alternative paradigms or models is needed to better understand the immune components of protection from campylobacteriosis.

Editor: Stefan Bereswill, Charité-University Medicine Berlin, Germany

Funding: This work was supported by the following grants: National Institute of Health National Center Research Resources 5M01RR000109 (http://www.nih.gov/about/almanac/organization/NCRR.htm) (support of General Clinical Research Center, UVM), the National Center for Research Resources (5P20RR021905-07) BK, the National Institute of General Medical Sciences (8 P20 GM103496-07) (http://www.nigms.nih.gov) from the National Institutes of Health BK, and the US Navy Medical Research Center work unit 6000.RAD1.DA3.A0308 (http://www.med.navy.mil/sites/nmrc/Pages/index.htm) BK. The funders had no role in study design, data collection and analysis, decision to publish, or preparation of the manuscript.

Competing Interests: The authors have declared that no competing interests exist.

* Email: kfimlaid@uvm.edu

Introduction

Campylobacter jejuni is among the most common enteric bacterial pathogens causing gastrointestinal disease. On a global scale, approximately 400-500 million people experience campylobacteriosis annually [1]. Ingestion of *C. jejuni*-contaminated food or water can cause a spectrum of disease symptoms, which include diarrhea, fever, and abdominal cramping [2,3]. While infection is self-limited in most healthy individuals, antibiotic therapy is necessary in severe cases and in immunocompromised individuals. A major concern associated with campylobacteriosis is the potential for post-infectious sequelae including the demyelinating neurologic disease, Guillain-Barré syndrome, reactive arthritis, and post-infectious irritable bowel syndrome [4,5]. Furthermore, increasing emergence of antibiotic resistant strains highlights the importance of the development of new therapeutics and prevention strategies which require a better understanding of the human immune response to *C. jejuni* infection [6].

Characterization of human immune responses that contribute to protection from clinical illness caused by *C. jejuni* has proven challenging. Information gathered from natural *C. jejuni* infection can only be cautiously interpreted, since inoculum and time from exposure is not known. Protection from clinical disease caused by *C. jejuni* also appears to vary with age, strain, and exposure history [7–10]. Further, the absence of a small animal model that shares characteristics of human disease has made mechanistic studies of the immune response to *C. jejuni* infection extremely difficult [11–14]. While important advances have been made, the human immune response to *C. jejuni* infection has not been fully characterized and more studies are needed to determine the immunologic responses that develop as a result of disease for vaccine design and drug development.

In human disease, the role of CD4+ T cells in adaptive immune responses to *C. jejuni* infection has not been characterized. Human *C. jejuni* experimental infection or 'challenge' models provide a unique opportunity to evaluate these immune responses.

Analysis from a previously performed human challenge and re-challenge model using *C. jejuni* strain 81-176 showed association between pre-infection levels of IFNγ and protection from clinical campylobacteriosis [13]. Cellular immune responses in other infection models have also been investigated. For example, human colonic explants infected with *C. jejuni* exhibited marked increases in IFNγ production following infection [14]. Additionally, in a *C. jejuni*-resistant C57BL/6 mouse model, *C. jejuni*-infected dendritic cells resulted in CD4$^+$ T$_H$1 polarization and IFNγ production [15].

In the present study, we used multiparameter flow cytometry to evaluate the T cell cytokine profiles from individuals infected with *C. jejuni* CG8421 in an experimental challenge and re-challenge model [12]. We sought to confirm that CD4$^+$ human T cells from *C. jejuni*-infected subjects produce IFNγ, following *ex vivo* stimulation. We asked whether these T cell responses were multifunctional (capable of producing multiple cytokines simultaneously) since multifunctional T cells have been associated with long-term immunity and protection from disease progression for a variety of bacterial, viral, and parasitic pathogens [16–18]. Our data demonstrate a consistent pattern of pro-inflammatory cytokine production by *C. jejuni*-specific CD4$^+$ T cells following primary infection, which included IFNγ, TNF-α, IL-2, and the chemokine, MIP-1β. Interestingly, upon re-infection, there was no enhancement of the CD4$^+$ cytokine response in any subject. Low quantities of multifunctional T cell responses were observed post infection, however a clear kinetic pattern was not distinguishable. One subject evaluated in this re-infection model was protected from clinical illness upon re-infection, and interestingly, this subject shared similar CD4$^+$ T cell profiles to study participants that were not protected from re-infection. Overall, this is the first detailed description of the human CD4$^+$ T cell response to primary and secondary *C. jejuni* infection and offers novel insights into the complexity of immune protection from campylobacteriosis.

Materials and Methods

C. jejuni CG8421 experimental infection trials

Peripheral blood mononuclear cells (PBMCs) used in this analysis were collected under two separate *C. jejuni* CG8421 inpatient trials as previously described [12]. Of note, volunteers were excluded if they had clinical or immunologic evidence (IgA or IFNγ production) of prior exposure to *C. jejuni*. Written informed consent was obtained from all subjects. Clinical protocols were approved by the Institutional Review Boards at University of Vermont and the Naval Medical Research Center. Clinical trials are registered as *Campylobacter jejuni* Challenge Model Development: Dose Ranging Study NCT00434798 (Trial 1) and *Campylobacter jejuni* Challenge Model Development: Assessment of Homologous Protection NCT01048112 (Trial 2).

PBMC collection and handling

Blood samples were collected in EDTA tubes; PBMCs were isolated using AccuSpin tubes within 4 hours of collection. Cells were cryopreserved in freezing media (Sigma) and were thawed in 37°C complete media [cRPMI-10FCS: RPMI-1640 (GIBCO), 10% fetal calf serum (HyClone), 1% penicillin/streptomycin (Sigma), 2 mM L-glutamine (GIBCO)], and 2.72 units DNase/mL media (NEB). Cells were pelleted (300xg, 10 min), and washed with cRPMI-10HS [RPMI-1640, 10% human serum (Gemini Bio-Products), 50 μM β-mercaptoethanol (Sigma), 2 mM L-glutamine, and 50 μg/mL gentamicin (GIBCO)]. Cells were resuspended in cRPMI-10HS and rested 12 hours at 5–10×10^6 cells/mL.

PBMCs were washed once with cRPMI-10HS, reconstituted to 1–1.5×10^7 cells/mL, and 100 μl was aliquoted into a 96-well tray well for each condition.

Campylobacter jejuni antigen preparation

C. jejuni antigen (CAg) used to stimulate PBMCs was prepared as follows: *C. jejuni* strain CG8421 was cultured under conditions used for human challenge [8], fixed with 4% formaldehyde, washed 3 times with PBS (10,000xg for 5 min, at 4°C), resuspended in 1 ml PBS, and sonicated on ice using a Fisher Scientific Sonic Dismembrator Model 100 (three 20 sec intervals, 100% power). Antigen was titrated and time courses were performed to optimize PBMC stimulation conditions utilizing PBMCs from individuals with confirmed natural exposure to *C. jejuni* or subjects from previous trials (data not shown).

Ex vivo PBMC stimulation

For all subjects and timepoints, PBMCs were assayed with the following negative control and stimulation conditions: i) negative control (PBS), ii) positive control [Staphylococcal enterotoxin B (SEB)], and iii) *C. jejuni* antigen (CAg). Each condition was incubated in cRPMI-10HS containing 1 μg/mL anti-CD28 and 1 μg/mL anti-CD49d for 24 hours at 37°C+5% CO$_2$. Brefeldin A (10 μg/mL) was added for the final 12 hours of incubation. Subject A from Trial 1, was evaluated at time-points: D0 (*C. jejuni* naïve sample), D28, D150 (day of re-challenge), D178, and D540. The 8 subjects from Trial 2 were evaluated on D0, D7, D14, D28, D98 (day of re-challenge), D105, D112, and D126 unless specified. Unless limited by PBMCs, technical replicates of the CAg condition were performed. All PBMCs evaluated were capable of producing IFNγ based on the positive control.

Staining procedure

After stimulation, 2 mM EDTA (final concentration) was added to each well for 10 min at room temperature (RT). A LIVE/DEAD Fixable Dead Cell Stain (blue fluorescent reactive dye; Invitrogen) was used to identify and exclude non-viable cells from the analysis. Cells were fixed (BD Lyse Solution) and permeabilized (BD Perm 2), according to manufacturer's instructions. Surface and intracellular staining were done simultaneously for 30 min at RT with the following pre-titered antibody panel: anti–CD3 PerCP Cy5.5 (UCHT1; BD), anti–CD8 V450 (RPA-T8; BD), anti–CD4 V500 (RPA-T4; BD), anti–IFNγ PE-Cy7 (B27; BD), anti–IL-2 PE (5344.111; BD), anti–TNFα FITC (6401.1111;BD), and anti–MIP-1β APC (D21-1351; BD). Cells were acquired using an LSRII flow cytometer (BD) within 24 hours and ≥200,000 total events were collected for each sample unless otherwise specified.

Flow Cytometry Analysis

FlowJo 9.3.1 software (Tree Star, Inc.) and SPICE V5.22β software were used for flow cytometry analysis [19]. PBMCs were analyzed as follows: singlets, lymphocytes, live/CD3$^+$ cells, CD4$^+$ and CD8$^+$ cell subsets. From the CD4$^+$ and CD8$^+$ cell subsets, cytokines were individually gated based on fluorescence minus one (FMO) data. GraphPad PRISM V5.0d was used for cytokine kinetic analyses. Boolean gating strategy and SPICE V5.22β were used for analysis of multifunctional cell subsets. All MFI values reported represent the median fluorescence intensity.

Statistics

T cell cytokines were analyzed and reported as the percent of cytokines produced in the antigen stimulation condition (CAg) minus the background (negative control). Single-group repeated measures analysis of variance based on the ranks of all values was used to examine cytokines or multifunctional T cells produced at each time point (the repeating factor) relative to a pre-challenge time-point [20]. Any statistically significant results were followed by post-hoc tests to examine day-specific differences from the pre-challenge time-point. Repeated measures analyses were performed using SAS, version 9.2; Wilcoxon rank sum tests were computed using SPICE v.5.22β. P values≤0.05 were considered significant.

Results

Clinical Subjects

Subjects B-I. Eight participants in an inpatient challenge model (Trial 2) (Subjects B-I) with no clinical or immunologic evidence of prior exposure to *C. jejuni* were evaluated for T cell responses associated with infection [21]. All eight subjects received an initial inoculum of 8.6×10^5 colony-forming units (CFU) of *C. jejuni* CG8421 and all experienced campylobacteriosis, as previously reported [21]. Following the same procedures, Subjects B-I underwent homologous rechallenge with the same strain 90 days after the initial inoculum, at a dose of 3.6×10^5 CFU. Subjects B-I experienced campylobacteriosis following re-challenge. As reported elsewhere, protection from clinical disease following first exposure was not observed nor was there a difference in the severity of clinical illness during Trial 2 after the first and second infections [21].

Subject A. One subject (Subject A), part of a separate trial (Trial 1), with no clinical or immunologic evidence of prior exposure to *C. jejuni*, underwent initial challenge with 1×10^5 CFU of *C. jejuni* CG8421 and homologous rechallenge 150 days later with the same strain dosed at a dose of 5×10^4 CFU [12]. While Trial 1 consisted of a large cohort of people, only Subject A underwent homologous re-challenge; Subject A did not experience diarrhea or any clinical signs or symtoms consistent with campylobacteriosis upon re-challenge.

Peripheral CD4+ and CD8+ T cells produce pro-inflammatory cytokines following primary challenge with *C. jejuni* CG8421 in naïve subjects

A representative flow cytometry gating scheme showing *C. jejuni* CG8421 antigen (CAg) compared to the negative control is shown in **Fig. S1**. PBMCs isolated from Subjects B-I were analyzed using the same *C. jejuni ex vivo* stimulation conditions, at pre- and post-primary infection time-points. Statistically significant increases in total percentages of CD4+IFNγ+, CD4+IL-2+, and CD4+TNFα+ T cells were detected post-infection relative to D0 (P<0.05, 0.01, and 0.05, respectively) following primary infection (**Fig. 1**). CD4+MIP-1β+ cells trended toward significance (P = 0.06) post-infection relative to pre-infection. Analysis of individual post-primary challenge days showed statistically significant increases in CD4+IFNγ+ cells on D7 and D14 relative to D0 (P<0.05 and P<0.01, respectively) (**Fig. 1A**). CD4+TNFα+ T cells were produced with similar kinetics as CD4+IFNγ+ T cells, exhibiting significant increases on D7, D14, and D28 relative to D0 (P<0.05 for all timepoints) (**Fig. 1B**). While CD4+IL-2+ T cell kinetics were delayed relative to those seen for CD4+IFNγ+ and CD4+TNFα+, significant levels were observed on D14 and D28 (P<0.01 and 0.01) (**Fig. 1C**). Lastly, CD4+MIP-1β+ cells were elevated at D7 compared to D0 (P<0.01) (**Fig. 1D**).

Analysis of CD8+ T cells showed modest increases in CD8+IFNγ+ and CD8+MIP-1β+ T cells at various time-points by subjects post initial infection, but no pattern was evident post initial infection (**Fig. S2A and S2B**). Following re-challenge, there

was no clear pattern of CD8+IFNγ+ and CD8+MIP-1β+ T cell profiles (**Fig. S2C and S2D**).

An enhanced CD4+ cytokine response is not observed following *C. jejuni* CG8421 re-challenge

To evaluate whether an enhanced T cell response occurred following homologous re-infection, suggestive of activation of a memory T cell response, we analyzed responses following re-exposure to *C. jejuni*. Analysis of the cytokine kinetics post re-exposure in subjects that did not have protection from clinical disease showed variable responses compared to what was seen after first exposure (**Fig. 2A-D**); PBMCs were not available for all subjects on all days during the re-challenge denoted by a missing square from the figure plane. Overall, the cytokine responses at time-points following re-challenge were not significantly different relative to day of re-challenge (D98) or D0 for any of the cytokines under investigation.

Mono-functional CD4+ T cells are the dominant T cell species produced following primary and secondary *C. jejuni* infections

Since we observed different T cell profiles between naïve and re-challenged subjects, we wanted to investigate the T cell functional diversity more closely. We used Boolean gating to evaluate the CD4+ T cell profiles; more specifically, to characterize whether responses were multifunctional or monofunctional, and to determine which cytokine patterns were prevalent. Although many of the cytokine-producing T cells were monofunctional CD4+IFNγ+ cells, statistically significant monofunctional populations included CD4+IL-2+ (D14 P<0.05), CD4+MIP-1β+ (D7 P<0.05), and CD4+TNFα+ (D7 P<0.05) (**Fig. 3A**). Monofunctional cytokine producing CD4+ T cells were more frequently produced over multifunctional cells for the overall study (P<0.0003). Low, but statistically significant percentages of multifunctional cells, were observed for the following T cell phenotypes and timepoints relative to pre-exposure: CD4+IFNγ+IL-2+TNFα+ (D14; P<0.05), CD4+IFNγ+MIP-1β+TNFα+ (D7, D14, D28, D105; P<0.01, 0.01, 0.05, and 0.05 respectively), CD4+IFNγ+IL-2+ (D14 and D98; P<0.05), and CD4+IL-2+TNFα+ (D28, D98, and D126; P<0.05) (**Fig. 3B**). CD4+IFNγTNFα+, CD4+IFNγ+IL-2+MIP-1β+, CD4+IFNγ+MIP-1β+, CD4+IFNγ+IL-2+MIP-1β+, CD4+IFNγ+-MIP-1β+, CD4+IL-2+MIP-1β+TNFα+, CD4+MIP-1β+TNFα+, CD4+IL-2+MIP-1β+, CD4+IFNγ+IL-2+MIP-1β+TNFα+, and CD4+IFNγ+IL-2+ multifunctional cells were not significant at any timepoint (Fig. 3B and Fig. 3C).

Protection after homologous rechallenge in a second challenge model

In a second Trial (Trial 2), using the same strain of *C. jejuni*, protection from clinical campylobacteriosis following homologous rechallenge was observed in one person. PBMCs isolated from Subject A one month after initial challenge (D28), were stimulated *ex vivo* using *C. jejuni* antigen and displayed increased numbers of IFNγ, TNFα, IL-2, and MIP-1β cytokine-producing CD4+ T cells relative to day of dosing, D0 (**Fig. 4**), suggesting a *C.jejuni* specific cellular immune response, similar to Trial 1. On the day of rechallenge (D150), TNFα, IL-2, and MIP-1β cytokine producing CD4+ T cells were back to baseline levels, however IFNγ CD4+ T cells were elevated relative to D0 (**Fig. 4**). Interestingly, there was a notable drop in IFNγ CD4+ T cells 28 days (D178) after re-challenge and further, all CD4+ T cells returned to baseline levels one year (D540) post re-challenge (**Fig. 4**). Subject A displayed

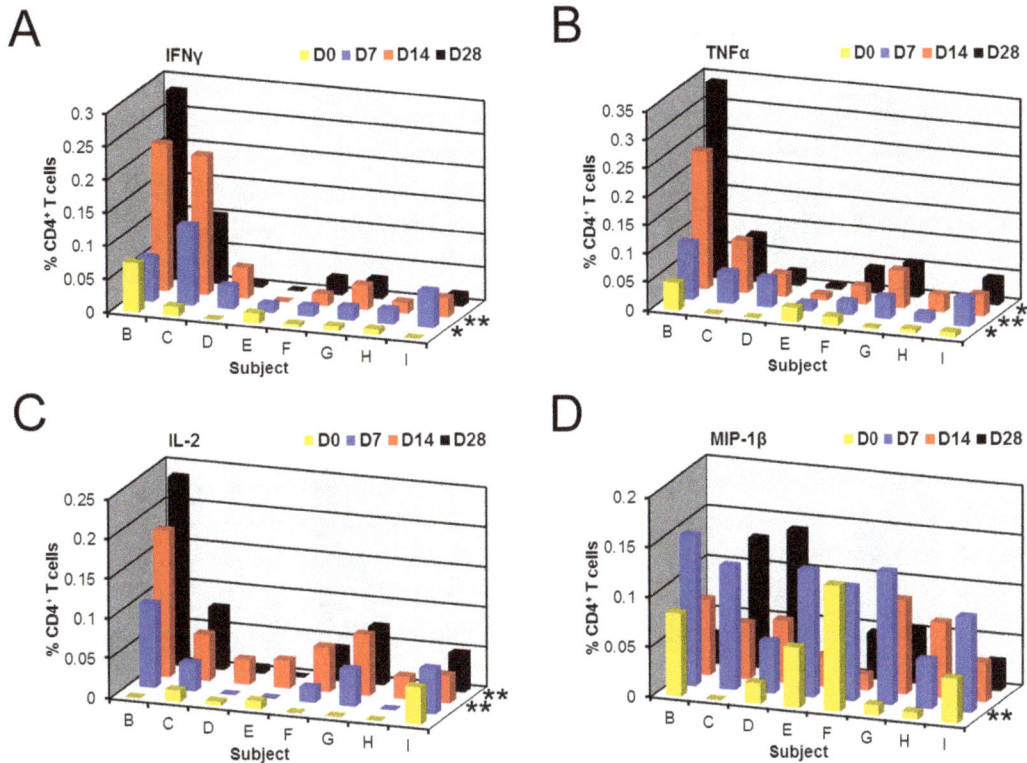

Figure 1. Proinflammatory cytokines and a chemokine are produced with specific kinetics post-primary infection with *C. jejuni*. We analyzed CD4$^+$ T cells for the production of IFNγ$^+$, TNFα$^+$, IL-2$^+$, and MIP-1β$^+$ for eight subjects challenged with *C. jejuni* at multiple timepoints pre- and post-primary infection. Responses shown are the percentage of cytokine positive CD4$^+$ T cells from CAg-stimulated PBMCs with the background percentage of cytokine-positive T cells in the negative control (PBS) subtracted. CD4$^+$ T cells producing each cytokine were reported for 3 time-points post-challenge: D7 (blue), D14 (red), and D28 (black). A) CD4$^+$IFNγ$^+$ T cells; B) CD4$^+$TNFα$^+$ T cells; C) CD4$^+$IL-2$^+$ T cells; and D) CD4$^+$MIP-1β$^+$ T cells. An asterisk denotes a significant difference between a response on a post-challenge day and D0 (yellow): * P<.05 and ** P<.01. Statistics were determined using repeated measures analysis of variance were not available for Subject B after re-infection.

similar monofunctional and multifunctional profiles to those from Trial 2 (data not shown).

C. jejuni specific CD4$^+$ IFNγ$^+$ T cell phenotype is not distinct between protected and non-protected subjects

Re-challenge T cell profiles from Subjects B-I (Trial 2) were compared to that of Subject A, who showed no clinical illness upon re-challenge (**Fig. S3**). As shown in **Fig. S3B**, CD4$^+$IFNγ$^+$ and CD4$^+$TNFα$^+$ appeared elevated on the day of re-challenge (D150 for Subject A) relative to D0 (**Fig. S3A**), while CD4$^+$IL-2$^+$ and CD4$^+$MIP-1β$^+$ cells trended lower. Analysis of Subjects B-I showed that CD4$^+$IFNγ$^+$ cells had fallen close to baseline at re-challenge (D98) (**Fig. S3A and Fig. S3B**) relative to D0 with the exception of two Subjects (C and D); we found significant differences only in CD4$^+$IL-2$^+$ T cells between first and second challenges (D0 and D98, P <0.05); we did not observe differences for CD4$^+$IFNγ$^+$, CD4$^+$TNFα$^+$, or CD4$^+$MIP-1β$^+$ T cells.

To investigate the variable clinical outcomes, we compared T cell cytokine profiles in greater depth between the protected Subject A and unprotected subjects from Trial 2. We compared the dominant T cell functional populations: CD4$^+$IFNγ$^+$, at D0, D28, and day of re-challenge D98 or D150 (Trial 1 and Trial 2, respectively). Analysis of the median fluorescent intensity (MFI) of the CD4$^+$IFNγ$^+$ populations suggests that the Subject A (protected) CD4$^+$IFNγ$^+$ cells produced more IFNγ at D28 than CD4$^+$IFNγ$^+$ cells from Subjects C and D at the same timepoint (**Fig.**

S4). Only 2 of the 8 subjects reached IFNγ levels comparable to those exhibited by Subject A after primary infection.

Discussion

To further investigate the previous observation that IFNγ production is associated with protection from campylobacteriosis, we performed the first kinetic evaluation of T cell cytokine responses following human *C. jejuni* infection [12]. We studied responses elicited by *C. jejuni* infection in a unique population of naïve human subjects (i.e. no prior history of campylobacteriosis), undergoing both primary and secondary infection (homologous re-challenge) with *C. jejuni* CG8421. We tested 8 subjects that experienced campylobacteriosis following primary and secondary infection to determine proinflammatory T cell profiles, and found that these subjects had an increase in pro-inflammatory T cells post primary infection but failed to boost upon secondary infection. Additionally, we tested a single subject that did not experience campylobacteriosis after re-infection and found that this subject had a similar pro-inflammatory T cell response post primary infection relative to the 8 subjects that experienced re-infection. Our data shows that following primary infection in all subjects, peripheral *C. jejuni*-specific CD4$^+$ T cells produce pro-inflammatory cytokines, including IFNγ and TNFα, peaking 7-14 days post-infection. Similarly, the production of the chemokine, MIP-1β, peaks at day 7 post infection, whereas the peak IL-2 response was detected 14-28 days post-infection, suggesting a

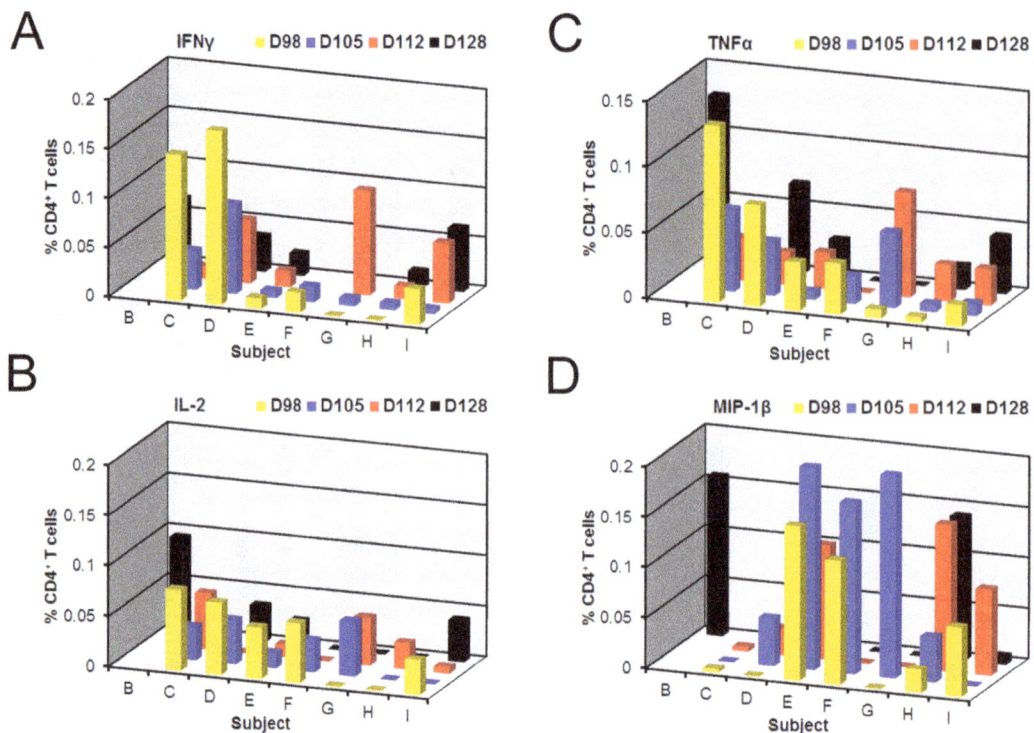

Figure 2. CD4+ T cell responses did not show a specific signature following re-challenge with the homologous *C. jejuni* strain. The effect of challenge on *C. jejuni* veterans shows a diverse T cell profile compared to naïve subjects. Eight subjects were re-dosed with the homologous *C. jejuni* CG8421 strain three months after initial infection. We examined CD4+ T cell responses for the production of IFNγ+, TNFα+, IL-2+, and MIP-1β at multiple timepoints pre- and post-re-infection. Responses shown are the percentage of cytokine positive CD4+ T cells from CAg-stimulated PBMCs with the background percentage of cytokine-positive T cells in the negative control (PBS) subtracted. D98 represents PBMCs from a blood drawn prior to re-infection. Bars represent percent of CD4+ T cells detected on specific days: D98 (day of re-dosing, yellow); D105 (blue); D112 (red); and D126 (black). No significant changes were observed post re-challenge compared to D98.

maturation of an effector cell response. Although the magnitude of cytokine responses varied between subjects, the timing and character of responses were similar. Lastly, we did not observe a clear pattern of cytokine responses by CD8+ populations, but this is likely because our assay was not optimized for CD8+ T cell stimulation due to the antigen used.

We anticipated that CD4+ cells would show a strong enhancement of cytokine production upon secondary exposure, particularly in the protected subject (Subject A), however this was not observed in any subject. While there were different dose amounts administered at rechallenge between Subject A and Subjects B-I, possibly explaining the lack of symptoms observed in Subject A, the percentage of CD4+ cells producing cytokines, including IFNγ, TNFα, and IL-2, appeared to fall or was unaltered in most subjects. Possible hypotheses that may explain these results include that i) memory T cells did not develop and thus were not present during secondary infection, as described in viral infections including HIV vaccine research [22]; ii) T cells may be unresponsive due to induction of tolerance or exhaustion [23]; iii) protective cells (Subject A) may reside in the gut and are not detectable in peripheral blood.

Our investigation of T cell heterogeneity showed that monofunctional CD4+ T cells were the primary phenotype observed after *C. jejuni* infection. More specifically, CD4+IFNγ+ T cells were the dominant cytokine-producing population following primary and secondary exposure, and did not correlate with clinical protection or severity of disease. As shown in **Fig. S4**, CD4+IFNγ+ T cells from the protected subject (Subject A)

demonstrated a higher MFI than unprotected subjects with similar cytokine patterns, even though all subjects had similar percentages of CD4+IFNγ+ cells on the day of re-challenge. Increases in monofunctional CD4+ cells producing IL-2, TNFα, or MIP-1β were also detected following primary exposure but a discernable pattern post-secondary exposure was not detected.

These unexpected results, characterized in a young, healthy adult population without previous *C.jejuni* exposure, highlight the difficulty in understanding the complex human immune responses to bacterial infections at mucosal surfaces. Complicating the analysis, *C. jejuni* has marked strain-to-strain variability, including phase variation in capsular expression [24,25]. Interestingly, our observation of recurrent campylobacteriosis following re-challenge with strain CG8421 was not observed in another challenge model using strain 81-176 (administered at a higher bacterial inoculum and displaying different capsular characteristics) [13]. The observation of a lack of a CD4+ cytokine response following secondary infection is consistent with the observation that IgA+ antibody secreting plasma cells also fail to boost after *C. jejuni* re-challenge [21]. It was previously noted that the serum IgG in these subjects boosted at Day 7 after initial challenge and displayed a drop after 3 months; interestingly, a boost after rechallenge was not observed [21]. Similarly a boost in serum IgA was noted at Day 7 post initial challenge which dropped almost to baseline after 3 months; a boost 7 days post rechallenge was observed but did not reach the titer observed after initial challenge before falling back to baseline [21]. In the context of the development of protective immunity, the detection of CD4+IFNγ+ monofunctional cells as

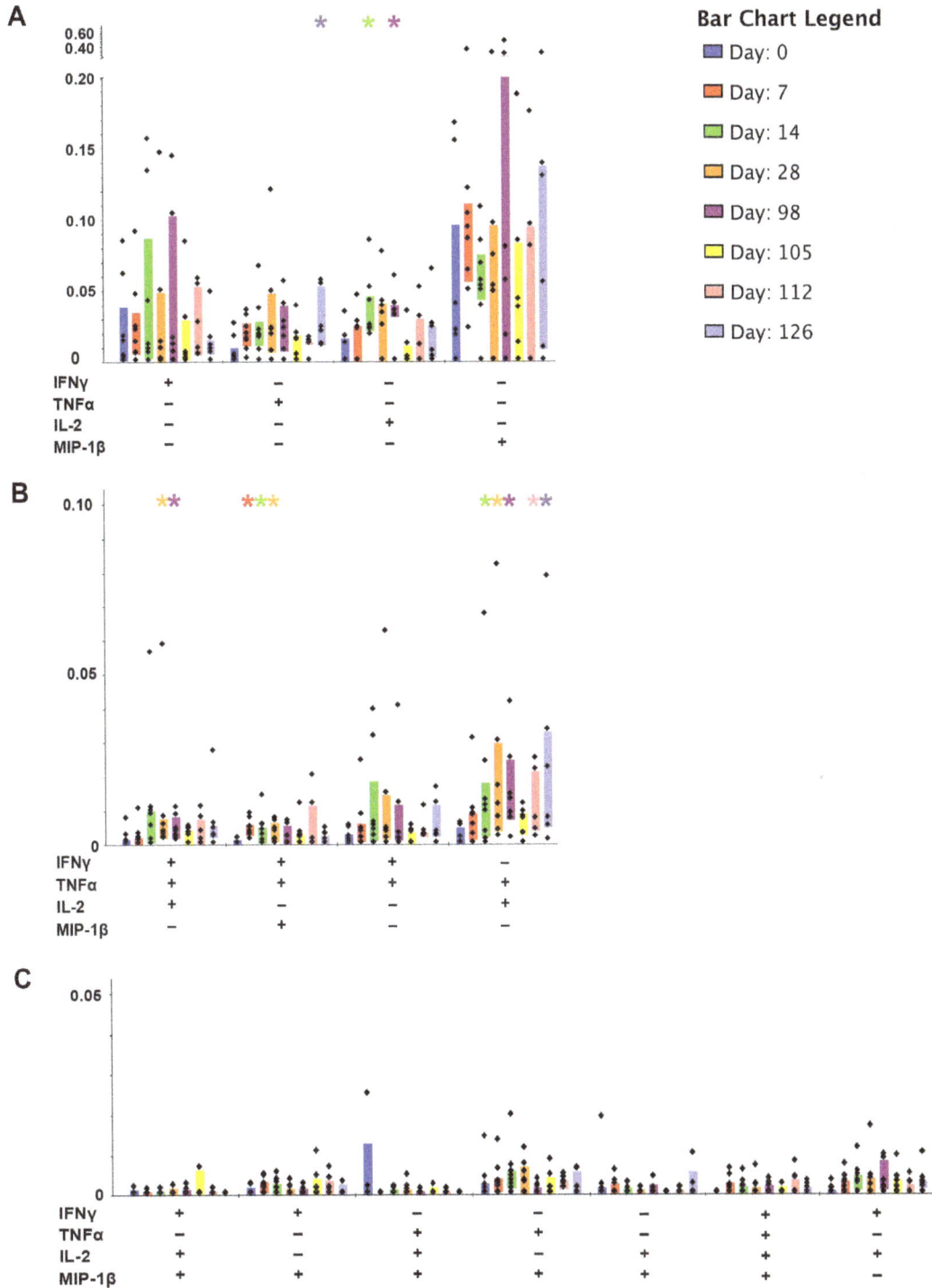

Figure 3. Monofunctional CD4$^+$ T cells from naïve and veterans post *C. jejuni* exposure are dominant over multifunctional cells. The kinetics of T cell responses are shown, separating CD4$^+$ phenotypes based on the combinations of cytokines they produced (designated by +/-) under the x-axis. X-axis shows the combinations of IFNγ, TNFα, IL-2, and MIP-1β producing cells. Each colored bar designates the interquartile range (IQR). Days evaluated include: D0, D7, D14, D28, D98, D105, D112, and D126. A) Monofunctional CD4$^+$ phenotypes. B and C) Multifunctional CD4$^+$ phenotypes relative to D0. Statistically significant days are relative to D0 (Wilcoxon ranked test) and P≤0.05 is designated by "*".

the dominant CD4$^+$ subset may be a marker of a poor quality immune response to primary infection, and may be less likely to lead to immunologic memory and protection [22]. Alternative hypotheses may explain our findings and will require further evaluation in future studies: Although not seen in our population,

multiple cytokine-producing effector cells may still be necessary for the generation of a protective and/or memory response to *C. jejuni*. IFNγ, which has been associated with protection, may be produced by other cell types. Protection may also be found in the

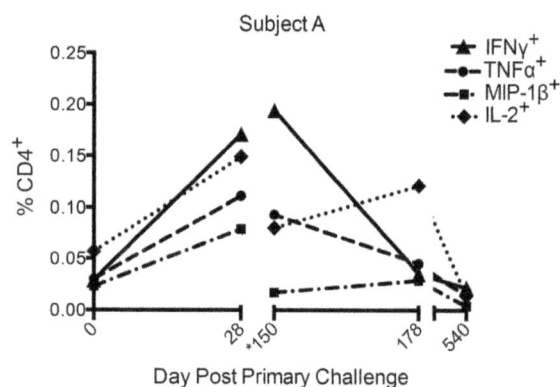

Figure 4. CD4⁺ T cells from protected Subject A produce proinflammatory cytokines following infection with live *C. jejuni*. PBMCs from pre-challenge (D0) and post-infection timeponts were stimulated with *C. jejuni* antigen in an *ex vivo* assay and assessed for CD4⁺ cytokine production by flow cytometry. Responses depicted represent the percentage of CD4⁺ T cells producing cytokine from CAg-stimulated PBMCs (CAg stimulation minus negative control). (*150 = Day of homologous re-challenge.)

setting of high and sustained levels of IFNγ not seen in our subjects.

Further study of CD8⁺ T cells, which are important in clearing intracellular infections, may also provide valuable clues to the immune response to *C. jejuni*. Recent investigations have shown that *C. jejuni*-containing endosomes avoid fusion with lysosomes in epithelial cells, a feature reminiscent of intracellular *Mycobacterium tuberculosis* and *Salmonella* Typhimurium [26–28]. Additionally, the mechanisms of epithelial cell invasion and intracellular survival are being elucidated, further suggesting that CD8⁺ T cell responses may be important in clearing infection [29,30]. While we investigated the CD8⁺ response and the chemokine MIP-1β, a chemokine important for recruitment of additional immune cells to sites on infection and produced by activated CD8⁺ and CD4⁺ cells, no clear patterns of CD8⁺ or MIP-1β responses were observed [31–33].

Further carefully constructed and detailed evaluations are needed to better understand the human immune response to *C. jejuni*. Although human challenge models are expensive and uncommon, future studies should address the role of different immune cell populations, including NK cells and Th17 cells, shown to be involved in a mouse model of *Campylobacter* infection [34]. Additionally, the importance of T cell priming by dendritic cells should be evaluated early post-infection, to characterize the initial development of *Campylobacter*-specific adaptive and memory responses and the expression of surface markers that regulate lymphocyte homing to the intestinal tract. Similarly, T cell phenotypes suggestive of the development of tolerance or T cell exhaustion following primary infection should be evaluated. Investigations into the acquisition of oral tolerance based on inoculum size will be particularly relevant. Given the global prevalence of this pathogen and its close associations with autoimmune post-infectious sequelae, further characterization of the human and mucosal immune responses to *C. jejuni* will be important to expand our ability to understand and control this clinically important pathogen.

Supporting Information

Figure S1   Flow cytometry analysis of T cells responding to CAg post *C. jejuni* infection. The representative gating scheme displays the raw data analysis for determining the T cell response using an *ex vivo* assay. After sample collection, PBMCs were gated for singlets, lymphocytes, and live CD3⁺ T cells (first three histograms). The CD3⁺ T cells were subdivided into CD4⁺CD8⁻ (CD4⁺) and CD4⁻CD8⁺ (CD8⁺) populations. CD4⁺ (represented above) and CD8⁺ populations were then analyzed for cytokine production including IFNγ, TNFα, IL-2, and MIP-1β, for all conditions run (negative control, positive control, and CAg). Gates were based on FMO data. Signal over background (percent positive T cells) was based on the mean of the CAg results minus the negative control.

Figure S2   CD8⁺ T cells from *C. jejuni* challenged subjects respond to CAg post infection. Increases in CD8⁺IFNγ⁺ and CD8⁺MIP-1β⁺ were observed after primary infection time-points. Responses shown are the percentage of cytokine positive CD8⁺ T cells from CAg-stimulated PBMCs with the background percentage of cytokine-positive T cells in the negative control (PBS) subtracted. CD8⁺ T cells analyzed post-challenge: D7 (blue), D14 (red), and D28 (black). A) CD8⁺IFNγ⁺ T cells; and B) CD8⁺MIP-1β⁺ T cells. CD8⁺ T cells analyzed post re-challenge: D105 (blue), D112 (red), and D126 (black). C) CD8⁺IFNγ⁺ T cells; and D) CD8⁺MIP-1β⁺ T cells.

Figure S3   Subjects C and D, not protected from re-infection, shared a similar cytokine profile to subject A. Nine *C. jejuni* veterans, one from Trial 1 and eight from Trial 2, underwent homologous re-challenge (150 days) and 98 days post initial challenge, respectively. A) D0 pre-challenge CD4⁺ T cell profiles display low levels of cytokine production. B) On day of re-challenge, Subject A reflected CD4⁺ cells making IFNγ, TNFα, and IL-2. Subjects C and D displayed similar cytokine profiles to Subject A. PBMCs were not available for Subject B after re-infection.

Figure S4   IFNγ⁺ producing CD4⁺T from protected Subject A cells have a higher median fluorescence intensity that those produced by unprotected Trial 2 Subjects C and D. Median Fluorescence Intensity (MFI) analysis for CD4⁺IFNγ⁺ T cells from timepoints including naïve D0, D28, and day of re-challenge (D150 and D98 for Trial 1 and Trial 2, respectively).

Acknowledgments

The authors would like to thank the study volunteers who participated in the clinical studies described.

Author Contributions

Conceived and designed the experiments: KF JL JB DT BK. Performed the experiments: KF. Analyzed the data: KF JL DT JB AM BK. Contributed reagents/materials/analysis tools: KF JL JB BK. Wrote the paper: KF JL BK. Obtained permission for use of samples: DT BK.

References

1. Ruiz-Palacios GM (2007) The health burden of Campylobacter infection and the impact of antimicrobial resistance: playing chicken. Clin Infect Dis 44: 701–703.

2. Dasti JI, Tareen AM, Lugert R, Zautner AE, Gross U (2010) Campylobacter jejuni: a brief overview on pathogenicity-associated factors and disease-mediating mechanisms. Int J Med Microbiol 300: 205–211.

3. Nachamkin I, Szymanski CM, Blaser MJ, editor (2008) *Campylobacter*. 3 ed. Washington, D.C.: ASM Press. 716 p.

4. Zilbauer M, Dorrell N, Wren BW, Bajaj-Elliott M (2008) Campylobacter jejuni-mediated disease pathogenesis: an update. Trans R Soc Trop Med Hyg 102: 123–129.

5. Garcia Rodriguez LA, Ruigomez A, Panes J (2006) Acute gastroenteritis is followed by an increased risk of inflammatory bowel disease. Gastroenterology 130: 1588–1594.

6. Kirkpatrick BD, Tribble DR (2011) Update on human Campylobacter jejuni infections. Curr Opin Gastroenterol 27: 1–7.

7. Buettner S, Wieland B, Staerk KD, Regula G (2010) Risk attribution of Campylobacter infection by age group using exposure modelling. Epidemiol Infect 138: 1748–1761.

8. Unicomb LE, Dalton CB, Gilbert GL, Becker NG, Patel MS (2008) Age-specific risk factors for sporadic Campylobacter infection in regional Australia. Foodborne Pathog Dis 5: 79–85.

9. Richardson NJ, Koornhof HJ, Bokkenheuser VD, Mayet Z, Rosen EU (1983) Age related susceptibility to Campylobacter jejuni infection in a high prevalance population. Arch Dis Child 58: 616–619.

10. Schonberg-Norio D, Sarna S, Hanninen ML, Katila ML, Kaukoranta SS, et al. (2006) Strain and host characteristics of Campylobacter jejuni infections in Finland. Clin Microbiol Infect 12: 754–760.

11. Baqar S, Tribble DR, Carmolli M, Sadigh K, Poly F, et al. (2010) Recrudescent Campylobacter jejuni infection in an immunocompetent adult following experimental infection with a well-characterized organism. Clin Vaccine Immunol 17: 80–86.

12. Tribble DR, Baqar S, Carmolli MP, Porter C, Pierce KK, et al. (2009) Campylobacter jejuni strain CG8421: a refined model for the study of Campylobacteriosis and evaluation of Campylobacter vaccines in human subjects. Clin Infect Dis 49: 1512–1519.

13. Tribble DR, Baqar S, Scott DA, Oplinger ML, Trespalacios F, et al. (2010) Assessment of the duration of protection in Campylobacter jejuni experimental infection in humans. Infect Immun 78: 1750–1759.

14. Edwards LA, Nistala K, Mills DC, Stephenson HN, Zilbauer M, et al. (2010) Delineation of the innate and adaptive T-cell immune outcome in the human host in response to Campylobacter jejuni infection. PLoS One 5: e15398.

15. Rathinam VA, Hoag KA, Mansfield LS (2008) Dendritic cells from C57BL/6 mice undergo activation and induce Th1-effector cell responses against Campylobacter jejuni. Microbes Infect 10: 1316–1324.

16. Betts MR, Nason MC, West SM, De Rosa SC, Migueles SA, et al. (2006) HIV nonprogressors preferentially maintain highly functional HIV-specific CD8+ T cells. Blood 107: 4781–4789.

17. Darrah PA, Patel DT, De Luca PM, Lindsay RW, Davey DF, et al. (2007) Multifunctional TH1 cells define a correlate of vaccine-mediated protection against Leishmania major. Nat Med 13: 843–850.

18. Caccamo N, Guggino G, Joosten SA, Gelsomino G, Di Carlo P, et al. (2010) Multifunctional CD4(+) T cells correlate with active Mycobacterium tuberculosis infection. Eur J Immunol 40: 2211–2220.

19. Roederer M, Nozzi JL, Nason MC (2011) SPICE: exploration and analysis of post-cytometric complex multivariate datasets. Cytometry A 79: 167–174.

20. Conover WJ, Iman RI (1981) Rank transformation as a bridge between parametric and nonparametric statistics. American Statistician 35: 124–128.

21. Kirkpatrick BD, Lyon CE, Porter CK, Maue AC, Guerry P, et al. (2013) Lack of Homologous Protection Against Campylobacter jejuni CG8421 in a Human Challenge Model. Clin Infect Dis. 57: 1106–1113.

22. Seder RA, Darrah PA, Roederer M (2008) T-cell quality in memory and protection: implications for vaccine design. Nat Rev Immunol 8: 247–258.

23. Weiner HL, da Cunha AP, Quintana F, Wu H (2011) Oral tolerance. Immunol Rev 241: 241–259.

24. Bacon DJ, Szymanski CM, Burr DH, Silver RP, Alm RA, et al. (2001) A phase-variable capsule is involved in virulence of *Campylobacter jejuni* 81-176. Mol Microbiol 40: 769–777.

25. Guerry P, Szymanski CM (2008) Campylobacter sugars sticking out. Trends Microbiol 16: 428–435.

26. Watson RO, Galan JE (2008) Campylobacter jejuni survives within epithelial cells by avoiding delivery to lysosomes. PLoS Pathog 4: e14.

27. Deretic V, Singh S, Master S, Harris J, Roberts E, et al. (2006) Mycobacterium tuberculosis inhibition of phagolysosome biogenesis and autophagy as a host defence mechanism. Cell Microbiol 8: 719–727.

28. Knodler LA, Steele-Mortimer O (2003) Taking possession: biogenesis of the Salmonella-containing vacuole. Traffic 4: 587–599.

29. Konkel ME, Samuelson DR, Eucker TP, Shelden EA, O'Loughlin JL (2013) Invasion of epithelial cells by Campylobacter jejuni is independent of caveolae. Cell Commun Signal 11: 100.

30. Bouwman LI, Niewold P, van Putten JP (2013) Basolateral invasion and trafficking of Campylobacter jejuni in polarized epithelial cells. PLoS One 8: e54759.

31. Hu L, Bray MD, Geng Y, Kopecko DJ (2012) Campylobacter jejuni-mediated induction of CC and CXC chemokines and chemokine receptors in human dendritic cells. Infect Immun 80: 2929–2939.

32. Hu L, Bray MD, Osorio M, Kopecko DJ (2006) Campylobacter jejuni induces maturation and cytokine production in human dendritic cells. Infect Immun 74: 2697–2705.

33. Castellino F, Huang AY, Altan-Bonnet G, Stoll S, Scheinecker C, et al. (2006) Chemokines enhance immunity by guiding naive CD8+ T cells to sites of CD4+ T cell-dendritic cell interaction. Nature 440: 890–895.

34. Maue AC, Mohawk KL, Giles DK, Poly F, Ewing CP, et al. (2012) The polysaccharide capsule of Campylobacter jejuni 81-176 modulates the host immune response. Infect Immun.

Peroxisome Proliferator-Activated Receptor γ Deficiency in T Cells Accelerates Chronic Rejection by Influencing the Differentiation of CD4+ T Cells and Alternatively Activated Macrophages

Xiaofan Huang[1][◗], Lingyun Ren[1][◗], Ping Ye[2], Chao Cheng[1], Jie Wu[1], Sihua Wang[3], Yuan Sun[1], Zheng Liu[1], Aini Xie[4], Jiahong Xia[1,5]*

1 Department of Cardiovascular Surgery, Union Hospital, Tongji Medical College, Huazhong University of Science and Technology, Wuhan, People's Republic of China, 2 Department of Cardiology, Central Hospital of Wuhan, Wuhan, People's Republic of China, 3 Department of Thoracic Surgery, Union Hospital, Tongji Medical College, Huazhong University of Science and Technology, Wuhan, People's Republic of China, 4 Division of Diabetes, Endocrinology and Metabolism, Department of Medicine, Baylor College of Medicine, Houston, Texas, United States of America, 5 Department of Cardiovascular Surgery, Central Hospital of Wuhan, Wuhan, People's Republic of China

Abstract

Background: In a previous study, activation of the peroxisome proliferator–activated receptor γ (PPARγ) inhibited chronic cardiac rejection. However, because of the complexity of chronic rejection and the fact that PPARγ is widely expressed in immune cells, the mechanism of the PPARγ - induced protective effect was unclear.

Materials and Methods: A chronic rejection model was established using B6.C-H-2^{bm12}KhEg (H-2^{bm12}) mice as donors, and MHC II-mismatched T-cell-specific PPARγ knockout mice or wild type (WT) littermates as recipients. The allograft lesion was assessed by histology and immunohistochemistry. T cells infiltrates in the allograft were isolated, and cytokines and subpopulations were detected using cytokine arrays and flow cytometry. Transcription levels in the allograft were measured by RT-PCR. In vitro, the T cell subset differentiation was investigated after culture in various polarizing conditions. PPARγ-deficient regularory T cells (Treg) were cocultured with monocytes to test their ability to induce alternatively activated macrophages (AAM).

Results: T cell-specific PPARγ knockout recipients displayed reduced cardiac allograft survival and an increased degree of pathology compared with WT littermates. T cell-specific PPARγ knockout resulted in more CD4+ T cells infiltrating into the allograft and altered the Th1/Th2 and Th17/Treg ratios. The polarization of AAM was also reduced by PPARγ deficiency in T cells through the action of Th2 and Treg. PPARγ-deficient T cells eliminated the pioglitazone-induced polarization of AAM and reduced allograft survival.

Conclusions: PPARγ-deficient T cells influenced the T cell subset and AAM polarization in chronic allograft rejection. The mechanism of PPARγ activation in transplantation tolerance could yield a novel treatment without side effects.

Editor: Josep Bassaganya-Riera, Virginia Tech, United States of America

Funding: This study was funded by the National Nature Science Foundation of China (Program No: 81070205, 81130056, 81100176 and 81373170). The funders had no role in study design, data collection and analysis, decision to publish, or preparation of the manuscript.

Competing Interests: The authors have declared that no competing interests exist.

* Email: jiahong.xia@mail.hust.edu.cn

◗ These authors contributed equally to this work.

Introduction

In end stage heart disease, heart transplantation is becoming the most important clinical treatment [1]. However, even with efficient immunosuppressive therapy to prevent acute rejection in the early stage after transplantation, chronic allograft rejection is the major obstacle to the long-term survival of heart transplant recipients [2]. The principal phenomena causing chronic allograft rejection are coronary allograft vasculopathy (CAV) [3] and leukocytes from recipients infiltrating into allografts [4]. Previous studies have demonstrated that an immune mechanism participates in chronic allograft rejection. Many studies have focused on CD4+ T helper cells and their subsets, such as Th1, Th2, Th17 and regulatory T cells (Treg), in the process of chronic allograft rejection. Th1 and Th17 secrete the pro-inflammatory cytokines interferon (IFN)-γ and IL-17A, which are known to promote chronic allograft rejection [5,6]. Th2 cells secrete IL-4, IL-5, IL-10, and IL-13, whereas Treg have an immunoregulatory function that has protective effects in numerous situations [7,8]. CD4+ T helper cells and their associated cytokines can influence the function and polarization of macrophages [9]. The classically activated macrophage (CAM)/alternatively activated macrophage (AAM) ratio in allografts has been considered to play a key role in the immune response to transplantation [10]. Within the complex mechanism of chronic allograft rejection, both T cells and macrophages participate in the lesion of allografts [3]. These cells are immunotherapy targets in chronic allograft rejection.

Peroxisome proliferator-activated receptor-γ (PPARγ) is a member of a nuclear receptor family that regulates glucose metabolism and lipogenesis. Recently, PPARγ and its agonists were found to have immunoregulatory functions in T cells and macrophages [11–13]. Given the anti-inflammatory effects of PPARγ agonists, we and other researchers have used them to treat both acute and chronic allograft rejection and have observed clear protective effects [14–16]. However, due to the complex pathological process of chronic rejection and the broad effects of PPARγ on multiple immune cells, details regarding the effects of PPARγ on immune cells in chronic allograft rejection are unclear.

To understand the mechanism of PPARγ and its agonists in chronic allograft rejection, we used B6.C-H-2^{bm12}KhEg (H-2^{bm12}) mice as donors and T cell specific PPARγ knockout (PPARγ fl/fl; Lck-Cre$^+$, T-cell-PPARγ^{ko}) mice or wild type (WT) littermates as recipients to establish a single major histocompatibility complex (MHC) class II-mismatched cardiac chronic allograft rejection model. We found that T cell-specific PPARγ deficiency impacted the differentiation of CD4+ T cell subsets and AAM bias in cardiac allografts. The protective effect of PPARγ agonists was eliminated in PPARγ deficiency in T cells.

Materials and Methods

Animals

B6.129-Ppargtm2Rev/J (H-2^b, in short PPARγ fl/fl) mice, B6.Cg-Tg (Lck-cre)548Jxm/J (H-2^b, in short Lck-Cre$^+$) mice and B6.C-H-2^{bm12}KhEg (H-2^{bm12}, in short bm12) mice were purchased from Jackson Laboratories Inc (Bar Harbor, ME, USA). C57BL/6 (H-2^b) mice were purchased from Tongji Medical College of Huazhong University of Science and Technology (HUST) (Wuhan, China). T cell-PPARγ^{ko} mice were generated by crossbreeding and verified by the standard PCR procedure recommended by Jackson Labs. PPARγ fl/fl; Lck-Cre$^+$ T cell-PPARγ^{ko} mice and PPARγ fl/fl; Lck-Cre$^-$ WT littermates were regarded as controls for each other. All of the experimental mice were male and 6 to 8 weeks old (18–25 g body weight). The animals were bred and maintained in a specific pathogen-free (SPF) barrier facility at Tongji Medical College (Wuhan, China). All animal experiments were approved by the Institutional Animal Care and Use Committee of Tongji Medical College. The protocol was approved by the Ethics Committee of Tongji Medical College, Huazhong University of Science and Technology (IORG No: IORG0003571). All surgery was performed under sodium pentobarbital anesthesia, and all efforts were made to minimize suffering.

Cardiac transplantation model and treatment

Heterotopic vascularized cardiac transplantation models were established as described previously [17]. Donor and recipient mice were anesthetized by intraperitoneal injection with ketamine at 1 mg/kg body weight. The donor hearts were transplanted into the abdomens of the recipients; the ascending aorta was connected to the recipient abdominal aorta and the pulmonary artery was sutured with the recipient inferior vena cava. The recipient mice were maintained on a thermal place until recovery from operation. Allograft function was monitored by daily palpation. At the

endpoint of experiments, mice were sacrificed by an over dose injection of ketamine and heart grafts were harvested for further detection. Pioglitazone (Ji'nan Zhongke Yitong Chemical Co., Ltd, Ji'nan, China) was provided in the chow (3 mg/kg*d) [15] starting at 1 day prior to the operation.

Histological analyses of allografts

Allografts from recipients were harvested 40 days after the operation. The allograft was embedded in paraffin for hematoxylin and eosin (H&E) and Masson trichrome staining. The severity of each allograft rejection was scored according to graft coronary artery disease (GAD) and parenchymal rejection (PR) grade [18,19]. A portion of the allograft was embedded in OCT (Sakura, Torrance, CA, USA) and subjected to immunohistochemical staining using anti-mouse CD4, CD8, and γδTCR antibodies (eBioscience, San Diego, CA).

Isolation of infiltrated lymphocytes from allografts and flow cytometry

The infiltrated lymphocytes were isolated as described previously [20]. The allografts were cut into pieces and digested with 2 mg/ml collagenase D (Worthington Bio, Lakewood, NJ) combined with 10% fecal calf serum in RPMI 1640 media for 2 h at 37°C. The suspensions were filtered with cell strainers (40 μm, BD Biosciences, San Diego, CA). The isolated cells were stained with FITC-anti-CD4, APC-Cy7-anti-CD11b, PerCP-Cy5.5-anti-IFN-γ, eFlour660-anti-IL-13, PE-anti-IL-17A, APC-anti-Foxp3, and 7-AAD (eBioscience, San Diego, CA) according to eBioscience's Best Protocols. The cells were assessed with a fluorescence activated cell sorter (FACS) Aria II (BD Biosciences, San Diego, CA) and analyzed using FCS Express 4 Plus (De Novo Software, Los Angeles, CA).

Immunoblots and enzyme-linked immunosorbent assay (ELISA)

To measure the cytokine secretion of the infiltrated CD4+ T cells, lymphocytes were sterilely isolated from allografts using a CD4+ T cell isolation kit (Miltenyi Biotec, Bergisch Gladbach, Germany) and cultured in neutral stimulate with plate-bound anti-CD3 (5 μm/ml, eBioscience) and anti-CD28 (10 μm/ml, eBioscience) antibodies. The supernatants were removed after 48 h, and cytokine levels were analyzed using a mouse cytokine antibody array (RayBiotech Inc., Norcross, GA).

Quantitative real-time PCR

Total RNA was extracted from allografts or cultured cells using TRIzol Reagent (Invitrogen, Carlsbad, CA) following the manufacturer's instructions. cDNA was prepared using the PrimeScript RT Master Mix reverse transcription kit (TaKaRa, Shiga, Japan). The PCR mixture was prepared using SYBR Premix EX Taq (TaKaRa, Shiga, Japan), and transcription levels were detected using a BioRad CFX96 (Bio-Rad Laboratories Inc., Hercules, CA). The relative expression levels were normalized to the expression of GAPDH using the ΔΔCt method. The primers used were as follows: T-bet, forward: 5'-CAACAACCCCTTTGC-GAAAG-3', reverse: 5'-TCCCCCAAGCAGTTGACAGT-3'; GATA-3, forward: 5'-AGCCACATCTCTCCCTTCAG-3', reverse: 5'-AGGGCTCTGCCTCTCTAACC-3'; RORγt, forward: 5'-TGCAAGACTCATCGACAAGG-3', reverse: 5'-AGGGGA-TTCAACATCAGTGC-3'; Foxp3, forward: 5'-ACTGGG-GTCTTCTCCCTCAA-3', reverse: 5'-GTGGGAAGGTGCAG-AGTAG-3'; iNOS, forward: 5'-GTTCTCAGCCCAACAATAC-AAGA-3', reverse: 5'-GTGGACGGGTCGATGTCA -3'; Arg1, forward: 5'-CTCCAAGCCAAAGTCCTTAGAG-3', reverse: 5'-GGAGCTGTCATTAGGGACATC-3'; Mrc1, forward: 5'-AAT-GAAGATCACAAGCGCTGC-3', reverse: 5'-TGACACCCAG-CGGAATTTCT-3', GAPDH, forward: 5'-TTCACCACCATG-GAGAAGGC-3', reverse: 5'-GGCATGGACTGTGGTCATG-A-3'.

Cell culture and monocyte/Treg coculture

Mouse splenic CD4+ T cells were purified with a CD4+ T cell isolation kit (Miltenyi Biotec, Bergisch Gladbach, Germany) and stimulated with plate-bound anti-CD3 (5 μm/ml, eBioscience) and anti-CD28 (10 μm/ml, eBioscience) antibodies together with IL-12 (10 ng/ml) for Th1 differentiation, IL-4 (10 ng/ml) for Th2 differentiation, TGF-β (5 ng/ml) and IL-6 (20 ng/ml) for Th17 differentiation, and TGF-β (5 ng/ml) alone for Treg differentiation. All cytokines were obtained from eBioscience. Monocytes and Treg were cocultured at a ratio of 2:1 according to a previously reported method [21]. Treg and monocytes were isolated from spleen using a CD4+CD25+ isolation kit or CD11b+ isolation kit (Miltenyi Biotec, Bergisch Gladbach, Germany). The purity of CD11b+ isolated monocytes is greater than 88% by flow cytometry. Cells were cocultured with RPMI 1640 and stimulated by anti-CD3 (5 μm/ml, eBioscience) and LPS (50 ng/ml, Sigma, St Louis, USA) for 36 h.

Statistical analysis

The data are expressed as the mean±SD, and comparisons between groups were conducted using unpaired Student's t tests. The allograft survival curve was plotted using the Kaplan-Meier method, and differences were determined using a log-rank test. All data were analyzed using Prism 5.0 (GraphPad Software, La Jolla, CA). P values less than 0.05 were considered statistically significant.

Results

PPARγ-deficient T cells exhibit significant decreases in cardiac allografts survival and aggravate chronic allograft rejection

We established a model of heterotrophic cardiac transplantation using an MHC class II - mismatched model. To investigate the contribution of PPARγ expression in T cells to chronic allograft rejection, we used T cell-PPARγ^{ko} mice as recipients. We evaluated allografts daily by palpation to detect their function. In WT littermates, a median allograft survival (MST) of 67 days was observed after transplantation; however, the MST in T cell-PPARγ^{ko} mice was only 48 days (Figure 1A). To detect lesions of chronic allograft rejection, HE and Masson staining were performed on the allografts 40 days after transplantation. In WT littermates, perivascular leukocytic infiltration, CAV and destruction of the cardiac muscle structure were observed, however, in T cell-PPARγ^{ko} mice, more intensive chronic allograft rejection signs were noted compared with the WT littermates. (Figure 1B). Consistent with these observations, the GAD and PR scores of T cell-PPARγ^{ko} mice were increased compared with WT littermates 40 days after transplantation (Figure 1C). These results suggested that recipients with PPARγ-deficient T cells exhibited decreased allograft survival and aggravated lesions of chronic allograft rejection.

T cell PPARγ deficiency increases CD4+ T cell infiltration in cardiac allografts

Leukocyte infiltration into allografts is a hallmark and pathogenic factor of chronic allograft rejection. Given that we identified more severe lesions in T cell-PPARγ^{ko} mice, we next detected the infiltration of T cell subsets into the allograft 40 days after transplantation. The CD4+, CD8+, and γδTCR+ T cell subsets in allografts were counted per high-power field (HPF) using immunohistochemical staining. Compared with the T cell subsets in the cardiac allografts of WT littermate recipients, a remarkable increase in infiltrated CD4+ T cells was observed in T cell-PPARγ^{ko} mice. In contrast, the numbers of CD8+ and γδTCR+ T cells did not differ between the groups (Figure 2A, B). As T cell-PPARγ^{ko} mice found to have CD4+, CD8+, γδTCR+ T cells and CD11b+ monocytes ratio comparable to those of C57BL/6 and WT littermate initiate before operation (Figure S1).

PPARγ-deficient T cells alter cytokine secretion and the polarization of CD4+ T cells in cardiac allografts

Most studies have focused on Th1 (secreting IFN-γ), Th2 (secreting IL-4/13) and Th17 (secreting IL-17) cells, which were considered the predominant contributors to chronic allograft rejection. Because we found increased CD4+ T cell infiltration in PPARγ-deficient T cell recipients in a previous study, we used a cytokine antibody array to detect cytokine secretion by infiltrated CD4+ T cells in vitro under the neutral stimulation conditions with anti-CD3/28 40 days after transplantation. We confirmed that in PPARγ-deficient T cell recipients, CD4+ T cells secreted higher levels of Th1-related IFN-γ and Th17-related IL-17. In contrast, Th2-related IL-5, IL-10 and IL-13 cytokine secretion decreased compared with WT littermates (Figure 3A). We also used RT-PCR to measure the mRNA levels of transcription factors specific for CD4+ T cells in the cardiac allografts. The cardiac allografts from PPARγ-deficient T cell recipients expressed higher levels of Th1- and Th17- related T-bet and RORγt and reduced levels of Th2- and Treg- related GATA-3 and Foxp3 (Figure 3B). The flow cytometry data on the infiltrated CD4+ T cells in the allograft revealed a variation trend consistent with the RT-PCR data (Figure 3C, D).

PPARγ-deficient CD4+ T cells enhance Th1 and Th17 polarization in vitro

Previous experiments indicated that CD4+ T cell subsets varied in PPARγ-deficient T cell allografts. We tested whether the PPARγ-deficient T cells exhibited altered polarization into Th1, Th2, Th17, and Treg cells. We isolated CD4+ T cells from the spleens of T cell-PPARγ^{ko} mice or WT littermates and cultured them under Th1/Th2/Th17/Treg-polarizing conditions for 4 days. Cells were then harvested, and intracellular cytokine levels were detected using flow cytometry with intracellular staining for IFN-γ, IL-13, IL-17A, and Foxp3. A remarkable increase in IFN-γ and IL-17A production was observed in the PPARγ-deficient CD4+ T cells. However, the percentage of CD4+IL-13+ and CD4+Foxp3+ T cells did not change (Figure 4A, B). These findings suggested increased differentiation into the Th1 and Th17 subsets in PPARγ-deficient CD4+ T cells. The decreased Th2 and Treg subsets in the allografts were likely attributed to the increase in Th1 and Th17 cells and not to a failure to differentiate.

The effect of T cell PPARγ deficiency on macrophage polarization in vivo and in vitro

Previous studies have suggested that macrophages participate in chronic allograft rejection and that T cell subsets may influence macrophage polarization [9,10,21]. Therefore, we next examined whether PPARγ-deficient T cells affect macrophage infiltration and polarization in cardiac allografts. Flow cytometry was performed to detect the amount of CD11b+ F4/80+ macrophage

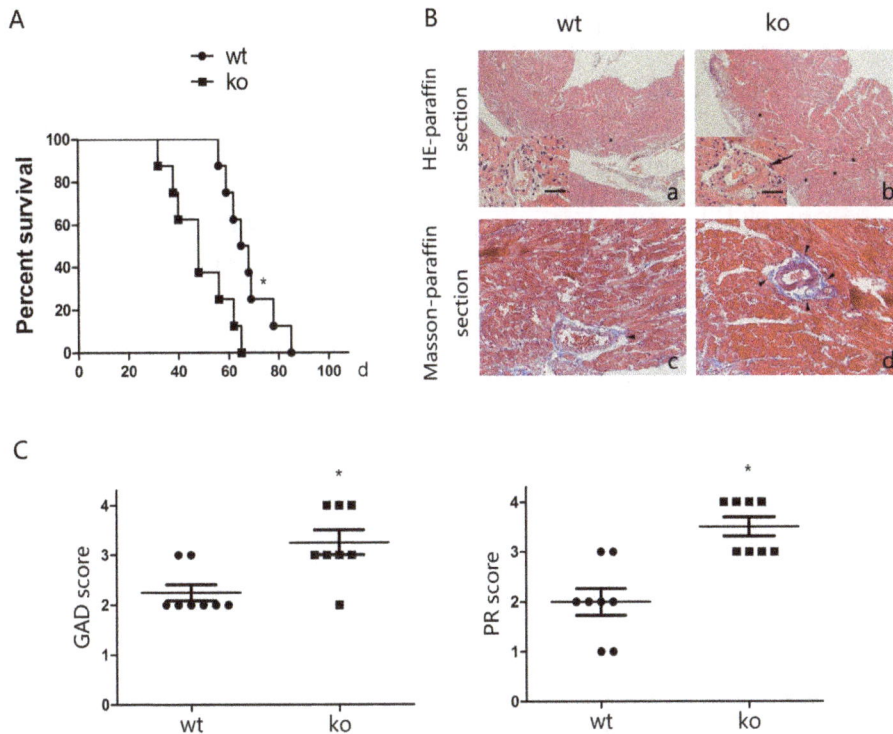

Figure 1. PPARγ-deficient T cells reduce survival and augment lesions associated with chronic rejection. A. The survival time of cardiac allografts in T cell-PPARγ^ko mice was significantly shorter than that of reduced compared with WT littermates. B. Cardiac allograft (bm12) sections of lesions 40 days after transplantation from T cell-PPARγ^ko mice (ko) or WT littermates. (a, b) HE staining, major view magnification 40×, left bottom view magnification 400×. Scale bars = 100 μm. (c, d) Masson trichrome staining, magnification 400×. T cell-PPARγ^ko mice exhibited severe lesions. Arrows indicate obvious intimal hyperplasia, asterisks indicate leukocytic infiltration, and filled arrowheads indicate collagen deposition. C. Graft coronary artery disease (GAD) and parenchymal rejection (PR) scores in T cell-PPARγ^ko mice were considerably increased compared with WT littermates. The data are presented as the mean±SD for each group (n = 8), *p<0.05.

infiltration at 7, 14, and 40 days after transplantation. In the cardiac allografts from T cell-PPARγ^ko mice, the number of macrophages was significantly increased compared with the WT littermates allografts (Figure 5A, B). To identify macrophage polarization into CAM and AAM, we measured the expression of CAM-related-iNOS, AAM-related-Arg1, and Mrc1 using RT-PCR at 7, 14, and 40 days after transplantation. Arg1 and Mrc1 mRNA levels did not increase in T cell-PPARγ^ko mice, whereas the levels were significantly elevated in WT littermates on days 14 and 40 post-grafting. In addition, no significant differences in the

mRNA levels of CAM-related-iNOS were noted in the two groups. Therefore, in T cell-PPARγ^ko recipients mice, macrophages failed to differentiate into AAM in local allografts. Because some studies have demonstrated that Treg can induce AAM polarization, we hypothesized that the PPARγ-deficient Treg failed to induce AAM polarization. We isolated autologous CD4+ CD25+ Treg from the spleens of T cell-PPARγ^ko mice or their WT littermates and cocultured these cells with CD11b monocytes from C57BL/6 mice. After 2 days, cells were collected for RT-PCR detection. Arg1 and Mrc1 transcription levels were reduced

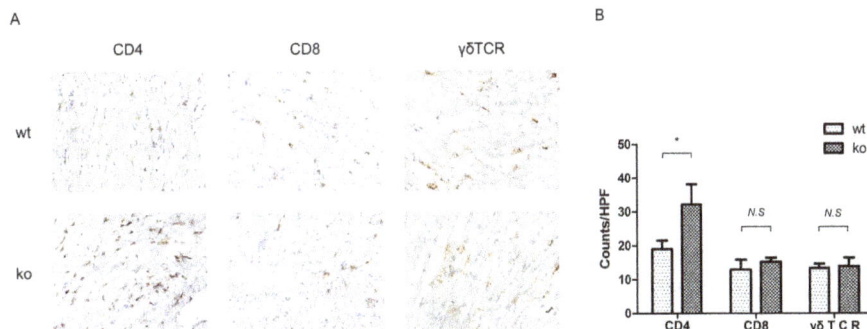

Figure 2. Infiltration CD4+, CD8+, and γδTCR+ cells in donor hearts from T cell-PPARγ^ko mice or WT littermates. A. Immunohistochemical staining of CD4+, CD8+, and γδTCR+ cells in allografts 40 days after transplantation. Top, allograft from T cell-PPARγ^ko mice (ko); bottom, allograft from WT littermates (wt). B. Quantitative analysis of CD4+, CD8+, and γδTCR+ cells in allografts counted per high power field (HPF). The data are presented as the mean±SD of 8 fields per group, *p<0.05.

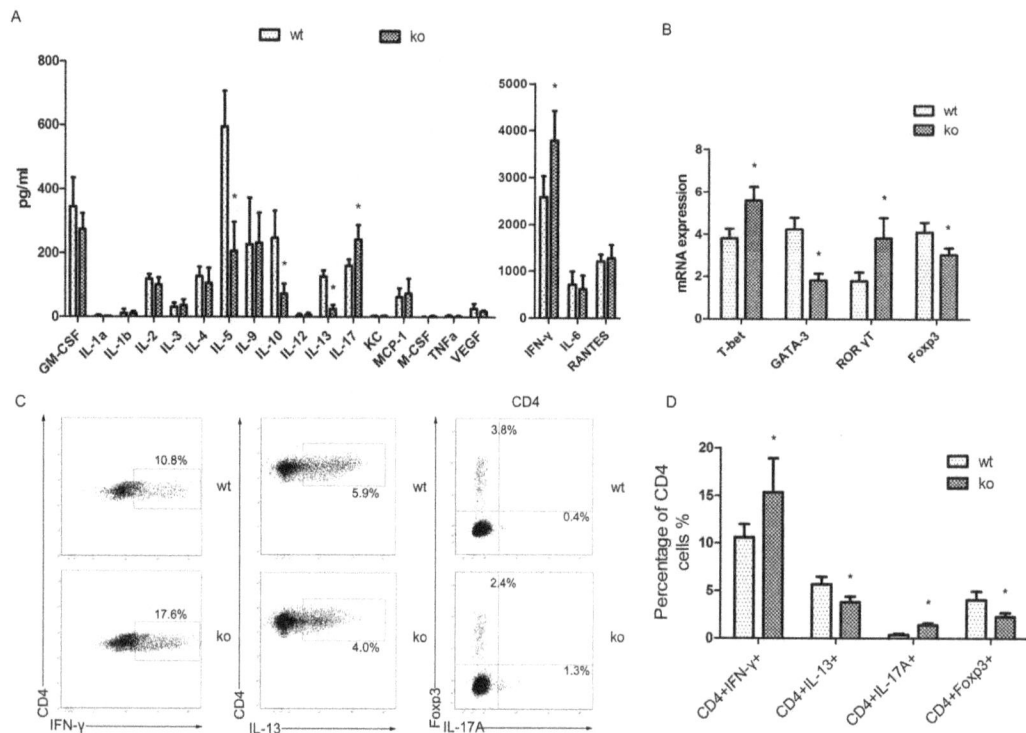

Figure 3. Cytokines and transcription factor expression in infiltrating CD4+ T cells in cardiac allografts. A. Analysis of cytokine secretion by infiltrating CD4+ T cells from T cell-PPARγ^ko mice (ko) and WT littermates (wt) using a cytokine antibody array 40 days after transplantation. B. The transcription levels of the transcription factors T-bet, GATA-3, RORγt, and Foxp3 in allografts were measured by RT-PCR 40 days after transplantation. C. Graft-infiltrating CD4+ T cells were isolated 40 days after transplantation. These cells were stained with CD45, CD4, and 7-AAD then intracellularly stained with IFN-γ, IL-13, IL-17A, and Foxp3 for assessment by flow cytometry. D. The percentage of CD4+IFN-γ+/CD4+IL-13+/CD4+IL-17A/CD4+ Foxp3+ cells in infiltrating CD4+ T cells was determined by flow cytometry. The data are presented as the mean±SD for each group (In panels A and B n = 10; in panels C and D n = 5), *p<0.05.

in PPARγ-deficient Treg cocultured with monocytes (Figure 6). All of the above results demonstrated that PPARγ-deficient T cells impact AAM polarization *in vivo* and *in vitro*.

PPARγ-deficient T cells abrogate the protective effect of a PPARγ agonist

In our prior study, we demonstrated that PPARγ-deficient T cells reduce the polarization of AAM. Other researchers have observed that PPARγ agonists enhance AAM differentiation [42]. We examined whether PPARγ-deficient T cells neutralize the protective effect of PPARγ agonists in chronic allograft rejection. After treatment with the PPARγ agonist pioglitazone, the median allograft survival significantly decreased in T cell-PPARγ^ko mice (Figure 7A). Moreover, Arg1 and Mrc1 transcription levels in allografts significantly decreased in T cell-PPARγ^ko groups compared with WT littermates administered pioglitazone 40 days after transplantation (Figure 7B).

Discussion

Several studies have demonstrated the protective role of PPARγ agonists in chronic allograft rejection [15,22,23]. In these studies, the allogeneic reactions of cell infiltration and proinflammatory cytokine secretion are suppressed by PPARγ agonists. However, the details regarding how PPARγ influences the immune response in chronic allograft rejection are unknown. Recent studies have reported that PPARγ plays an important immunoregulatory function in autoimmune diseases, such as experimental autoim-

mune encephalomyelitis (EAE) [24], allergic airway inflammation [25], trinitrobenzene sulfonic acid-induced colitis [26], and insulin resistance [27]. In these disease models, PPARγ is the key factor promoting the differentiation of CD4+ T cells and macrophages. Our previous study found that PPARγ activation with eicosapentaenoic acid can impact the balance between Th17/Treg cells and protect cardiac allografts [14], consistent with its effect on autoimmune diseases. Therefore, we hypothesize that PPARγ controls T cell subset polarization in chronic allograft rejection and influences tolerance to allografts after transplantation.

In this study, we established a MHC class II-mismatched chronic allograft rejection model. To eliminate confusion due to non-selective PPARγ agonists in the entire immune system, we used B6 background PPARγ fl/fl; Lck-Cre+ T cell-specific PPARγ knockout mice and WT littermates as recipients. In the T cell-PPARγ^ko group, leukocyte infiltration and CAV were aggravated, and allograft survival decreased compared with WT littermates. These results confirmed that although PPARγ influences both T cells and macrophages [28], in chronic allograft rejection, T cells expressing PPARγ may participate in the primary function of transplant tolerance. Previous studies have suggested that CD4+, CD8+, and γδTCR+ T cells infiltrated into the allografts and contributed to allograft rejection [19,29]. We used immunohisto-chemical staining to detect infiltrated T cells in cardiac allografts 40 days after transplantation. The number of infiltrated CD4+ T cells was significantly increased in allografts in T cell-PPARγ^ko recipients. This result suggested that the infiltration of CD4+ T

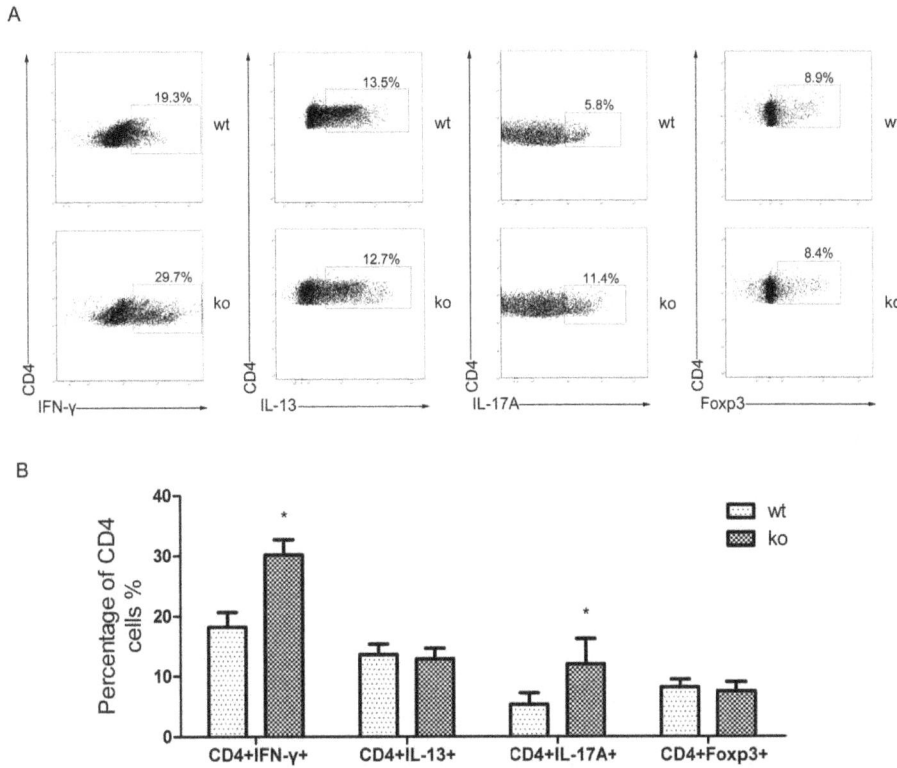

Figure 4. T cell-specific-PPARγ knockout changes CD4+ T cell subsets differentiation. A. CD4+ T cells were isolated from T cell-PPARγ[ko] mice (ko) and WT littermates (wt) spleens and then cultured in protocols that induce T cell polarization into Th1, Th2, Th17, and Treg. After 4 days of culture, these cells were assessed by flow cytometry. B. The percentage of CD4+IFN-γ+/CD4+IL-13+/CD4+IL-17A/CD4+Foxp3+ cells in each cultured group of total CD4+ cells. The data are presented as the mean±SD for each group (n = 5), *p<0.05.

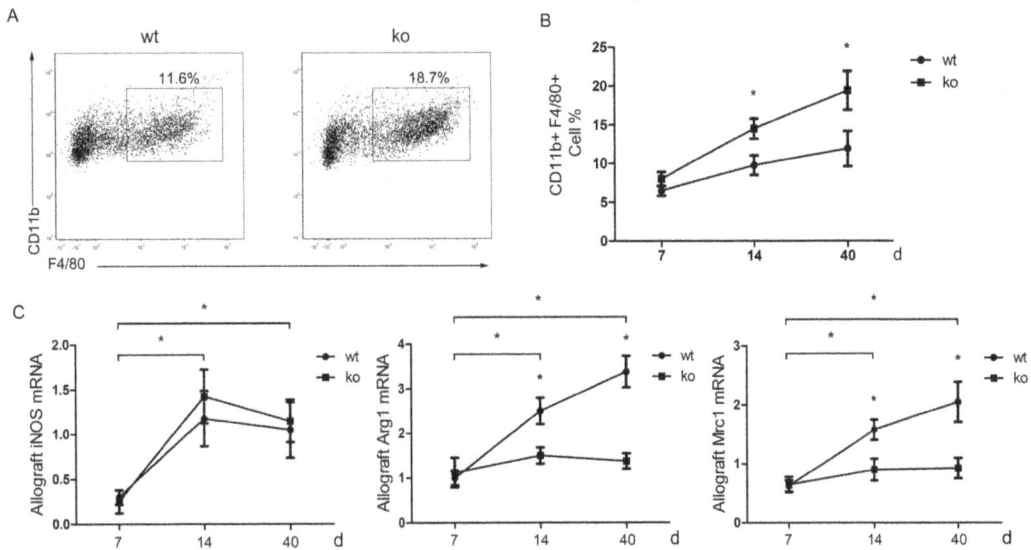

Figure 5. Analysis of macrophage infiltration and polarization in cardiac allografts. A. Flow cytometry analyses of the proportion of CD11b+ F4/80+ macrophages infiltrating cardiac allografts 40 days after transplantation. B. Dynamic analyses of the proportion of infiltrated macrophages in the total mononuclear cells in allografts at 7, 14, and 40 days after transplantation. C. iNOS, Arg1 and Mrc1 transcription levels in allografts were measured by RT-PCR at 7, 14 and 40 days after transplantation. The data are presented as the mean±SD for each group (n = 5), *p< 0.05.

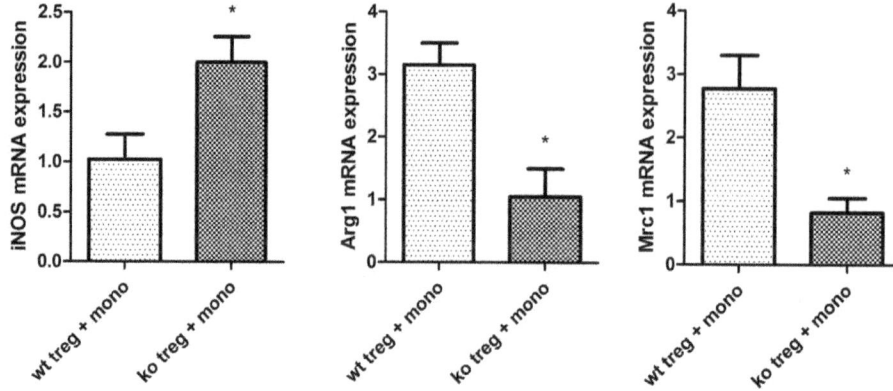

Figure 6. PPARγ^ko Treg fail to induce AAM in a monocyte and T cell coculture. CD4+CD25+ T cells were isolated from the spleens of T cell-PPARγ^ko mice (ko) and WT littermates (wt) and cocultured with CD11b+ monocytes from PBMC C57BL/6 mice. The transcription level of iNOS, Arg1, and Mrc1 was assessed in monocytes after 48 h of coculture by RT-PCR. The data are presented as the mean±SD for each group (n = 5), *p<0.05.

cells in allografts increased with PPARγ knockout and caused the intensive lesion.

CD4+ T cells and their secretion of various cytokines participate in allogeneic rejection [30]. We isolated infiltrated CD4+ T cells in allografts and examined their secreted cytokines. Based on RT-PCR and flow cytometry, the percentage of Th1 and Th17 increased, whereas Th2 and Treg decreased in the T cell-PPARγ^ko group. These results implied that PPARγ knockout altered the subsets of CD4+ T cells. We next examined T cell differentiation *in vitro*. In contrast to the allografts, Th1 and Th17 differentiated more efficiently when PPARγ was knocked out, whereas Th2 and Treg differentiation remained unchanged. These results are consistent with those of previous studies that also used conditional PPARγ knockout mice cells [24,26]. Other laboratories using PPARγ agonists reached similar conclusions. Augstein et al. used the PPARγ agonist troglitazone to reduce T cell production of IFN-γ in an autoimmune diabetes model [31]. In an allergic airway inflammation model, a PPARγ agonist decreased NF-κB activity and reduced IL-17 release [25]. We concluded that the number of Th1 and Th17 cells infiltrated into allografts increased remarkably and led to a relative decrease in Th2 and Treg cells. Th1 is a classic proinflammatory cell and has been shown to be principally responsible for chronic allograft rejection [32]. Yuan et al. demonstrated that Th17 secretion of the proinflammatory cytokine IL-17A resulted in CAV when T-bet

was knocked out [6]. Th2 and Treg cells have always been recognized as elements that prolong allograft survival [33,34] and were present at a lower ratio in allografts than in WT littermates. Their protective effect was limited with PPARγ deficiency.

Recent studies have reported that macrophages are a major component in the immune response involved in allograft rejection [35,36]. CAM accelerate the immune response, whereas AAM have repair and anti-inflammatory abilities [37]. Moreover, PPARγ agonists skewed monocytes toward AAM polarization [13]. We have observed that without PPARγ in T cells, PPARγ agonists cannot exert protective function on macrophages. In additional studies, we investigated macrophage polarization in T cell-PPARγ^ko mice. Previous studies have indicated that IL-4 and IL-13 binding to IL-4Rα and IL-13Rα1 resulted in downstream phosphorylation of STAT6, thereby causing macrophage polarization [38–40]. More recently, Szanto et al. proposed that PPARγ plays a critical role in these path ways because IL-4 signaling activates PPARγ through STAT6 interactions with PPARγ and promotes their binding to PPRE [41]. Indeed, the IL-4/13-STAT6-KLF4-PPARγ axis is regarded as an essential regulator of CAM/AAM polarization and function [42]. In our experiments, the ratio of Th2 decreased, and Th2-related cytokine production was reduced. The AAM markers Arg1 and Mrc1 were down-regulated after T cell specific knockout of PPARγ. Additionally, Tiemessen et al indicated that Treg have the ability

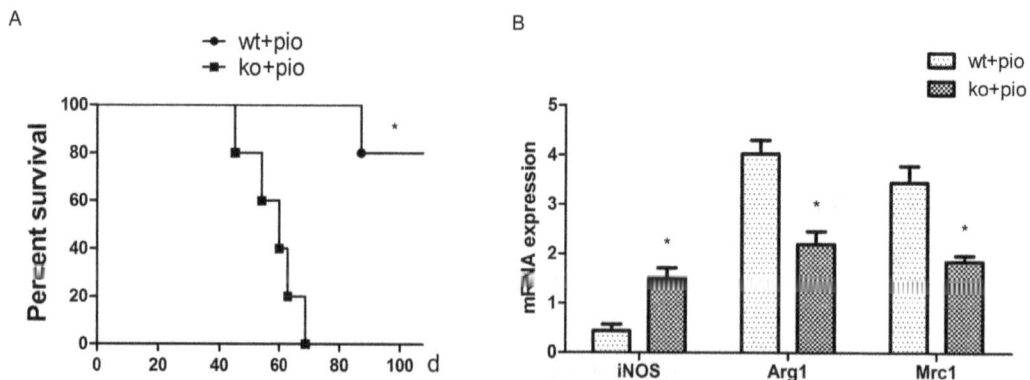

Figure 7. The beneficial effects of pioglitazone on the survival of cardiac allografts were counteracted in T cell-PPARγ^ko. A. T cell-PPARγ^ko mice (ko) abrogate the protective effect of pioglitazone on the survival curve. B. iNOS, Arg1, and Mrc1 transcription levels in allografts were measured by RT-PCR 40 days after transplantation. The data are presented as the mean±SD for each group (n = 5), *p<0.05.

to induce AAM *in vitro* [21]. Thus, we employed the same method to demonstrate that PPARγ-deficient Treg failed to induce AAM polarization. The reduced Th2-related cytokine release together with the elimination of the ability of Treg to induce AAMs indicated that the decline in number of AAMs in PPARγ-deficient allografts might be the cause of the severity of chronic rejection. To confirm that T cells influenced by PPARγ were the primary cause of AAM polarization in transplantation tolerance, we administered a PPARγ agonist to T-cell-PPARγ^ko mice and WT littermate recipients. Indeed, PPARγ-deficient T cells significantly reduced the survival of allografts and suppressed AAM polarization in the pioglitazone-treated groups.

In conclusion, the present study demonstrated that PPARγ expression is important for maintaining subsets of CD4+ T cells and macrophages in transplantation tolerance. The protective effect of a PPARγ agonist in allograft rejection potentially functions through these immune processes. However, one of the remarkable features in chronic rejection is CAV, whose pathologic lesions occasionally appear similar to atherosclerosis but occur through a unique mechanism [43]. Vladimir et al. reported that macrophage-specific PPARγ knockout increased atherosclerosis [44]. PPARγ expression in macrophages requires further investigation. Although PPARγ agonists have effective immunoregulatory capacity in many autoimmune diseases and transplant rejection animal models, the side effects of conventional thiazolidinedione drugs (TZD) have been reported in recent clinical studies [12]. Because the mechanism of the protective effect of PPARγ in chronic rejection has been demonstrated, we expect that PPARγ-targeted therapeutics might serve as a novel method to promote transplant tolerance.

Supporting Information

Figure S1 T cell-PPARγ^ko mice have normal T cell and monocyte subpopulations. Flow cytometry analyzing the proportion of T cell and monocyte subpopulations from T cell-PPARγ^ko mice are normally comparable to those of C57BL/6 mice and WT littermate before operation in the spleens. The data are presented as the mean±SD for each group (n = 5).

Acknowledgments

The authors of this manuscript have certified that they comply with the Principles of Ethical Publishing in the *PLOS ONE*.

Author Contributions

Conceived and designed the experiments: XH JW SW AX JX. Performed the experiments: XH LR PY CC. Analyzed the data: XH. Wrote the paper: XH. Revised the manuscript: YS ZL.

References

1. Stehlik J, Edwards LB, Kucheryavaya AY, Benden C, Christie JD, et al. (2012) The registry of the international society for heart and lung transplantation: 29th official adult heart transplant report-2012. J Heart Lung Transplant 31: 1052–1064.
2. Schmauss D, Weis M (2008) Cardiac allograft vasculopathy: recent developments. Circulation 117: 2131–2141.
3. Suzuki J-i, Isobe M, Morishita R, Nagai R (2010) Characteristics of Chronic Rejection in Heart Transplantation. Circ J 74: 233–239.
4. El-Sawy T, Fahmy NM, Fairchild RL (2002) Chemokines: directing leukocyte infiltration into allografts. Curr Opin Immunol 14: 562–568.
5. Piccotti JR, Li K, Chan SY, Eichwald EJ, Bishop DK (1999) Cytokine Regulation of Chronic Cardiac Allograft Rejection: Evidence Against A Role for Th1 in the Disease Process1. Transplantation 67: 1548–1555.
6. Yuan X, Paez-Cortez J, Schmitt-Knosalla I, D'Addio F, Mfarrej B, et al. (2008) A novel role of CD4 Th17 cells in mediating cardiac allograft rejection and vasculopathy. J Exp Med 205: 3133–3144.
7. Tay SS, Plain KM, Bishop GA (2009) Role of IL-4 and Th2 responses in allograft rejection and tolerance. Curr Opin Organ Transplant 14: 16–22.
8. Moraes-Vieira PM, Bassi EJ, Larocca RA, Castoldi A, Burghos M, et al. (2013) Leptin deficiency modulates allograft survival by favoring a Th2 and a regulatory immune profile. [corrected] Am J Transplant 13: 36–44.
9. Martinez FO, Helming L, Gordon S (2009) Alternative activation of macrophages: an immunologic functional perspective. Annu Rev Immunol 27: 451–483.
10. Mannon RB (2012) Macrophages: contributors to allograft dysfunction, repair, or innocent bystanders? Curr Opin Organ Transplant 17: 20–25.
11. da Rocha Junior LF, Dantas AT, Duarte AL, de Melo Rego MJ, Pitta Ida R, et al. (2013) PPARgamma Agonists in Adaptive Immunity: What Do Immune Disorders and Their Models Have to Tell Us? PPAR Res 2013: 519724.
12. Ahmadian M, Suh JM, Hah N, Liddle C, Atkins AR, et al. (2013) PPARgamma signaling and metabolism: the good, the bad and the future. Nat Med 19: 557–566.
13. Bouhlel MA, Derudas B, Rigamonti E, Dievart R, Brozek J, et al. (2007) PPARgamma activation primes human monocytes into alternative M2 macrophages with anti-inflammatory properties. Cell Metab 6: 137–143.
14. Ye P, Li J, Wang S, Xie A, Sun W, et al. (2012) Eicosapentaenoic acid disrupts the balance between Tregs and IL-17+ T cells through PPARgamma nuclear receptor activation and protects cardiac allografts. J Surg Res 173: 161–170.
15. Kosuge H, Haraguchi G, Koga N, Maejima Y, Suzuki J, et al. (2006) Pioglitazone prevents acute and chronic cardiac allograft rejection. Circulation 113: 2613–2622.
16. Tobiasova Z, Zhang L, Yi T, Qin L, Manes TD, et al. (2011) Peroxisome proliferator-activated receptor-gamma agonists prevent in vivo remodeling of human artery induced by alloreactive T cells. Circulation 124: 196–205.
17. Corry RJ, Winn HJ, Russell PS (1973) Primarily vascularized allografts of hearts in mice. The role of H-2D, H-2 K, and non-H-2 antigens in rejection. Transplantation 16: 343–350.
18. Furukawa Y, Libby P, Stinn JL, Becker G, Mitchell RN (2002) Cold ischemia induces isograft arteriopathy, but does not augment allograft arteriopathy in non-immunosuppressed hosts. The American journal of pathology 160: 1077–1087.
19. Wang S, Xu X, Xie A, Li J, Ye P, et al. (2012) Anti-interleukin-12/23p40 antibody attenuates chronic rejection of cardiac allografts partly via inhibition gammadeltaT cells. Clin Exp Immunol 169: 320–329.
20. Itoh S, Kimura N, Axtell RC, Velotta JB, Gong Y, et al. (2011) Interleukin-17 accelerates allograft rejection by suppressing regulatory T cell expansion. Circulation 124: S187–196.
21. Tiemessen MM, Jagger AL, Evans HG, van Herwijnen MJ, John S, et al. (2007) CD4+CD25+Foxp3+ regulatory T cells induce alternative activation of human monocytes/macrophages. Proc Natl Acad Sci U S A 104: 19446–19451.
22. Chen Y, Liu Y, Yuan Z, Tian L, Dallman MJ, et al. (2007) Rosiglitazone suppresses cyclosporin-induced chronic transplant dysfunction and prolongs survival of rat cardiac allografts. Transplantation 83: 1602–1610.
23. Chen Y, Li D, Tsang JY, Niu N, Peng J, et al. (2011) PPAR-gamma signaling and IL-5 inhibition together prevent chronic rejection of MHC Class II-mismatched cardiac grafts. J Heart Lung Transplant 30: 698–706.
24. Klotz L, Burgdorf S, Dani I, Saijo K, Flossdorf J, et al. (2009) The nuclear receptor PPAR gamma selectively inhibits Th17 differentiation in a T cell-intrinsic fashion and suppresses CNS autoimmunity. J Exp Med 206: 2079–2089.
25. Park SJ, Lee KS, Kim SR, Min KH, Choe YH, et al. (2009) Peroxisome proliferator-activated receptor gamma agonist down-regulates IL-17 expression in a murine model of allergic airway inflammation. J Immunol 183: 3259–3267.
26. Hontecillas R, Bassaganya-Riera J (2007) Peroxisome proliferator-activated receptor γ is required for regulatory CD4+ T cell-mediated protection against colitis. The Journal of Immunology 178: 2940–2949.
27. Odegaard JI, Ricardo-Gonzalez RR, Goforth MH, Morel CR, Subramanian V, et al. (2007) Macrophage-specific PPARgamma controls alternative activation and improves insulin resistance. Nature 447: 1116–1120.
28. Glass CK, Saijo K (2010) Nuclear receptor transrepression pathways that regulate inflammation in macrophages and T cells. Nat Rev Immunol 10: 365–376.
29. Fischbein MP, Yun J, Laks H, Irie Y, Fishbein MC, et al. (2001) CD8+ lymphocytes augment chronic rejection in a MHC class II mismatched model. Transplantation 71: 1146–1153.
30. Liu Z, Fan H, Jiang S (2013) CD4(+) T-cell subsets in transplantation. Immunol Rev 252: 183–191.
31. Augstein P, Dunger A, Heinke P, Wachlin G, Berg S, et al. (2003) Prevention of autoimmune diabetes in NOD mice by troglitazone is associated with modulation of ICAM-1 expression on pancreatic islet cells and IFN-γ expression in splenic T cells. Biochem Biophys Res Commun 304: 378–384.
32. Koglin J, Glysing-Jensen T, Gadiraju S, Russell ME (2000) Attenuated cardiac allograft vasculopathy in mice with targeted deletion of the transcription factor STAT4. Circulation 101: 1034–1039.

33. He XY, Chen J, Verma N, Plain K, Tran G, et al. (1998) Treatment with interleukin-4 prolongs allogeneic neonatal heart graft survival by inducing T helper 2 responses. Transplantation 65: 1145–1152.

34. Ge W, Jiang J, Liu W, Lian D, Saito A, et al. (2010) Regulatory T Cells Are Critical to Tolerance Induction in Presensitized Mouse Transplant Recipients Through Targeting Memory T Cells. Am J Transplant 10: 1760–1773.

35. Wyburn KR, Jose MD, Wu H, Atkins RC, Chadban SJ (2005) The role of macrophages in allograft rejection. Transplantation 80: 1641–1647.

36. Magil AB (2009) Monocytes/macrophages in renal allograft rejection. Transplant Rev (Orlando) 23: 199–208.

37. Gordon S, Martinez FO (2010) Alternative Activation of Macrophages: Mechanism and Functions. Immunity 32: 593–604.

38. Heller NM, Qi X, Junttila IS, Shirey KA, Vogel SN, et al. (2008) Type I IL-4Rs selectively activate IRS-2 to induce target gene expression in macrophages. Sci Signal 1: ra17.

39. Martinez-Nunez RT, Louafi F, Sanchez-Elsner T (2011) The interleukin 13 (IL-13) pathway in human macrophages is modulated by microRNA-155 via direct targeting of interleukin 13 receptor α1 (IL13Rα1). J Biol Chem 286: 1786–1794.

40. Dhakal M, Hardaway JC, Guloglu FB, Miller MM, Hoeman CM, et al. (2013) IL-13Ralpha1 is a surface marker for M2 macrophages influencing their differentiation and function. Eur J Immunol.

41. Szanto A, Balint BL, Nagy ZS, Barta E, Dezso B, et al. (2010) STAT6 transcription factor is a facilitator of the nuclear receptor PPARgamma-regulated gene expression in macrophages and dendritic cells. Immunity 33: 699–712.

42. Liu G, Yang H (2013) Modulation of macrophage activation and programming in immunity. J Cell Physiol 228: 502–512.

43. Rahmani M, Cruz RP, Granville DJ, McManus BM (2006) Allograft vasculopathy versus atherosclerosis. Circ Res 99: 801–815.

44. Babaev VR, Yancey PG, Ryzhov SV, Kon V, Breyer MD, et al. (2005) Conditional knockout of macrophage PPARgamma increases atherosclerosis in C57BL/6 and low-density lipoprotein receptor-deficient mice. Arterioscler Thromb Vasc Biol 25: 1647–1653.

Tumor Induced Hepatic Myeloid Derived Suppressor Cells Can Cause Moderate Liver Damage

Tobias Eggert[1], José Medina-Echeverz[1], Tamar Kapanadze[1,2], Michael J. Kruhlak[3], Firouzeh Korangy[1], Tim F. Greten[1]*

1 Gastrointestinal Malignancy Section, Center for Cancer Research, National Cancer Institute, National Institutes of Health, Bethesda, Maryland, United States of America, **2** Department of Gastroenterology, Hepatology and Endocrinology, Hannover Medical School, Hannover, Germany, **3** Experimental Immunology Branch, Center for Cancer Research, National Cancer Institute, National Institutes of Health, Bethesda, Maryland, United States of America

Abstract

Subcutaneous tumors induce the accumulation of myeloid derived suppressor cells (MDSC) not only in blood and spleens, but also in livers of these animals. Unexpectedly, we observed a moderate increase in serum transaminases in mice with EL4 subcutaneous tumors, which prompted us to study the relationship of hepatic MDSC accumulation and liver injury. MDSC were the predominant immune cell population expanding in livers of all subcutaneous tumor models investigated (RIL175, B16, EL4, CT26 and BNL), while liver injury was only observed in EL4 and B16 tumor-bearing mice. Elimination of hepatic MDSC in EL4 tumor-bearing mice using low dose 5-fluorouracil (5-FU) treatment reversed transaminase elevation and adoptive transfer of hepatic MDSC from B16 tumor-bearing mice caused transaminase elevation indicating a direct MDSC mediated effect. Surprisingly, hepatic MDSC from B16 tumor-bearing mice partially lost their damage-inducing potency when transferred into mice bearing non damage-inducing RIL175 tumors. Furthermore, MDSC expansion and MDSC-mediated liver injury further increased with growing tumor burden and was associated with different cytokines including GM-CSF, VEGF, interleukin-6, CCL2 and KC, depending on the tumor model used. In contrast to previous findings, which have implicated MDSC only in protection from T cell-mediated hepatitis, we show that tumor-induced hepatic MDSC themselves can cause moderate liver damage.

Editor: Salvatore Papa, Institute of Hepatology - Birkbeck, University of London, United Kingdom

Funding: The underlying research reported in the study was funded by the National Institutes of Health intramural research program. The funders had no role in study design, data collection and analysis, decision to publish, or preparation of the manuscript.

Competing Interests: The authors have declared that no competing interests exist.

* Email: tim.greten@nih.gov

Introduction

Infections, toxins, radiation, neoplasms, ischemia and trauma cause liver injury. The degree of liver injury depends on both, direct (agent dependent) and indirect (immune mediated) effects, since different cells of the innate immune system are rapidly recruited to the site of liver injury, where they aggravate liver damage [1–3]. On a molecular level, there are different mechanisms that can cause liver injury. For instance, detoxification of exogenous substances renders the liver susceptible to oxidative stress, which is produced during metabolism of toxic exogenous substances [4]. Acetaminophen [5] and alcohol [4] have been shown to exert a direct toxic effect through reactive oxygen species (ROS) or intermediate metabolites on hepatocytes. However, in addition to these mechanisms these agents also cause immune-mediated liver injury.

The contribution of the innate immune system to liver injury is universally acknowledged and has been extensively reviewed [6–10]. Not only the innate immune system in general, but more specifically the accumulation of neutrophils and macrophages can cause liver damage [8,11]. In alcoholic liver disease, activated Kupffer cells produce TNF-α, which induces apoptosis in

hepatocytes through TNF-α receptor binding [12]; thereby contributing to hepatocyte cell death and hepatic inflammation [13,14]. This sterile cell death can trigger Kupffer cells to secrete the acute inflammatory response cytokine IL-1 [15], which can lead to recruitment of neutrophils to the liver. In acetaminophen induced liver injury, the depletion of these infiltrating neutrophils protects mice from severe hepatotoxicity [1]. These cells also play a pivotal role not only in drug-induced liver injury as described above, but also in liver damage caused by obesity, i.e. non-alcoholic steatohepatitis. In mouse models of dietary-induced non-alcoholic steatohepatitis, liver inflammation was aggravated by accumulation of immature myeloid cells or macrophages [16,17].

Immature myeloid cells with immune suppressive ability are also termed myeloid-derived suppressor cells (MDSC). These MDSC were initially found to accumulate in tumor bearing hosts [18]. More recently, they have also been identified in trauma and chronic infections [19]. MDSC are a heterogeneous population of immature myeloid cells and comprise myeloid progenitors at different stages of the differentiation, such as precursors of granulocytes, macrophages and dendritic cells (DC). They can be found as tumor infiltrating cells, in blood, bone marrow, spleen and liver. In tumor-bearing mice, MDSC are identified by their co-expression of CD11b and Gr-1. The hallmark of MDSC is their ability to suppress both adaptive and innate immune responses through multiple mechanisms. Their accumulation in livers has been shown to protect from liver injury and to dampen T cell mediated-hepatitis [20–23].

Recently, our group investigated antibody-mediated hepatic MDSC depletion [24]. In addition to the finding, that anti-Gr-1 antibody failed to deplete MDSC in the liver, we observed an increase in alanine aminotransferase (ALT) and aspartate aminotransferase (AST) in EL4 subcutaneous tumor bearing mice. Therefore, we set out to study the effect of hepatic MDSC in different models of subcutaneous tumor-bearing mice in more detail. Here, we provide evidence that hepatic MDSC accumulation in tumor bearing mice can causes mild liver damage. MDSC-induced liver damage was tumor specific as not all tumor models investigated caused liver injury, although MDSC expansion was observed in all models.

Materials and Methods

Mice and cell lines

8–10 week-old female C57BL/6 and BALB/c were obtained from NCI/Frederick (Frederick, USA). EL4 (lymphoma), RIL175 (hepatocellular carcinoma [25]) and B16 (melanoma) tumor cell lines on C57BL/6 background and CT26 (colon carcinoma) and BNL (hepatocellular carcinoma) tumor cell lines on BALB/c background were used for subcutaneous tumor models. EL4 [26], B16 [27] and CT26 [28] cell lines were a kind gift of Dr. Drew Pardoll (The Johns Hopkins University, Baltimore, USA), The BNL cell line was generously provided by Dr. Jesus Prieto (University of Navarra, Spain; [29]) and the RIL175 cell line was obtained from Dr. Lars Zender (University Hospital of Tübingen, Germany; [25,30]). All experiments were performed according to the institutional guidelines and approved by the National Cancer Institute Bethesda Animal Care and Use Committee (Bethesda, MD, USA).

Animal experiments

1×10^6 tumor cells were injected subcutaneously into the left flank of 8–10 week-old female mice. Mice were sacrificed, when subcutaneous tumors reached 15 mm or 20 mm mean diameter. ALT and AST levels were determined in mouse sera and livers were collected for immune cell analysis or fixed in 10% Formaldehyde for histology and TUNEL assays. TUNEL stainings were performed using the ApopTag Peroxidase In Situ Apoptosis Detection Kit (Millipore, Billerica, USA) according to manufacturer's instructions. Mouse testis served as control tissue. Liver histology slides stained with TUNEL were analyzed by counting TUNEL positive cells in 20 non-overlapping visual fields from individual specimens of 2 livers per group. Immunohistochemistry images were collected using a Zeiss AxioObserver Z1 microscope equipped a 10× plan-apochromat (N.A. 0.45) objective lens and a AxioCam MRc5 color CCD camera (Carl Zeiss Microscopy, llc., Thornwood, NY, USA).

MDSC depletion was achieved as described previously [31]. Briefly, mice were treated with 5 FU (50 µg/g body weight) when EL4 tumor surface was approximately 100 mm². Saline treated mice served as controls.

For hepatic MDSC transfer, a single cell suspension was prepared from B16 subcutaneous tumor-bearing mouse livers by density gradient centrifugation (Percoll; Fisher Scientific, Pittsburgh, USA) and red blood cell lysis (ACK Lysis Buffer; Quality Biologicals), subsequently MACS-sorted using CD11b microbeads (Miltenyi Biotec Inc., San Diego, USA) and injected (5×10^7 cells)

intravenously into female C57BL/6 mice. Accumulation of transferred cells in livers of recipient mice was confirmed in a pilot experiment by transferring hepatic CD45.1+CD11b+ cells from tumor-bearing mice into naïve C57BL/6 (CD45.2+) mice and detection of CD45.1+CD11b+Gr-1+ cells in the recipient mouse liver via flow cytometry. Purity of MACS-sorted cells was assessed by flow cytometry. >95% of cells for transfer were CD11b+ and 75% were CD11b+Gr1+. Mice were sacrificed 16 h after transfer and serum ALT and AST levels were analyzed.

Flow cytometry analysis

Single cell suspensions were prepared as described earlier [24]. Briefly, livers were homogenized, passed through a nylon mesh and liver-infiltrating cells were isolated by isotonic Percoll (Fisher Scientific, Pittsburgh, USA) centrifugation. RBCs were lysed using ACK lysis buffer (Quality Biological, Gaithersburg, USA). Cells were stained with the following mouse antibodies against: CD11b (Clone M1/70), Ly6G (1A8), Ly6C (HK1.4) CD3 (17A2), CD4 (GK1.5), CD8 (53–6.7), NK1.1 (PK136), CD19 (eBio1D3), CD11c (N418), B220 (RA3-6B2) and CD244 (eBio244F4) (all from eBioscience Inc., San Diego, USA) and Gr-1 (RB6-8C5; BioLegend, San Diego, USA). Flow cytometry was performed on BD FACS Calibur using BD CellQuest Pro software or LSRII using BD FACSDiva software (BD Biosciences, San Diego, USA). Data were analyzed using FlowJo software (Tree Star Inc., Ashland, USA). MDSC were defined as CD11b+Gr-1+, monocytic MDSC (M-MDSC) as CD11b+Ly6G−Ly6C^{high}, granulocytic MDSC (PMN-MDSC) as CD11b+Ly6G+Ly6C^{low}, Macrophages as CD11b+Gr-1−F4/80+, conventional DC as CD11c+CD11b+, plasmacytoid DC as CD11c+CD11b−B220+, CD4 T cells as CD3^{high}CD4+, CD8 T cells as CD3+CD4+, NK cells as NK1.1+CD3−, NKT cells as NK1.1+CD3^{low} and B cells as CD19+CD3−.

Cytokine assay

Mouse serum samples and tumor-conditioned media, derived from in vitro cultured tumor cell lines, were analyzed by Mouse Cytokine/Chemokine Magnetic bead panel (Millipore, Billerica, USA) according to manufacturer's instructions. Serum samples from tumor-bearing mice were normalized to naïve wild-type mice.

Statistical analysis

Data were analyzed for statistical significance using Student's t test to compare two groups. When one control group was compared to multiple groups, One-way ANOVA was used. (Prism software; GraphPad); $p < 0.05$ was considered to be statistically significant.

Results

Tumor-bearing mice suffer from mild liver damage

To investigate liver damage in subcutaneous tumor-bearing mice, we analyzed ALT and AST serum levels of BALB/c or C57BL/6 mice bearing tumors of ectodermal (B16), mesodermal (EL4) and endodermal (RIL175, BNL, CT26) origin (Figure 1A, B). B16 and EL4 tumor bearing mice had elevated levels of both liver enzymes, ALT and AST, whereas only subtle statistically not significant ALT and AST elevation were noticed in mice with other tumors. The highest increase was observed in B16 tumor-bearing mice. Both macroscopic and microscopic evaluation of livers from B16 and EL4 subcutaneous tumor-bearing mice indicated no signs for the presence of liver metastasis as a possible cause for elevated ALT and AST levels (data not shown). TUNEL assays were performed to demonstrate that the increase in ALT and AST levels in subcutaneous tumor-bearing mice was due to hepatocyte injury, i.e. apoptosis. Indeed, more apoptotic hepatocytes were seen on sections from B16 tumor-bearing mice compared to tumor-free controls (Figure 1C, D). Together, these results show that subcutaneous growth of certain tumors causes mild liver damage.

Subcutaneous tumors induce primarily expansion of MDSC among liver immune cell subsets

Since immune cells are capable of exacerbating liver injury, we hypothesized that the increase in ALT and/or AST in subcutaneous tumor-bearing mice is mediated by an accumulation of immune cells in the liver. To this end, we analyzed the hepatic immune subsets in mice with the highest (B16 and EL4) increase in liver enzymes in C57BL/6 mice (Figure 2). In all tumor-bearing mice the frequency and number of cells of the myeloid compartment increased compared to naïve mice (Figure 2A, B and D). Of all myeloid cells, the strongest increase was seen in MDSC. On the other hand, cells of the lymphoid compartment did not increase in frequency and only slightly increased in cell number (Figure 2B). To confirm that $CD11b^+Gr-1^+$ cells represent MDSC rather than neutrophils in our tumor-bearing mice, we studied whether $CD11b^+Gr-1^+$ cells were also positive for CD244, which has been proposed as a marker to distinguish neutrophils from granulocytic MDSC [32]. Indeed, $CD11b^+Gr1^+$ cells were also positive for CD244 in livers of B16 and RIL175 tumor-bearing mice (Figure 2C). Next, we analyzed the cell number of MDSC and non-MDSC in all tumor models used (Figure 2E). The increase of MDSC in tumor bearing vs. naïve mice was higher than the increase of non-MDSC. In summary, MDSC were the predominant immune subset expanding in livers of mice with subcutaneous tumors.

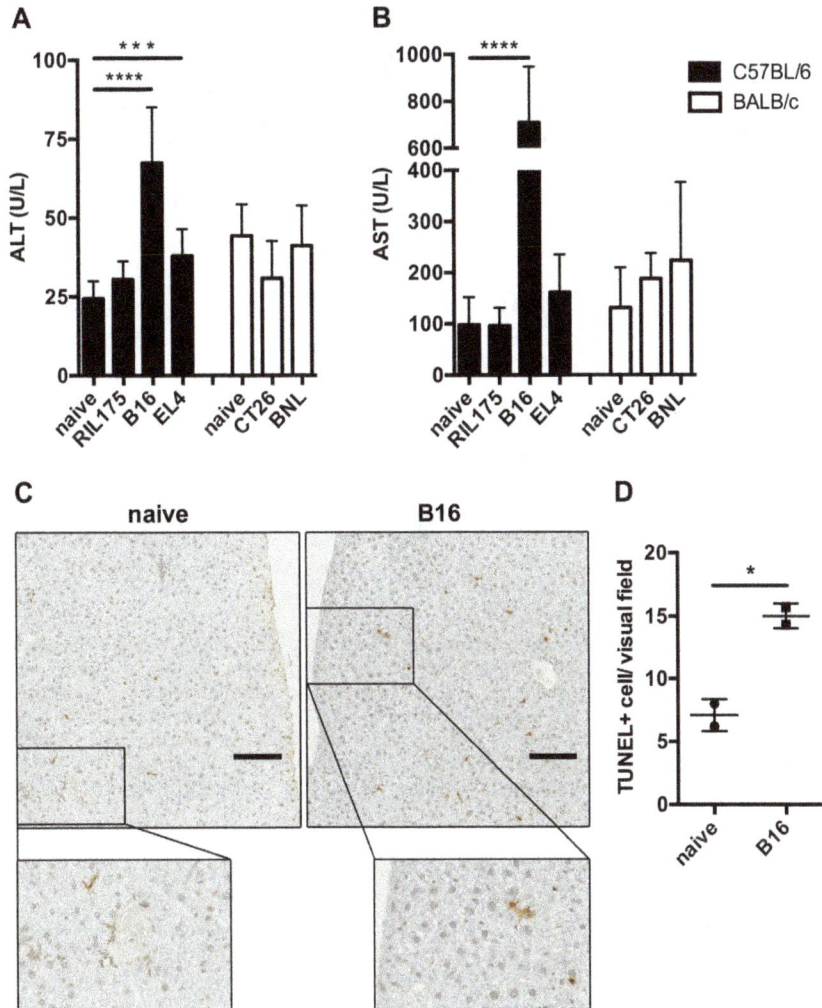

Figure 1. Melanoma and lymphoma subcutaneous tumor-bearing mice suffer from mild liver damage. C57BL/6 and BALB/c mice bearing indicated subcutaneous tumors were sacrificed, when tumor diameter reached 15 mm. ALT (A) and AST (B) levels were analyzed in mouse serum (N≥8 mice per tumor, N≥6 naïve mice, 3 independent experiments). Naïve C57BL/6 mice (C, left image) or mice bearing B16 subcutaneous tumors (C, right image) were sacrificed, when tumor diameter reached 20 mm. TUNEL assays were performed on liver specimen (C; scale bar = 100 μm; N = 2 mice per group, total of 5 TUNEL assays per group) and TUNEL positive cells were counted in 20 non-overlapping visual fields. Means of TUNEL positive cells per liver section were plotted (D). C, Representative examples of visual fields are shown. Data are expressed as mean ±SEM. *p<0.05, ***p<0.001, ****p<0.0001 (by One-way ANOVA).

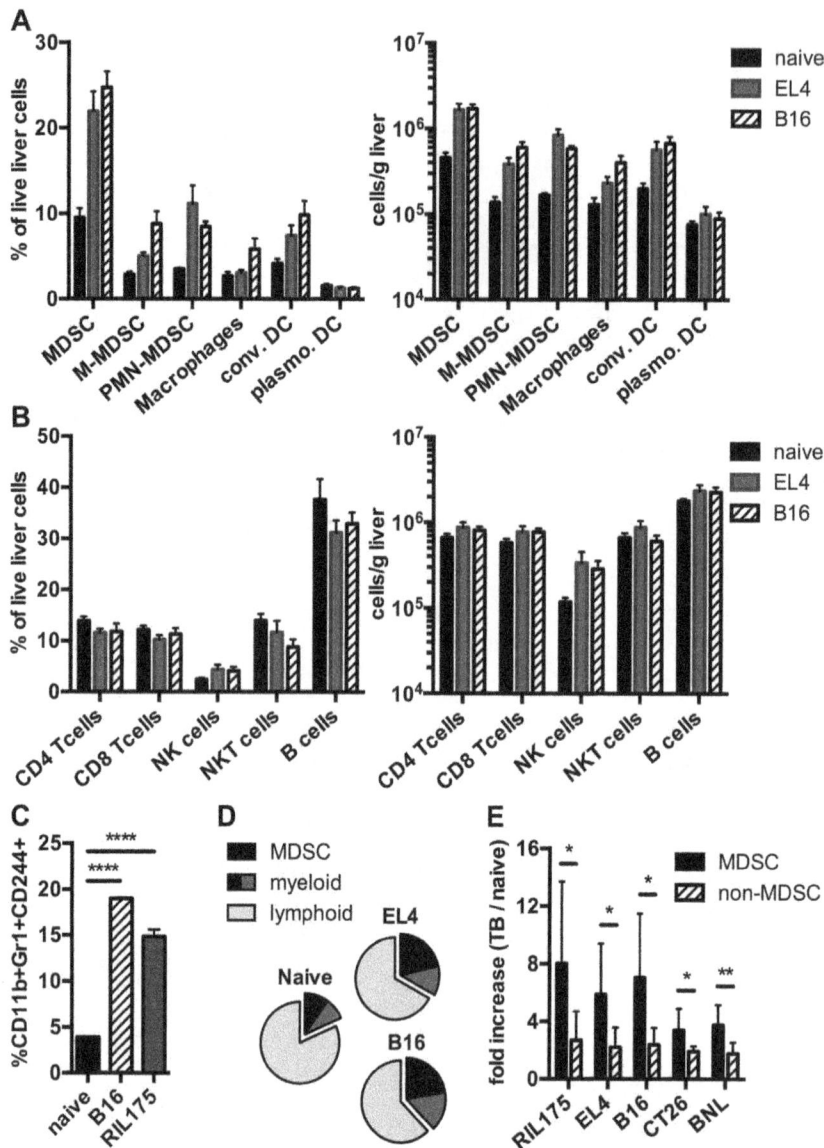

Figure 2. Analysis of hepatic immune cells in mice with subcutaneous tumors. C57BL/6 naïve mice or mice bearing EL4 or B16 tumors were sacrificed, when tumor diameter reached 15 mm. Hepatic immune cells were analyzed by flow cytometry and frequency and absolute cell number per gram liver were calculated for the myeloid compartment (A) and the lymphoid compartment (B) (N = 5 mice per tumor). C, Frequencies of CD11b$^+$Gr-1$^+$CD244$^+$ cells in livers of naïve mice or mice bearing indicated tumors (N = 3 mice per group). D, Change of frequency of myeloid (including MDSC) and lymphoid cells in naïve vs. EL4 or B16 tumor-bearing mice. E, fold increase of absolute numbers of MDSC (CD11b$^+$Gr-1$^+$ cells) or non-MDSC (total number of liver leukocytes minus number of CD11b$^+$Gr-1$^+$ cells) in tumor bearing vs. naïve mice (N = 8 mice per tumor). Data are expressed as mean ±SEM. *$p<0.05$, **$p<0.01$ (C was analyzed by One-way ANOVA. E was analyzed by two-tailed Student's t test).

Liver damage in subcutaneous tumor-bearing mice is MDSC mediated

To determine whether the elevation of liver enzymes in our subcutaneous tumor models was MDSC mediated, we treated EL4 tumor-bearing mice with low dose 5-FU, which had been shown to deplete MDSC in tumor-bearing mice successfully [31]. As expected, the frequency of hepatic MDSC dropped significantly compared to saline treated control mice. Depletion was more prominent in the granulocytic than in the monocytic MDSC population (Figure 3A). ALT values also significantly fell; suggesting that depletion of hepatic MDSC alleviated liver damage in subcutaneous tumor bearing mice (Figure 3A). To further corroborate our result, we adoptively transferred CD11b$^+$ cells

from livers of liver damage-inducing B16 tumor-bearing mice into naïve C57BL/6 mice. Transferred CD11b$^+$Gr-1$^+$CD45.1$^+$ MDSC were successfully detected in livers of recipient mice 1 and 16 h after injection, demonstrating hepatic recruitment of MDSC upon transfer (Figure S1). ALT and AST levels increased significantly 16 h after cell transfer compared to naïve mice (Figure 3B), supporting our hypothesis that hepatic MDSC were the cause of liver injury in this model.

Subcutaneous tumors shape the potency of MDSC to cause liver damage

Since mice bearing RIL175 tumors did not have increased ALT and AST levels, we investigated the liver damage-inducing ability

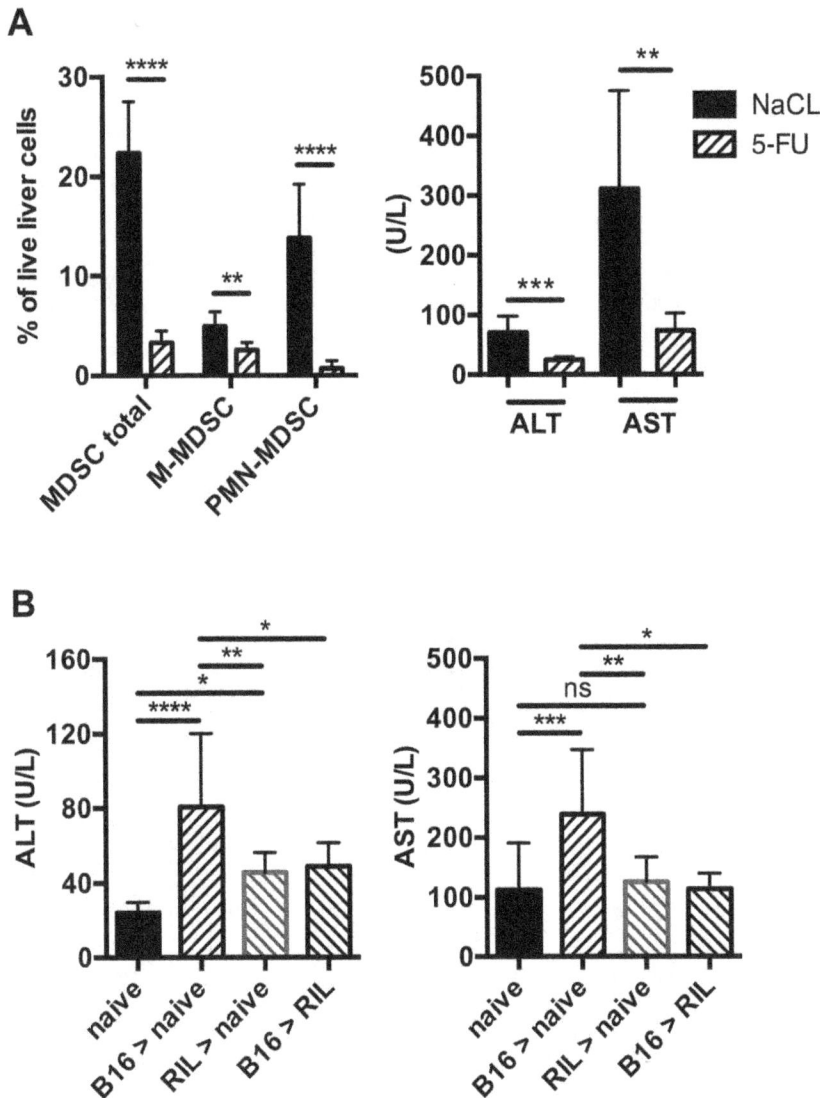

Figure 3. Liver injury depends on the presence of hepatic MDSC with damage-inducing potency. EL4 tumor-bearing mice were treated with 5-FU or saline. Liver immune cells were analyzed for MDSC and MDSC subsets and mouse serum was analyzed for ALT and AST levels (A) (N = 6 mice per treatment group, 2 independent experiments). B, 5×10^7 CD11b$^+$ cells isolated from livers of indicated untreated subcutaneous tumor-bearing mice were injected intravenously into naïve or RIL175 tumor-bearing recipient mice and ALT and AST serum levels were analyzed 16 h after transfer (N≥6 recipient mice, 2 independent experiments). Data are expressed as mean ±SEM. **$p<0.01$, ***$p<0.001$, ****$p<0.0001$ (A was analyzed by two-tailed Student's t test. B was analyzed by One-way ANOVA).

of MDSC from these livers by transferring hepatic CD11b$^+$ cells from RIL175 tumor-bearing mice into naïve mice (Figure 3B). The recipient mice showed an ALT increase, but no increase in AST over naïve mice levels. Compared to the transfer of CD11b$^+$ from B16 tumor-bearing mice, the ALT increase was lower when CD11b$^+$ cell from RIL175 tumor-bearing mice were transferred, indicating less liver damage inducing potency of MDSC from RIL175 tumor-bearing mice. Furthermore, transfer of hepatic CD11b$^+$ cells from B16 tumor-bearing mice into RIL175 tumor-bearing mice almost completely abolished the ALT and AST increase observed upon transfer into naïve mice (Figure 3B). Thus, MDSC partially loose their potency to cause liver damage when transferred into a host bearing a non-liver damage-inducing tumor. Together our data show, that the MDSC-inducing tumor determines the potency of MDSC to cause liver damage.

Cytokine analysis

In order to determine the mechanism leading to MDSC accumulation and consecutive hepatotoxicity in tumor bearing mice with liver damage (B16 and EL4) and without (RIL175 and CT26), we next screened tumor-conditioned media (Figure 4A) and serum (Figure 4B) of tumor-bearing animals for cytokines and chemokines that have been described to expand MDSC [19] including interleukin-6, CCL-2, GM-CSF, M-CSF, KC and VEGF. The highest interleukin-6 concentration was detected in B16 tumor conditioned media, which also contained M-CSF. M-CSF was also secreted by CT26. RIL175 tumor-conditioned media contained significant amounts of a wide range of cytokines. EL4 tumor cells secreted VEGF (Figure 4A). Additionally, EL4 also secreted interleukin-4, interleukin-10 and interleukin-17 (Figure S2).

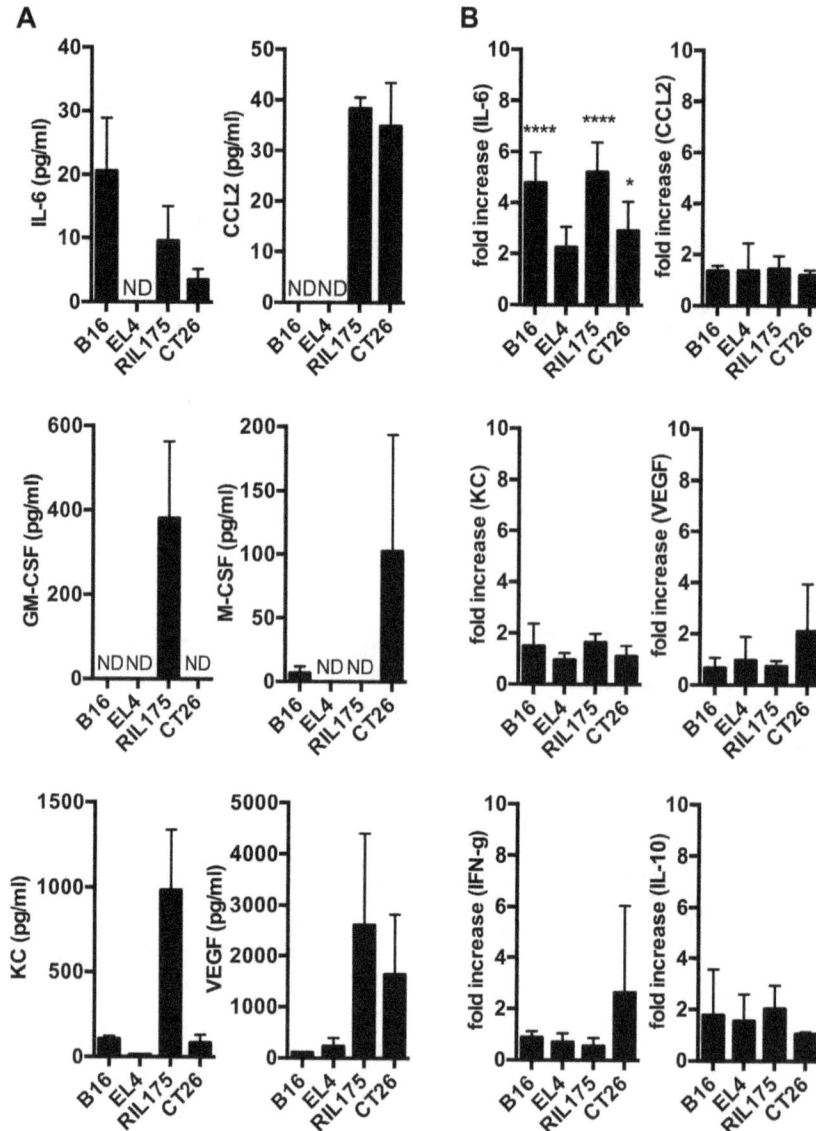

Figure 4. Cytokine secretion profiles of different tumor models. Duplicates of tumor-conditioned media (A, N = 4–6 media samples per tumor cell line culture) or serum samples from tumor-bearing mice (B, N = 4–6 serum samples per group) were analyzed for interleukin-6, CCL-2, GM-CSF, M-CSF, KC and VEGF (A) or interleukin-6, CCL-2, KC, VEGF, IFN-γ and interleukin 10 (B). Serum samples from tumor-bearing mice were normalized to serum from naïve wild-type mice. ND = not detected. Data are expressed as mean ±SEM. *$p<0.05$, **$p<0.01$, ***$p<0.001$ (by One-way ANOVA).

In serum of tumor-bearing mice on the other hand, interleukin-6 was elevated in all tumor models compared to tumor-free mice (Figure 4B). In contrast to our results from tumor-conditioned media, GM-CSF and M-CSF did not increase in tumor-bearing mice compared to naïve mice (data not shown). In addition to the cytokines that are known to induce MDSC accumulation, we also found an increase in serum levels of IFNγ and IL-10 in several tumor models. Serum TNF-α, interleukin-12p70, interleukin-4 and interleukin-17 remained unchanged compared to naïve mice (data not shown). In summary, each tumor cell line secreted distinct types as well as different amounts of cytokines that are known to induce MDSC accumulation. However, no increase in serum levels was found for most cytokines, which were increased in supernatants from tumor cells.

Frequency of hepatic MDSC correlate with amount of serum transaminases

We wondered whether increasing tumor burden in our subcutaneous model would also increase the number of hepatic MDSC and subsequently, the degree of liver damage. To this end, we analyzed hepatic MDSC numbers and liver enzymes in mice bearing tumors with two different sizes. We chose the two tumor models that induced (B16 and EL4) and two models that did not induce (RIL175 and CT26) liver damage. The number of MDSC per gram liver increased significantly in all mice bearing large tumors compared to mice bearing small tumors (Figure 5A). However, the ALT values only increased further in mice bearing liver damage-inducing B16 and EL4 tumors, indicating that a mere expansion of MDSC per se does not suffice to cause or aggravate liver damage (Figure 5B–C). Hence, these data confirmed our previous finding, that the MDSC potency to cause liver damage varied between tumor cell lines and was tumor specific. Furthermore, continued expansion of liver damage-inducing MDSC aggravated liver injury. Since total MDSC as well as the granulocytic and monocytic subset expanded similarly, we could not attribute the MDSC mediated liver damage to a specific subset.

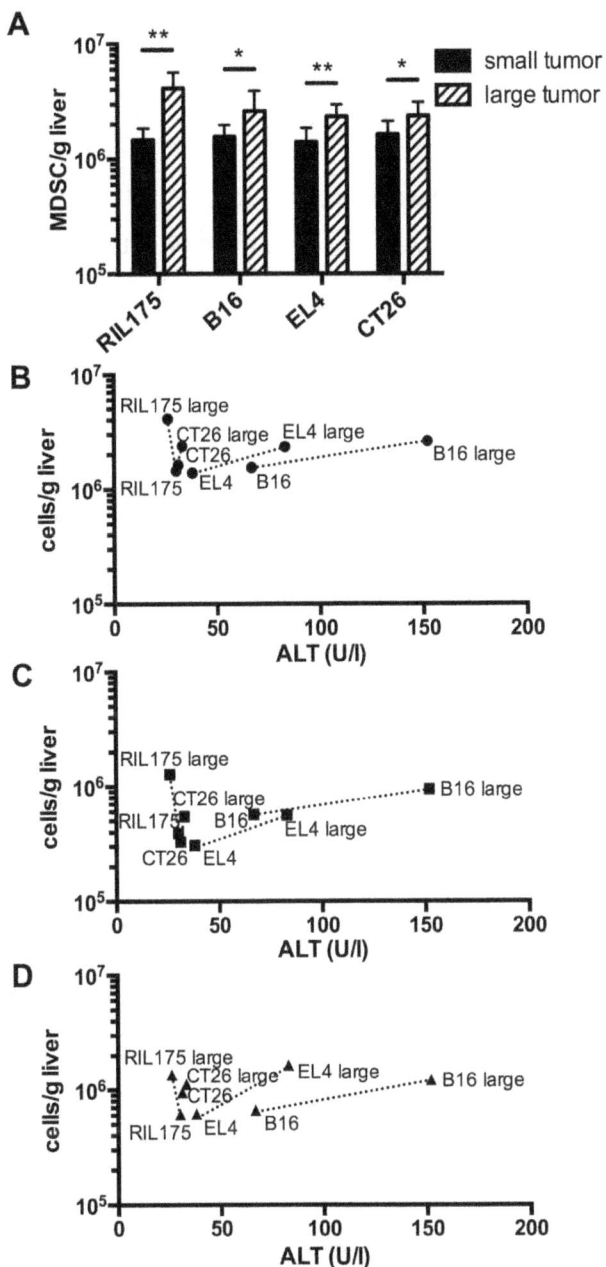

Figure 5. Increased expansion of liver damage-inducing MDSC exacerbates liver damage. Mice with different size subcutaneous tumors were analyzed for absolute numbers of hepatic MDSC (A and B), M-MDSC or (C), PMN-MDSC (D) and serum ALT levels (B–D). B–D, graphs correlate ALT levels with absolute numbers of MDSC and MDSC subsets. (N = 6–9 mice per tumor, 3 independent experiments). Data are expressed as mean ±SEM. *$p<0.05$, **$p<0.01$ (by two-tailed Student's t test).

Discussion

Accumulation of MDSC in blood and secondary lymphoid organs of tumor-bearing mice, in which MDSC co-express CD11b and Gr-1, and cancer patients has long been recognized. The finding that CD11b$^+$Gr-1$^+$ cells also accumulate in disease-free livers of subcutaneous tumor-bearing mice is relatively new [33] and has also been confirmed in mice with intra-abdominal tumors [34]. More recently our group has shown, that hepatic CD11b$^+$Gr-1$^+$ cells in subcutaneous tumor-bearing mice actually do suppress T cell proliferation; hence, they represent MDSC [25]. In our present study, we show, that MDSC not only accumulate, but rather constitute the predominant expanding cell population in livers of subcutaneous tumor-bearing mice and that these MDSC can cause tumor-dependent mild liver damage. Furthermore, we show a correlation between liver damage-inducing hepatic MDSC numbers and severity of liver injury.

Immune cells, more specifically myeloid cells, are known to be involved in exacerbating liver injury caused by drugs, toxins, alcohol, and obesity. The degree of liver damage in these settings is aggravated by myeloid cells that are attracted to the liver through cytokines, secreted in response to hepatocyte cell death [1–3,16,17]. However, in subcutaneous tumor-bearing mice, myeloid cells accumulated in livers without initial hepatocyte insult. Among these myeloid cells, primarily MDSC accumulated and their expansion was significantly greater than the expansion of all other immune cells. Furthermore, in our melanoma and lymphoma models, hepatic MDSC triggered liver injury and the degree of liver injury increased with further expansion of these MDSC.

We established a causal link between MDSC accumulation and liver damage by depleting or transferring MDSC. Administration of anti-Gr-1 antibody is a common and widely used approach to deplete MDSC in blood and spleens of tumor-bearing mice [1,2,35,36]. However, anti-Gr-1 antibody depletion does not successfully eliminate MDSC in the liver, because MDSC repopulate the liver immediately after treatment [24]. On the other hand, 5-FU treatment has been shown to selectively deplete MDSC in EL4 tumor-bearing mice [31] and was indeed successful to deplete hepatic MDSC in this study. It is noteworthy however, that treatment with 5-FU also decreases tumor sizes, which is attributed to CD8$^+$ T cell activation through loss of immunosuppressive MDSC [31]. Consequently, hepatic immune cell numbers and frequencies might change. Moreover, a hypothetical direct liver damaging effect of tumor-released molecules could have been reduced with shrinking tumors and potentially could have led to the misinterpretation, that MDSC depletion alone alleviated liver damage. Indeed, cytokines might also cause hepatocyte death and liver injury directly, without harnessing immune cells as effector cells. TNF-α can bind to its receptor on hepatocytes and initiate apoptosis through pathways including ROS production and caspase-8 activation [12,14,37]. In our study however, TNF-α was not secreted by any of the tumor models investigated. We cannot rule out, that other tumor-secreted cytokines had a direct effect on hepatocytes, but with the data presented here, it is rather unlikely that this could have been a major contributor of liver damage, because our transfer experiments in conjunction with the depletion experiments established a direct link between MDSC and liver damage.

Production of ROS is believed to be the main mechanism by which infiltrating myeloid cells cause liver damage in settings with initial hepatic insult [7,8,11,38]. Since MDSC also produce ROS [39], this mechanism could be responsible for the MDSC-mediated liver damage in our study, where an initial hepatic insult was absent. Among MDSC subsets, PMN-MDSC are the predominant subset and produce more ROS than their monocytic counterpart [40]. Accordingly, in mice with growing tumor burden and increasing ALT levels, we saw an expansion of this MDSC subset. Nevertheless, M-MDSC expanded as well, suggesting that this subtype might also contribute to MDSC-mediated liver damage. MDSC not only produce ROS, but are also known to produce a plethora of other immune suppressive factors, e.g. transforming growth factor-β (TGF-β) [18,41]. However, TGF-β has also been recognized to induce apoptosis in hepatocytes [42–44] and macrophage-derived TGF-β has been shown to cause hepatocellular injury [45], providing another potential mechanism by which MDSC might cause liver damage. In summary, MDSC are equipped with means that have the potential to cause hepatocyte injury.

Several cytokines and chemokines like IL-6, CCL2, GM-CSF, M-CSF, KC and VEGF have been implicated in MDSC expansion and migration [20,25,46–51]. In our study, every tumor cell line secreted at least one of the aforementioned factors and IL-6 elevation could also be detected in the serum of tumor-bearing mice compared to tumor free controls. The combination and secreted amount of these factors varied between all cell lines; therefore, each cell line possessed an individual cytokine secretion profile. Still, each individual cytokine profile was capable of inducing hepatic MDSC expansion. Nevertheless, it is important to distinguish between mechanisms of MDSC expansion and MDSC activation, as factors that induce MDSC accumulation do not necessarily confer functional activity [19]. Cytokines whose signaling pathways converge on the transcription factor STAT3 have been reported to be the key mechanism of MDSC expansion [52,53], while STAT1 and STAT6 signaling has been shown to be important for MDSC activity [54–56]. Moreover, it has been shown that the combination of GM-CSF with either G-CSF or interleukin-6 gave rise to a more immunosuppressive phenotype of MDSC than each cytokine alone, indicating that a secretion pattern of different cytokines rather than one specific cytokine is important for the function and activity of these cells [57]. Indeed, our transfer experiments showed, that the liver damage-inducing potency of MDSC was tumor-specific and our cytokine analysis revealed, that each tumor had an individual cytokine secretion profile, suggesting that these cytokine profiles determined the liver damage-inducing potency. In summary, all tumor-specific cytokine profiles in our study were capable of expanding hepatic MDSC, yet with differing potencies to cause liver damage. However, we could not establish a correlation between the accumulation of liver damage-inducing MDSC and a specific cytokine. Future experiments should dissect the role of candidate cytokines in inducing MDSC with liver damaging potency.

The hallmark of MDSC is their immune suppressive function. Therefore, it is not surprising that various studies provide evidence of MDSC-mediated liver protection [20–23]. In these studies, the immune cells causing liver injury were T cells and the degree of liver damage was much more severe than in our study, where MDSC only cause tumor-specific mild liver damage. Naturally, the T cell mediated liver injury could be prevented through MDSC-mediated T cell suppression. Therefore, we argue that the moderate liver damage caused by hepatic MDSC accumulation observed here is 'collateral damage', triggered by the same mechanisms that are actually in place to prevent severe forms of liver injury mediated by other immune cells.

Supporting Information

Figure S1   Adoptively transferred CD11b⁺ cells accumulate in livers of recipient mice. 5×10^7 MACS-sorted hepatic CD45.1⁺CD11b⁺ cells from tumor-bearing mice were injected intravenously into naïve C57BL/6 (CD45.2⁺) mice. Accumulation of transferred cells in the liver of recipient mice was confirmed via detection of CD45.1⁺CD11b⁺Gr-1⁺ cells in the recipient mouse liver via flow cytometry. (N = 2 recipient mice per time point). Data are expressed as mean ±SEM.

Figure S2   Cytokine secretion profiles of different tumor models. Duplicates of tumor-conditioned media (N = 4–6 media samples per tumor cell line culture) were analyzed for interleukin-4, interleukin-10 and interleukin-17 (A). ND = not detected. Data are expressed as mean ±SEM.

Acknowledgments

We would like to thank Dr. Leigh Samsel (National Heart, Lung, and Blood Institute) for technical assistance with the luminex cytokine assays.

Author Contributions

Conceived and designed the experiments: TE JME FK TG. Performed the experiments: TE TK. Analyzed the data: TE MJK. Contributed reagents/materials/analysis tools: MJK. Wrote the paper: TE TG.

References

1. Liu ZX, Han D, Gunawan B, Kaplowitz N (2006) Neutrophil depletion protects against murine acetaminophen hepatotoxicity. Hepatology 43: 1220–1230.
2. Bonder CS, Ajuebor MN, Zbytnuik LD, Kubes P, Swain MG (2004) Essential role for neutrophil recruitment to the liver in concanavalin A-induced hepatitis. Journal of immunology 172: 45–53.
3. Jaeschke H, Hasegawa T (2006) Role of neutrophils in acute inflammatory liver injury. Liver international: official journal of the International Association for the Study of the Liver 26: 912–919.
4. Wu D, Cederbaum AI (2009) Oxidative stress and alcoholic liver disease. Seminars in liver disease 29: 141–154.
5. Nelson SD (1990) Molecular mechanisms of the hepatotoxicity caused by acetaminophen. Seminars in liver disease 10: 267–278.
6. Eksteen B, Afford SC, Wigmore SJ, Holt AP, Adams DH (2007) Immune mediated liver injury. Seminars in liver disease 27: 351–366.
7. Schwabe RF, Brenner DA (2006) Mechanisms of Liver Injury. I. TNF-alpha-induced liver injury: role of IKK, JNK, and ROS pathways. American journal of physiology Gastrointestinal and liver physiology 290: G583–589.
8. Jaeschke H (2006) Mechanisms of Liver Injury. II. Mechanisms of neutrophil-induced liver cell injury during hepatic ischemia-reperfusion and other acute inflammatory conditions. American journal of physiology Gastrointestinal and liver physiology 290: G1083–1088.
9. Corazza N, Badmann A, Lauer C (2009) Immune cell-mediated liver injury. Seminars in immunopathology 31: 267–277.
10. Adams DH, Ju C, Ramaiah SK, Uetrecht J, Jaeschke H (2010) Mechanisms of immune-mediated liver injury. Toxicological sciences: an official journal of the Society of Toxicology 115: 307–321.
11. Jaeschke H, Smith CW (1997) Mechanisms of neutrophil-induced parenchymal cell injury. Journal of leukocyte biology 61: 647–653.
12. Faubion WA, Gores GJ (1999) Death receptors in liver biology and pathobiology. Hepatology 29: 1–4.
13. Adachi Y, Bradford BU, Gao W, Bojes HK, Thurman RG (1994) Inactivation of Kupffer cells prevents early alcohol-induced liver injury. Hepatology 20: 453–460.
14. Iimuro Y, Gallucci RM, Luster MI, Kono H, Thurman RG (1997) Antibodies to tumor necrosis factor alfa attenuate hepatic necrosis and inflammation caused by chronic exposure to ethanol in the rat. Hepatology 26: 1530–1537.
15. Kono H, Karmarkar D, Iwakura Y, Rock KL (2010) Identification of the cellular sensor that stimulates the inflammatory response to sterile cell death. Journal of immunology 184: 4470–4478.
16. Deng ZB, Liu Y, Liu C, Xiang X, Wang J, et al. (2009) Immature myeloid cells induced by a high-fat diet contribute to liver inflammation. Hepatology 50: 1412–1420.
17. Miura K, Yang L, van Rooijen N, Ohnishi H, Seki E (2012) Hepatic recruitment of macrophages promotes nonalcoholic steatohepatitis through CCR2. American journal of physiology Gastrointestinal and liver physiology 302: G1310–1321.

18. Gabrilovich DI, Ostrand-Rosenberg S, Bronte V (2012) Coordinated regulation of myeloid cells by tumours. Nature reviews Immunology 12: 253–268.

19. Gabrilovich DI, Nagaraj S (2009) Myeloid-derived suppressor cells as regulators of the immune system. Nature reviews Immunology 9: 162–174.

20. Cheng L, Wang J, Li X, Xing Q, Du P, et al. (2011) Interleukin-6 induces Gr-1+ CD11b+ myeloid cells to suppress CD8+ T cell-mediated liver injury in mice. PloS one 6: e17631.

21. Conrad E, Resch TK, Gogesch P, Kalinke U, Bechmann I, et al. (2014) Protection against RNA-induced liver damage by myeloid cells requires type I interferon and IL-1 receptor antagonist in mice. Hepatology 59: 1555–1563.

22. Sarra M, Cupi ML, Bernardini R, Ronchetti G, Monteleone I, et al. (2013) IL-25 prevents and cures fulminant hepatitis in mice through a myeloid-derived suppressor cell-dependent mechanism. Hepatology 58: 1436–1450.

23. Zuo D, Yu X, Guo C, Wang H, Qian J, et al. (2013) Scavenger receptor A restrains T-cell activation and protects against concanavalin A-induced hepatic injury. Hepatology 57: 228–238.

24. Ma C, Kapanadze T, Gamrekelashvili J, Manns MP, Korangy F, et al. (2012) Anti-Gr-1 antibody depletion fails to eliminate hepatic myeloid-derived suppressor cells in tumor-bearing mice. Journal of leukocyte biology 92: 1199–1206.

25. Kapanadze T, Gamrekelashvili J, Ma C, Chan C, Zhao F, et al. (2013) Regulation of accumulation and function of myeloid derived suppressor cells in different murine models of hepatocellular carcinoma. Journal of hepatology 59: 1007–1013.

26. Gorer PA, Kaliss N (1959) The effect of isoantibodies in vivo on three different transplantable neoplasms in mice. Cancer research 19: 824–830.

27. Fidler IJ (1975) Biological behavior of malignant melanoma cells correlated to their survival in vivo. Cancer research 35: 218–224.

28. Griswold DP, Corbett TH (1975) A colon tumor model for anticancer agent evaluation. Cancer 36: 2441–2444.

29. Drozdzik M, Qian C, Xie X, Peng D, Bilbao R, et al. (2000) Combined gene therapy with suicide gene and interleukin-12 is more efficient than therapy with one gene alone in a murine model of hepatocellular carcinoma. Journal of hepatology 32: 279–286.

30. Zender L, Xue W, Cordon-Cardo C, Hannon GJ, Lucito R, et al. (2005) Generation and analysis of genetically defined liver carcinomas derived from bipotential liver progenitors. Cold Spring Harbor symposia on quantitative biology 70: 251–261.

31. Vincent J, Mignot G, Chalmin F, Ladoire S, Bruchard M, et al. (2010) 5-Fluorouracil selectively kills tumor-associated myeloid-derived suppressor cells resulting in enhanced T cell-dependent antitumor immunity. Cancer research 70: 3052–3061.

32. Youn JI, Collazo M, Shalova IN, Biswas SK, Gabrilovich DI (2012) Characterization of the nature of granulocytic myeloid-derived suppressor cells in tumor-bearing mice. Journal of leukocyte biology 91: 167–181.

33. Ilkovitch D, Lopez DM (2009) The liver is a site for tumor-induced myeloid-derived suppressor cell accumulation and immunosuppression. Cancer research 69: 5514–5521.

34. Connolly MK, Mallen-St Clair J, Bedrosian AS, Malhotra A, Vera V, et al. (2010) Distinct populations of metastases-enabling myeloid cells expand in the liver of mice harboring invasive and preinvasive intra-abdominal tumor. Journal of leukocyte biology 87: 713–725.

35. Li H, Han Y, Guo Q, Zhang M, Cao X (2009) Cancer-expanded myeloid-derived suppressor cells induce anergy of NK cells through membrane-bound TGF-beta 1. Journal of immunology 182: 240–249.

36. Xia S, Sha H, Yang L, Ji Y, Ostrand-Rosenberg S, et al. (2011) Gr-1+ CD11b+ myeloid-derived suppressor cells suppress inflammation and promote insulin sensitivity in obesity. The Journal of biological chemistry 286: 23591–23599.

37. Kaplowitz N (2002) Biochemical and cellular mechanisms of toxic liver injury. Seminars in liver disease 22: 137–144.

38. Teufelhofer O, Parzefall W, Kainzbauer E, Ferk F, Freiler C, et al. (2005) Superoxide generation from Kupffer cells contributes to hepatocarcinogenesis: studies on NADPH oxidase knockout mice. Carcinogenesis 26: 319–329.

39. Corzo CA, Cotter MJ, Cheng P, Cheng F, Kusmartsev S, et al. (2009) Mechanism regulating reactive oxygen species in tumor-induced myeloid-derived suppressor cells. Journal of immunology 182: 5693–5701.

40. Youn JI, Nagaraj S, Collazo M, Gabrilovich DI (2008) Subsets of myeloid-derived suppressor cells in tumor-bearing mice. Journal of immunology 181: 5791–5802.

41. Terabe M, Matsui S, Park JM, Mamura M, Noben-Trauth N, et al. (2003) Transforming growth factor-beta production and myeloid cells are an effector mechanism through which CD1d-restricted T cells block cytotoxic T lymphocyte-mediated tumor immunosurveillance: abrogation prevents tumor recurrence. The Journal of experimental medicine 198: 1741–1752.

42. Black D, Lyman S, Qian T, Lemasters JJ, Rippe RA, et al. (2007) Transforming growth factor beta mediates hepatocyte apoptosis through Smad3 generation of reactive oxygen species. Biochimie 89: 1464–1473.

43. Shima Y, Nakao K, Nakashima T, Kawakami A, Nakata K, et al. (1999) Activation of caspase-8 in transforming growth factor-beta-induced apoptosis of human hepatoma cells. Hepatology 30: 1215–1222.

44. Schrum LW, Bird MA, Salcher O, Burchardt ER, Grisham JW, et al. (2001) Autocrine expression of activated transforming growth factor-beta(1) induces apoptosis in normal rat liver. American journal of physiology Gastrointestinal and liver physiology 280: G139–148.

45. Hori Y, Takeyama Y, Ueda T, Shinkai M, Takase K, et al. (2000) Macrophage-derived transforming growth factor-beta1 induces hepatocellular injury via apoptosis in rat severe acute pancreatitis. Surgery 127: 641–649.

46. Bunt SK, Yang L, Sinha P, Clements VK, Leips J, et al. (2007) Reduced inflammation in the tumor microenvironment delays the accumulation of myeloid-derived suppressor cells and limits tumor progression. Cancer research 67: 10019–10026.

47. Huang B, Lei Z, Zhao J, Gong W, Liu J, et al. (2007) CCL2/CCR2 pathway mediates recruitment of myeloid suppressor cells to cancers. Cancer letters 252: 86–92.

48. Filipazzi P, Valenti R, Huber V, Pilla L, Canese P, et al. (2007) Identification of a new subset of myeloid suppressor cells in peripheral blood of melanoma patients with modulation by a granulocyte-macrophage colony-stimulation factor-based antitumor vaccine. Journal of clinical oncology: official journal of the American Society of Clinical Oncology 25: 2546–2553.

49. Serafini P, Carbley R, Noonan KA, Tan G, Bronte V, et al. (2004) High-dose granulocyte-macrophage colony-stimulating factor-producing vaccines impair the immune response through the recruitment of myeloid suppressor cells. Cancer research 64: 6337–6343.

50. Menetrier-Caux C, Montmain G, Dieu MC, Bain C, Favrot MC, et al. (1998) Inhibition of the differentiation of dendritic cells from CD34(+) progenitors by tumor cells: role of interleukin-6 and macrophage colony-stimulating factor. Blood 92: 4778–4791.

51. Gabrilovich D, Ishida T, Oyama T, Ran S, Kravtsov V, et al. (1998) Vascular endothelial growth factor inhibits the development of dendritic cells and dramatically affects the differentiation of multiple hematopoietic lineages in vivo. Blood 92: 4150–4166.

52. Nefedova Y, Huang M, Kusmartsev S, Bhattacharya R, Cheng P, et al. (2004) Hyperactivation of STAT3 is involved in abnormal differentiation of dendritic cells in cancer. Journal of immunology 172: 464–474.

53. Nefedova Y, Nagaraj S, Rosenbauer A, Muro-Cacho C, Sebti SM, et al. (2005) Regulation of dendritic cell differentiation and antitumor immune response in cancer by pharmacologic-selective inhibition of the janus-activated kinase 2/signal transducers and activators of transcription 3 pathway. Cancer research 65: 9525–9535.

54. Kusmartsev S, Nagaraj S, Gabrilovich DI (2005) Tumor-associated CD8+ T cell tolerance induced by bone marrow-derived immature myeloid cells. Journal of immunology 175: 4583–4592.

55. Bronte V, Serafini P, De Santo C, Marigo I, Tosello V, et al. (2003) IL-4-induced arginase 1 suppresses alloreactive T cells in tumor-bearing mice. Journal of immunology 170: 270–278.

56. Rutschman R, Lang R, Hesse M, Ihle JN, Wynn TA, et al. (2001) Cutting edge: Stat6-dependent substrate depletion regulates nitric oxide production. Journal of immunology 166: 2173–2177.

57. Marigo I, Bosio E, Solito S, Mesa C, Fernandez A, et al. (2010) Tumor-induced tolerance and immune suppression depend on the C/EBPbeta transcription factor. Immunity 32: 790–802.

The Ratio of Circulating Regulatory T Cells (Tregs)/Th17 Cells Is Associated with Acute Allograft Rejection in Liver Transplantation

Ying Wang[1,2,9], Min Zhang[2,9], Zhen-Wen Liu[2], Wei-Guo Ren[3], Yan-Chao Shi[1,2], Yan-Ling Sun[2], Hong-Bo Wang[2], Lei Jin[4], Fu-Sheng Wang[4], Ming Shi[1,2]*

1 Research Center for Liver Transplantation, Beijing 302 Hospital, Peking University Health Science Center, Beijing, China, **2** Research Centre for Liver Transplantation, Beijing 302 Hospital, Beijing, China, **3** The Third Xiangya Hospital of Central South University, Changsha, China, **4** Research Center for Biological Therapy, Beijing 302 Hospital, Beijing, China

Abstract

$CD4^+CD25^+FoxP3^+$ regulatory T cells (Tregs) and Th17 cells are known to be involved in the alloreactive responses in organ transplantation, but little is known about the relationship between Tregs and Th17 cells in the context of liver alloresponse. Here, we investigated whether the circulating Tregs/Th17 ratio is associated with acute allograft rejection in liver transplantation. In present study, thirty-eight patients who received liver transplant were enrolled. The patients were divided into two groups: acute allograft rejection group (Gr-AR) (n = 16) and stable allograft liver function group (Gr-SF) (n = 22). The frequencies of circulating Tregs and circulating Th17 cells, as well as Tregs/Th17 ratio were determined using flow cytometry. The association between Tregs/Th17 ratio and acute allograft rejection was then analyzed. Our results showed that the frequency of circulating Tregs was significantly decreased, whereas the frequency of circulating Th17 cells was significantly increased in liver allograft recipients who developed acute rejection. Tregs/Th17 ratio had a negative correlation with liver damage indices and the score of rejection activity index (RAI) after liver transplantation. In addition, the percentages of $CTLA-4^+$, $HLA-DR^+$, $Ki67^+$, and $IL-10^+$ Tregs were higher in Gr-SF group than in Gr-AR group. Our results suggested that the ratio of circulating Tregs/Th17 cells is associated with acute allograft rejection, thus the ratio may serve as an alternative marker for the diagnosis of acute rejection.

Editor: Valquiria Bueno, UNIFESP Federal University of São Paulo, Brazil

Funding: This work was supported by Project of Research on The Application of Capital, Clinical Characteristics (Z111107058811069); The Key Project of Medical Science and Technology of PLA (BWS11J075) of China. The funders had no role in study design, data collection and analysis, decision to publish, or preparation of the manuscript.

Competing Interests: The authors have declared that no competing interests exist.

* Email: shiming302@sina.com

9 These authors contributed equally to this work.

Introduction

Despite the use of potent immunosuppressive agents, acute rejection (AR) remains a major cause of early allograft loss and an obstacle for long-term allograft survival. The hallmarks of acute rejection include infiltration of T lymphocytes, monocytes, and other inflammatory cells [1,2]. Laboratory and clinical investigations have indicated that $CD4^+CD25^+FoxP3^+$ regulatory T cells (Tregs) are one of the major cell types responsible for the immune responses to alloantigens. Tregs activation is involved in the prevention of rejection, the induction and maintenance of peripheral tolerance of the allograft [3], and the support of allograft survival [4–6]. Several other studies indicated that Tregs are an essential element of the immunoregulatory pathway which induces peripheral allograft tolerance [7,8], that the frequency of circulating Tregs is significantly decreased during acute rejection [9], and that the transfer of Tregs pre-stimulated *in vitro* can protect skin and cardiac allografts from acute and chronic rejection [10,11]. In clinical transplantation, T cells with the phenotypic characteristics of regulatory cells are detected in both the peripheral blood and within the graft itself [3,12,13]. In renal transplant recipients, grafts infiltrated with more Tregs display much longer survival [7,14]. Pediatric patients who acquired operational tolerance after liver transplantation showed increased levels of circulating Tregs compared with patients who received immunosuppression [12]. Allograft tolerance in liver transplant recipients may be partly attributable to a higher frequency of circulating Tregs [9]. Therefore, an increased level of circulating Tregs may be beneficial for allograft survival.

Th17 cells are a subset of T helper cells which is characterized by the production of IL-17. Th17 cells have been suggested to play a role in allograft rejection in the context of organ transplantation [15–18]. A study reported that cardiac allografts infiltrated with Th17 cells underwent accelerated vascular rejection in Tbet−/− mice model [19]. IL-17, a potent proinflammatory cytokine, has been demonstrated to participate in allograft rejection [20–23]. It promotes cardiac allograft rejection by inducing the maturation, antigen presentation, and co-stimulatory capabilities of dendritic cells in mice [20]. In a corneal transplant model, mice with deficient IL-17 experienced delayed graft rejection compared to wild-type mice [24]. Blocking IL-17 promoted the maturation of dendritic cells, inhibited the proliferation of alloreactive T cells *in vitro*, and prolonged the survival time of vascularized cardiac allografts *in vivo* [19,20]. IL-17 neutralization inhibits acute, but not chronic, vascular rejection in mice [17,25]. Clinical evidence showed that the level of IL-17 in the blood is positively correlated with acute allograft rejection in the renal [21,26] and the liver [22] transplant recipients. Graft infiltrated with Th17 cells is associated with a faster destruction of allograft in renal transplant patients [27,28].

The aforementioned evidence suggests that Tregs cells have a protective effect against graft rejection, whereas Th17 cells play an essential role in promoting graft rejection. The differentiation pathways of Tregs and Th17 cells are known to be antagonistic [29,30], and Tregs can be converted into Th17 cells under inflammatory conditions [31]. However, the relationship between Tregs and Th17 cells is yet to be fully understood in the context of transplant alloresponse. Further validation is necessary to determine whether the balance between circulating Tregs and Th17 cells may be used as a predictor for the outcome of transplantation. This study is aimed to investigate the dynamics of Tregs/Th17 ratio in liver transplant recipients with or without post-operative rejection, and to assess whether Tregs/Th17 ratio may serve as an alternative marker for the diagnosis of acute rejection.

Materials and Methods

Patients

The study protocol was approved by the institutional review board of Beijing 302 hospital. All participants provided written informed consent to participate in this study. Thirty-eight patients were enrolled in our hospital for this study. All participants received a first cadaveric liver transplantation with an identical or compatible blood-group graft. Based on clinical and biochemical indicators as well as pathologic diagnosis, the patients were divided into two groups: acute allograft rejection group (Gr-AR, n = 16) and stable allograft liver function group (Gr-SF, n = 22). The histopathologic diagnosis of acute allograft rejection was defined according to Banff criteria [32]. Acute rejection and stable allograft liver function were defined as previously described [33]. All patients received conventional immunosuppressive agents after liver transplantation, such as tacrolimus, steroids (prednisolone) and mycophenolate mofetil (MMF). The dose of tacrolimus was adjusted when acute rejection was diagnosed. Patients with HBV infection received prophylactic therapies with hepatitis B immune globulin (HBIG) plus nucleos(t)ide analogues (NAs). The blood samples were obtained from all patients prior to transplant and at the following timepoints after transplantation: 1, 2, 3, 4, 8, 12 weeks. In addition, the blood samples and allograft biopsy tissues were obtained at the time of presenting worsening liver function test results and/or symptoms suggestive of acute rejection after liver transplantation. The clinical characteristics of these subjects were listed in Table 1.

Flow cytometric analysis

The phycoerythrin (PE)-conjugated anti-IL-17A and fluorescein isothiocyanate (FITC)-conjugated anti-FoxP3 were purchased from eBioscience (San Diego, CA), and all other antibodies used in flow cytometry were from BD Biosciences (San Jose, CA). For immunostaining of intracellular IL-17A, two samples of freshly heparinized peripheral blood (200 μL each) were incubated for 6 hours with phorbol-12-myristate-13-acetate (PMA, 300 ng/mL,

Sigma-Aldrich, St. Louis, MO) and ionomycin (1 μL/mL, Sigma-Aldrich) in 800 μL of RPMI 1640 medium supplemented with 10% fetal calf serum. Monensin (0.4 μM, BD PharMingen) was added during the first hour of incubation. Then cytofix/cytoperm kit (BD PharMingen), anti-CD3, anti-CD8, anti-IL17, and anti-IFN-γ antibody (mAb) were used in one sample, whereas anti-CD4, anti-CD25, and anti- FoxP3 mAb were used in the other sample according to the manufacturers' protocols. For Tregs analysis, anti-CD4, anti-CD25, and anti-HLA-DR mAb were added to 200 μL freshly heparinized blood sample, and then the sample was permeabilized and fixed using fix/perm kit (eBioscience) according to the manufacturer's instructions. After permeabilization, cells were incubated with anti-FoxP3, anti-CTLA-4, and anti-Ki67 mAb. The stained cells were acquired on a FACSCalibur (BD Biosciences) and analyzed using FlowJo software (Tritar, USA).

Immunohistochemistry

Biopsy specimens from 16 patients with acute rejection were collected and used in immunochemical staining with antiFoxP3 (eBioscience) and anti-IL-17 (R&D Systems). Formalin-fixed, paraffin-embedded liver tissues were cut into 5 μm sections and placed on polylysine-coated slides. Antigen retrieval was achieved via pressure cooking for 10 min in citrate buffer (pH 6.0). Endogenous peroxidase activity was blocked with 0.3% H_2O_2. The sections were then incubated with anti-FoxP3 or anti-IL-17 antibodies for overnight at 4°C. 3-amino-9-ethyl-carbazole (red color) was used as a substrate, and hematoxylin was used in the subsequent counterstaining.

Statistical analysis

SPSS 16.0 software (SPSS, Chicago, IL, USA) was used for all statistical analyses. The data were presented as means ± SD. Mann-Whitney nonparametric U-test was applied to comparisons between 2 groups. Spearman's rank test was used to analyze the association between the severity of allograft tissue injury and Tregs frequency, Th17 cell frequency, or Tregs/Th17 ratio. Chi-square-test was used to assess the difference among clinical data. A value of $P<0.05$ was considered to be statistically significant.

Results

The patterns of Tregs and Th17 cell frequencies and Tregs/Th17 ratio in transplant recipients with acute rejection

We investigated Tregs and Th17 cell frequencies and Tregs/Th17 ratio in all participants after liver transplantation. We collected the values of Tregs, Th17 cells and Tregs/Th17 ratio in Gr-SF and Gr-AR in the period prior to a rejection or at the onset of acute rejection after liver transplantation, and compared the values in Gr-SF group to those in Gr-AR group. Flow cytometry was used to analyze Tregs and Th17 frequencies in peripheral blood in all patients after liver transplantation. The results showed that during the period preceding rejection, the frequencies of Tregs, Th17 cells, and the Tregs/Th17 ratio have not significant differences between two groups. At the period onset of acute rejection, however, the frequency of Tregs was significantly higher in Gr-SF than in Gr-AR ($P<0.01$), but the frequency of Th17 was significantly lower in Gr-SF than in Gr-AR ($P<0.01$), yielding a significantly higher Tregs/Th17 ratio in Gr-SF than in Gr-AR ($P<0.01$). In addition, the frequency of IL-17/IFN-γ producing CD4$^+$ T cells (IL-17$^+$IFN-γ$^+$) was higher in Gr-AR than that in Gr-SF ($P<0.05$) (Fig. 1A, B).

Table 1. Characteristics of participants.

Parameters	Gr-AR	Gr-SF
	n = 16	n = 22
Age (Mean±SD)	51±9	49±11
Gender (M/F)	11/5	15/7
Primary etiology		
HBV	10	15
HCV	2	3
HBV+HCV	1	2
Alcohol	3	2

To investigate the distribution patterns of Tregs and Th17 cells in acute rejection allografts, we next examined the infiltration of Tregs and Th17 cells in biopsy samples obtained from allografts in patients with acute rejection. Immunohistochemical staining was performed using anti-FoxP3$^+$ and anti-IL-17 antibodies on paraffin embedded sections. Our results demonstrated an extensive infiltration of Tregs and Th17 cells in the acute reject allograft liver tissue (Fig. 1C). These findings, along with previously published data [34], suggested that Tregs may be involved in the regulation of alloreactive response in liver allograft tissue, but might be deficient in some patients. One representative patient with acute allograft rejection was followed up for 12 months after liver transplantation. The dynamics of Tregs and Th17 cell frequencies during the follow-up period was depicted in Figure 1D. The Th17 cell frequency exhibited a trend opposite to that of Tregs or Tregs/Th17 ratio. At the onset of acute rejection, Tregs frequency and Tregs/Th17 ratio were sharply decreased, whereas Th17 cell frequency was dramatically increased. Interestingly, as the rejection subsided, the frequencies of Tregs and Th17 cells were both restored to levels close to those before rejection.

The correlation between Tregs/Th17 ratio and the biochemical indices of liver damage

Little is known about the association between the balance of Tregs/Th17 and the liver damage in liver transplant recipients. Therefore, we analyzed the correlation of Tregs/Th17 ratio and the biochemical indices of liver damage, such as alanine amino transferase (ALT), aspartate amino transferase (AST), alkaline phosphatase (ALP) and gamma-glutamyl transpeptidase (GGT), in the 16 patients during the acute allograft rejection episode. Negative correlations were observed between Tregs/Th17 ratio and the levels of ALT (r = -0.668, P = 0.005), AST (r = -0.541, P = 0.031), ALP (r = -0.518, P = 0.039), and GGT (r = -0.764, P = 0.001) (Fig. 2). These results indicated that Tregs/Th17 ratio may be used as an alternative indicator for the diagnosis of liver damage in liver transplant recipients.

Tregs frequency, Th17 cell frequency, and Tregs/Th17 ratio is correlated with rejection activity index (RAI)

To confirm whether Tregs and Th17 cells were associated with liver allograft rejection, we analyzed the correlation between the rejection activity index (RAI) and the frequencies of circulating Tregs and Th17 cells. We found that Tregs/Th17 ratio (r = -0.859, P<0.001) and the level of Tregs (r = -0.867, P<0.001) had a negative correlation with RAI, whereas the level of Th17

cells showed a positive correlation with RAI (r = 0.890, P<0.001) (**Fig. 3**). These results suggested that Tregs/Th17 ratio may serve as a biomarker for the diagnosis of acute rejection.

The phenotypes of CTLA-4$^+$, HLA-DR$^+$, Ki67$^+$ Tregs in liver transplant patients

To better understand the mechanism by which Tregs function in liver transplant recipients, some important molecules that regulate Tregs were analyzed. CTLA-4 is expressed by human Tregs and is also upregulated in T cells upon activation. We characterized the patterns of CTLA-4 expression in Tregs in all patients. The percentage of CTLA-4$^+$ Tregs was calculated as the percentage in total Tregs. The results showed that the frequency of CTLA-4$^+$ Tregs was higher in Gr-SF group (35.5±18.9%) than in Gr-AR group (23.7±12.8%) (P<0.05). We also evaluated the activated (HLA-DR$^+$) and proliferating (Ki67$^+$) Tregs in peripheral blood in all patients. We found that the percentages of HLA-DR$^+$ Tregs and Ki67$^+$ Tregs were higher in Gr-SF (26.8±17.2%, 30.6±15.8%, respectively) than in Gr-AR (17.2±11.6%, 20.3±10.9%, respectively) (P<0.05) (**Fig. 4**). Such data suggested that more Tregs were in active and proliferating state in Gr-SF than in Gr-AR, and may facilitate the suppression of alloreactive responses in liver transplant recipients.

Discussion

Many studies have demonstrated that CD4$^+$CD25$^+$FoxP3$^+$ Tregs and Th17 cells are involved in the tolerance or rejection response in organ transplantation [17,34–37]. The current study is designed to investigate the relationship between Tregs and Th17 cells in the context of alloresponse in liver transplant patients. The major finding of our study is that Tregs/Th17 ratio is associated with alloresponse after liver transplantation. Our data confirm that the frequency of circulating Tregs is significantly decreased, whereas the frequency of Th17 cells is significantly increased in liver allograft recipients with acute rejection, and that Tregs/Th17 ratio has a negative correlation with liver damage. To our knowledge, this is the first study to demonstrate an association between Tregs/Th17 imbalance and allografts rejection. These findings suggest that the ratio of circulating Tregs/Th17 may serve as an alternative marker for the diagnosis of acute rejection and for the evaluation of the immune status in liver transplant recipients.

Tregs are a unique subset of CD4$^+$ T helper cells in that they control the responses of effector T-cells to prevent autoimmune reactions. Several studies show that Tregs can prevent rejection and promote the long-term survival of skin grafts in a mouse model [6,38]. In clinical, Tregs have been reported to be

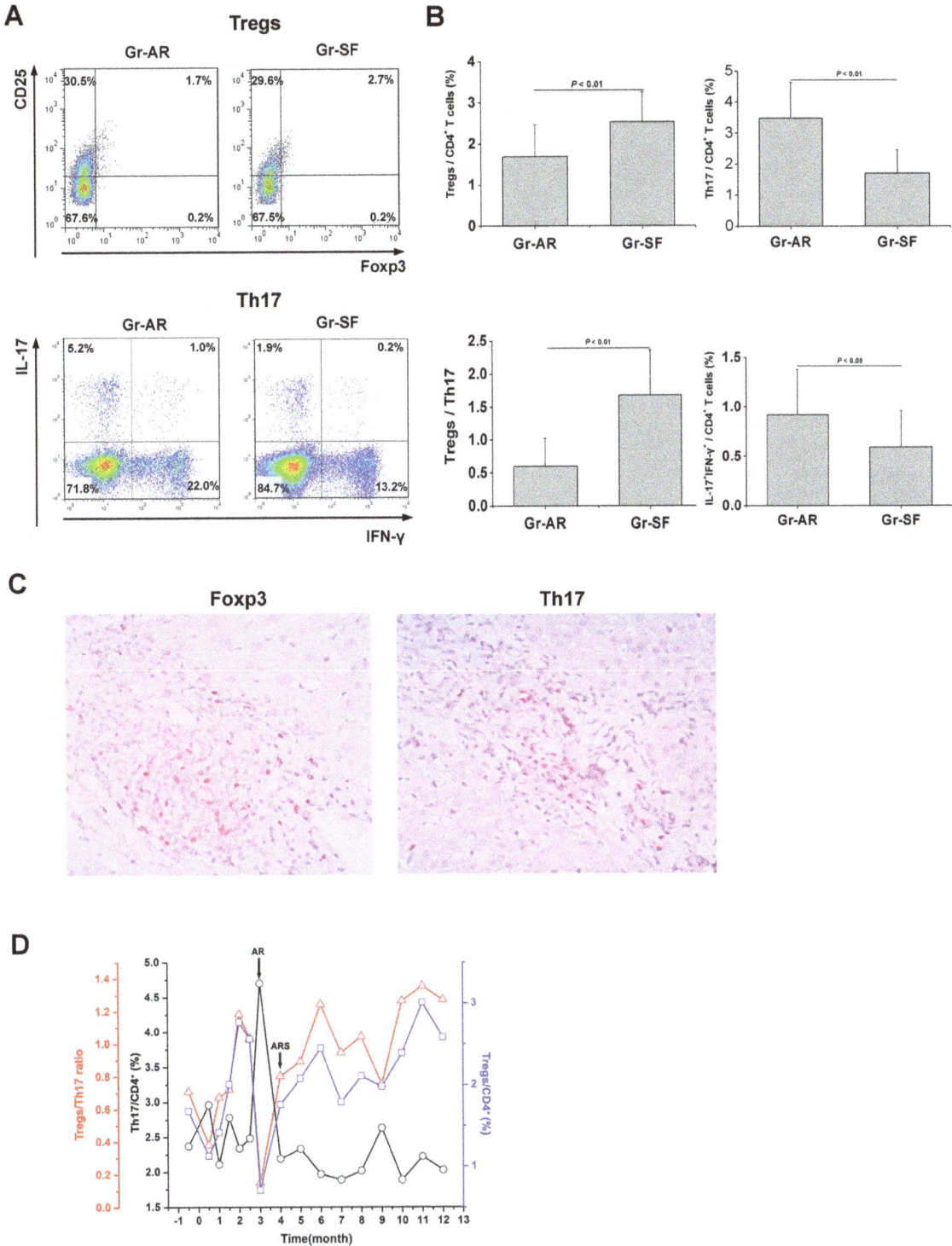

Figure 1. The distribution of Tregs and Th17 cells in the peripheral blood and in the grafts of patients with acute allograft rejection.
(A) Representative profiles of Tregs and Th17 cells in peripheral blood collected using fluorescence-activated cell sorter (FACS). (B) The frequency of Tregs and Tregs/Th17 ratio were significantly higher in Gr-SF than in Gr-AR. On the contrary, the frequency of Th17 cells was significantly lower in Gr-SF than in Gr-AR. In addition, the frequency of IL-17$^+$IFN-γ^+ cells was lower in Gr-SF than in Gr-AR. (C) To evaluate the distribution pattern of Tregs and Th17 cells in allografts with acute rejection, we examined the infiltration of Tregs and Th17 cells using immunohistochemical staining. Anti-FoxP3$^+$ and anti-IL-17 antibodies were used on paraffin embedded biopsy samples which were obtained from allograft with acute rejection. The results showed extensive infiltration of Tregs (red) and Th17 cells (red). Original magnification, ×400. (D) One representative patient with acute allograft rejection was followed-up for 12 months after liver transplantation. The dynamics of Tregs and Th17 cell frequencies were depicted during the follow-up period (the black line represents Th17 cells frequency; the blue line the Tregs frequency; and the red line Tregs/Th17 ratio). ARS: Acute rejection subsided.

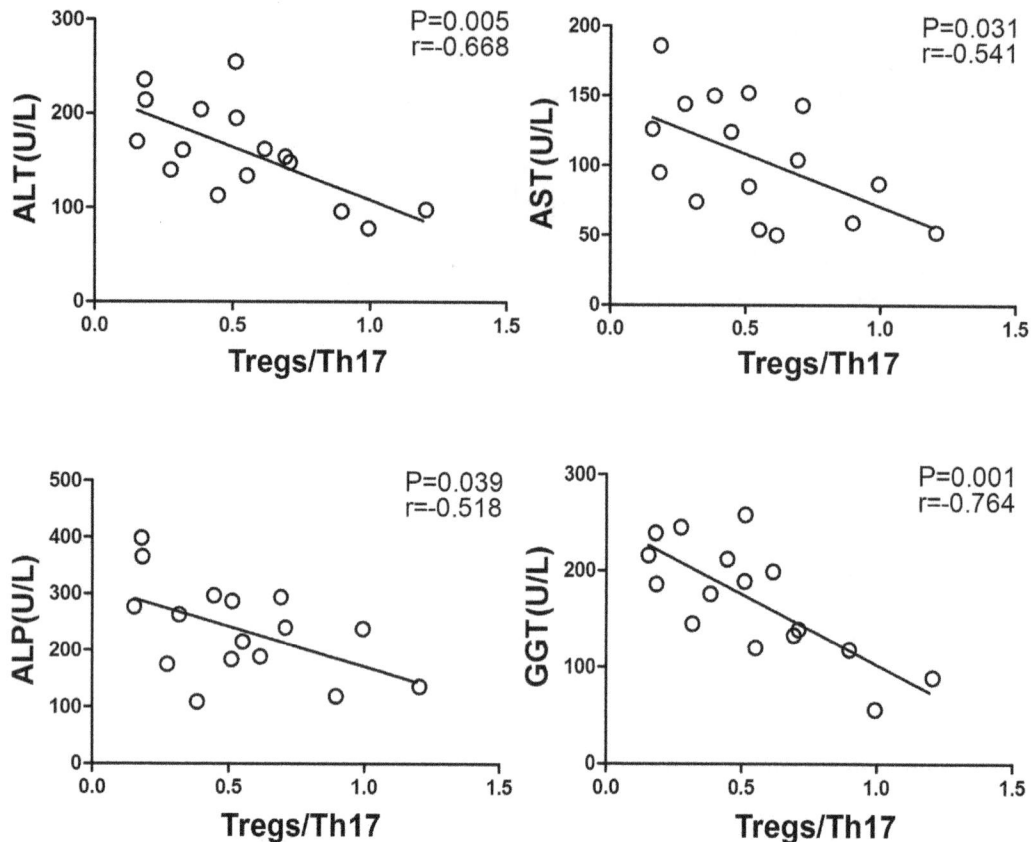

Figure 2. Tregs/Th17 ratio is correlated with the serum levels of ALT, AST, ALP and GGT. We analyzed the correlation between the ratio of circulating Tregs/Th17 and the biochemical indices for liver damage, ALT, AST, ALP and GGT, in the 16 patients with acute allograft rejection. Negative correlations were found between the ratio of circulating Tregs/Th17 and the levels of ALT, AST, ALP, and GGT (*P*<0.05).

associated with allograft tolerance in liver transplant recipients [9,12]. The Th17 subset is involved in mediating autoimmune responses and regulating allograft rejection both in rat renal transplant models and human renal transplantation [39,40]. In lung and heart transplantation, IL-17 has also been reported to be involved in allograft acute rejection [41,42]. A recent study reported that the levels of circulating CD4+IL−17+ T cells are substantially higher in rejection group than in non-rejection group in liver transplant recipients, and the frequency of CD4+IL−17+ cells in peripheral blood is positively correlated with the rejection activity index [43]. Recent researches reported that a new subpopulation of CD161+ Treg is able to produce IL-17 and has both inflammatory and suppressive potentials [44,45]. The functional and phenotypic characteristics of this subset in alloreactive response are worth further study.

The frequency of Tregs in Gr-AR is significantly lower; on the contrary, the frequency of Th17 cells in Gr-AR is significantly higher than that in Gr-SF. In addition, the frequency of circulating Tregs has a negative correlation with RAI, whereas the frequency of circulating Th17 cells has a positive correlation with RAI. These data indicate that the decreased levels of Tregs and increased levels of Th17 cells may be involved in the acute rejection episodes in liver transplantation. Histopathological results demonstrate that the allograft tissue with acute rejection is extensively infiltrated with Tregs and Th17 cells. These findings are consistent with that from Stenard's study, which revealed increased intragraft Tregs during acute rejection [34]. Such data suggest that Tregs are mobilized to the site of immune activation and may participate in

the regulation of alloreactive responses. However, the observation that acute allograft rejection can occur, even in the presence of Tregs, indicates that at least under some circumstances the mobilization of Tregs to the site is insufficient to effectively down-modulate the alloreactivity.

Next, we suggest the mechanism by which Tregs are involved in the rejection episodes. CTLA-4 is an inhibitory receptor expressed by both activated T cells and Tregs, and may be crucial for their activity. HLA-DR is a marker for T cell activation. Ki67 is a marker of T cell proliferation. In our results, the percentages of CTLA-4 and HLA-DR+ Tregs are significantly higher in Gr-SF than in Gr-AR. In addition, the level of Ki67+ Tregs is significantly higher in Gr-SF than in Gr-AR. In general, the increase in the frequencies of CTLA-4+ Tregs, HLA-DR+ Tregs, and Ki67+ Tregs following the alloreactive immunosuppression may facilitate Tregs to exert their suppressive function, and may reflect the restoration of their functions because these changes occurred in parallel with stable liver functions. However, we have not assessed the suppressive function of Tregs in stable versus acutely rejecting subjects, so cannot draw any conclusions about the functional relevance of these cells in preventing/ameliorating rejection and impacting transplant outcomes.

In conclusion, maintaining an appropriate balance between Tregs and Th17 cells is indispensable for the maintenance of stable liver function in transplant recipients. Tilting Tregs-Th17 equilibrium toward Tregs dominance may promote transplant tolerance. However, we carried out a small-scale observation study that is underpowered to draw firm conclusions about cause and

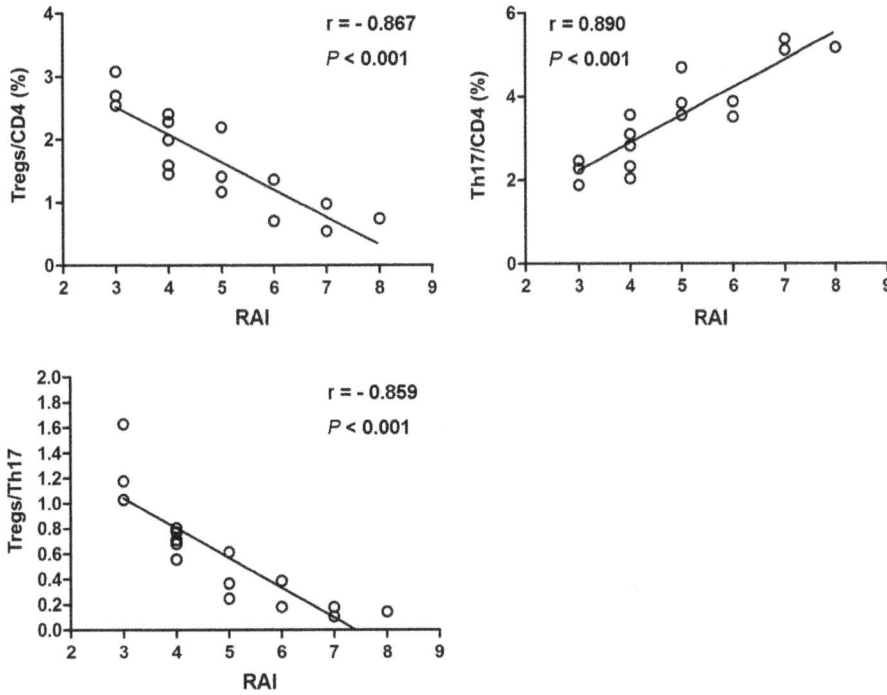

Figure 3. The frequency of Tregs, the frequency of Th17 cells, and Tregs/Th17 ratio are correlated with RAI. To confirm whether Tregs, Th17 cells and Tregs/Th17 were associated with the liver allograft rejection, we analyzed the correlation between RAI and the frequency of circulating Tregs, the frequency of circulating Th17 cells, and Tregs/Th17 ratio. We found that the Tregs level and Tregs/Th17 ratio had a negative correlation with RAI, whereas the Th17 cell level showed a positive correlation with RAI ($P<0.01$).

effect between Treg/Th17 ratio and acute rejection. These findings should be the subject of further inquiry through a carefully conducted, larger, prospective study to determine whether Tregs/Th17 ratio can be used as a diagnosis marker and whether it may serve as a potential therapeutic target to manage the acute rejection of liver allografts.

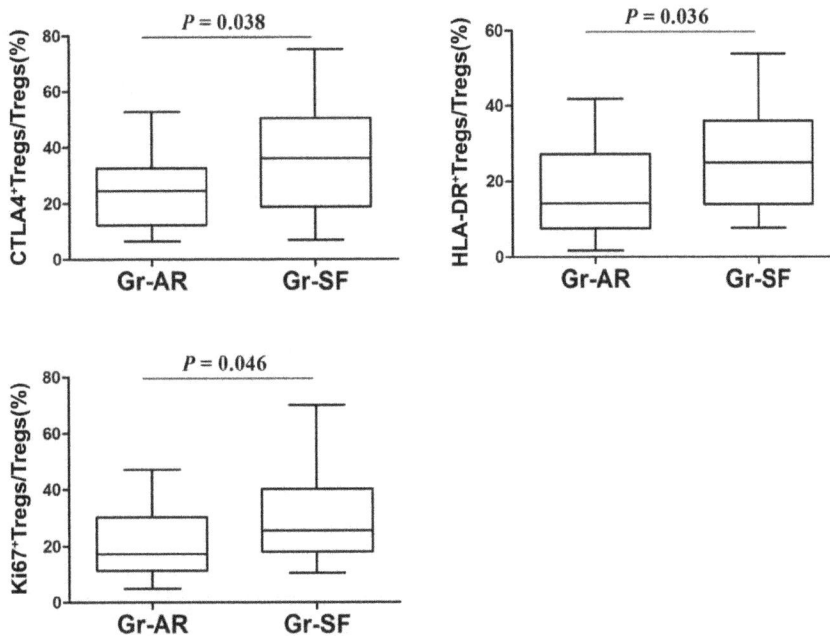

Figure 4. The phenotypes of CTLA-4$^+$, HLA-DR$^+$, Ki67$^+$ Tregs in liver transplant patients. The activated and proliferative molecules on Tregs were detected in liver transplant patients. The results showed that the frequencies of CTLA-4$^+$, HLA-DR$^+$, and Ki67$^+$ Tregs were higher in Gr-SF than in Gr-AR (all $P<0.05$). The above data suggested more Tregs were active and proliferating in Gr-SF than in Gr-AR in liver transplant recipients.

Author Contributions

Conceived and designed the experiments: YW MZ ZWL FSW MS. Performed the experiments: YW WGR YCS YLS HBW LJ MS. Analyzed the data: YW MZ MS. Contributed reagents/materials/analysis tools: MZ ZWL FSW MS. Contributed to the writing of the manuscript: MS.

References

1. O'Leary JG, Lepe R, Davis GL (2008) Indications for liver transplantation. Gastroenterology 134: 1764–1776.

2. Blöcher S, Wilker S, Sucke J, Pfeil U, Dietrich H, et al. (2007) Acute rejection of experimental lung allografts: characterization of intravascular mononuclear leukocytes. Clin Immunol 124: 98–108.

3. Wood KJ (2011) Regulatory T Cells in Transplantation. Transpl Proc 43: 2135–2136.

4. Keller MR, Burlingham WJ (2011) Loss of tolerance to self after transplant. Semin Immunopathol 33: 105–110.

5. Long E, Wood KJ (2009) Regulatory T cells in transplantation: transferring mouse studies to the clinic. Transplantation 88: 1050–1056.

6. Issa F, Hester J, Goto R, Nadig SN, Goodacre TE, et al. (2010) Ex Vivo-Expanded Human Regulatory T Cells Prevent the Rejection of Skin Allografts in a Humanized Mouse Model. Transplantation 90: 1321–1327.

7. Sakaguchi S, Yamaguchi T, Nomura T, Ono M (2008) Regulatory T cells and immune tolerance. Cell 133: 775–787.

8. Gorantla VS, Schneeberger S, Brandacher G, Sucher R, Zhang D, et al. (2010) T Regulatory Cells and Transplantation Tolerance. Transplant Rev 24: 147–159.

9. He Q, Fan H, Li JQ, Qi HZ (2011) Decreased Circulating CD4+CD25 highFoxp3+ T Cells During Acute Rejection in Liver Transplant Patients. Transpl Proc 43: 1696–1700.

10. Joffre O, Santolaria T, Calise D, Saati TA, Hudrisier D, et al. (2008) Prevention of acute and chronic allograft rejection with CD4+CD25+Foxp3+ regulatory T lymphocytes. Nat Med 14: 88–92.

11. Zhang X, Li M, Lian D, Zheng X, Zhang ZX, et al. (2008) Generation of therapeutic dendritic cells and regulatory T cells for preventing allogeneic cardiac graft rejection. Clin Immunol 127: 313–321.

12. Li Y, Koshiba T, Yoshizawa A, Yonekawa Y, Masuda K, et al. (2004) Analyses of peripheral blood mononuclear cells in operational tolerance after pediatric living donor liver transplantation. Am J Transplant 4: 2118–2125.

13. Li Y, Zhao X, Cheng D, Haga H, Tsuruyama T, et al. (2008) The presence of Foxp3 expressing T cells within grafts of tolerant human liver transplant recipients. Transplantation 86: 1837–1843.

14. Zuber J, Brodin-Sartorius A, Lapidus N, Patey N, Tosolini M, et al. (2009) FOXP3-enriched infiltrates associated with better outcome in renal allografts with inflamed fibrosis. Nephrol Dial Transplant 24: 3847–3854.

15. Heidt S, Segundo DS, Chadha R, Wood KJ (2010) The impact of TH17 cells on transplant rejection and the induction of tolerance. Curr Opin Organ Transplant 15: 456–461.

16. Hammerich L, Heymann F, Tacke F (2011) Role of IL-17 and Th17 cells in liver diseases. Clin Dev Immunol 2011: 1–12.

17. Burrell BE, Bishop DK (2010) Th17 cells and transplant acceptance. Transplantation 90: 945–948.

18. Kim HY, Cho ML, Jhun JY, Byun JK, Kim EK, et al. (2013) The imbalance of T helper 17/regulatory T cells and memory B cells during the early post-transplantation period in peripheral blood of living donor liver transplantation recipients under calcineurin inhibitor-based immunosuppression. Immunology 138: 124–133.

19. Yuan X, Paez-Cortez J, Schmitt-Knosalla I, D'Addio F, Mfarrej B, et al. (2008) A novel role of CD4 Th17 cells in mediating cardiac allograft rejection and vasculopathy. J Exp Med 205: 3133–3144.

20. Antonysamy MA, Fanslow WC, Fu F, Li W, Qian S, et al. (1999) Evidence for a role of IL-17 in organ allograft rejection: IL-17 promotes the functional differentiation of dendritic cell progenitors. J Immunol 162: 577–584.

21. Loong CC, Hsieh HG, Lui WY, Chen A, Lin CY (2002) Evidence for the early involvement of interleukin 17 in human and experimental renal allograft rejection. J Pathol 197: 322–332.

22. Fabrega E, Lopez-Hoyos M, San Segundo D, Casafont F, Pons-Romero F (2009) Changes in the serum levels of interleukin-17/interleukin-23 during acute rejection in liver transplantation. Liver Transpl 15: 629–633.

23. Vanaudenaerde BM, Dupont LJ, Wuyts WA, Verbeken EK, Meyts I, et al. (2006) The role of interleukin-17 during acute rejection after lung transplantation,. Eur Respir J 27: 779–787.

24. Chen H, Wang W, Xie H, Xu X, Wu J, et al. (2009) A pathogenic role of IL-17 at the early stage of corneal allograft rejection. Transpl Immunol 21: 155–161.

25. Tang JL, Subbotin VM, Antonysamy MA, Troutt AB, Rao AS, et al. (2001) Interleukin-17 antagonism inhibits acute but not chronic vascular rejection. Transplantation 72: 348–350.

26. Crispim JC, Grespan R, Martelli-Palomino G, Rassi DM, Costa RS, et al. (2009) Interleukin-17 and kidney allograft outcome. Transplant Proc 41: 1562–1564.

27. Abadja F, Atemkeng S, Alamartine E, Berthoux F, Mariat C (2011) Impact of Mycophenolic Acid and Tacrolimus on Th17-Related Immune Response. Transplantation 92: 396–403.

28. Deteix C, Attuil-Audenis V, Duthey A, Patey N, McGregor B, et al. (2010) Intragraft Th17 infiltrate promotes lymphoid neogenesis and hastens clinical chronic rejection. J Immunol 184: 5344–5351.

29. Korn T, Bettelli E, Oukka M, Kuchroo VK (2009) IL-17 and Th17 Cells. Annu Rev Immunol 27: 485–517.

30. Bettelli E, Carrier Y, Gao W, Korn T, Strom TB, et al. (2006) Reciprocal developmental pathways for the generation of pathogenic effector TH17 and regulatory T cells. Nature 441: 235–238.

31. Deknuydt F, Bioley G, Valmori D, Ayyoub M (2009) IL-1beta and IL-2 convert human Treg into T(H)17 cells. Clin Immunol 131: 298–307.

32. (1997) Banff schema for grading liver allograft rejection: an international consensus document. Hepatology 25: 658–663.

33. Yu X, Liu ZW, Wang Y, Wang HB, Zhang M, et al. (2013) Characteristics of Vδ1+ and Vδ2+ γδ T cell subsets in acute liver allograft rejection. Transpl Immunol 29: 118–122.

34. Stenard F, Nguyen C, Cox K, Kambham N, Umetsu DT, et al. (2009) Decreases in circulating CD4+CD25hiFOXP3+ cells and increases in intragraft FOXP3+ cells accompany allograft rejection in pediatric liver allograft recipients. Pediatr Transplant 13: 70–80.

35. Koshiba T, Li Y, Takemura M, Wu Y, Sakaguchi S, et al. (2007) Clinical, immunological, and pathological aspects of operational tolerance after pediatric living-donor liver transplantation. Transpl Immunol 17: 94–97.

36. Li J, Lai X, Liao W, He Y, Liu Y, et al. (2011) The dynamic changes of Th17/Treg cytokines in rat liver transplant rejection and tolerance. Int Immunopharmacol 11: 962–967.

37. Hanidziar D, Koulmanda M (2010) Inflammation and the balance of Treg and Th17 cells in transplant rejection and tolerance. Curr Opin Organ Transplant 15: 411–415.

38. Feng G, Wood KJ, Bushell A (2008) Interferon-gamma conditioning ex vivo generates CD25+CD62L+Foxp3+ regulatory T cells that prevent allograft rejection: Potential avenues for cellular therapy. Transplantation 86: 578–589.

39. Afzali B, Lombardi G, Lechler RI, Lord GM (2007) The role of T helper 17 (Th17) and regulatory T cells (Treg) in human organ transplantation and autoimmune disease. Clin Exp Immunol 148: 32–46.

40. Loong CC, Hsieh HG, Lui WY, Chen A, Lin CY (2002) Evidence for the early involvement of interleukin 17 in human and experimental renal allograft rejection. J Pathol 197: 322–332.

41. Yoshida S, Haque A, Mizobuchi T, Iwata T, Chiyo M, et al. (2006) Anti-type V collagen lymphocytes that express IL-17 and IL-23 induce rejection pathology in fresh and well-healed lung transplants. Am J Transplant 6: 724–735.

42. Li J, Simeoni E, Fleury S, Dudler J, Fiorini E, et al. (2006) Gene transfer of soluble interleukin-17 receptor prolongs cardiac allograft survival in a rat model. Eur J Cardiothorac Surg 29: 779–783.

43. Fan H, Li LX, Han DD, Kou JT, Li P, et al. (2012) Increase of peripheral Th17 lymphocytes during acute cellular rejection in liver transplant recipients. Hepatobiliary Pancreat Dis Int 11: 606–611.

44. Afzali B, Mitchell PJ, Edozie FC, Povoleri GAM, Dowson SE, et al. (2013) CD161 expression characterizes a subpopulation of human regulatory T cells that produces IL-17 in a STAT3-dependent manner. Eur J Immunol 43: 2043–2054.

45. Pesenacker AM, Bending David, Ursu S, Wu Qi, Nistala K, et al. (2013) CD161 defines the subset of FoxP31 T cells capable of producing proinflammatory cytokines. Blood 121: 2647–2658.

Pharmacological Inhibition of the Chemokine CXCL16 Diminishes Liver Macrophage Infiltration and Steatohepatitis in Chronic Hepatic Injury

Alexander Wehr[1], Christer Baeck[1], Florian Ulmer[2], Nikolaus Gassler[3], Kanishka Hittatiya[4], Tom Luedde[1], Ulf Peter Neumann[2], Christian Trautwein[1], Frank Tacke[1]*

1 Department of Medicine III, RWTH University-Hospital, Aachen, Germany, 2 Department of General, Visceral and Transplant Surgery, RWTH University-Hospital, Aachen, Germany, 3 Institute of Pathology, RWTH University-Hospital, Aachen, Germany, 4 Department of Pathology, Rheinische Friedrich-Wilhelms-University, Bonn, Germany

Abstract

Non-alcoholic fatty liver disease (NAFLD) is a major cause of morbidity and mortality in developed countries, resulting in steatohepatitis (NASH), fibrosis and eventually cirrhosis. Modulating inflammatory mediators such as chemokines may represent a novel therapeutic strategy for NAFLD. We recently demonstrated that the chemokine receptor CXCR6 promotes hepatic NKT cell accumulation, thereby controlling inflammation in experimental NAFLD. In this study, we first investigated human biopsies (n = 20), confirming that accumulation of inflammatory cells such as macrophages is a hallmark of progressive NAFLD. Moreover, CXCR6 gene expression correlated with the inflammatory activity (ALT levels) in human NAFLD. We then tested the hypothesis that pharmacological inhibition of CXCL16 might hold therapeutic potential in NAFLD, using mouse models of acute carbon tetrachloride (CCl$_4$)- and chronic methionine-choline-deficient (MCD) diet-induced hepatic injury. Neutralizing CXCL16 by i.p. injection of anti-CXCL16 antibody inhibited the early intrahepatic NKT cell accumulation upon acute toxic injury *in vivo*. Weekly therapeutic anti-CXCL16 administrations during the last 3 weeks of 6 weeks MCD diet significantly decreased the infiltration of inflammatory macrophages into the liver and intrahepatic levels of inflammatory cytokines like TNF or MCP-1. Importantly, anti-CXCL16 treatment significantly reduced fatty liver degeneration upon MCD diet, as assessed by hepatic triglyceride levels, histological steatosis scoring and quantification of lipid droplets. Moreover, injured hepatocytes up-regulated CXCL16 expression, indicating that scavenging functions of CXCL16 might be additionally involved in the pathogenesis of NAFLD. Targeting CXCL16 might therefore represent a promising novel therapeutic approach for liver inflammation and steatohepatitis.

Editor: Anna Alisi, Bambino Gesu' Children Hospital, Italy

Funding: This work was supported by the German Research Foundation (DFG Ta434/2-1 to F.T., DFG SFB/TRR 57) and by the Interdisciplinary Center for Clinical Research (IZKF) Aachen. The funders had no role in study design, data collection and analysis, decision to publish, or preparation of the manuscript.

Competing Interests: The authors have declared that no competing interests exist.

* Email: frank.tacke@gmx.net

Introduction

Non-alcoholic fatty liver disease (NAFLD) is defined as the accumulation of liver fat exceeding 5% of hepatocytes in the absence of significant alcohol intake (20 g/d for men, 10 g/d for women), viral infection, or any other specific etiology of liver disease. NAFLD has an increasing prevalence worldwide and is now the leading cause of liver diseases in Western countries [1]. The prevalence rate of NAFLD is reported to be 14–44% in the general population in Europe or the US and even 42.6–69.5% in people with type 2 diabetes [2,3]. Patients with NAFLD, particularly those with non-alcoholic steatohepatitis (NASH), have a higher prevalence and incidence of clinically manifested cardiovascular disease as well and a 10-fold increased liver-related mortality owing to liver cirrhosis and hepatocellular carcinoma [3]. In a Danish study, after adjustment for sex, diabetes and cirrhosis at baseline, NAFLD-associated age-adjusted standardized mortality ratios (SMR) were 2.3 (95% CI 2.1–2.6) for all causes, 19.7 (95% CI 15.3–25.0) for hepatobiliary disease, and 2.1 (95%

CI 1.8–2.5) for cardiovascular disease (CVD) [4]. Due to the lack of effective therapeutic measures and due to the epidemic of obesity and metabolic syndrome (affecting nearly 33% of the population in the US), NAFLD is projected to become the leading indication for liver transplantation in the next several years [5].

The progression of NAFLD, from hepatic lipid overload, steatosis, to non-alcoholic steatohepatitis (NASH) and to its complications liver fibrosis, cirrhosis or hepatocellular carcinoma, is causally linked to a massive inflammatory response in the liver [6]. However, despite the fact that the extent of hepatic inflammation is the predominant factor determining disease progression in NAFLD [7], no specific anti-inflammatory interventional approaches have entered clinical practice yet. There is a growing body of evidence that chemokines fulfill essential functions in regulating liver inflammation and NAFLD progression, thereby emerging as potential attractive targets for future therapeutic approaches [8].

Work from our laboratory has recently identified a yet unrecognized pathway promoting inflammation in experimental steatohepatitis in mice. Using mice either deficient for the chemokine receptor CXCR6 or transgenic for a fluorescent protein in one of the CXCR6 alleles, the accumulation of natural killer T (NKT) cells was identified as a rapid response to hepatocyte injury [9]. $Cxcr6^{-/-}$ mice lacking type-I NKT cells were protected against acute- and chronic liver failure in two independent models of liver fibrosis, showed significantly attenuated hepatic inflammation and reduced levels of pro-inflammatory cytokines like tumor necrosis factor (TNF), monocyte chemoattractant protein-1 (MCP-1) and interferon-γ (IFNγ). The adoptive transfer of wildtype (WT) NKT cells into $Cxcr6$-deficient mice in a model of steatohepatitis restored inflammation and liver fibrosis [9].

Our experimental data indicated that hepatic NKT cells specifically utilize its receptor CXCR6 for the rapid accumulation in injured livers, where they produce and release cytokines like interleukin 4 (IL-4) and IFNγ that act on macrophages (Kupffer cells) and possibly other hepatic cell compartments to initiate and perpetuate inflammation [9,10]. We thus reasoned that inhibiting the cognate ligand for CXCR6, CXCL16, might hold therapeutic potential in steatohepatitis. Whereas in human inflamed livers CXCR6 is expressed by CD4 as well as CD8 T cells, NK cells and NKT cells the chemokine CXCL16 exists in a soluble and transmembrane form and is expressed by liver sinusoids, possibly allowing NKT cells to patrol hepatic vessels [11–13]. CXCL16 is also expressed by hepatic macrophages, likely favoring interactions between NKT and Kupffer cells [9]. Importantly, CXCL16 expression is up-regulated in acute or chronic liver injury in mice, but also in chronic liver diseases in humans [9]. In this study, we investigated the pharmacological inhibition of CXCL16 using a monoclonal antibody as a novel therapeutic approach in experimental steatohepatitis in mice.

Materials and Methods

Human liver samples

Liver biopsies of patients (n = 20) with NAFLD were collected and processed as described previously [14]. All liver biopsies were scored by an experienced pathologist, who was blinded to any experimental data, according to the NAS score [15]. Tissue from healthy patients (n = 3) with resections of hepatic hemangioma and normal ALT serum activity served as controls.

Mice

C57bl/6 wild-type mice (B6-mice) were purchased from Janvier (Le Genest-Saint-Isle Saint-Berthevin Cedex, France) and were housed in a specific pathogen-free environment. All experiments were performed with male animals at 6 weeks of age under ethical conditions approved by the appropriate authorities according to German legal requirements.

Induction of acute or chronic liver injury and anti-CXCL16 treatment

To induce acute liver injury, mice received 0.6 ml/kg body weight carbon tetrachloride (CCl₄, Merck, Darmstadt, Germany) mixed with corn oil intraperitoneally and were sacrificed 6 h thereafter. The control population of animals received the same volume of vehicle (corn oil) intraperitoneally. For induction of steatohepatitis and fibrosis, mice were fed with a methionine and choline deficient (MCD) diet for 6 weeks (MP Biomedicals, Cat.#390439, Solon, OH, USA) [9]. In order to block CXCL16, mice received 100 μg of monoclonal rat anti-mouse CXCL16 neutralizing antibody (R&D Systems, Clone #142417, Germany) intraperitoneally, whereas the control group received 100 μg of

Bovine-Serum-Albumin (Sigma-Aldrich, St. Louis, MO, USA). Mice were either pre-treated 4 hours before acute CCl₄ injury or received weekly injections during weeks 4–6 of a 6-week course of MCD diet. The i.p. route of antibody administration was chosen, because earlier studies had revealed a similar biodistribution in healthy as well as in diseased tissue compared to i.v. injections, and the i.p. administration was considered more reproducible in repetitive injections during the chronic injury model [16–19].

Liver enzymes, histology and immunohistochemistry

Alanine (ALT) activities (UV test at 37°C) were measured from serum (Roche Modular preanalytics system, Rotkreuz Switzerland). Conventional H&E, Sirius red, and Ladewig staining were performed according to standard protocols [20]. Steatosis was scored by an experienced pathologist blinded to experimental data, as previously described [9,15]. Liver sections from fixed paraffin blocks were immunohistochemically stained according to standard procedures using anti-mouse F4/80 and anti-human CD68 (Serotec), respectively [21]. CD68 and H&E pictures were analysed by quantifying the area fraction using imaging software in a blinded fashion (ImageJ).

Isolation of primary hepatic cell populations

B6 mice were either treated with CCl₄ or with corn oil three times per week for 2 weeks to induce liver fibrosis. Primary hepatocytes were isolated from murine livers by convential collagenase perfusion methodology as described before [22].

Isolation of intrahepatic leukocytes

For the analysis of the intrahepatic leukocytes livers were perfused with 25 ml of phosphate buffered saline (PBS), minced with scissors and finally digested for 30 min with collagenase type IV (Worthington, Lakewood, NJ, USA) at 37°C. Digested extracts were pressed through 70 μm cell strainers. A small aliquot was stained with CD45 to assess the relative amount of intrahepatic leukocytes (CD45⁺) among all liver cells. The remaining liver cells were subjected to density gradient centrifugation (LSM-1077, PAA, Pasching, Austria) at 2000 rpm for 20 min at 25°C. Leukocytes were collected from the interface after centrifugation, washed twice with Hank's balanced salt solution containing 2% BSA and 0.1 mM EDTA, and subjected to FACS [9].

Flow cytometry

Six-color staining was conducted using combinations of following monoclonal antibodies: F4/80 (Serotec, Raleigh, NC, USA); CD4, CD11b (both eBioscience, San Diego, CA, USA); CD45, Gr1/Ly6C, Ly6G, CD19, NK1.1, CD8 and CD3 (all BD); CD1d tetramer loaded with αGalCer (ProImmune, Oxford, UK). Dead cells were excluded by Hoechst 33258 dye (Sigma-Aldrich, St. Louis, USA). Flow cytometric analysis was performed on a FACS-Canto (BD) and analysed with FlowJo (Tree Star, Ashland, OR, USA).

Gene expression analysis

Liver tissue was shock frozen in liquid nitrogen and stored at 80°C. RNA was purified from frozen liver samples by pegGOLD (peqLab, Erlangen, Germany), and cDNA was generated from 1 μg of RNA using a cDNA synthesis kit (Roche). Quantitative real-time PCR (qPCR) was performed using SYBR Green Reagent (Invitrogen, Carlsbad, CA, USA). Reactions were done twice in triplicate, and ß-actin values were used to normalize gene expression [9]. Primer sequences are available upon request.

Hydroxyproline, cytokine and triglyceride measurements

The hepatic hydroxyproline content (reflecting total collagen) was measured as described before [23]. Tumor-necrosis-factor-α (TNFα) and monocyte chemoattractant protein-1 (MCP-1) were measured from protein extracts of liver by Elisa (eBioscience) [9]. Total protein content was quantified by photometric assay (Biorad, Hercules, Ca USA). The intrahepatic triglyceride content was measured by TG liquicolor mono (Human Diagnostics, Wiesbaden, Germany) according to the manufacturer's instructions from homogenised snap-frozen liver samples.

Statistical analysis

All experimental data are expressed as mean$\pm$SD. Differences between groups of mouse experiments were assessed by two-tailed unpaired Student t-test. Correlations between variables were asses by Pearson rank correlation test.

Results

Macrophage infiltration is a hallmark feature of steatohepatitis in humans

Experimental rodent models of fatty liver diseases revealed that intrahepatic macrophages massively increase in response to hepatic lipid overload and promote the progression of liver fibrosis as an aberrant wound-healing response [6]. We examined liver biopsies of 10 patients with NAFLD undergoing bariatric surgery in comparison to healthy liver tissue obtained from patients undergoing resections of benign liver lesions (i.e. hemangioma). NAFLD was characterized by steatosis, hepatocyte ballooning and a pronounced infiltrate of mononuclear cells (Fig. 1A), as reflected by the NAFLD Activity Score (NAS) (Fig. 1B). Upon immuno-histochemical staining for the macrophage marker CD68, the accumulation of macrophages, especially around portal fields, was identified as a hallmark feature of NAFLD (Fig. 1C–D), in line with current literature [24]. Additionally, the hepatic macrophage content as quantified by CD68 immunohistochemistry significant-ly correlated with the NAS (Fig. 1E). In some of the patients, NAFLD was associated with moderate to severe hepatic fibrosis, characterized by extracellular matrix deposition around and partially bridging between portal fields (Fig. 1F).

Following our hypothesis that the CXCR6-dependent recruit-ment of NKT cells might contribute to enhanced macrophage accumulation in NAFLD, we assessed hepatic gene expression levels for CXCR6 by quantitative PCR. Hepatic CXCR6 expression showed a significant correlation with elevated serum ALT levels in patients suffering from NAFLD (Fig. 1G). These data prompted the current study to address on a functional level in mouse models whether inhibition of the CXCL16-CXCR6 pathway might be suitable to inhibit steatohepatitis and macro-phage accumulation in NAFLD.

Anti-CXCL16 antibody sufficiently blocks early hepatic NKT cell accumulation upon acute liver injury

Our prior experiments, using intravital multiphoton-imaging of Cxcr6$^{+/gfp}$ transgenic mice and FACS phenotyping of CXCR6$^+$ immune cells, indicated that hepatic NKT cells accumulate very early after injury - e.g., at a maximum as early as 6 hours after injection of the hepatotoxin CCl$_4$ - in the liver in a CXCR6-dependent manner [9]. We therefore hypothesized that inhibition of CXCL16, the specific ligand for CXCR6, could efficiently block this early NKT-dependent step in the initiation of the hepatic inflammatory response. Therefore, c57bl/6 wildtype mice were treated with anti-CXCL16 antibody (αCXCL16) or Bovine-

Serum-Albumin (BSA) as control i.p., followed by CCl$_4$ injection 4 hours later (Fig. 2A). Six hours after CCl$_4$, the liver showed initial signs of injury with cellular swelling, some necrosis and inflammatory cell infiltration in histology (Fig. 2A+B). In the CCl$_4$ injury model, massive necrosis of hepatocytes and even further inflammatory infiltration peaks at around 24 hours after injury (Fig. S1A) [23]. Serum ALT levels are mildly elevated at 6 hours as a measure for early acute liver injury (Fig. 2C). Notably, liver injury appeared slightly attenuated in αCXCL16-treated mice at this early time-point (Fig. 2B–C), as indicated by moderately reduced ALT levels in αCXCL16-treated mice.

To investigate the infiltrating immune cells, intrahepatic leukocytes were phenotypically characterized by FACS at 6 hours after CCl$_4$, and NKT cells were identified as CD45$^+$CD4$^+$NK1.1$^+$ cells. Interestingly, the early NKT cell accumulation could be efficiently blocked by administration of αCXCL16, as hepatic NKT cell numbers were reduced to the level of non-injured control mice due to αCXCL16 treatment (Fig. 2D–E). Mice that received BSA did not show the altered hepatic NKT cell accumulation, thereby excluding an unspecific protein reaction. Moreover, the effect of αCXCL16 treatment appeared specific to NKT cells, as other lymphocytes, which also express the chemokine receptor CXCR6 like CD4 and NK cells [9], were not affected by the antibody injection.

Therapeutic administration of αCXCL16 inhibits macrophage infiltration and hepatic inflammation in experimental steatohepatitis

Our experiments indicated that the administration of αCXCL16 effectively blocked the early accumulation of hepatic NKT cells in response to hepatocyte injury, thus possibly allowing to dampen the subsequent inflammatory response in the liver. In order to test this, B6-mice were subjected to a methionine-choline deficient (MCD) diet over 6 weeks of time. The lack of the amino acids methionine and choline leads to hepatic inflammation induced by accumulation of fatty acids and pro-inflammatory immune cells [25]. During the last three weeks of progressing steatohepatitis in a 6 weeks course of MCD diet, mice were treated with 100 µg αCXCL16 or BSA i.p. once per week (Fig. 3A). In line with our hypothesis, αCXCL16-treated mice showed a significant reduction of pro-inflammatory macrophages as evi-denced by immunohistological stainings for F4/80 and FACS analysis of intrahepatic leukocytes (Fig. 3B–D). Of note, hepatic NKT cell numbers were very low in all groups fed with MCD diet (data not shown), due to the rapid activation induced cell death (AICD) of NKT in hepatic injury [9,26]. The strong reduction of hepatic macrophages upon αCXCL16 administration during the MCD diet was accompanied by a trend towards reduced intrahepatic levels of pro-inflammatory cytokines like TNFα and MCP-1 (Fig. 3E).

Therapeutic administration of αCXCL16 attenuates steatosis development in experimental steatohepatitis

We next analyzed whether pharmacological inhibition of CXCL16 might represent a successful therapeutic approach to limit disease progression in experimental steatohepatitis. Treat-ment with αCXCL16 (experimental design as in Fig. 3A) did not significantly affect hepatic fibrosis in the MCD-induced chronic liver injury, as assessed by collagen deposition in Sirius red histological stainings (Fig. 4A), by serum ALT levels (Fig. 4B) or by quantification of the hepatic hydroxyproline content (Fig. 4C) as a sensitive measure for collagen fibers in the liver. However, already by conventional H&E stainings from liver histology, it was

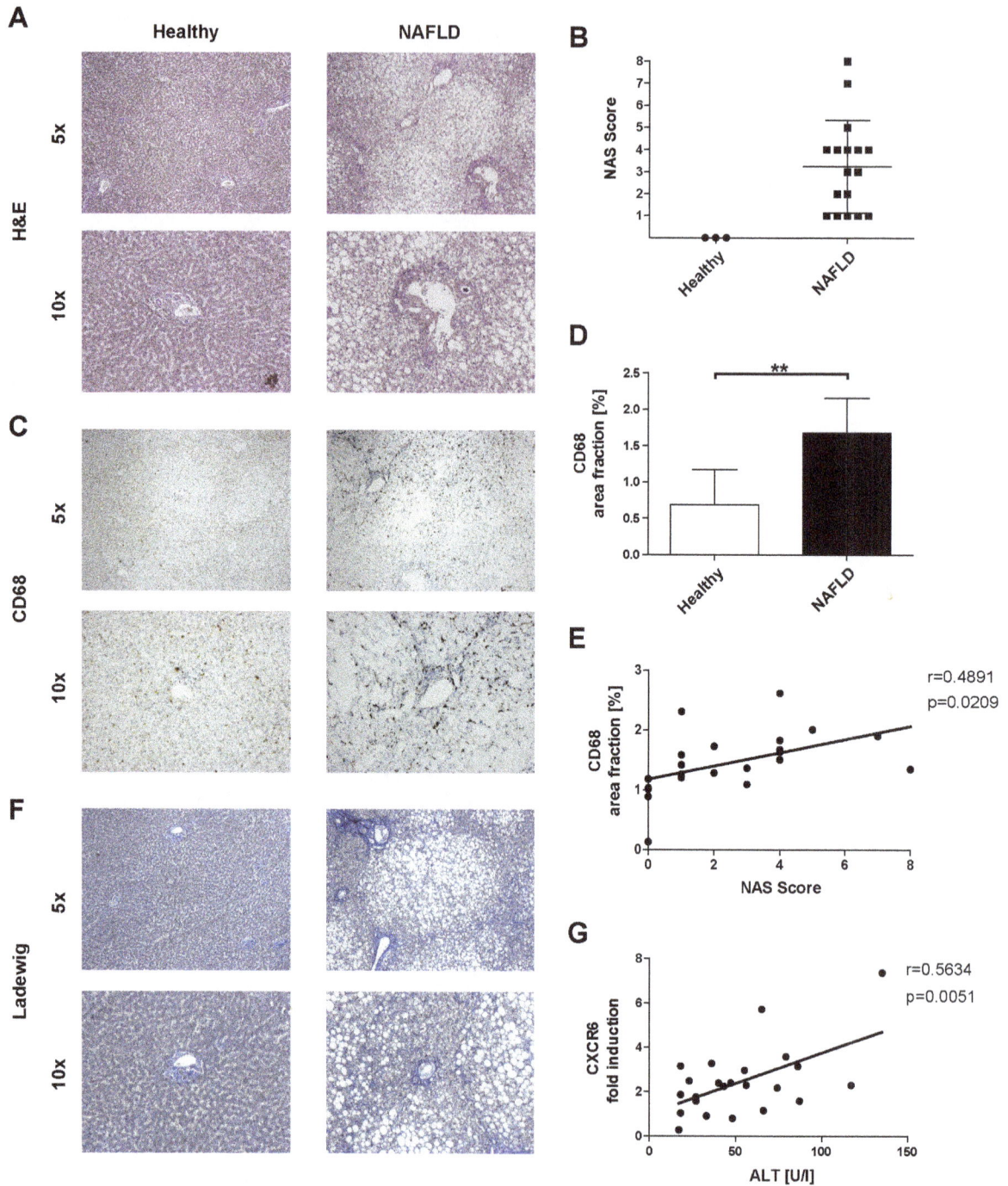

Figure 1. Hepatic macrophage infiltration is increased in liver of patients with non-alcoholic-steatohepatitis and accompanied by slightly enhanced CXCR6 expression. Liver biopsies of patients with NAFLD (n=20) and healthy controls (n=3) were analyzed. (**A–B**) Hematoxylin-Eosin stainings (H&E) of liver paraffin sections demonstrated steatosis development in patients with NAFLD compared to healthy controls. NAFLD severity was scored according to the NAS-Kleiner-Score. (**C–D**) CD68 immunohistochemical stainings showed a significant increase of intrahepatic macrophages in livers of NAFLD patients compared to healthy controls. (**E**) Hepatic macrophages (CD68 positive) significantly correlated with the NAS. (**F**) Patients with NAFLD developed fibrosis, as evidenced by collagen deposition (blue) in Ladewig staining of liver biopsies. (**G**) High CXCR6 expression correlated with elevated serum ALT levels. P-values and correlation coefficients are given in the figure. All data are expressed as mean ± SD. *p<0.05, **p<0.005, ***p<0.001.

apparent that αCXCL16 administration not only reduced the inflammatory infiltrate, but also the numbers of lipid droplets in hepatocytes (Fig. 4A). Measurement of the hepatic triglyceride content as well as histological quantification of lipid droplets confirmed significantly attenuated steatosis development, if MCD-fed mice received αCXCL16 during the last 3 weeks of a 6-week MCD diet-induced metabolic injury (Fig. 4D–E). In agreement

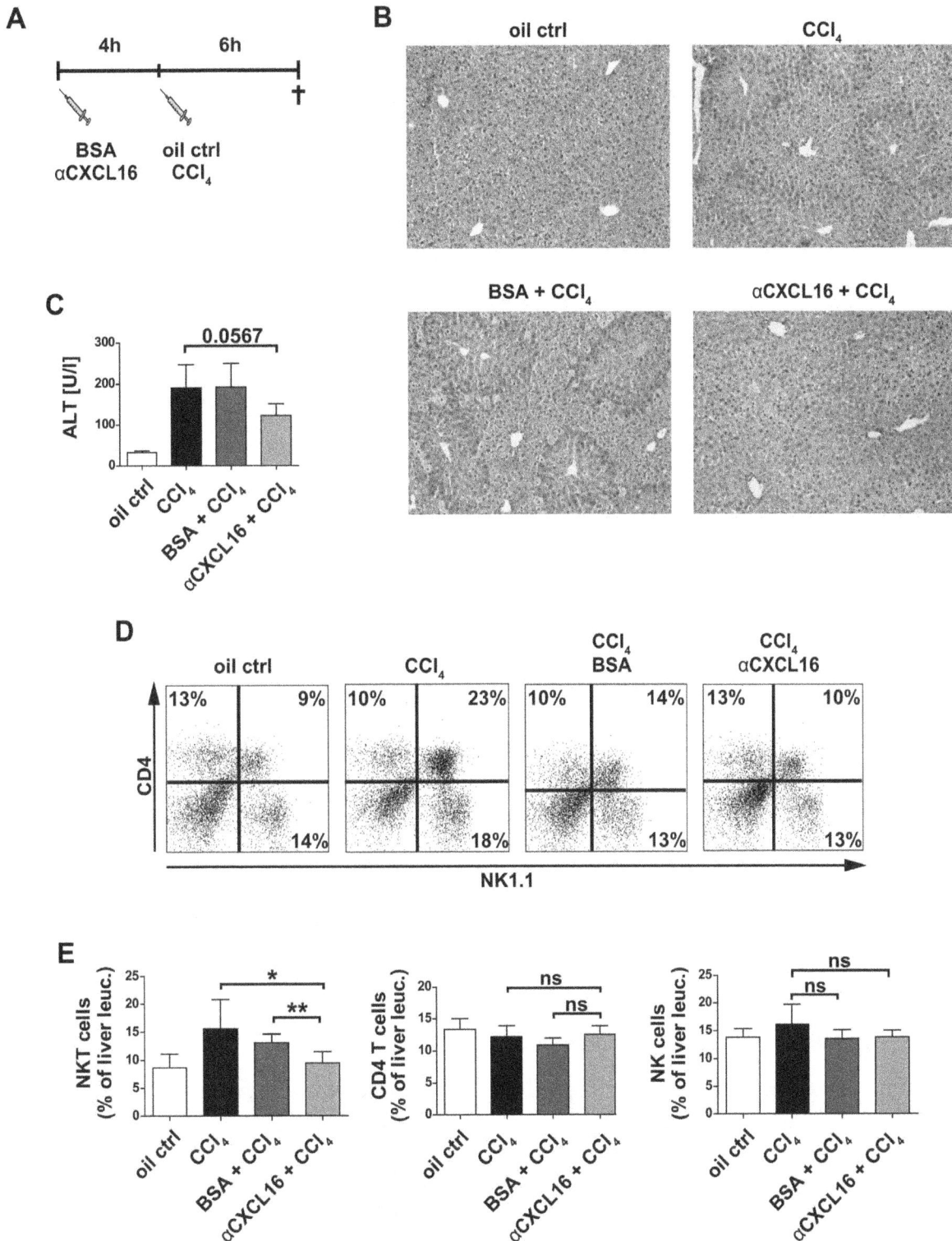

Figure 2. Anti-CXCL16 antibody sufficiently blocks early hepatic NKT cell accumulation upon acute liver injury. (**A**) B6-mice received a singular intraperitoneal application of either αCXCL16 or BSA (unspecific protein control) 4 hours before injection of carbon tetrachloride (CCl$_4$). Mice were sacrificed 6 hours after CCl$_4$ application. (**B–C**) As evidenced by H&E stainings and serum ALT activity, αCXCL16 treated mice showed reduced toxic liver damage *in vivo* compared to BSA treated mice. (**D–E**) Flow cytometric analysis of intrahepatic leukocytes (representative FACS plots in D, statistical analyses in E) showed a significant decrease of hepatic NKT cells in mice that received αCXCL16 compared to controls. Other CXCR6 expressing cells like CD4 T- and NK cells were not altered with respect to their migration behavior into the injured liver upon αCXCL16 injection. All data are expressed as mean ± SD from three independent experiments, summarizing n = 6 animals per group. *p<0.05, **p<0.005, ***p<0.001.

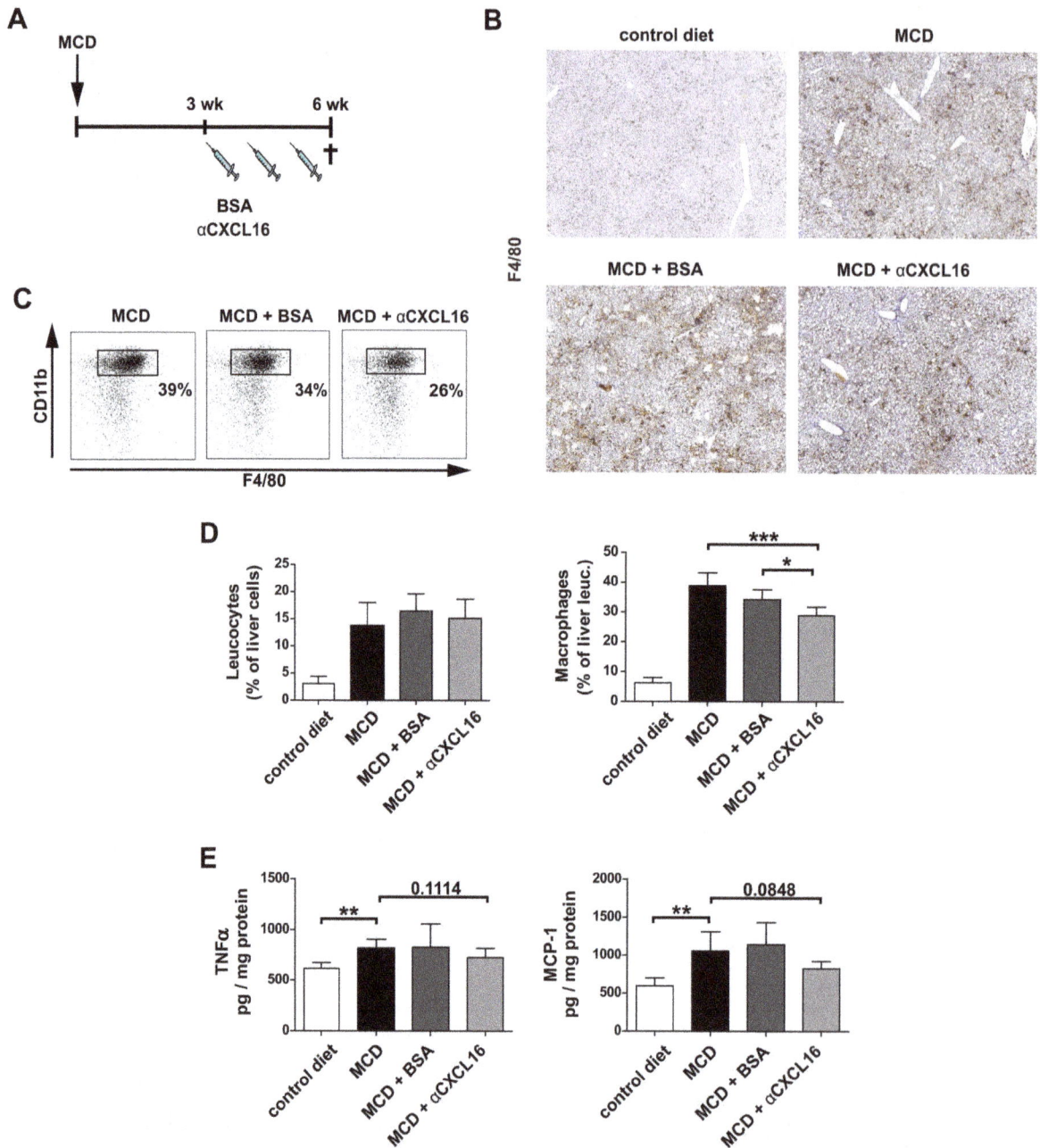

Figure 3. Therapeutic administration of αCXCL16 inhibits macrophage infiltration and hepatic inflammation in experimental steatohepatitis. (A) B6-mice were subjected to a methionine-choline deficient (MCD) diet over 6 weeks. During the last three weeks of progressing steatohepatitis, mice were treated with αCXCL16 or BSA i.p. once per week. **(B–D)** F4/80 immunohistochemical staining of liver tissue (B) and flow cytometric analysis of intrahepatic leukocytes (representative plots, C; statistical analysis, D) showed a significant reduction of infiltrating CD11b⁺F4/80⁺ macrophages in αCXCL16 treated mice compared to controls. **(E)** Pro-inflammatory cytokines like TNFα and MCP-1 were slightly decreased in liver tissue of mice that received weekly αCXCL16 injections compared to controls during MCD diet. All data are expressed as mean ± SD from three independent experiments, summarizing n = 6 animals per group. *p<0.05, **p<0.005, ***p<0.001.

with these data, the fatty degeneration score was also significant decreased in mice treated with αCXCL16 (Fig. 4F).

Discussion

Non-alcoholic fatty liver disease is a raising health burden in Western countries, which affect about 30% of the general adult population, is associated with an increased mortality and promote several medical complications like hepatocarcinogenesis in hu-

mans [3,27]. Within the liver, hepatocyte apoptosis, ER stress and oxidative stress are key contributors to hepatocellular injury. Moreover, lipotoxic mediators and danger signals activate the hepatic macrophage pool, mainly Kupffer cells, which are critical for the initiation and perpetuation of the inflammatory response and release several inflammatory mediators [6]. Such mediators, mainly cytokines and chemokines, attract inflammatory cells and activate parenchymal as well as non-parenchymal liver cells during

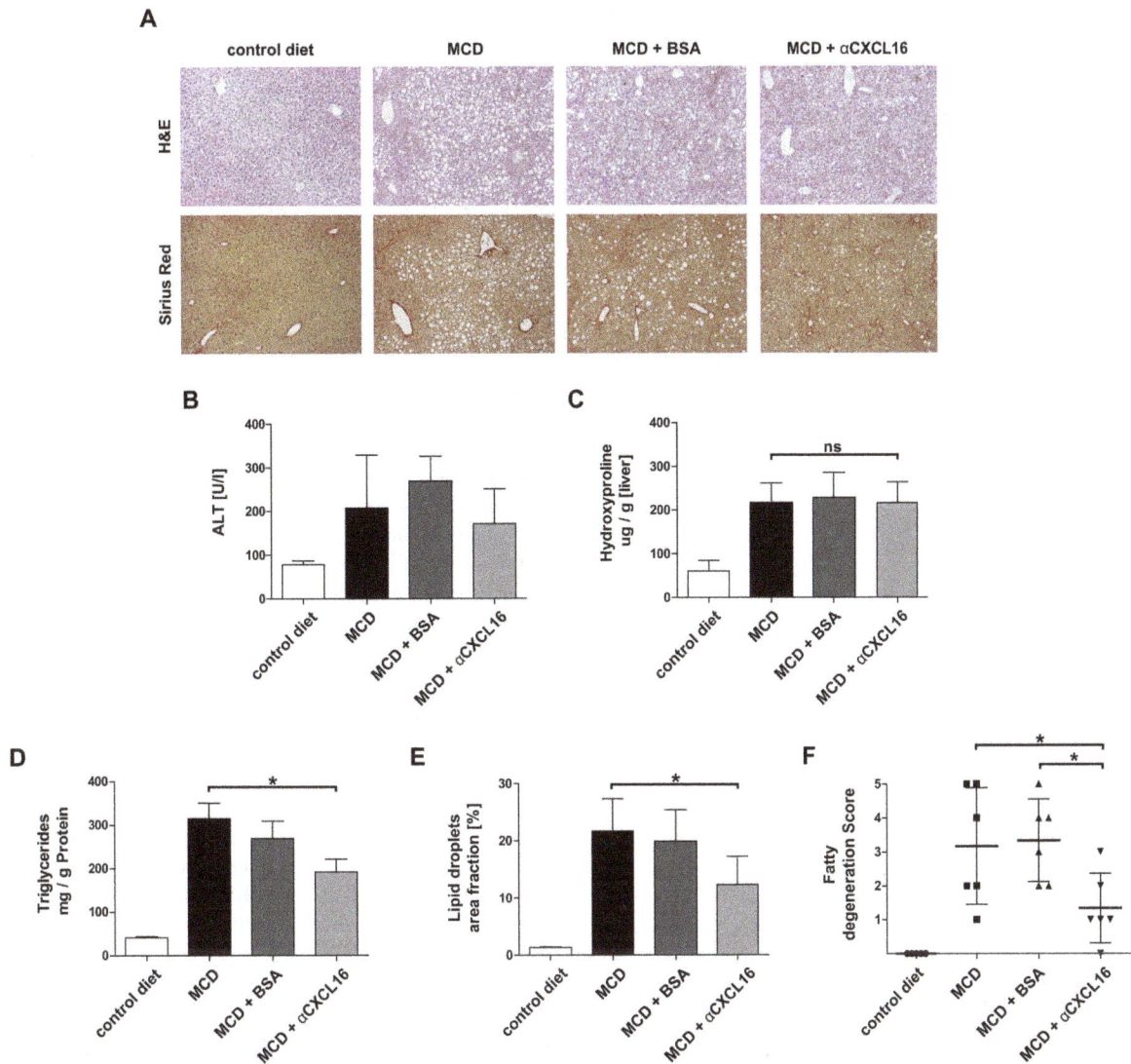

Figure 4. Therapeutic administration of αCXCL16 attenuates steatosis development in experimental steatohepatitis. (A) Liver histology showed no altered fibrosis development, but a clear reduction of lipid accumulation in injured livers of αCXCL16 treated mice compared to controls as evidenced by H&E- and Sirius red stainings. **(B–C)** Serum ALT activity and hydroxyproline content were not affected by the administration of αCXCL16. **(D–E)** Intrahepatic triglyceride content and periportal lipid droplets were significant reduced in mice that received weekly αCXCL16 injections compared to controls during MCD diet. **(F)** Fatty degeneration score was significantly decreased in αCXCL16 treated mice compared to controls. All data are expressed as mean ± SD from three independent experiments, summarizing n=6 animals per group. *p<0.05, **p<0.005, ***p<0.001.

NAFLD progression [21]. In our study, we provide experimental evidence that interfering with the CXCR6-CXCL16 pathway might hold therapeutic potential in NAFLD. The administration of an anti-CXCL16 antibody blocked the rapid accumulation of patrolling hepatic NKT cells in response to acute hepatocyte injury. In line, therapeutic administration of this antibody in experimental chronic metabolic injury attenuated hepatic macrophage infiltration, pro-inflammatory cytokine levels and steatosis development in mice.

On the one hand, our experiments using αCXCL16 revealed that blocking this chemokine pathway almost completely abolished the rapid accumulation of hepatic NKT cells in response to an acute injury. This is well in line with a prior *in vitro* experiment from our group, demonstrating that CXCR6 is specifically required by NKT, but not other CXCR6-expressing lymphocytes,

to migrate towards CXCL16 [9]. Moreover, it had been reported that CXCL16 neutralization reduced accumulation of mature NK1.1[+], but not immature NK1.1[−] NKT cell recent thymic emigrants in the liver in homeostatic conditions *in vivo* [28]. NKT cells display a unique population of unconventional T cells that express both a T cell receptor (Vα-14-Jα18 in mice; Vα24-Jα18 in humans) and NK1.1 receptor from NK cells [10,29]. There are different types of NKT cell subsets that are defined by the ability of recognizing α-galactosylceramide (α-GalCeramide) presented by the non-classical MHC-like molecule CD1d [10], termed type-I classical, type-II non classical and CD1d-independent NK1.1[+] NKT cells. Especially the type-I NKT cells, which the by far largest subset in the liver, have the ability to secrete various types of cytokines within a very short time period after activation, including IL-4 and IFNγ [9,10]. In line, mice that are deficient for the CXCL16 chemokine displayed a reduced number of liver NKT cells, decreased production of IFNγ and IL-4 by administration of α-GalCeramide and impaired (Th1-type) inflammatory responses against *Propionibacterium acnes*-infections *in vivo* [30].

On the other hand, our experiments indicate that αCXCL16 could be an interesting therapeutic strategy in hepatic inflammation and steatohepatitis. Importantly, the same αCXCL16 antibody had been tested as an interventional approach for severe inflammatory conditions before. In a murine immunological liver injury induced by Bacille Calmette-Guerin and lipopolysaccharide, mice treated with αCXCL16 showed reduced liver injury, inflammation and improved survival [31]. Administration of αCXCL16 also reduced colonic inflammation in mouse models of on dextran sodium sulfate- and trinitrobenzene sulfonic acid-induced colitis [32]. In our hands, therapeutic administration of αCXCL16 during the last three weeks of a 6-weeks course of MCD diet in mice significantly reduced the number of hepatic macrophages, alongside minor reductions in intrahepatic levels of pro-inflammatory cytokines, and steatosis development. The link between macrophages and progression of fatty liver degeneration is well established, as macrophages release many inflammatory mediators that not only attract additional immune cells, but also drive oxidative stress and intrahepatocytic lipid accumulation [6,25,33]. Our experiments now indicate that blocking CXCL16 effectively reduces pro-inflammatory macrophages in experimental steatohepatitis. As macrophages do not express CXCR6 [9] (and data not shown), the effects of αCXCL16 on hepatic macrophages are likely the result on inhibiting NKT cell accumulation early in the course of injury. In fact, reducing the additional pro-inflammatory effects of NKT cells in injured liver was shown before to significantly ameliorate the extent of chronic hepatic inflammation and macrophage activation [9,26,34–38]. Our study now emphasizes that this can be sufficiently achieved by targeting the CXCR6/CXCL16 chemokine axis.

However, an alternative explanation for the effects of inhibiting CXCL16 needs to be considered. It has been shown previously that CXCL16 can act as a scavenging receptor for oxidized low density lipoprotein (oxLDL) [39–41]. In order to explore whether CXCL16 might act as a scavenger for lipids or lipid-protein complexes on hepatocytes in conditions of NAFLD, we have isolated hepatocytes from normal and from chronically injured B6 mice. In fact, CXCL16 gene expression was about 7-fold up-regulated in hepatocytes from injured mice (Fig. S1B). Thus, it is possible that inhibiting CXCL16 by an antibody not only affects immune cell migration and function, but has additional effects on the lipid accumulation in hepatocytes. Further studies are needed to investigate the relevance of scavenging functions by CXCL16 for NAFLD progression.

Importantly, although steatosis development was attenuated upon αCXCL16 in the MCD diet model, hepatic fibrosis progression was not significantly affected. Several factors might explain this observation. First, we have chosen a relatively low dose of the antibody (100 μg) and only three injections (once per week); in experimental models of murine colitis, mice were subjected to 500 μg of αCXCL16 i.p. every day for the total of 7 days [32]. Thus, different doses and more frequent applications should be considered for future studies. Second, the MCD diet model is characterized by a rather scattered deposition of collagen in the liver and a rather mild fibrosis, especially when mice are analyzed after 6 weeks of diet [25]. Thus, in order to address the possible impact of αCXCL16 on fibrosis, 'classical' fibrosis models,

modifications of the metabolic injury model or mice with a more fibrosis-prone genetic background (e.g., Balb/c instead of B6) should be investigated [33,42]. Third, it is currently unclear to which extent infiltrating vs. resident hepatic macrophages contribute to progression of liver fibrosis [43]. Based on the flow cytometric characterization in our study, αCXCL16 primarily affected the $CD11b^+F4/80^+$ macrophage population, which is mainly derived from infiltrating inflammatory $Ly-6C^+$ ($Gr1^+$) monocytes [23]. As shown before by selectively blocking $Ly-6C^+$ monocyte influx in chronic liver injury models, this macrophage subset appeared functionally essential for steatohepatitis, but less relevant for fibrosis progression [25]. In line, a recent study demonstrated a crucial role of inflammatory $CD11b^+$ macrophages in CCl_4 induced acute liver injury. The hepatic injury was driven by macrophage-derived TNFα and Fas-Ligand (FasL), as inhibition of TNFα and FasL dampened the hepatic injury induced by a single CCl_4 injection. Interestingly, CD1d-deficient mice lacking both type I and II NKT cells, did not show significant differences in the progression of acute liver injury compared with control mice in this study [44]. However, this study was conducted in Balb/c mice. A similar study with CD1d-deficient mice on a c57bl/6 background showed that NKT-cell-deficient mice were protected from acute toxic liver injury [35], in well agreement with our previous [9] and the current study. Possibly, these data might indicate that hepatic NKT cells are especially relevant in Th1-prone inflammatory conditions.

Taken together, our study provides experimental evidence that targeting the chemokine CXCL16 is a promising strategy in fatty liver diseases. The inhibition of CXCR6-dependent NKT cell accumulation as an important inflammatory cell component ameliorated the extent of hepatic inflammation, macrophage activation and steatosis development in experimental metabolic injury. Future studies should address the optimal dose and administration schedule and should aim at translating these findings into novel approaches for human NAFLD.

Supporting Information

Figure S1 (A) Kinetics of necrosis development in CCl_4 injured B6 mice. Six hours after CCl_4 injection, the liver showed initial signs of injury with cellular swelling, some necrosis and inflammatory cell infiltration. Massive necrosis of hepatocytes and even further inflammatory infiltration peaks at around 24 hours after injury. **(B) CXCL16 mRNA expression in primary hepatocytes.** CXCL16 is highly up-regulated in primary hepatocytes isolated from chronically injured mouse livers compared to primary hepatocytes from control livers.

Acknowledgments

We thank Karina Kreggenwinkel and Aline Roggenkamp for excellent technical assistance.

Author Contributions

Conceived and designed the experiments: AW CB TL CT FT. Performed the experiments: AW CB FU NG KH UPN. Analyzed the data: AW CB NG KH. Contributed reagents/materials/analysis tools: FU NG KH TL UPN. Contributed to the writing of the manuscript: AW CB TL UPN CT FT.

References

1. Schuppan D, Schattenberg JM (2013) Non-alcoholic steatohepatitis: pathogenesis and novel therapeutic approaches. J Gastroenterol Hepatol 28 Suppl 1: 68–76.

2. Blachier M, Leleu H, Peck-Radosavljevic M, Valla DC, Roudot-Thoraval F (2013) The burden of liver disease in Europe: a review of available epidemiological data. J Hepatol 58: 593–608.

3. Bhala N, Jouness RI, Bugianesi E (2013) Epidemiology and natural history of patients with NAFLD. Curr Pharm Des 19: 5169–5176.

4. Jepsen P, Vilstrup H, Mellemkjaer L, Thulstrup AM, Olsen JH, et al. (2003) Prognosis of patients with a diagnosis of fatty liver–a registry-based cohort study. Hepatogastroenterology 50: 2101–2104.

5. Agopian VG, Kaldas FM, Hong JC, Whittaker M, Holt C, et al. (2012) Liver transplantation for nonalcoholic steatohepatitis: the new epidemic. Ann Surg 256: 624–633.

6. Marra F, Lotersztajn S (2013) Pathophysiology of NASH: perspectives for a targeted treatment. Curr Pharm Des 19: 5250–5269.

7. Argo CK, Northup PG, Al-Osaimi AM, Caldwell SH (2009) Systematic review of risk factors for fibrosis progression in non-alcoholic steatohepatitis. J Hepatol 51: 371–379.

8. Marra F, Tacke F (2014) Roles for Chemokines in Liver Disease. Gastroenterology 147: 577–594 e571.

9. Wehr A, Baeck C, Heymann F, Niemietz PM, Hammerich L, et al. (2013) Chemokine receptor CXCR6-dependent hepatic NK T Cell accumulation promotes inflammation and liver fibrosis. J Immunol 190: 5226–5236.

10. Godfrey DI, MacDonald HR, Kronenberg M, Smyth MJ, Van Kaer L (2004) NKT cells: what's in a name? Nat Rev Immunol 4: 231–237.

11. Tuncer C, Oo YH, Murphy N, Adams DH, Lalor PF (2013) The regulation of T-cell recruitment to the human liver during acute liver failure. Liver Int 33: 852–863.

12. Boisvert J, Kunkel EJ, Campbell JJ, Keeffe EB, Butcher EC, et al. (2003) Liver-infiltrating lymphocytes in end-stage hepatitis C virus: subsets, activation status, and chemokine receptor phenotypes. J Hepatol 38: 67–75.

13. Geissmann F, Cameron TO, Sidobre S, Manlongat N, Kronenberg M, et al. (2005) Intravascular immune surveillance by CXCR6+ NKT cells patrolling liver sinusoids. PLoS Biol 3: e113.

14. Zimmermann HW, Seidler S, Nattermann J, Gassler N, Hellerbrand C, et al. (2010) Functional contribution of elevated circulating and hepatic non-classical CD14CD16 monocytes to inflammation and human liver fibrosis. PLoS One 5: e11049.

15. Kleiner DE, Brunt EM, Van Natta M, Behling C, Contos MJ, et al. (2005) Design and validation of a histological scoring system for nonalcoholic fatty liver disease. Hepatology 41: 1313–1321.

16. Mattes MJ (1987) Biodistribution of antibodies after intraperitoneal or intravenous injection and effect of carbohydrate modifications. J Natl Cancer Inst 79: 855–863.

17. Wahl RL, Barrett J, Geatti O, Liebert M, Wilson BS, et al. (1988) The intraperitoneal delivery of radiolabeled monoclonal antibodies: studies on the regional delivery advantage. Cancer Immunol Immunother 26: 187–201.

18. Yoshida K, Fujikawa T, Yoshizawa G, Tanabea A, Sakurai K (1992) Biodistribution of radiolabeled monoclonal antibody after intraperitoneal administration in nude mice with hepatic metastasis from human colon cancer. Surg Today 22: 155–158.

19. Barrett JS, Wagner JG, Fisher SJ, Wahl RL (1991) Effect of intraperitoneal injection volume and antibody protein dose on the pharmacokinetics of intraperitoneally administered IgG2a kappa murine monoclonal antibody in the rat. Cancer Res 51: 3434–3444.

20. Malato Y, Sander LE, Liedtke C, Al-Masaoudi M, Tacke F, et al. (2008) Hepatocyte-specific inhibitor-of-kappaB-kinase deletion triggers the innate immune response and promotes earlier cell proliferation during liver regeneration. Hepatology 47: 2036–2050.

21. Zimmermann HW, Tacke F (2011) Modification of chemokine pathways and immune cell infiltration as a novel therapeutic approach in liver inflammation and fibrosis. Inflamm Allergy Drug Targets 10: 509–536.

22. Hammerich L, Bangen JM, Govaere O, Zimmermann HW, Gassler N, et al. (2014) Chemokine receptor CCR6-dependent accumulation of gammadelta T-cells in injured liver restricts hepatic inflammation and fibrosis. Hepatology 59: 630–42.

23. Karlmark KR, Weiskirchen R, Zimmermann HW, Gassler N, Ginhoux F, et al. (2009) Hepatic recruitment of the inflammatory Gr1+ monocyte subset upon liver injury promotes hepatic fibrosis. Hepatology 50: 261–274.

24. Tannapfel A, Denk H, Dienes HP, Langner C, Schirmacher P, et al. (2011) Histopathological diagnosis of non-alcoholic and alcoholic fatty liver disease. Virchows Arch 458: 511–523.

25. Baeck C, Wehr A, Karlmark KR, Heymann F, Vucur M, et al. (2012) Pharmacological inhibition of the chemokine CCL2 (MCP-1) diminishes liver macrophage infiltration and steatohepatitis in chronic hepatic injury. Gut 61: 416–426.

26. Park O, Jeong WI, Wang L, Wang H, Lian ZX, et al. (2009) Diverse roles of invariant natural killer T cells in liver injury and fibrosis induced by carbon tetrachloride. Hepatology 49: 1683–1694.

27. Baffy G, Brunt EM, Caldwell SH (2012) Hepatocellular carcinoma in non-alcoholic fatty liver disease: an emerging menace. J Hepatol 56: 1384–1391.

28. Germanov E, Veinotte L, Cullen R, Chamberlain E, Butcher EC, et al. (2008) Critical role for the chemokine receptor CXCR6 in homeostasis and activation of CD1d-restricted NKT cells. J Immunol 181: 81–91.

29. Bendelac A, Savage PB, Teyton L (2007) The biology of NKT cells. Annu Rev Immunol 25: 297–336.

30. Shimaoka T, Seino K, Kume N, Minami M, Nishime C, et al. (2007) Critical role for CXC chemokine ligand 16 (SR-PSOX) in Th1 response mediated by NKT cells. J Immunol 179: 8172–8179.

31. Xu HB, Gong YP, Cheng J, Chu YW, Xiong SD (2005) CXCL16 participates in pathogenesis of immunological liver injury by regulating T lymphocyte infiltration in liver tissue. World J Gastroenterol 11: 4979–4985.

32. Uza N, Nakase H, Yamamoto S, Yoshino T, Takeda Y, et al. (2011) SR-PSOX/CXCL16 plays a critical role in the progression of colonic inflammation. Gut 60: 1494–1505.

33. Galastri S, Zamara E, Milani S, Novo E, Provenzano A, et al. (2012) Lack of CC chemokine ligand 2 differentially affects inflammation and fibrosis according to the genetic background in a murine model of steatohepatitis. Clin Sci (Lond) 123: 459–471.

34. Syn WK, Agboola KM, Swiderska M, Michelotti GA, Liaskou E, et al. (2012) NKT-associated hedgehog and osteopontin drive fibrogenesis in non-alcoholic fatty liver disease. Gut 61: 1323–1329.

35. Ishikawa S, Ikejima K, Yamagata H, Aoyama T, Kon K, et al. (2011) CD1d-restricted natural killer T cells contribute to hepatic inflammation and fibrogenesis in mice. J Hepatol 54: 1195–1204.

36. Jin Z, Sun R, Wei H, Gao X, Chen Y, et al. (2011) Accelerated liver fibrosis in hepatitis B virus transgenic mice: involvement of natural killer T cells. Hepatology 53: 219–229.

37. Syn WK, Oo YH, Pereira TA, Karaca GF, Jung Y, et al. (2010) Accumulation of natural killer T cells in progressive nonalcoholic fatty liver disease. Hepatology 51: 1998–2007.

38. Wang H, Feng D, Park O, Yin S, Gao B (2013) Invariant NKT cell activation induces neutrophil accumulation and hepatitis: Oppositely regulated by IL-4 and IFN-gamma. Hepatology.

39. Gutwein P, Abdel-Bakky MS, Schramme A, Doberstein K, Kampfer-Kolb N, et al. (2009) CXCL16 is expressed in podocytes and acts as a scavenger receptor for oxidized low-density lipoprotein. Am J Pathol 174: 2061–2072.

40. Gutwein P, Abdel-Bakky MS, Doberstein K, Schramme A, Beckmann J, et al. (2009) CXCL16 and oxLDL are induced in the onset of diabetic nephropathy. J Cell Mol Med 13: 3809–3825.

41. Postea O, Koenen RR, Hristov M, Weber C, Ludwig A (2008) Homocysteine up-regulates vascular transmembrane chemokine CXCL16 and induces CXCR6+ lymphocyte recruitment in vitro and in vivo. J Cell Mol Med 12: 1700–1709.

42. Mederacke I (2013) Liver fibrosis - mouse models and relevance in human liver diseases. Z Gastroenterol 51: 55–62.

43. Tacke F (2012) Functional role of intrahepatic monocyte subsets for the progression of liver inflammation and liver fibrosis in vivo. Fibrogenesis Tissue Repair 5 Suppl 1: S27.

44. Sato A, Nakashima H, Nakashima M, Ikarashi M, Nishiyama K, et al. (2014) Involvement of the TNF and FasL produced by CD11b Kupffer cells/macrophages in CCl4-induced acute hepatic injury. PLoS One 9: e92515.

Longitudinal Analysis of T and B Cell Phenotype and Function in Renal Transplant Recipients with or without Rituximab Induction Therapy

Elena G. Kamburova[1], Hans J. P. M. Koenen[1], Martijn W. F. van den Hoogen[2], Marije C. Baas[2], Irma Joosten[1◊], Luuk B. Hilbrands[2*◊]

1 Department of Laboratory Medicine - Medical Immunology, Radboud University Medical Centre, Nijmegen, The Netherlands, 2 Department of Nephrology, Radboud University Medical Centre, Nijmegen, The Netherlands

Abstract

Background: Prevention of rejection after renal transplantation requires treatment with immunosuppressive drugs. Data on their in vivo effects on T- and B-cell phenotype and function are limited.

Methods: In a randomized double-blind placebo-controlled study to prevent renal allograft rejection, patients were treated with tacrolimus, mycophenolate mofetil (MMF), steroids, and a single dose of rituximab or placebo during transplant surgery. In a subset of patients, we analyzed the number and phenotype of peripheral T and B cells by multiparameter flow cytometry before transplantation, and at 3, 6, 12, and 24 months after transplantation.

Results: In patients treated with tacrolimus/MMF/steroids the proportion of central memory CD4$^+$ and CD8$^+$ T cells was higher at 3 months post-transplant compared to pre-transplant levels. In addition, the ratio between the percentage of central memory CD4$^+$ and CD4$^+$ regulatory T cells was significantly higher up to 24 months post-transplant compared to pre-transplant levels. Interestingly, treatment with tacrolimus/MMF/steroids resulted in a shift toward a more memory-like B-cell phenotype post-transplant. Addition of a single dose of rituximab resulted in a long-lasting B-cell depletion. At 12 months post-transplant, the small fraction of repopulated B cells consisted of a high percentage of transitional B cells. Rituximab treatment had no effect on the T-cell phenotype and function post-transplant.

Conclusions: Renal transplant recipients treated with tacrolimus/MMF/steroids show an altered memory T and B-cell compartment post-transplant. Additional B-cell depletion by rituximab leads to a relative increase of transitional and memory-like B cells, without affecting T-cell phenotype and function.

Trial Registration: ClinicalTrials.gov NCT00565331

Editor: Ray Borrow, Public Health England, United Kingdom

Funding: This study was supported by research funding from the Dutch Kidney Foundation (nr C09-2301). The funders had no role in study design, data collection and analysis, decision to publish, or preparation of the manuscript.

Competing Interests: The authors of this manuscript have read the journal's policy and have the following competing interests: LBH has received research funds from Roche, the manufacturer of rituximab. The other authors have declared that no competing interests exist.

* Email: Luuk.Hilbrands@radboudumc.nl

◊ These authors contributed equally to this work.

Introduction

Life-long use of immunosuppressive drugs is required to prevent rejection after renal transplantation. Nevertheless, the continuous use of immunosuppressive drugs does not preclude the development of chronic rejection, which is a major cause of long-term allograft loss [1]. T cells play an important role in the pathogenesis of rejection via the recognition of alloantigens, resulting in T-cell activation, proliferation, and differentiation into CD8$^+$ cytotoxic T cells and CD4$^+$ T helper cells [2]. Therefore, the most commonly used immunosuppressive drugs in transplantation are directed against T cells to inhibit these processes [3]. On the other hand, regulatory T cells are able to suppress the immune response and prevent allograft rejection [4]. The balance between memory and regulatory T cells during the course after transplantation can be used to predict renal graft rejection following the reduction of immunosuppressive therapy [5]. Next to T cells, B cells can be involved in graft rejection [6]. The presence of B-cell clusters in renal grafts during acute rejection or the presence of anti-HLA antibodies before transplantation is associated with poorer graft survival [7–9]. Notably, B cells can induce alloimmune responses by acting as professional antigen presenting cells, or by the production of various (pro-)inflammatory cytokines [10]. Therefore, depletion of B cells in renal transplant recipients might help to prevent allograft rejection. Current immunosuppressive regimens consisting of steroids, a calcineurin-inhibitor, and mycophenolate mofetil (MMF) inhibit B-cell function directly due to inhibition of their proliferation and indirectly via the inhibition of T-cell help. B cells can also be selectively depleted by rituximab (RTX), an anti-CD20 monoclonal antibody. RTX is successfully used in the treatment of B-cell malignancies and autoimmune disorders mediated by T and B cells [11,12]. Although the major target of RTX-based treatment was to reduce the levels of circulating autoantibodies, additional B-cell functions may be affected, such as antigen presentation and cytokine production [13]. Furthermore induction of regulatory T cells (T_{REGS}) was reported after RTX treatment in patients with lupus nephritis [14]. Therefore, next to its effect on B cells, RTX might decrease the chance of rejection after transplantation by affecting the T-cell compartment. Remarkably little is known about the effects of the currently used immunosuppressive strategies on the phenotype and function of T and B cells during the course after renal transplantation. Advancements in multiparameter flow cytometry have made it possible to analyze the effects of immunosuppressive agents on various T- and B-cell subsets in more detail. We had the opportunity to study the effects of standard immunosuppression (tacrolimus, MMF and steroids), with or without the addition of RTX induction therapy on the phenotype and function of T and B cells over time in renal transplant recipients participating in a randomized placebo-controlled trial, studying the efficacy and safety of RTX added to standard immunosuppression. To avoid bias by other immunological events as much as possible, we analyzed only Cytomegalovirus (CMV) seronegative patients who received a kidney from a CMV seronegative donor, did not experience a rejection episode, and were not treated with additional immunosuppressive drugs during the follow-up period.

Materials and Methods

Patients

Patients were selected from participants of a clinical trial with RTX in renal transplantation at our hospital (ClinicalTrials.gov, NCT00565331). This study investigated the effectiveness and safety of RTX for prophylaxis of acute rejection after renal transplantation. Patients were randomized between treatment with a single dose of RTX (375 mg/m^2) or placebo during transplant surgery. Concomitant immunosuppression consisted of tacrolimus, MMF, and steroids. Patients received 100 mg of prednisolone intravenously during the first 3 days after transplantation and subsequently an oral dose of 15–25 mg/day, tapered to a maintenance dose of 0.1 mg/kg/day. Tacrolimus was started at 0.2 mg/kg/day and the dose was subsequently adjusted to achieve whole-blood trough levels of 15–20 ng/ml during the first 2 weeks, 10–15 ng/ml during weeks 3–6, and 5–10 ng/ml from week 7. MMF was administered at 1000 mg twice daily with a dose reduction to 750 mg twice daily at 2 weeks after transplantation, and discontinued after 6 months.

The current study was carried out as preplanned side study of the clinical trial. To create a homogeneous study population without disturbing immunological events, we selected patients who did not meet the primary end point of the clinical trial (biopsy-proven acute rejection). Moreover, we investigated only Cytomegalovirus (CMV) seronegative patients who received a kidney from a CMV seronegative donor (and thus did not develop CMV infection), and we excluded patients in whom the immunosuppressive treatment was changed during the follow-up period. After

applying these selection criteria, all remaining patients were included: 14 patients in the group treated with tacrolimus, MMF and steroids, and 12 patients in the group additionally treated with RTX (Figure S1). Peripheral blood mononuclear cells (PBMCs) of 4 standard-treated patients and 3 RTX-treated patients were not available at 24 months after transplantation. Table 1 summarizes the characteristics of all patients. The study was approved by the Institutional review board of the Radboudumc Nijmegen. Written informed consent was obtained from all participants.

Cells

Peripheral blood samples were obtained before transplantation, and up to 24 months after transplantation. Whole blood counts were performed and PBMCs were isolated by density gradient centrifugation using Lymphoprep (Lucron, Dieren, The Netherlands). PBMCs were cryopreserved in liquid nitrogen until analysis. For each patient longitudinal flow cytometric analysis was performed for all available samples at the same time.

Flow cytometry

For cell surface staining, the following fluorochrome-conjugated monoclonal antibodies were used CD3(UCHT1), CD4(13B8.2), CD8(B9.11), CD19(J3-119), CD24(ALB9), CD38(LS198-4-3), CD45(J.33), CD45RO(UCHL1), CD127(R34.34) and IgD(IADB6) (all from Beckman-Coulter, Mijdrecht, The Netherlands), CD25(M-A251), CCR4(1G1), CCR6(11A9) and CXCR3(1C6/CXR3) (BD Biosciences, Erembodegem, Belgium), and BAFF-R(11C1) (BioLegend, Uithoorn, The Netherlands). Intracellular analysis of IL-2(MQ1-17H12) (BD Biosciences), IL-4(8D4-8), IL-17(EBIO64CAP17), IFNγ(4S.B3) (eBioscience, San Diego, CA, USA), and TNFα(Mab11) (Dako, Glostrup, Denmark) was performed after fixation and permeabilization, using Fix and Perm reagent (eBioscience). Before intracellular cytokine measurement, the cells were stimulated for 4 hours with PMA (12.5 ng/ml), ionomycin (500 ng/ml) and Brefeldin A (5 µg/ml; Sigma-Aldrich, Zwijndrecht, The Netherlands).

The cell phenotype was analyzed by five-color (FC500) or ten-color flow cytometry (Navios), and data were analyzed using Kaluza software (all from Beckman-Coulter). Isotype controls or unstained cells were used for gate settings. Cell populations >0.1% of the CD45$^+$ lymphocyte population with a threshold of more than 50 cells were considered reliable.

Statistical analysis

Continuous data are expressed as box plots displaying the median, 25th and 75th percentiles as the box, and the 5th and 95th percentiles as whiskers. Wilcoxon signed rank test was used to test differences between each follow-up and pre-transplantation value within the triple immunosuppression-treated group. Statistical testing between RTX- and placebo-treated patients was performed according to distribution and type of data (unpaired T test, Mann-Whitney U, or Fisher's exact tests). P<0.05 was considered statistically significant. Statistical analysis was performed using GraphPad Prism 5.03 (GraphPad Software Inc., La Jolla, CA, USA).

Results

Phenotype and function of T cells in renal transplant recipients after treatment with tacrolimus, MMF and steroids

CD4$^+$ and CD8$^+$ T cells can be divided into naive, central and effector memory, and highly differentiated memory cells based on

Table 1. Patient characteristics.

	Triple IS	Triple IS + rituximab	P
N	14	12	
Median age at Tx, years (range)	50 (20–73)	57 (25–66)	0.440
Sex, no. male (%)	11 (79%)	7 (58%)	0.401
Type of dialysis			0.446
- Hemodialysis	6	5	
- Peritoneal dialysis	2	4	
- None	6	3	
Median PRA, % (range)	0 (0–58)	0 (0–10)	0.852
Living donor, no. (%)	13 (93%)	8 (67%)	0.217
HLA mismatches total, median (range)	4 (2–6)	3 (1–5)	0.224

IS: immunosuppression.

CD27 and CD45RO expression. [15]. The absolute numbers of $CD4^+$ and $CD8^+$ T cells in peripheral blood did not change during the use of triple drug immunosuppression after transplantation (Figure 1A–C). However, the percentages of central memory (T_{CM}; $CD27^+CD45RO^+$) $CD4^+$ and $CD8^+$ T cells were significantly higher at 3 months after transplantation compared to before transplantation, while the percentages of effector memory (T_{EM}; $CD27^-CD45RO^+$) $CD4^+$ and $CD8^+$ T cells, and regulatory (T_{REGS}; $CD25^{hi}FOXP3^+$) $CD4^+$ T cells were significantly decreased. The percentages of naive (T_N; $CD27^+CD45RO^-$) and highly differentiated memory (T_{EMRA}; $CD27^-CD45RO^-$) $CD4^+$ and $CD8^+$ T cells were comparable to pre-transplant levels. Next to the T-cell subset distribution, the ratio between memory and regulatory T cells might be an important determinant of the risk of rejection [16]. Interestingly, the $CD4^+$ T_{CM}/$CD4^+$ T_{REGS} ratio significantly increased from 3 months after transplantation and remained elevated compared to the pre-transplant ratio (Figure 1D). The $CD4^+$ T_{EM}/$CD4^+$ T_{REGS} ratio after transplantation was comparable to pre-transplant levels. Finally, we determined the expression of chemokine receptors associated with T helper (Th) 1 (CXCR3), Th2 (CCR4), and Th17 (CCR6) cells (Figure 1E). The percentage of $CXCR3^+$ and $CCR6^+$ $CD4^+$ T cells increased during immunosuppressive treatment, whereas triple drug immunosuppression did not affect the percentage of $CCR4^+$ $CD4^+$ T cells.

Although triple drug immunosuppression had minimal effects on the phenotype of peripheral T cells, this did not preclude an effect on functional capacities. To assess the cytokine producing capacity of circulating T cells, PBMCs were *ex vivo* stimulated for 4 hours with PMA, ionomycin and Brefeldin A. Effector cytokine production was assessed using intracellular cytokine staining in both $CD4^+$ and $CD8^+$ T cells. The percentage of IL-2, IL-4, IL-17, and TNFα producing $CD4^+$ cells decreased at 3 months after transplantation compared to pre-transplant levels. Hereafter, the production of all cytokines but TNFα returned to baseline levels within 24 months after transplantation (Figure 2). Ex vivo IFNγ production was not affected by triple drug immunosuppression, nor was cytokine producing capacity of $CD8^+$ T cells. Taken together, within the T-cell compartment, the most notable changes were found in the effector $CD4^+$ T-cell pool.

Under treatment with tacrolimus, MMF and steroids, renal transplant recipients develop a memory-like B-cell phenotype

During immunosuppressive treatment, the absolute B-cell numbers in peripheral blood were comparable to pre-transplant levels up to 24 months after transplantation (Figure 3A). To define whether the composition of the peripheral B-cell compartment was affected, we characterized $CD19^+$ B cells using the Bm1-Bm5 classification [17]. Compared to pre-transplant levels, the percentages of naive Bm2 (IgD^+CD38^+) and transitional Bm2' (IgD^+CD38^{++}) $CD19^+$ cells were lower, and the percentage of late memory Bm5 (IgD^-CD38^-) cells was higher after transplantation (Figure 3B–C). This shift to a more memory-like phenotype was accompanied by an increase in the percentage of virgin naive Bm1 cells, probably needed for B-cell renewal. Accordingly, using an alternative terminology for B cells, the percentages of transitional $CD24^{++}CD38^{++}$, mature $CD24^+CD38^+$, and naive IgD^+CD27^- B cells were decreased, while there was a relative increase in $CD24^{++}CD38^-$ memory and IgD^-CD27^+ switched memory B cells (Figure S2). At 12 and 24 months after transplantation, there was a higher percentage of $CD80^+$ and $CD95^+$ B cells as compared to before transplantation, supporting the more complete differentiation towards memory cells within the B-cell compartment (Figure 3D). The majority of B cells remained positive for B-cell activating factor receptor (BAFF-R) after transplantation. Interestingly, the expression level of BAFF-R increased after transplantation, as documented by an increase in median fluorescence intensity (MFI; Figure 3E–F). Overall, renal transplant recipients treated with tacrolimus, MMF and steroids developed a more memory-like B-cell phenotype.

A single dose of RTX results in a long lasting B-cell depletion in peripheral blood without affecting the T-cell compartment

The participation of renal transplant recipients in a randomized double-blind placebo-controlled study evaluating the efficacy and safety of RTX when added to triple drug immunosuppression gave us the opportunity to study the effects of additional B-cell depletion on the phenotype and function of T and B cells. RTX treatment resulted in a nearly complete depletion of B cells from the peripheral lymphocyte population up to 12 months after transplantation. Remarkably, the B-cell depletion after a single dose of RTX was long lasting. The absolute numbers of B cells

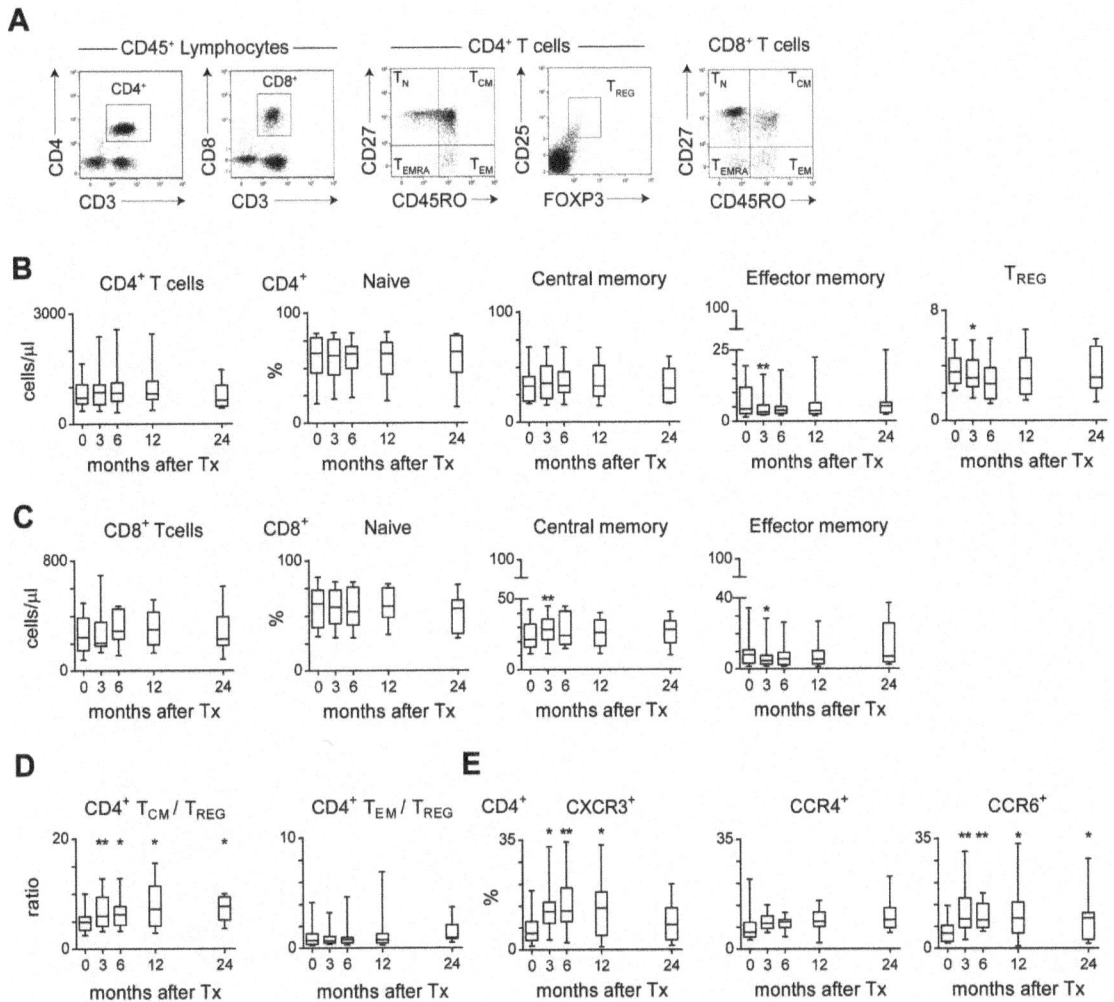

Figure 1. Subset distribution of circulating T cells in renal transplant recipients after treatment with tacrolimus, MMF and steroids over time. (A) Representative dot plots for a renal transplant recipient showing $CD3^+CD4^+$ and $CD3^+CD8^+$ T cells within the $CD45^+$ lymphocyte population. Circulating $CD4^+$ and $CD8^+$ T cells can be characterized as naive (T_N; $CD27^+CD45RO^-$), central memory (T_{CM}; $CD27^+CD45RO^+$), effector memory (T_{EM}; $CD27^-CD45RO^+$) and highly differentiated memory (T_{EMRA}; $CD27^+CD45RO^-$) cells. Furthermore, $CD4^+$ T cells can be characterized as regulatory T cells (T_{REGS}; $CD25^{hi}FOXP3^+$). (B) Shown are the absolute numbers of $CD4^+$ T cells and the percentages of T_N, T_{CM} and T_{EM} within the $CD4^+$ T-cell population for 14 triple immunosuppression-treated patients before transplantation (t=0) and at 3, 6, 12 and 24 months after transplantation (n=10 at 24 m). (C) As described under B, for $CD8^+$ T cells. (D) The ratio between the percentage of $CD4^+$ T_{CM} or T_{EM} and the percentage of T_{REGS}. (E) Longitudinal analysis of the percentages of $CXCR3^+$, $CCR4^+$, and $CCR6^+$ cells within the $CD4^+$ T-cell population of 14 triple immunosuppression-treated patients (n=10 at 24 m). Results are shown as box plots displaying the median, 25th and 75th percentiles as the box, and the 5th and 95th percentiles as whiskers. Significant differences are indicated compared to pre-transplant levels: *$P<0.05$, **$P<0.01$.

remained quite low at 24 months after RTX treatment with a median of 9.7 B cells/μl (range 3.0–294.8) compared to a median of 116.4 B cells/μl (range 49.7–379.7) in patients not treated with RTX (Figure 4A–B). Interestingly, at 12 months the percentage of Bm2' ($IgD^{++}CD38^{++}$) and Bm3+4 (IgD^-CD38^{++}) cells was significantly higher in RTX-treated patients, while the percentages of Bm1 (IgD^+CD38^-) and Bm2 (IgD^+CD38^+) cells were lower in RTX-treated patients. (Figure 4C). Accordingly, the percentages of $CD24^{++}CD38^{++}$ transitional and IgD^-CD27^+ switched memory B cells were higher in RTX-treated patients, while the percentages of IgD^+CD27^- naïve B cells were lower in RTX-treated patients (Figure S3A). Fitting with the relative increase of Bm3+4 (IgD^-CD38^{++}) cells, there was an increase in the percentage of $CD80^+$ and $CD95^+$ B cells at 12 and/or 24 months after transplantation (Figure 4D). Remarkably, the percentage of $BAFF-R^+$ B cells was lower in RTX-treated patients at 3 and 12

months after transplantation. In addition, the BAFF-R expression (MFI) on B cells of RTX-treated patients was lower up to 24 months after transplantation (Figure 4D).

Next, we analyzed whether the long-lasting B-cell depletion with a relative increase of transitional B cells resulted in changes in the T-cell compartment. There was no significant effect of RTX treatment on the absolute numbers and percentages of $CD4^+$ and $CD8^+$ T cells or on the subset distribution and phenotype of these cells (Figure S3B). In addition, *in vivo* B-cell depletion with RTX had no effect on the production of IL-2, IL-4, IL-17, IFNγ and TNFα by *ex vivo* stimulated T cells (Figure S3C).

Discussion

Despite the extensive clinical experience with currently used immunosuppressive drug regimens, there are limited data

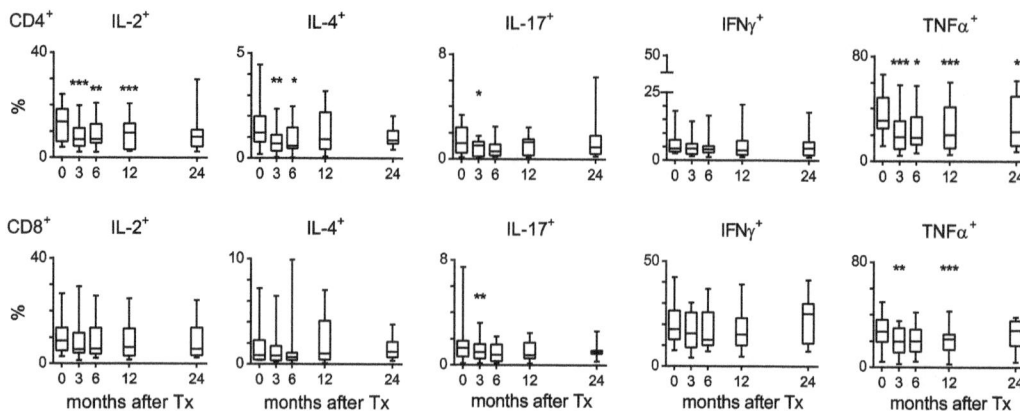

Figure 2. *Ex vivo* **cytokine production by circulating T cells in renal transplant recipients after treatment with tacrolimus, MMF and steroids.** Peripheral blood mononuclear cells (PBMCs) were stimulated for 4 hours in the presence of PMA, ionomycin and Brefeldin A. Shown are the percentages IL-2, IL-4, IL-17, IFNγ or TNFα-producing cells within the $CD4^+$ or $CD8^+$ T-cell population of 14 triple immunosuppression-treated patients before transplantation (t = 0) and at 3, 6, 12, and 24 months after transplantation (n = 10 at 24 m). Results are shown as box plots displaying the median, 25th and 75th percentiles as the box, and the 5th and 95th percentiles as whiskers. Significant differences are indicated compared to pre-transplant levels: *$P<0.05$, **$P<0.01$, ***$P<0.001$.

available regarding their effects on the peripheral lymphocyte compartment after kidney transplantation. One study describes the effects of cyclosporine, MMF, steroids, and anti-CD25

monoclonal antibody therapy on T and B cells of mainly CMV seropositive renal transplant recipients at 6, 24, and 60 months after transplantation [18]. This therapy resulted in an increased

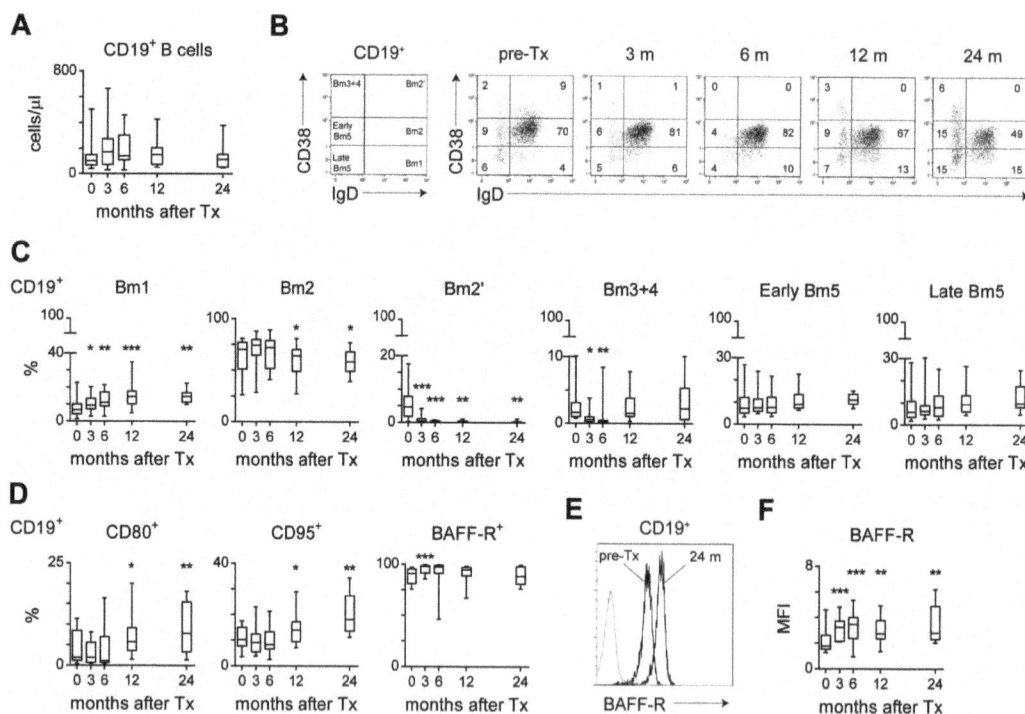

Figure 3. Longitudinal analysis of circulating B cells in renal transplant recipients after treatment with tacrolimus, MMF and steroids. (A) Shown are the absolute numbers of $CD19^+$ B cells of 14 triple immunosuppression-treated patients before transplantation (t = 0) and at 3, 6, 12, and 24 months after transplantation (n = 10 at 24 m). (B) Representative dot plots for a renal transplant recipient over time using the Bm1-Bm5 classification: Bm1 (IgD^+CD38^-), Bm2 (IgD^+CD38^+), Bm2' (IgD^+CD38^{++}), Bm3+4 (IgD^-CD38^{++}), Early Bm5 (IgD^-CD38^+) and Late Bm5 (IgD^-CD38^-) cells within the $CD19^+$ B-cell population. (C) Shown are the percentages of the different B-cell subsets using the Bm1-Bm5 classification over time. (D) Shown are the percentages of $CD80^+$, $CD95^+$, and BAFF-receptor$^+$ (BAFF-R) cells within the $CD19^+$ B-cell population. (E) Overlay plot of the BAFF-R expression (MFI: median fluorescence intensity) within the $CD19^+$ B-cell population of one patient before transplantation (pre-Tx) and 24 months (24 m) after transplantation under treatment with tacrolimus, MMF and steroids. Gray line shows unstained cells. (F) Summary graph showing the BAFF-R MFI of 14 triple immunosuppression-treated patients before over time (n = 10 at 24 m). Results are shown as box plots displaying the median, 25th and 75th percentiles as the box, and the 5th and 95th percentiles as whiskers. Significant differences are indicated compared to pre-transplant (pre-Tx; t = 0) levels: *$P<0.05$, **$P<0.01$, ***$P<0.001$.

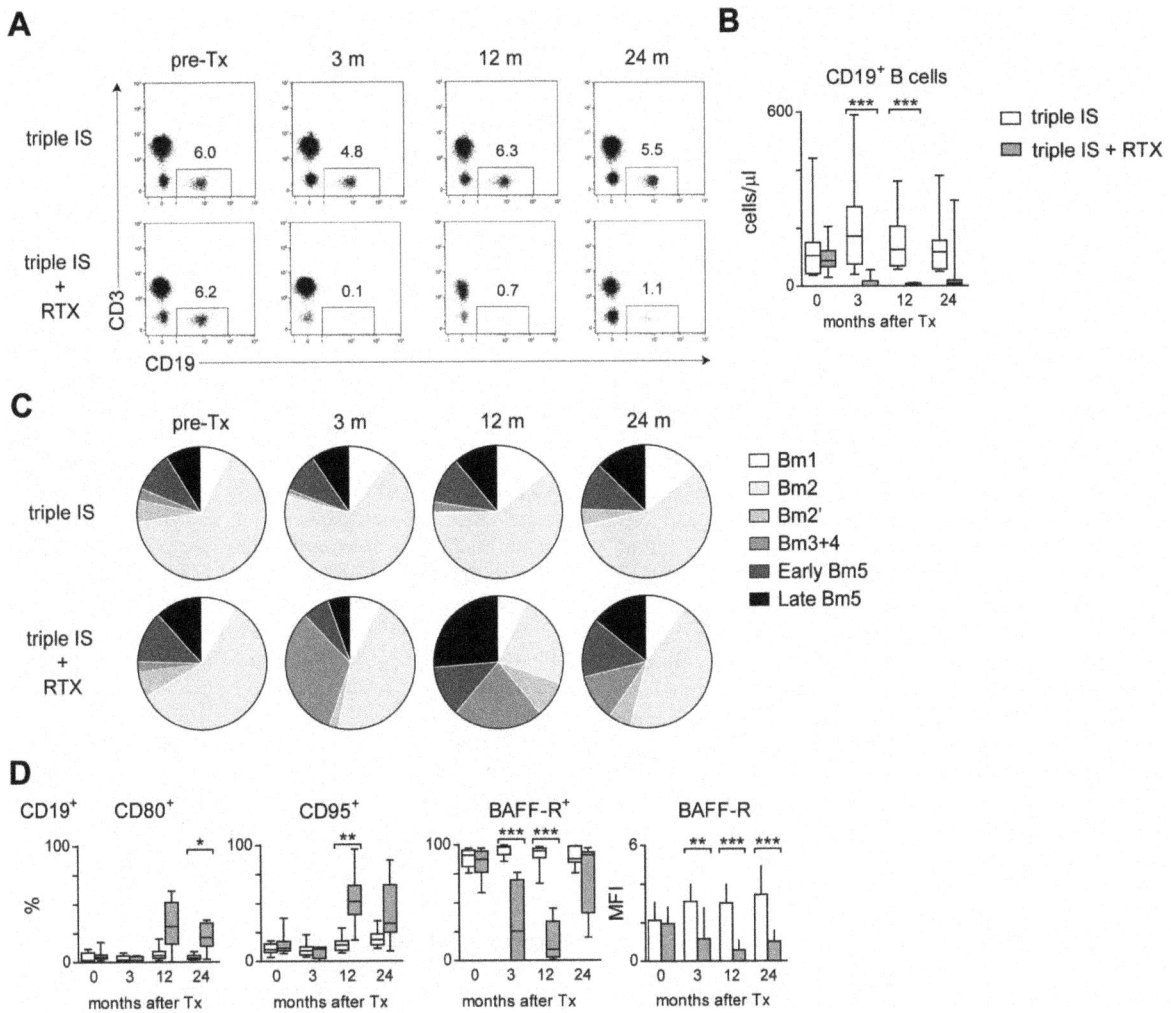

Figure 4. Longitudinal analysis of circulating B cells in renal transplant recipients after treatment with tacrolimus, MMF and steroids, and a single dose of rituximab (RTX) during transplant surgery. (A) Representative dot plots of CD19+ B cells within the CD45+ lymphocyte population for a RTX-treated and a triple immunosuppression (IS)-treated patient before transplantation (pre-Tx) and at 3, 12, and 24 months after transplantation. (B) Shown are the absolute numbers of CD19+ B cells for RTX-(gray, n = 12) and triple IS-treated (white, n = 14) patients before transplantation (t = 0) and up to 24 months after transplantation (n = 10 and n = 9 at t = 24 m, respectively). (C) Pie charts depicting the distribution the different B cells subsets over time using the Bm1-Bm5 classification as depicted in Figure 3B: Bm1 (IgD+CD38−), Bm2 (IgD+CD38+), Bm2' (IgD+CD38++), Bm3+4 (IgD−CD38++), Early Bm5 (IgD−CD38+) and Late Bm5 (IgD−CD38−) cells within the CD19+ B-cell population. Data are represented as means of 14 triple IS+RTX-treated and 12 IS-treated patients before transplantation (pre-Tx) and at 3, 12, and 24 months after transplantation (n = 10 and n = 9 at t = 24 m, respectively). (D) Shown are the percentages of CD80+, CD95+ and BAFF-R+ cells within the CD19+ B-cell population for RTX- (gray, n = 12) and triple IS-treated (white, n = 14) patients before transplantation (t = 0) and up to 24 months after transplantation. Results are shown as box plots displaying the median, 25th and 75th percentiles as the box, and the 5th and 95th percentiles as whiskers. Significant differences are indicated by asterisks: **P<0.01.

percentage of CD4+CD25+ T_{REGS} and CD27+ memory B cells in renal transplant recipients compared to healthy donors [18], but the data were not compared with pre-transplant levels. In contrast, we performed a longitudinal analysis of T- and B-cell phenotype and function in CMV seronegative patients who received a kidney from a CMV seronegative donor and did not experience a rejection episode up to 24 months after transplantation. In this homogeneous patient population, not affected by major immunological events, we showed that treatment with the combination of tacrolimus, MMF and steroids had no effects on the total number of T and B cells. Nevertheless, these patients had a higher proportion of central memory CD4+ and CD8+ T cells at 3 months after transplantation compared to pre-transplant levels. Interestingly, the triple drug immunosuppression resulted in a shift

toward a more memory-like phenotype in the B-cell population. Addition of a single dose of RTX resulted not only in a long-lasting B-cell depletion, but also in a higher percentage of transitional B cells upon B-cell recovery at 12 months post-transplant. The additional RTX treatment had no effect on the T-cell phenotype.

Although tacrolimus, MMF, and steroids mainly target T-cell activation, proliferation, and differentiation [3,19], we found that treatment with a combination of tacrolimus, MMF, and steroids, induced only marginal changes in the peripheral T-cell phenotype. These changes were mainly present within the first 6 months after transplantation, which suggests a role for MMF, as this drug was discontinued at 6 months after transplantation. *Ex vivo*, the T cells collected from patients treated with triple immunosuppressive therapy were functional, suggesting that they are only suppressed when the drug is present (during treatment). In addition, we found that the ratio between CD4+ central memory and T_{REGS} was increased under triple drug immunosuppressive therapy. Concomitantly, we observed a relative increase of CXCR3+ and CCR6+ CD4+ T cells, chemokine receptors associated with memory or activated Th1 and Th17 cells, respectively. This expression enables them to migrate toward inflammatory sites that express their cognate chemokines [20], such as observed in the graft during rejection [21] and on activated human primary tubular epithelial cells [22].

With respect to B cells, mycophenolic acid, but not tacrolimus, has been shown to inhibit the proliferation and immunoglobulin production *in vitro* [23]. However, in patients with systemic lupus erythematosus who were treated with MMF, the number and phenotype of B cells were similar to that in controls without immunosuppressive therapy [24]. In our cohort, discontinuation of MMF at 6 months after transplantation resulted in a relative increase of virgin naive Bm1 cells, while naive Bm2 cells were decreased compared to pre-transplant levels. Transitional Bm2 cells remained low up to 24 months after transplantation, suggesting that their development is mainly suppressed by treatment with tacrolimus and/or steroids. Finally, following the discontinuation of MMF, the percentage of memory B cells became comparable to levels before transplantation. Steroids were also found to have clear effects on B cells; *ex vivo* immunoglobulin production by PBMC was decreased during treatment with a high dose of prednisolone (60 mg) while a lower dose (30 mg) resulted in an increased production after stimulation [25]. Others have described that steroids have an effect on B-cell activation, while proliferation and activation are less affected [26]. Under combined treatment with tacrolimus, MMF, and steroids, our renal transplant recipients had a more memory-like B-cell phenotype compared to before transplantation. This relative increase of memory B cells was also found in a patient cohort treated with cyclosporine, MMF, steroids, and an anti-CD25 monoclonal antibody [18]. The observed memory-like B-cell phenotype was accompanied by an increased percentage of CD80+ and CD95+ B cells, which may be explained by the preferential expression of these molecules on memory-like B cells [17].

Treatment with RTX provides a highly efficient means for the (temporary) depletion of B cells, with potential suppression of B cell-associated anti-graft responses. Adding a single dose of RTX to the combination of tacrolimus, MMF, and steroids in our patients indeed resulted in a long lasting B-cell depletion in peripheral blood. A remarkable characteristic of the returning B cells was a decreased expression of the receptor for B-cell activating factor (BAFF), an essential growth factor for B cells [27]. The decreased percentage of BAFF-R+ B cells after RTX treatment, which was also found in patients with rheumatoid arthritis [28] may be due to a relative increase of memory-like B cells, which have lower or no BAFF-R expression [27]. In addition, treatment with B-cell depleting agents has previously been shown to elevate BAFF levels [29–31], and increased BAFF levels in turn were inversely correlated with BAFF-R expression during B-cell repopulation [30,32]. Another interesting observation was an increase in the percentage of transitional B cells at 12 months after treatment with RTX compared to triple immunosuppression therapy alone. Interestingly, BAFF-R deficiency in patients with common variable immunodeficiency (CVID) was associated with B-cell lymphopenia and a relative increase in the number of transitional B cells [33]. Taken together, an increase in BAFF level, reduced BAFF-R expression, and an increase in the

proportion of transitional B cells appear to be interrelated phenomena which are associated with RTX treatment.

Upon activation, B cells are able to proliferate, produce various cytokines and process antigen for presentation to T cells [34–36]. Previously, we showed that *in vitro* RTX treatment can affect B-cell phenotype and function, resulting in an altered outcome of B-T-cell interaction upon stimulation [37]. However, in contrast, we did not observe any changes in the T-cell compartment in our patients treated with RTX. In another *ex vivo* study, we neither were able to show that RTX influenced the production of IL-17 and other monocyte- and T-cell-derived cytokines by PBMCs [38]. It should be noted however that we only analyzed peripheral blood T cells. From a previous study in renal transplant patients, we know that a single dose of RTX leads a to nearly complete B-cell depletion in peripheral blood, but not in secondary lymphoid organs, and that these remaining B cells have different functional capacities [39]. From our current data, it seems that this population of mostly memory type B cells residing in lymphoid organs does not noticeably affect the peripheral blood T-cell compartment as compared to transplant recipients on triple immunosuppression without RTX. Interestingly, several studies on patients with autoimmune disease revealed that the T-cell compartment was affected upon RTX treatment [12,40,41]. However, in most of these patients the cumulative dose of RTX was higher than in our patients, who received only a single, relatively low dose [40].

In summary, we have demonstrated that treatment of renal transplant recipients with tacrolimus, MMF and steroids leads to alterations in the T- and B-cell compartments. This detailed longitudinal analysis provides more insight into the immune status of renal transplant recipients with stable graft function and may be used as a reference in the monitoring of renal transplant patients.

Supporting Information

Figure S1 Patient selection for the side study of the clinical trial. CMV, Cytomegalovirus; D, donor; R, recipient.

Figure S2 Longitudinal analysis of circulating B cells in renal transplant recipients after treatment with tacrolimus, MMF and steroids. Shown are the percentages of transitional CD24++CD38++, mature CD24+CD38+, memory CD24++CD38−, naive IgD+CD27− and switched memory IgD+CD27− B cells within the CD19+ B-cell population. Results are shown as box plots displaying the median, 25th and 75th percentiles as the box, and the 5th and 95th percentiles as whiskers. Significant differences are indicated compared to pre-transplant (t = 0) levels: *P<0.05, **P<0.01, ***P<0.001.

Figure S3 Longitudinal analysis of circulating B and T cells in renal transplant recipients after treatment with tacrolimus, MMF and steroids, and a single dose of rituximab (RTX) during transplant surgery. (A) Shown are the percentages of transitional CD24++CD38++, naive IgD+CD27− and switched memory IgD+CD27− B cells within the CD19+ B-cell population for RTX- (gray, n = 14) and triple IS-treated (white, n = 12) patients before transplantation (t = 0) and up to 24 months after transplantation (n = 10 and n = 9 at t = 24 m, respectively). (B) The percentage of regulatory T cells (T_{REGS}; CD25hiCD127lo), central memory (T_{CM}; CD27+CD45RO+), effector memory (T_{EM}; CD27−CD45RO+), CXCR3+ and CCR6+ within the CD4+ T-cell population in

RTX- (gray, n = 12) and triple IS-treated (white, n = 14) patients before transplantation (t = 0) and up to 24 months after transplantation (n = 10 and n = 9 at t = 24 m, respectively). (C) Peripheral blood mononuclear cells (PBMCs) were stimulated for 4 hours in the presence of PMA, ionomycin and Brefeldin A. Shown are the percentages IL-2, IL-4, IL-17, IFNγ or TNFα-producing cells within the CD4$^+$ T-cell population in RTX- (gray, n = 12) and triple IS-treated (white, n = 14) patients before transplantation (t = 0) and up to 24 months after transplantation (n = 10 and n = 9 at t = 24 m, respectively). Results are shown as box plots displaying the median, 25th and 75th percentiles as the box, and the 5th and

95th percentiles as whiskers. Significant differences are indicated by asterisks: **$P < 0.01$.

Author Contributions

Conceived and designed the experiments: EGK HJPMK MWFvdH MCB IJ LBH. Performed the experiments: EGK. Analyzed the data: EGK HJPMK MCB IJ LBH. Contributed to the writing of the manuscript: EGK HJPMK MCB IJ LBH. Provided patient data: MWFvdH LBH.

References

1. Chapman JR, O'Connell PJ, Nankivell BJ (2005) Chronic renal allograft dysfunction. J Am Soc Nephrol 16: 3015–3026.
2. Safinia N, Afzali B, Atalar K, Lombardi G, Lechler RI (2010) T-cell alloimmunity and chronic allograft dysfunction. Kidney International 78 Suppl 119: S2–12.
3. Kahan BD (2003) Individuality: the barrier to optimal immunosuppression. Nat Rev Immunol 3: 831–838.
4. Wood KJ, Bushell A, Hester J (2012) Regulatory immune cells in transplantation. Nat Rev Immunol 12: 417–430.
5. Kreijveld E, Koenen HJ, van Cranenbroek B, van Rijssen E, Joosten I, et al. (2008) Immunological monitoring of renal transplant recipients to predict acute allograft rejection following the discontinuation of tacrolimus. PLoS One 3: e2711.
6. Zarkhin V, Chalasani G, Sarwal MM (2010) The yin and yang of B cells in graft rejection and tolerance. TransplantRev(Orlando) 24: 67–78.
7. Hippen BE, DeMattos A, Cook WJ, Kew CE, Gaston RS (2005) Association of CD20+ infiltrates with poorer clinical outcomes in acute cellular rejection of renal allografts. Am J Transplant 5: 2248–2252.
8. Zarkhin V, Kambham N, Li L, Kwok S, Hsieh SC, et al. (2008) Characterization of intra-graft B cells during renal allograft rejection. Kidney International 74: 664–673.
9. Otten HG, Verhaar MC, Borst HP, Hene RJ, van Zuilen AD (2012) Pretransplant donor-specific HLA class-I and -II antibodies are associated with an increased risk for kidney graft failure. Am J Transplant 12: 1618–1623.
10. Jordan SC, Kahwaji J, Toyoda M, Vo A (2011) B-cell immunotherapeutics: emerging roles in solid organ transplantation. Curr Opin Organ Transplant 16: 416–424.
11. Thurlings RM, Vos K, Wijbrandts CA, Zwinderman AH, Gerlag DM, et al. (2008) Synovial tissue response to rituximab: mechanism of action and identification of biomarkers of response. Annals of the Rheumatic Diseases 67: 917–925.
12. Bar-Or A, Fawaz L, Fan B, Darlington PJ, Rieger A, et al. (2010) Abnormal B-cell cytokine responses a trigger of T-cell-mediated disease in MS? Annals of Neurology 67: 452–461.
13. Piccio L, Naismith RT, Trinkaus K, Klein RS, Parks BJ, et al. (2010) Changes in B- and T-lymphocyte and chemokine levels with rituximab treatment in multiple sclerosis. Archives of Neurology 67: 707–714.
14. Vigna-Perez M, Hernandez-Castro B, Paredes-Saharopulos O, Portales-Perez D, Baranda L, et al. (2006) Clinical and immunological effects of Rituximab in patients with lupus nephritis refractory to conventional therapy: a pilot study. Arthritis Res Ther 8: R83.
15. Sallusto F, Geginat J, Lanzavecchia A (2004) Central memory and effector memory T cell subsets: function, generation, and maintenance. Annu Rev Immunol 22: 745–763.
16. Lechler RI, Garden OA, Turka LA (2003) The complementary roles of deletion and regulation in transplantation tolerance. NatRevImmunol 3: 147–158.
17. Bohnhorst JO, Bjorgan MB, Thoen JE, Natvig JB, Thompson KM (2001) Bm1-Bm5 classification of peripheral blood B cells reveals circulating germinal center founder cells in healthy individuals and disturbance in the B cell subpopulations in patients with primary Sjogren's syndrome. JImmunol 167: 3610–3618.
18. van de Berg PJ, Hoevenaars EC, Yong SL, van Donselaar-van de Pant KA, van Tellingen A, et al. (2012) Circulating lymphocyte subsets in different clinical situations after renal transplantation. Immunology 136: 198–207.
19. Koenen HJ, Michielsen EC, Verstappen J, Fasse E, Joosten I (2003) Superior T-cell suppression by rapamycin and FK506 over rapamycin and cyclosporine A because of abrogated cytotoxic T-lymphocyte induction, impaired memory responses, and persistent apoptosis. Transplantation 75: 1581–1590.
20. Sallusto F, Lanzavecchia A, Mackay CR (1998) Chemokines and chemokine receptors in T-cell priming and Th1/Th2-mediated responses. Immunology Today 19: 568–574.
21. Matz M, Beyer J, Wunsch D, Mashreghi MF, Seiler M, et al. (2006) Early post-transplant urinary IP-10 expression after kidney transplantation is predictive of short- and long-term graft function. Kidney Int 69: 1683–1690.
22. Demmers MW, Baan CC, van Beelen E, Ijzermans JN, Weimar W, et al. (2013) Differential effects of activated human renal epithelial cells on T-cell migration. PLoS One 8: e64916.
23. Heidt S, Roelen DL, Eijsink C, van Kooten C, Claas FH, et al. (2008) Effects of immunosuppressive drugs on purified human B cells: evidence supporting the use of MMF and rapamycin. Transplantation 86: 1292–1300.
24. Eickenberg S, Mickholz E, Jung E, Nofer JR, Pavenstadt HJ, et al. (2012) Mycophenolic acid counteracts B cell proliferation and plasmablast formation in patients with systemic lupus erythematosus. Arthritis Res Ther 14: R110.
25. Hanson RG, Peters MG, Hoofnagle JH (1986) Effects of immunosuppressive therapy with prednisolone on B and T lymphocyte function in patients with chronic type B hepatitis. Hepatology 6: 173–179.
26. Cupps TR, Gerrard TL, Falkoff RJ, Whalen G, Fauci AS (1985) Effects of in vitro corticosteroids on B cell activation, proliferation, and differentiation. J Clin Invest 75: 754–761.
27. Pieper K, Grimbacher B, Eibel H (2013) B-cell biology and development. J Allergy Clin Immunol 131: 959–971.
28. de ITI, Moura RA, Leandro MJ, Edwards J, Cambridge G (2010) B-cell-activating factor receptor expression on naive and memory B cells: relationship with relapse in patients with rheumatoid arthritis following B-cell depletion therapy. Annals of the Rheumatic Diseases 69: 2181–2188.
29. Vallerskog T, Heimburger M, Gunnarsson I, Zhou W, Wahren-Herlenius M, et al. (2006) Differential effects on BAFF and APRIL levels in rituximab-treated patients with systemic lupus erythematosus and rheumatoid arthritis. Arthritis Res Ther 8: R167.
30. Zarkhin V, Li L, Sarwal MM (2009) BAFF may modulate the rate of B-cell repopulation after rituximab therapy for acute renal transplant rejection. Transplantation 88: 1229–1230.
31. Bloom D, Chang Z, Pauly K, Kwun J, Fechner J, et al. (2009) BAFF is increased in renal transplant patients following treatment with alemtuzumab. AmJTransplant 9: 1835–1845.
32. Lehnhardt A, Dunst F, van Husen M, Loos S, Oh J, et al. (2012) Elevated serum levels of B-cell activating factor in pediatric renal transplant patients. Pediatr Nephrol 27: 1389–1395.
33. Warnatz K, Salzer U, Rizzi M, Fischer B, Gutenberger S, et al. (2009) B-cell activating factor receptor deficiency is associated with an adult-onset antibody deficiency syndrome in humans. Proc Natl Acad Sci U S A 106: 13945–13950.
34. Duddy ME, Alter A, Bar-Or A (2004) Distinct profiles of human B cell effector cytokines: a role in immune regulation? JImmunol 172: 3422–3427.
35. Harris DP, Haynes L, Sayles PC, Duso DK, Eaton SM, et al. (2000) Reciprocal regulation of polarized cytokine production by effector B and T cells. NatImmunol 1: 475–482.
36. Janeway CA, Jr., Ron J, Katz ME (1987) The B cell is the initiating antigen-presenting cell in peripheral lymph nodes. JImmunol 138: 1051–1055.
37. Kamburova EG, Koenen HJ, Boon L, Hilbrands LB, Joosten I (2012) In vitro effects of rituximab on the proliferation, activation and differentiation of human B cells. Am J Transplant 12: 341–350.
38. Smeekens SP, van den Hoogen MW, Kamburova EG, van de Veerdonk FL, Joosten I, et al. (2013) The effects of in vivo B-cell depleting therapy on ex-vivo cytokine production. Transpl Immunol 28: 183–188.
39. Kamburova EG, Koenen HJ, Borgman KJ, ten Berge IJ, Joosten I, et al. (2013) A single dose of rituximab does not deplete B cells in secondary lymphoid organs but alters phenotype and function. Am J Transplant 13: 1503–1511.
40. Iwata S, Saito K, Tokunaga M, Yamaoka K, Nawata M, et al. (2011) Phenotypic changes of lymphocytes in patients with systemic lupus erythematosus who are in longterm remission after B cell depletion therapy with rituximab. Journal of Rheumatology 38: 633–641.
41. Stasi R, Cooper N, Del Poeta G, Stipa E, Laura Evangelista M, et al. (2008) Analysis of regulatory T-cell changes in patients with idiopathic thrombocytopenic purpura receiving B cell-depleting therapy with rituximab. Blood 112: 1147–1150.

23

Fingolimod Increases CD39-Expressing Regulatory T Cells in Multiple Sclerosis Patients

Nathalie Muls[1], Hong Anh Dang[1], Christian J. M. Sindic[1,2], Vincent van Pesch[1,2]*

1 Neurochemistry Unit, Institute of Neuroscience, Université catholique de Louvain, Brussels, Belgium, **2** Cliniques Universitaires Saint-Luc, Brussels, Belgium

Abstract

Background: Multiple sclerosis (MS) likely results from an imbalance between regulatory and inflammatory immune processes. CD39 is an ectoenzyme that cleaves ATP to AMP and has been suggested as a novel regulatory T cells (Treg) marker. As ATP has numerous proinflammatory effects, its degradation by CD39 has anti-inflammatory influence. The purpose of this study was to explore regulatory and inflammatory mechanisms activated in fingolimod treated MS patients.

Methods and Findings: Peripheral blood mononuclear cells (PBMCs) were isolated from relapsing-remitting MS patients before starting fingolimod and three months after therapy start. mRNA expression was assessed in *ex vivo* PBMCs. The proportions of CD8, B cells, CD4 and CD39-expressing cells were analysed by flow cytometry. Treg proportion was quantified by flow cytometry and methylation-specific qPCR. Fingolimod treatment increased mRNA levels of CD39, AHR and CYP1B1 but decreased mRNA expression of IL-17, IL-22 and FOXP3 mRNA in PBMCs. B cells, CD4$^+$ cells and Treg proportions were significantly reduced by this treatment, but remaining CD4$^+$ T cells were enriched in FOXP3$^+$ cells and in CD39-expressing Tregs.

Conclusions: In addition to the decrease in circulating CD4$^+$ T cells and CD19$^+$ B cells, our findings highlight additional immunoregulatory mechanisms induced by fingolimod.

Editor: Martin Sebastian Weber, Klinikum rechts der Isar der Technischen Universitaet Muenchen, Germany

Funding: This work was financially supported by the Fonds pour la formation à la Recherche dans l'Industrie et dans l'Agriculture, Bayer educational grants (www.fnrs.be/), the Belgian Charcot Foundation (www.fondation-charcot.org/) and the Walloon Region "Désordres Inflammatoires dans les Affections Neurologiques" project (http://recherche-technologie.wallonie.be/). The funders had no role in study design, data collection and analysis, decision to publish, or preparation of the manuscript.

Competing Interests: VvP has served on advisory boards for Biogen Idec, Novartis Pharma and Genzyme; has received travel grants and speaking honoraria from Biogen Idec, Bayer Schering, Teva, Sanofi Aventis, Merck Serono and Novartis Pharma. NM and HD have no competing interests. CS has received honoraria for consultancy, lectures, educational and research grants, from Bayer-Schering, Biogen Idec, GSK Biological Vaccines, Merck Serono, Novartis Pharma, Sanofi-Aventis and Teva.

* Email: vincent.vanpesch@uclouvain.be

Introduction

Multiple sclerosis (MS) is a chronic inflammatory disease of the central nervous system (CNS) characterized by demyelination and neurodegeneration. A key event in MS pathogenesis is the peripheral activation of autoreactive lymphocytes. These cells damage the blood-brain barrier (BBB), enter the CNS and cause local inflammation.

Disease-modifying treatments are designed to slow down disease progression by reducing the relapse rate and the accumulation of new lesions on MRI. Fingolimod (Gilenya, Novartis), a sphingosine analogue, was the first once-daily oral drug approved for the treatment of relapsing-remitting MS (RRMS). Both sphingosine and fingolimod are phosphorylated to their active forms by intracellular sphingosine kinases. Phosphorylated fingolimod (fingolimod-P) mimics the activity of sphingosine-1-phosphate (S1P) and acts as an agonist on 4 out of its 5 receptors [1]. Thanks to their S1P receptors, acting as sensors, lymphocytes follow the S1P gradient to exit secondary lymphoid organs and reach the blood flow. Prolonged binding of fingolimod-P to its receptors induces their internalization and degradation [2]. Fingolimod therefore reversibly retains most lymphocytes subsets within the lymph nodes. In MS patients, fingolimod reduces the proportion of pro-inflammatory T helper (Th) cells producing interleukin-17 (IL-17), in the circulating blood [3]. The effects of fingolimod on T regulatory cells (Tregs) are still incompletely described. Animal studies have shown that fingolimod induces the conversion of CD4$^+$FOXP3$^-$ cells into CD4$^+$FOXP3$^+$ cells [4,5]. In contrast, one report supports that fingolimod decreases the immunosuppressive activity of Tregs in the context of graft-versus-host disease [6].

CD4$^+$CD25^{hi}FOXP3$^+$ regulatory T cells are a subset of cells specialized in the suppression of activation and proliferation of effector T cells. Therefore, this subset is of particular importance in limiting autoimmunity. Tregs are characterized by the expression of the cellular marker CD25 and the transcription factor FOXP3. However, in humans, these two markers are not specific for Tregs as they are also expressed on effector T cells after stimulation. Therefore, it remains uneasy to distinguish natural Tregs and recently activated T cells. Analysing the methylation status of the *FOXP3* locus might be of particular interest to quantify these cells. Indeed, the first intron of *FOXP3* (*FOXP3i1*) shows complete demethylation in natural Tregs (nTregs) [7]. CD39 is an immunoregulatory molecule expressed by effector/memory-like Tregs (T$_{REM}$) that decreases the extracellular level of ATP, converting it into AMP [8]. Under certain conditions, its expression can be regulated by the transcription factor Aryl Hydrocarbon Receptor (AHR) [9]. CD39-expressing Tregs are of particular interest in MS as they have been shown to specifically inhibit Th17 cells [10].

The aim of our study was to investigate the effects of fingolimod on pro- and anti-inflammatory Th17- and Treg-related immune markers, by analysing their *ex vivo* expression profile in treated MS patients. We then analysed the effects of fingolimod therapy on the proportions of various cell subsets, notably of CD39-expressing cells.

Materials and Methods

Subjects and sample collection

Blood samples were obtained from 16 patients with RRMS before starting fingolimod therapy, and after 3 months of treatment (0.5 mg daily). The study was approved by the local ethics committee and written informed consent was obtained from all patients. Peripheral blood mononuclear cells (PBMCs) were also collected from ten age- and sex-matched healthy controls (HC). Basic demographic features are summarized in Table S1. All patients displayed the expected lymphocyte count reduction three months after starting fingolimod treatment.

Methylation Specific-qPCR (MethylS-qPCR) for FOXP3i1

Genomic DNA (gDNA) was prepared from frozen pellets containing 10^6 total PBMCs with the PureLink DNA Mini Kit (Invitrogen). One µg of gDNA was treated with sodium bisulfite using the EpiTect Plus DNA Bisulfite Kit (Qiagen). Real-Time PCR amplification of methylated and demethylated *FOXP3i1* sequences was performed in a final volume of 25 µl with the Rotor-Gene Probe PCR Kit (Qiagen), 300 nM of each primer and 100 mM of probe in a 72-well rotor on Rotor-Gene PCR 6000 Realtime Analyser (Corbett Life Science). Two-step thermal cycling was started with a first denaturation at 95°C for 3 minutes followed by 45 cycles at 95°C for 3 seconds and 64°C for 30 seconds. Sequences of primers and probes are indicated in Table S2. The percentage of demethylated sequences is calculated as follows: 2^(Ct methylated −Ct demethylated)/[2^(Ct methylated −Ct demethylated)+1]*100.

Fluorescence activated cell sorting (FACS)

Thawed PBMCs were resuspended in PBS with 1% foetal calf serum and 2 mM EDTA. Cells were stained for surface antigens with anti-human CD4 (eBioscience), CD8, CD19, CD39 and CD25 (BioLegend) antibodies, then fixed and permeabilized overnight prior to FOXP3 staining (clone 236A/E7, eBioscience). Lymphocytes were gated according to their FSC/SSC (forward/side scatter) profile. Median fluorescent intensity (MFI) was analysed on the FOXP3 channel for CD4$^+$ cells and on the CD39 channel for CD4$^+$CD25^{hi}FOXP3$^+$ cells. Acquisition was performed on a BD LSR Fortessa instrument (BD Biosciences). All data were analysed using FlowJo software (Tree Star Inc.). Conditions were assayed in duplicate.

cDNA analysis and qPCR experiments

RNA from PBMCs was isolated using the miRNeasy mini kit (Qiagen) according to the manufacturer's protocol and reverse transcribed to cDNA using Superscript Reverse Transcriptase

(Invitrogen). Quantitative PCR (qPCR) assays were performed using Absolute qPCR SYBR Green mix (Thermo Scientific) on a Rotor-Gene 6000 (Corbett Life Science). The relative amount of transcripts was determined by normalizing for Abelson gene (ABL) using the comparative Ct method ($2^{-\Delta\Delta C_t}$) [11]. Results are expressed relative to the mean of the healthy control patients (HC) set at 1. Sequences of primers are detailed in Table S3.

Statistical analysis

Statistical analysis was performed using the GraphPad Prism 5 software. To test for differences before and after ivMP treatment, a non-parametric Wilcoxon's signed rank test was performed. MS patients and HC were compared using the non-parametric Mann Whitney test. P-values ≤0.05 were considered as statistically significant.

Results

Ex vivo mRNA expressions of IL-17, IL-22, CD39, FOXP3, AHR and CYP1B are affected by fingolimod in PBMC

In comparison to HC, the only significant difference was an increase of CD39 mRNA level in MS patients (Figure 1). Indeed, median mRNA level was 70% higher in MS patients (p = 0.0002). The mRNA expression levels of CD39 (p = 0.0033), as well as of AHR (p = 0.007) and CYP1B1, an AHR-induced gene (p<0.0001) were increased after fingolimod treatment. On the contrary, fingolimod reduced the mRNA levels of IL-17, IL-22 and FOXP3. The most dramatic decrease was observed for IL-17 mRNA, which was undetectable after therapy in most patients (n = 11/16) (p = 0.024).

CD4$^+$ T and B cell proportions are reduced in circulating lymphoid cells after fingolimod treatment

As fingolimod inhibits the egress of lymphocytes from lymph nodes, we wanted to further quantify cellular subsets present in PBMCs. The proportion of B cells, characterised by the CD19 surface marker, was reduced by 50% with fingolimod treatment (p = 0.0012). Before therapy, CD19$^+$ B cells represented 11.45% of the circulating lymphoid cells. This proportion was reduced to 5.9% under treatment (Figure 2, Table 1). In contrast, the proportion of CD8$^+$ T cells did not show a significant decrease.

Fingolimod decreased the proportion of CD4$^+$ T cells by 7-fold (p = 0.0006) (Figure 2). Before treatment, CD4$^+$ T cells accounted for 46% of the circulating lymphoid cells, but only for 6.5% after three months of fingolimod therapy. In contrast, the proportion of FOXP3-expressing CD4$^+$ cells was increased in 12 out of 16 patients (p = 0.04, Figure 3A). This was associated with a median increase of 40% in the FOXP3 MFI values (p = 0.0005, Fig. 3B).

Regulatory T cells proportion is decreased in PBMCs after fingolimod treatment

As regulatory T cells play a central role in maintaining self-tolerance, we then analysed the Treg proportion within total PBMCs or CD4$^+$ T cells. Natural Tregs were quantified by analysing the epigenetic status of the first intron of *FOXP3* using methylation specific PCR (Figure 4A). CD4$^+$CD25^{hi}FOXP3$^+$ Treg phenotype was also examined by flow cytometry (Figure 4B). Using both MethylS-qPCR (p = 0.041) and flow cytometry (p = 0.0029), we showed that the proportion of Tregs among total PBMCs was decreased by the treatment. However, the proportion of CD25^{hi}Foxp3$^+$ Tregs within the CD4$^+$ cell population increased in 12 patients out of 16 (Figure 4C, Table 1). Only 3 patients displayed a reduction in their Treg proportion while on treatment

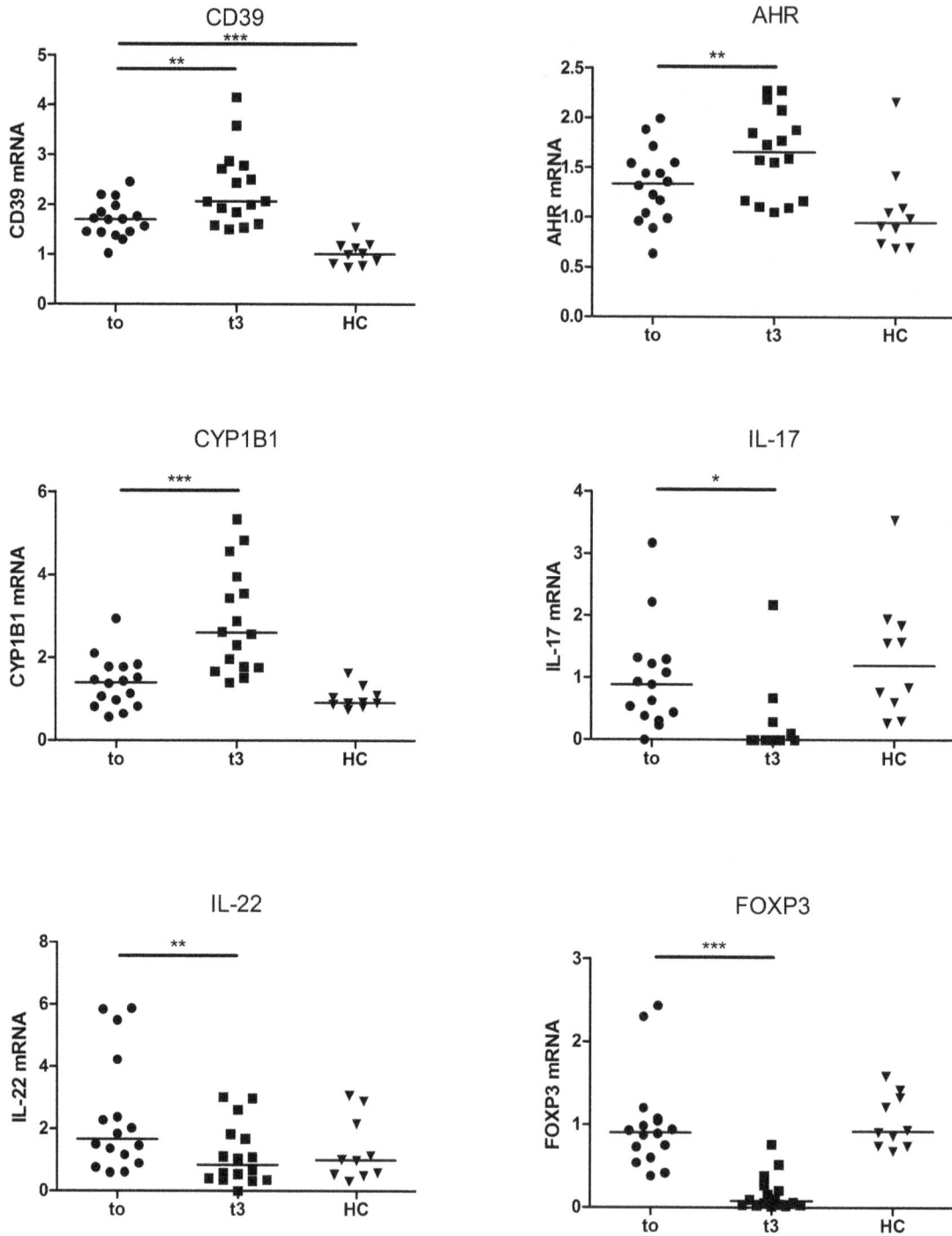

Figure 1. *Ex vivo* mRNA expression in total PBMCs from fingolimod-treated patients. Scatter dot plots show relative mRNA expression levels in PBMCs from MS patients before (t0) or after 3 months (t3) of treatment by fingolimod, and healthy controls (HC) analysed by q-PCR. For each target, individual mRNA levels were expressed as relative values to the mean level of the control group. The mRNA expression levels of CD39 (p = 0.0033), as well as of AHR (p = 0.007) and CYP1B1, an AHR-induced gene (p<0.0001) were increased after fingolimod treatment. On the contrary, fingolimod reduced the mRNA levels of IL-17, IL-22 and FOXP3. Horizontal lines represent the median value in all subgroups. *, ** and *** indicate p-values of <0.05, <0.01 and <0.001 respectively.

by fingolimod and one patient did not show change in this parameter.

CD39+ Tregs increase after fingolimod

CD39+ Tregs have been shown to specifically inhibit IL-17 producing cells. Since Th17 cells exert pathogenic effect in MS, we quantified CD39+ Tregs after treatment by fingolimod. The proportion of CD39-expressing CD4+CD25hiFOXP3+ Tregs was

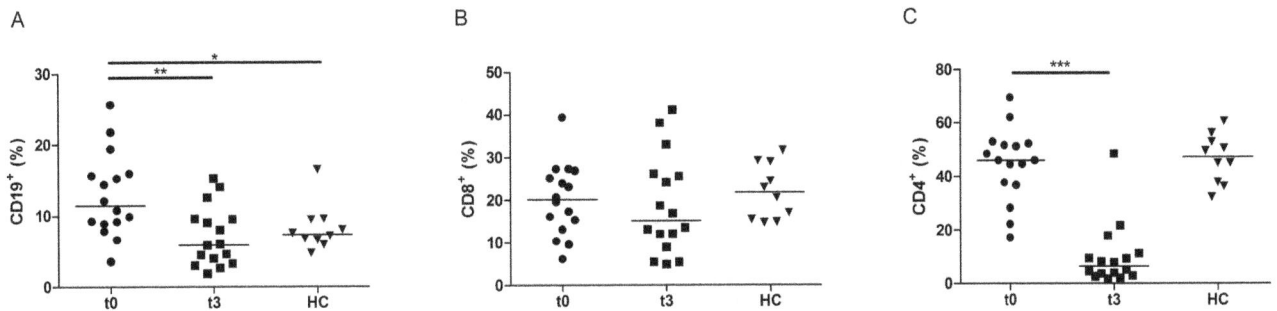

Figure 2. Circulating T and B cell proportions in patients treated by fingolimod. PBMCs of MS patients before (t0, n = 16) or after three months of treatment by fingolimod (t3, n = 16) and healthy controls (HC, n = 10) were analysed *ex vivo* by flow cytometry. The percentage of (A) CD19+ B cells, (B) CD8+ and (C) CD4+ T cells within lymphoid cells is shown. The proportion of B cells and CD4+ T cells decreased after fingolimod while the proportion of CD8+ T cells was not significantly modified. The horizontal lines represent the median value in all subgroups. *, ** and *** indicate p-values of ≤0.05, ≤0.01 and ≤0.001 respectively.

increased in MS patients in comparison to HC (43.4% *versus* 26.9%; p = 0.009). After three months of fingolimod treatment, the proportion of CD39+ Tregs further increased from 43.4% to 76.2%, representing a median increase of 77%. This was associated with an increase in the MFI of CD39 (Figure 5A and 5B and Table 1). The proportion of CD4+FOXP3−CD39+ cells was affected to a lesser extent after fingolimod treatment rising from 5.1% to 7.2% (median increase of 41%). On the contrary, within the CD8+ and CD19+ populations, the proportion of CD39+ cells and the CD39 MFI were not increased by the treatment (Figure S1).

Discussion

MS is a demyelinating disease of the CNS thought to be mediated in part by autoreactive lymphocytes. The role of proinflammatory responses in MS has been largely investigated and the implication of the Th17 lineage has been demonstrated in animal and human studies [12–14]. Fingolimod has been approved as a disease-modifying drug in the treatment of RRMS. Fingolimod may participate to various immunoregulatory processes other than lymphocytes retention as the S1P$_1$ signalling is involved in many other physiological responses [15].

Here, we show that fingolimod significantly reduces the mRNA level of IL-17 in total PBMCs. This result is in agreement with the finding that fingolimod decreases the amount of circulating IL-17 producing cells [3]. A similar effect is shown for IL-22. This IL-10

cytokine family member plays both protective and pathogenic roles in autoimmune diseases but its involvement in MS is still matter of debate. [16–18] IL-22 is not crucial in the development of the murine experimental model of MS [19]. However, *IL22RA2* is a susceptibility gene for MS [20,21].

Interestingly, mRNA levels of CD39, AHR and CYP1B1, an AHR-induced gene are increased in fingolimod-treated patients. CD39 is an ectonucleotidase that hydrolyses ATP to AMP. Since ATP acts as an inducer of proinflammatory cytokines, its cleavage has anti-inflammatory consequences [22]. CD39 has been described as a novel functional marker of regulatory effector/ memory-like T (T$_{REM}$) cells [8]. AHR is a member of the family of basic helix-loop-helix transcription factors. Upon binding of exogenous agents, AHR mediates transcriptional responses of a wide variety of genes, named AHR gene battery, which includes CYP1B1 [23]. AHR has also been demonstrated to influence the expression of IL-22 and CD39 [9,24]. In this study, we show an increase in the mRNA expression levels of CD39 and CYP1B1. Thus, AHR activation might be an additional anti-inflammatory mechanism induced by fingolimod. AHR activation was shown to exacerbate or to suppress EAE depending on its ligand [24,25]. EAE suppression by AHR was associated with expansion of Treg cells. Therefore, the effects of fingolimod on AHR might have functional relevance, in addition to its effects on the redistribution of circulating immune cells.

We have also shown that the *ex vivo* levels of FOXP3 mRNA in PBMCs are drastically reduced in contrast to the increase in the

Table 1. Immune cell subpopulations in MS patients before (t0) or after three months of fingolimod treatment (t3) and healthy controls analysed by *ex vivo* flow cytometry.

	t0	t3	p-value (t0 vs t3)	HC	p-value (t0 vs HC)
CD4 (%of lymphoid cells)	46.03 (17.2–69.6)	6.4 (1.7–48.5)	**0.0006**	47.3 (32.3–60.6)	0.770
CD8 (%of lymphoid cells)	20.1 (6.2–39.4)	15.18 (4.9–41.1)	0.4851	21.73 (14.7–31.5)	0.544
CD19 (%of lymphoid cells)	11.45 (3.6–25.7)	5.9 (1.8–15.25)	**0.0012**	7.36 (4.7–16.5)	**0.025**
FOXP3+ (%of CD4+)	7.92 (3.46–11.2)	11.78 (1.35–20.6)	**0.0411**	5.45 (2.93–10.6)	0.087
CD4+CD25hiFOXP3+ (%of lymphoid cells)	3.2 (1.67–8.26)	0.68 (0.06–4.34)	**0.0029**	2.63 (1.98–5.01)	0.580
CD25hiFOXP3+ (%of CD4+)	8.33 (3.73–11.9)	11.45 (1.17–19.75)	0.0929	6.27 (4.4–10.95)	0.087
CD39+ (%of CD4+CD25hiFOXP3+)	43.4 (17.9–77.3)	76.2 (29.9–93.6)	**0.0005**	26.9 (10.1–53.15)	**0.0425**

The median and range are shown. Lymphoid cells were gated according to their FSC/SSC profile.

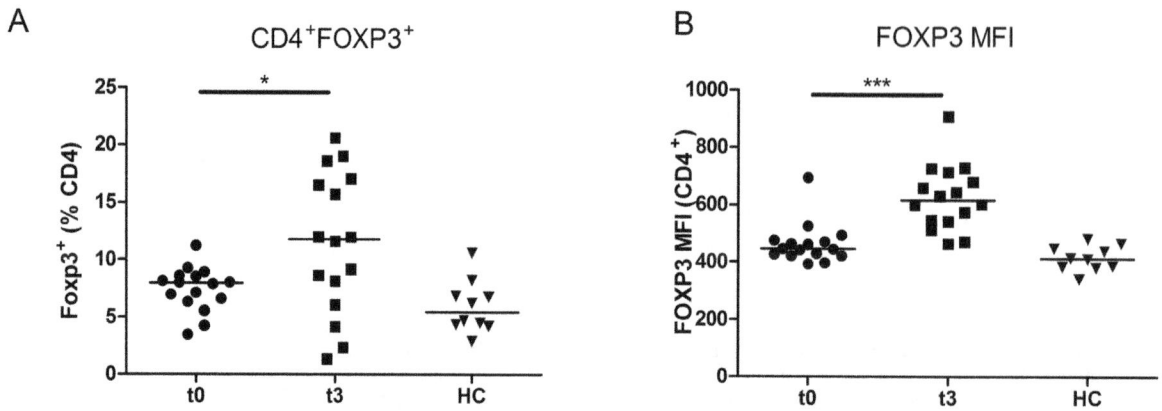

Figure 3. FOXP3 expression by CD4$^+$ T cells of fingolimod-treated MS patients before (t0, n = 16) or after three months of treatment by fingolimod (t3, n = 16) and healthy controls (HC, n = 10) analysed *ex vivo* by flow cytometry. (A) The percentage of FOXP3-expressing CD4$^+$ cells was increased in 12 out of 16 patients and associated with an increase (B) of FOXP3 MFI values. * and *** indicate p-values of ≤0.05 and ≤ 0.001 respectively.

proportion of FOXP3$^+$ cells within CD4$^+$ T cells in fingolimod-treated patients. FOXP3 is the transcription factor of Tregs but is also transiently expressed upon activation of effector T cells. Therefore, its decreased mRNA level is likely due to the large reduction of CD4$^+$ cell count observed by flow cytometry. Indeed, in agreement with previous studies, CD4$^+$ and B cells proportions are decreased by fingolimod while CD8$^+$ T cells are less affected [26,27]. This is consistent with the observation that T$_{EM}$ cells, which are mainly CD8$^+$ cells, are not retained in lymph nodes in the presence of fingolimod, in contrast to T$_{CM}$ cells, which are predominantly CD4$^+$ cells [28].

Divergent findings have been published regarding the effects of fingolimod on the proportion of Tregs [29,30]. Due to the lack of specific cell surface Treg markers in humans, we used *FOXP3i1* demethylation to assess the effect of fingolimod on circulating natural Tregs. By flow cytometry, we confirm that the proportion of Tregs within lymphoid cells is reduced by fingolimod. However, the proportion of CD25^{hi}Foxp3$^+$ cells within the CD4$^+$ subpopulation increases in 12 treated patients out of 16. It has been suggested that fingolimod induces FOXP3 expression in CD4$^+$FOXP3$^-$ T cells and causes an increase in FOXP3$^+$ Treg cells [4,5]. Here, we show an increase in the proportion of FOXP3$^+$ cells within the CD4$^+$ cell population, as well as an

increase in median FOXP3 expression level, as indicated by higher MFI values.

Beneficial effects of fingolimod might be additionally mediated by modulating the function of Tregs. In order to investigate this, we analysed the expression of CD39 by Tregs. The proportion of CD39$^+$ Tregs is significantly increased by fingolimod. Surface expression of CD39 in Tregs is also increased by the treatment. It has been suggested that CD39$^+$ Tregs specifically inhibit Th17 cells. Therefore, their increased number might be an additional mechanism by which fingolimod attenuates inflammation and mediates its therapeutic benefits.

In summary, we have shown that CD39, AHR and CYP1B1 mRNA levels are increased in PBMCs following fingolimod treatment while IL-17 mRNA is decreased. Fingolimod induces a large decrease of B and CD4$^+$ cells but remaining CD4$^+$ T cells are enriched in FOXP3$^+$ cells. Furthermore, the proportion of CD39-expressing Tregs within the CD4$^+$ subpopulation is increased by the treatment, thereby possibly providing an additional therapeutic benefit of this drug. Indeed, apart from its effects on lymphocyte egress from lymph nodes, experimental data points towards an effect of fingolimod on Treg development. Signalling through the S1P1 receptor has been shown to inhibit Foxp3$^+$ Treg differentiation, by down-regulating SMAD3 activity [31]. This consequently counteracts TGF-β receptor-mediated signalling,

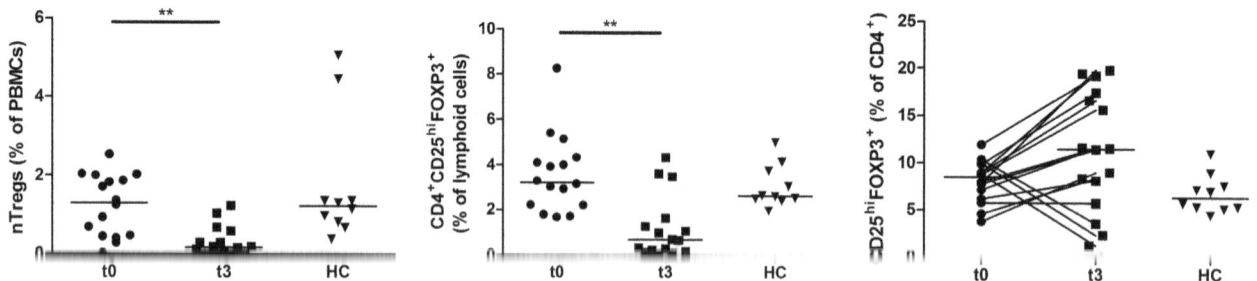

Figure 4. Regulatory T cells in PBMCs of fingolimod-treated patients. Regulatory T cells of MS patients before (t0, n = 16) or after three months of treatment by fingolimod (t3, n = 16) and healthy controls (HC, n = 10) were analysed *ex vivo* by MethylS-qPCR (A) to quantify nTregs with demethylated *FOXP3i1*. The proportion of circulating CD4$^+$CD25^{hi}FOXP3$^+$ Tregs was also measured by flow cytometry and expressed as a percentage of lymphoid cells (B). The proportion of CD25^{hi}FOXP3$^+$ cells was also expressed as a percentage of CD4$^+$ T cells (C). nTreg proportion among total PBMCs was decreased by the treatment, as well as the proportion of Tregs within lymphoid cells. CD25^{hi}FOXP3$^+$ Tregs were however enriched within the CD4$^+$ cell population in 12 out of 16 patients. The horizontal lines represent the median value in all subgroups. ** indicates a p-value of ≤0.01.

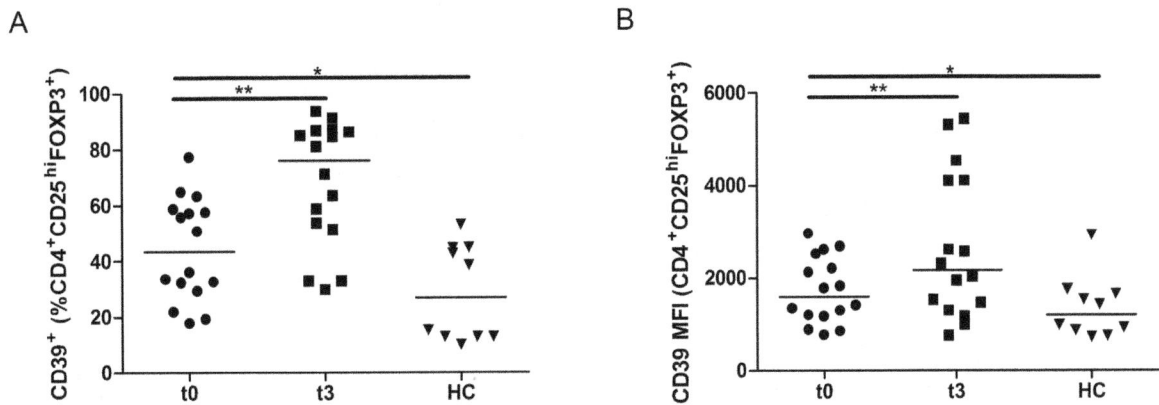

Figure 5. Proportion of CD39-expressing cells within CD4⁺CD25ʰⁱFOXP3⁺ T cells of fingolimod-treated patients. (A) The percentage of CD39 expression within the population CD4⁺CD25ʰⁱFOXP3⁺ T cells of MS patients before (t0, n = 16) or after three months of treatment by fingolimod (t3, n = 16) and healthy controls (HC, n = 10) was analysed *ex vivo* by flow cytometry. The proportion of CD39-expressing Tregs was increased after three months of fingolimod treatment and was associated with (B) an increase in the MFI of CD39. The horizontal lines represent the median value in all subgroups. * and ** indicate p-values of ≤0.05 and ≤0.01 respectively.

which is required for Treg differentiation. Inhibition of S1P1 signalling by fingolimod might therefore regulate the balance towards Treg development, as observed in our study. It has also been shown that treatment with fingolimod induces TGF-β in splenocyte cell cultures, which could also be a mechanism involved in the increased proportion of CD39-expressing Tregs in fingolimod-treated patients [32]. Finally, our data showing an induction of CYP1B1 mRNA following treatment by fingolimod suggests that AHR, another transcription factor involved in Treg differentiation and CD39 expression is activated, providing an alternative hypothesis for our observations [9,25]. Studies are ongoing regarding the mechanisms by which fingolimod induces CD39-expressing cells.

Supporting Information

Figure S1   CD39-expressing cells within other cell subpopulations. CD39 expression was analysed by flow cytometry in CD4⁺FOXP3⁻ T cells (A), CD19⁺ B cells (B) and CD8⁺ T cells (C). The proportion of CD4⁺FOXP3⁻CD39⁺ cells increases slightly following treatment by fingolimod. The treatment did not increase the proportion of CD39⁺ cells within the CD8⁺ and CD19⁺ populations. The horizontal lines represent the median value in all

subgroups. * and ** indicate p-values of ≤0.05 and ≤0.01 respectively.

Table S1   Main demographic features of patient and healthy control groups.

Table S2   Primers and probes sequences for MS-qPCR amplification.

Table S3   Primer sequences for qPCR amplification.

Acknowledgments

We thank Professor S. Lucas and N. Dauguet for invaluable discussions (de Duve Institute, Brussels).

Author Contributions

Conceived and designed the experiments: VvP CS NM. Performed the experiments: NM HD. Analyzed the data: VvP NM CS HD. Contributed reagents/materials/analysis tools: VvP NM CS HD. Wrote the paper: VvP CS NM HD.

References

1. Brinkmann V, Davis MD, Heise CE, Albert R, Cottens S, et al. (2002) The immune modulator FTY720 targets sphingosine 1-phosphate receptors. J Biol Chem 277: 21453–21457.

2. Graler MH, Goetzl EJ (2004) The immunosuppressant FTY720 down-regulates sphingosine 1-phosphate G-protein-coupled receptors. Faseb j 18: 551–553.

3. Mehling M, Lindberg R, Raulf F, Kuhle J, Hess C, et al. (2010) Th17 central memory T cells are reduced by FTY720 in patients with multiple sclerosis. Neurology 75: 403–410.

4. Sun Y, Wang W, Shan B, Di J, Chen L, et al. (2011) FTY720-induced conversion of conventional Foxp3- CD4+ T cells to Foxp3+ regulatory T cells in NOD mice. Am J Reprod Immunol 66: 349–362.

5. Kimss MG, Lee SY, Ko YS, Lee HY, Jo SK, et al. (2011) CD4+ CD25+ regulatory T cells partially mediate the beneficial effects of FTY720, a sphingosine-1-phosphate analogue, during ischaemia/reperfusion-induced acute kidney injury. Nephrol Dial Transplant 26: 111–124.

6. Wolf AM, Eller K, Zeiser R, Durr C, Gerlach UV, et al. (2009) The sphingosine 1-phosphate receptor agonist FTY720 potently inhibits regulatory T cell proliferation in vitro and in vivo. J Immunol 183: 3751–3760.

7. Baron U, Floess S, Wieczorek G, Baumann K, Grutzkau A, et al. (2007) DNA demethylation in the human FOXP3 locus discriminates regulatory T cells from activated FOXP3(+) conventional T cells. Eur J Immunol 37: 2378–2389.

8. Borsellino G, Kleinewietfeld M, Di Mitri D, Sternjak A, Diamantini A, et al. (2007) Expression of ectonucleotidase CD39 by Foxp3+ Treg cells: hydrolysis of extracellular ATP and immune suppression. Blood 110: 1225–1232.

9. Gandhi R, Kumassr D, Burns EJ, Nadeau M, Dake B, et al. (2010) Activation of the aryl hydrocarbon receptor induces human type 1 regulatory T cell-like and Foxp3(+) regulatory T cells. Nat Immunol 11: 846–853.

10. Fletcher JM, Lonergan R, Costelloe L, Kinsella K, Moran B, et al. (2009) CD39+Foxp3+ regulatory T Cells suppress pathogenic Th17 cells and are impaired in multiple sclerosis. J Immunol 183: 7602–7610.

11. Beillard E, Pallisgaard N, van der Velden VH, Bi W, Dee R, et al. (2003) Evaluation of candidate control genes for diagnosis and residual disease detection in leukemic patients using 'real-time' quantitative reverse-transcriptase polymerase chain reaction (RQ-PCR) - a Europe against cancer program. Leukemia 17: 2474–2486.

12. Muls N, Jnaoui K, Dang HA, Wauters A, Van Snick J, et al. (2012) Upregulation of IL-17, but not of IL-9, in circulating cells of CIS and relapsing MS patients. Impact of corticosteroid therapy on the cytokine network. J Neuroimmunol 243: 73–80.

13. Komiyama Y, Nakae S, Matsuki T, Nambu A, Ishigame H, et al. (2006) IL-17 plays an important role in the development of experimental autoimmune encephalomyelitis. J Immunol 177: 566–573.

14. Kebir H, Kreymborg K, Ifergan I, Dodelet-Devillers A, Cayrol R, et al. (2007) Human TH17 lymphocytes promote blood-brain barrier disruption and central nervous system inflammation. Nat Med 13: 1173–1175.

15. Garris CS, Blaho VA, Hla T, Han MH (2014) Sphingosine-1-phosphate receptor 1 signalling in T cells: trafficking and beyond. Immunology 142: 347–353.

16. Wolk K (2006) IL-22 regulates the expression of genes responsible for antimicrobial defense, cellular differentiation, and mobility in keratinocytes: a potential role in psoriasis. Eur J Immunol 36: 1309–1323.

17. Radaeva S, Sun R, Pan H-n, Hong F, Gao B (2004) Interleukin 22 (IL-22) plays a protective role in T cell-mediated murine hepatitis: IL-22 is a survival factor for hepatocytes via STAT3 activation. Hepatology 39: 1332–1342.

18. Brand S, Beigel F, Olszak T, Zitzmann K, Eichhorst ST, et al. (2006) IL-22 is increased in active Crohn's disease and promotes proinflammatory gene expression and intestinal epithelial cell migration. Am J Physiol Gastrointest Liver Physiol 290: G827–838.

19. Kreymborg K, Etzensperger R, Dumoutier L, Haak S, Rebollo A, et al. (2007) IL-22 is expressed by Th17 cells in an IL-23-dependent fashion, but not required for the development of autoimmune encephalomyelitis. J Immunol 179: 8098–8104.

20. Beyeen AD, Adzemovic MZ, Ockinger J, Stridh P, Becanovic K, et al. (2010) IL-22RA2 associates with multiple sclerosis and macrophage effector mechanisms in experimental neuroinflammation. J Immunol 185: 6883–6890.

21. Sawcer S, Hellenthal G, Pirinen M, Spencer CC, Patsopoulos NA, et al. (2011) Genetic risk and a primary role for cell-mediated immune mechanisms in multiple sclerosis. Nature 476: 214–219.

22. Martinon F, Mayor A, Tschopp J (2009) The inflammasomes: guardians of the body. Annu Rev Immunol 27: 229–265.

23. Tijet N, Boutros PC, Moffat ID, Okey AB, Tuomisto J, et al. (2006) Aryl Hydrocarbon Receptor Regulates Distinct Dioxin-Dependent and Dioxin-Independent Gene Batteries. Molecular Pharmacology 69: 140–153.

24. Veldhoen M, Hirota K, Westendorf AM, Buer J, Dumoutier L, et al. (2008) The aryl hydrocarbon receptor links TH17-cell-mediated autoimmunity to environmental toxins. Nature 453: 106–109.

25. Quintana FJ, Basso AS, Iglesias AH, Korn T, Farez MF, et al. (2008) Control of T(reg) and T(H)17 cell differentiation by the aryl hydrocarbon receptor. Nature 453: 65–71.

26. Mehling M, Brinkmann V, Antel J, Bar-Or A, Goebels N, et al. (2008) FTY720 therapy exerts differential effects on T cell subsets in multiple sclerosis. Neurology 71: 1261–1267.

27. Miyazaki Y, Niino M, Fukazawa T, Takahashi E, Nonaka T, et al. (2014) Suppressed pro-inflammatory properties of circulating B cells in patients with multiple sclerosis treated with fingolimod, based on altered proportions of B-cell subpopulations. Clin Immunol 151: 127–135.

28. Sallusto F, Geginat J, Lanzavecchia A (2004) Central memory and effector memory T-cell subsets: function, generation, and maintenance. Annu Rev Immunol 22: 745–763.

29. Brinkmann V, Raulf F, Vedrine C, Allard C (2012) Fingolimod Treatment Reduces Circulating CD4+ Regulatory T Cells and Th17 Cells in Blood of Patients with Multiple Sclerosis. Neurology Meeting abstracts.

30. Serpero LD, Filaci G, Parodi A, Battaglia F, Kalli F, et al. (2013) Fingolimod modulates peripheral effector and regulatory T cells in MS patients. J Neuroimmune Pharmacol 8: 1106–1113.

31. Liu G, Burns S, Huang G, Boyd K, Proia RL, et al. (2009) The receptor S1P1 overrides regulatory T cell-mediated immune suppression through Akt-mTOR. Nat Immunol 10: 769–777.

32. Sehrawat S, Rouse BT (2008) Anti-inflammatory effects of FTY720 against viral-induced immunopathology: role of drug-induced conversion of T cells to become Foxp3+ regulators. J Immunol 180: 7636–7647.

24

BDC12-4.1 T-Cell Receptor Transgenic Insulin-Specific CD4 T Cells Are Resistant to *In Vitro* Differentiation into Functional Foxp3⁺ T Regulatory Cells

Ghanashyam Sarikonda[1]❂, Georgia Fousteri[1]❂¤, Sowbarnika Sachithanantham[1], Jacqueline F. Miller[1], Amy Dave[1], Therese Juntti[1], Ken T. Coppieters[2], Matthias von Herrath[1,2]*

1 Diabetes Center, La Jolla Institute for Allergy and Immunology, La Jolla, California, USA, **2** Type 1 Diabetes R&D center, Novo Nordisk Inc., Seattle, Washington, USA

Abstract

The infusion of ex vivo-expanded autologous T regulatory (Treg) cells is potentially an effective immunotherapeutic strategy against graft-versus-host disease (GvHD) and several autoimmune diseases, such as type 1 diabetes (T1D). However, *in vitro* differentiation of antigen-specific T cells into functional and stable Treg (iTreg) cells has proved challenging. As insulin is the major autoantigen leading to T1D, we tested the capacity of insulin-specific T-cell receptor (TCR) transgenic CD4⁺ T cells of the BDC12-4.1 clone to convert into Foxp3⁺ iTreg cells. We found that *in vitro* polarization toward Foxp3⁺ iTreg was effective with a majority (>70%) of expanded cells expressing Foxp3. However, adoptive transfer of Foxp3⁺ BDC12-4.1 cells did not prevent diabetes onset in immunocompetent NOD mice. Thus, *in vitro* polarization of insulin-specific BDC12-4.1 TCR transgenic CD4⁺ T cells toward Foxp3⁺ cells did not provide dominant tolerance in recipient mice. These results highlight the disconnect between an *in vitro* acquired Foxp3⁺ cell phenotype and its associated *in vivo* regulatory potential.

Editor: Ciriaco A. Piccirillo, McGill University Health Center, Canada

Funding: This work was supported by a U01 (DK078013) National Institute of Diabetes and Digestive and Kidney (NIDDK) grant to MvH and a subaward from the University of Colorado, Denver (UCD) to LIAI, issued under NIH award number 5U19AI050864-08 to UCD under the direction of Dr. George S. Eisenbarth. The funders had no role in study design, data collection and analysis, decision to publish, or preparation of the manuscript.

Competing Interests: Two of the authors, Matthias von Herrath and Ken Coppieters are affiliated with Novo Nordisk Inc. NovoNordisk Inc. was not involved in this study and has no vested or other interests in the work.

* Email: matthias@liai.org

¤ Current address: San Raffaele Scientific Institute, Diabetes Research Institute, Milan, Italy

❂ These authors contributed equally to this work.

Introduction

Type 1 diabetes (T1D) is a chronic autoimmune disease characterized by gradual destruction of insulin-producing beta cells in pancreatic islets. In the non-obese diabetic (NOD) mouse model of T1D, insulin is an essential autoantigen (reviewed in [1]) and mice with certain mutations in the insulin gene do not develop diabetes [2]. In NOD mice CD4⁺ T cell infiltration into islets can be detected as early as 3-4 weeks of age. However, disease onset appears later in life between 10-24 weeks of age suggesting that there are two phases of the disease, the initiation phase, characterized by monocyte infiltration, and the propagation phase, where CD4⁺ and CD8⁺ T effector (Teff) cells accumulate leading to loss of >80% beta cell mass, coinciding with disease onset. The majority of CD4⁺ T cells that infiltrate pancreas are insulin-specific [3], reacting against the 15-amino acid region 9-23 of the insulin B-chain (InsB:9-23) [4]. Despite such restricted T-cell receptor (TCR) reactivity, insulin specific CD4⁺ T cells exhibit diverse TCR-α/β chain usage [5]. Several insulin reactive T cell clones have been generated, some from the pancreas of prediabetic NOD mice (i.e., the BDC12-4.1 [5]) and some from the pancreatic lymph nodes (PLN) (i.e., the 2H6 [6]). While a significant proportion of the clones appear to be pathogenic,

including the BDC12-4.1 clone, some, e.g. the 2H6 T cell clone, are protective.

The presence of InsB:9-23 reactive CD4⁺ T cells in the periphery of NOD mice has historically been attributed to incomplete negative thymic selection [7,8]. It was recently shown that negative selection mechanisms per se are in fact not critically impaired in NOD mice [9] but rather that InsB:9-23-reactive CD4⁺ T cells escape selection due to limited presentation of peptide in the thymus due to low affinity binding mode of the peptide to the I-A^{g7} major histocompatibility molecule [10].

Two different TCR transgenic (Tg) mouse lines, BDC12-4.1 [11] and 2H6 [12], both specific for InsB:9-23 peptide were established independently. BDC12-4.1 TCR Tg mice develop spontaneous insulitis but no diabetes in F1 mice (FVB x NOD), whereas diabetes manifests in NOD.RAG^{KO} (backcross 1 generation) but with only 40% penetrance [11]. We recently described that both effector and Foxp3⁺ Treg cells are generated in the periphery of BDC12-4.1.RAG^{KO} mice, where the latter account for the reduced penetrance of T1D in this mouse line [13]. On the other hand, 2H6 Tg mice (2H6.NOD or 2H6.NOD.SCID) have almost no signs of insulitis and do not develop diabetes [12]. We initially set out to assess the permissiveness of insulin-specific T cells from both strains toward *in vitro* iTreg cell induction. We found that 2H6 T cells did not expand *in vitro* in an antigen specific manner. Whereas BDC12-4.1 T cells expanded upon antigen-specific activation and moreover differentiated into Foxp3$^+$ Treg in *in vitro* polarizing conditions (iTreg), they did not protect from diabetes onset upon adoptive transfer in prediabetic NOD mice. This data shows that the demonstrated *in vivo* ability of BDC12-4.1 insulin-specific T cells to differentiate into functional Foxp3$^+$ Treg occurs inefficiently under *in vitro* conditions, despite acquisition of key phenotypic markers.

Results

Insulin recognition by BDC12-4.1 and 2H6 TCR transgenic T-cells

To confirm the insulin recognition properties of the two InsB:9-23 specific T cells, we assessed their proliferative capacity in response to peptide stimulation. BDC12-4.1 T-cells exhibited robust proliferation in a dose-dependent manner (Fig. 1A). Exposure to R22E mimotope [14] of the InsB:9-23 peptide resulted in an enhanced dose-dependent proliferation. These results confirm the recognition of InsB:9-23 peptide as the cognate antigen for BDC12-4.1 T cells. On the other hand, we could not obtain convincing evidence of insulin-specific responses from 2H6 T cells. Addition of antigen presenting cells (APCs) to 2H6 TCR Tg cells in the absence of antigen resulted in non-specific proliferation. Such proliferation did not increase in magnitude upon the addition of the native InsB:9-23 peptide or the R22E mimotope (Fig. 1B). Further, although 2H6 T cells exhibited Ca^{+2} mobilization in response to InsB:9-23 stimulation, in some but not all of our experiments, (Fig. S1), they did not bind to I-A^{g7} tetramer (data not shown) loaded with the modified InsB:9-23 peptide [15]. Taken together, these results show that only T cells from the BDC12-4.1 clone respond to cognate antigen-specific stimulation and therefore we focused on generating iTregs only from BDC12-4.1 TCR Tg mice.

BDC12-4.1 T cells expand in the periphery and display activated-memory and Treg phenotypes

Few BDC12-4.1 T cells escape thymic deletion [2] and undergo positive selection. Surprisingly, we found that CD4$^+$CD8$^+$ double positive thymocytes from BDC12-4.1 mice also express elevated levels of CD69 suggesting that some antigen-specific recognition is ongoing during positive selection (data not included). We previously showed that the majority of BDC12-4.1 TCR Tg cells acquire memory and Foxp3$^+$ Treg phenotype in the spleen and PLN. Here, we also examined the number of total CD4$^+$ T cells and found that in both spleen (Fig. 2A) and PLN (Fig. 2B) CD4$^+$ T cells show a trend to expand with age. Prior to *in vitro* polarization into Foxp3 Treg, we evaluated the presence of CD44^{hi}CD62L^{low} effector memory and Foxp3$^+$ Treg cells in the spleens of the donor mice. As depicted in Fig. 2C and D, on average, 60% of CD4$^+$ splenocytes displayed activated-memory phenotype and 5% expressed Foxp3. Whereas this data confirm our previous observations, it also shows that the starting CD4$^+$ T cell population in the *in vitro* T cell cultures contains a great amount of already differentiated CD4$^+$ T cells. Subsequently, we tested whether these cells can be polarized into functional Foxp3$^+$ Treg cells.

Cytokine production increases with age in BDC12-14.1 T cells

Before testing the plasticity of BDC12-4.1 T cells to differentiate into functional Foxp3$^+$ Treg cells, we evaluated whether continuous antigen (insulin) exposure affects their functional properties. We found that BDC12-4.1 T-cells responded to InsB:9-23 stimulation by producing high amounts of IFN-γ, IL-4 and IL-2 cytokines (Fig. 3A), while the detection of other cytokines such as IL-10 and IL-17 was not as evident (data not shown). Interestingly, and in concordance with the rise in CD4$^+$ T cell number cell with increasing age (Fig. 2), the number of cells producing IFN-γ in response to InsB:9-23 stimulation also increased (Fig. 3B). These results suggest that despite omnipresent *in vivo* antigen exposure,

A.

B.

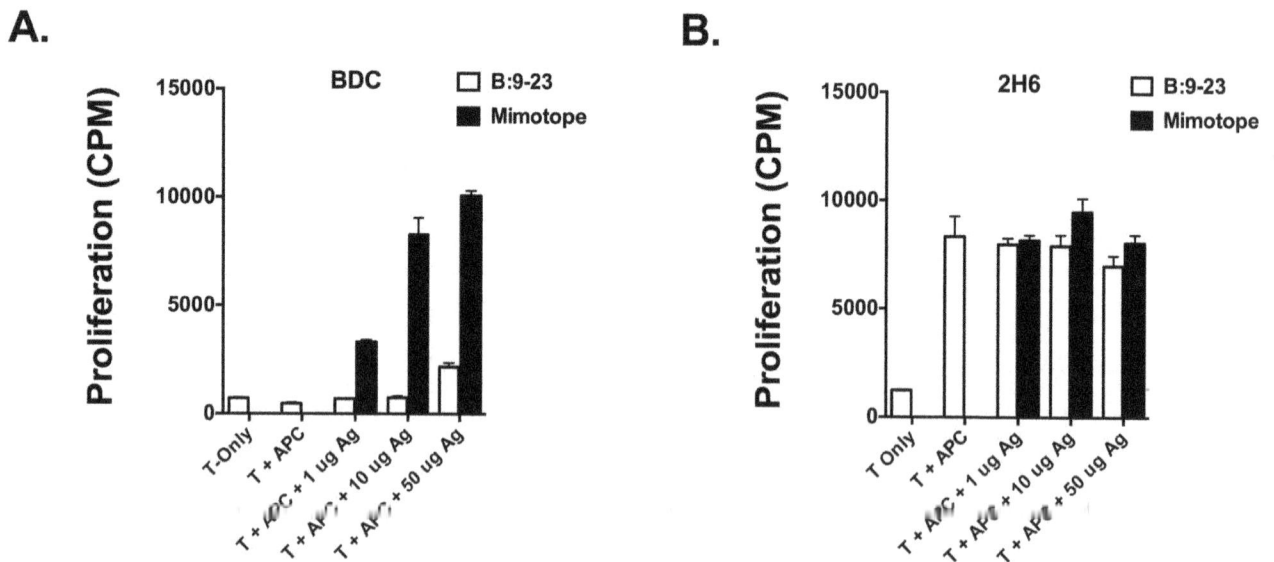

Figure 1. BDC12-4.1 TCR transgenic T cells exhibit robust insB:9-23-specific responses. CD4$^+$ T cells purified from splenocytes of BDC12-4.1/RAG^{KO} or 2H6 mice were plated in triplicate, in round-bottom 96-well plates. 5–10×10^4 T cells per well were incubated with an equal number of APCs for 48 hours. Native InsB:9-23 peptide (open bars) or R22E mimotope ([14]) of the InsB:9-23 peptide (filled bars) were used at the indicated concentration. T cells incubated alone or with only APCs (without added antigen) served to measure spontaneous proliferation. Mean and SEM values for average of the triplicate wells derived from pooled mice (n = 3) is shown.

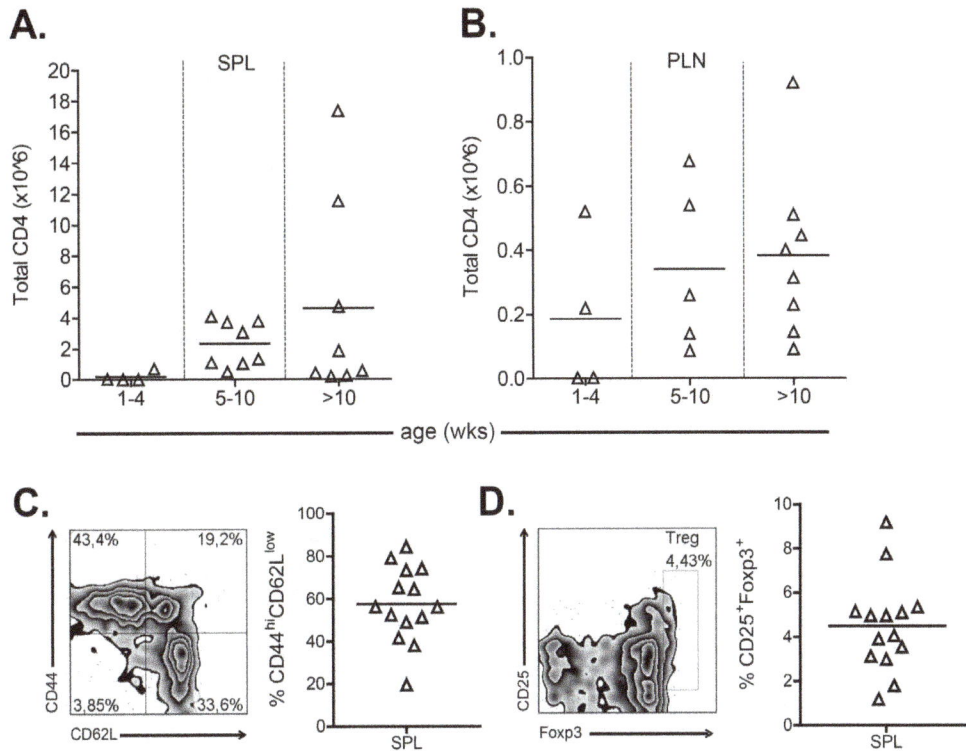

Figure 2. BDC12-4.1 T cells expand and display memory and Treg cell phenotypes in the periphery. (A and B) Age-associated increases in total CD4$^+$ T cell numbers in the spleen and PLN of BDC12-4.1.RAG^{KO} mice. Splenocytes and PLN lymphocytes from BDC12-4.1.RAG^{KO} mice were analyzed at different ages by flow cytometry for the frequency of CD4$^+$Vβ2$^+$ T cells. The percentage of CD4$^+$Vβ2$^+$ cells was multiplied with the total number of cells isolated from the spleen or PLN to calculate the total number of CD4$^+$ T cells. Trypan blue was used for the exclusion of dead cells prior to counting. (C and D) Representative FACS plots and data for activated T cells, CD44^{hi}CD62L^{low}, and Treg cells, CD25$^+$Foxp3$^+$, from the spleens of donor mice that were used to generate Foxp3$^+$ Treg cells in vitro are shown.

BDC12-4.1 T-cells remain functionally active and do not achieve an anergic state.

In vivo polarized Foxp3$^+$ cells from BDC12-4.1 mice do not protect recipient NOD mice from diabetes onset

To assess whether pre-differentiated BDC12-4.1 T cells in peripheral tissues can be converted to protective iTregs, purified CD4$^+$CD25$^-$ T cells from BDC12-4.1 mice were cultured under *in vitro* Treg polarizing conditions with anti-CD3 or the cognate peptide antigen. In the presence of TGF-β and IL-2, BDC12-4.1 T cells readily differentiated into CD25$^+$Foxp3$^+$CD127^{lo} iTreg cells (Fig. 4A, phenotypically *bona-fide* Treg cells). To determine whether these *in vitro* polarized Foxp3$^+$ cells could alter ongoing diabetogenic process we adoptively transferred them into fully

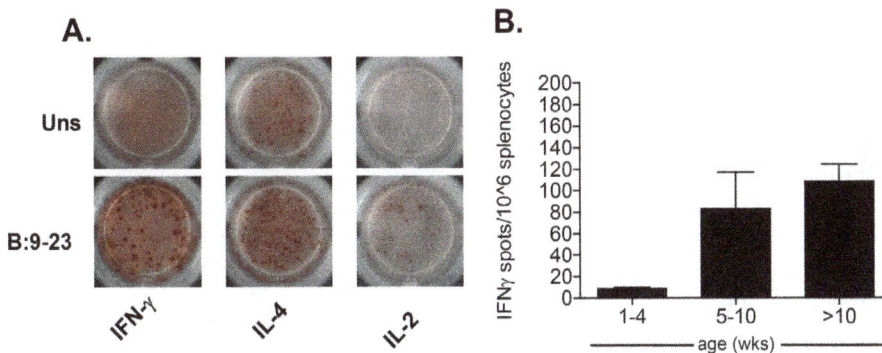

Figure 3. T cells with InsB:9-23 specific responses increase in frequencies with age. Total splenocytes from BDC12-4.1.RAG^{KO} mice were obtained at different ages. 250,000 splenocytes per well were incubated with or without native InsB:9-23 peptide in triplicates. Following 3-day incubation, IFN-γ, IL-2, and IL-4 production were determined by ELISpot assay. Representative images of cytokine production from BDC12-4.1.RAG^{KO} T-cells with (bottom row) or without antigen (top row) stimulation is shown in A. Background (media) subtracted IFN-γ spot numbers produced in response to antigen stimulation, from BDC12-4.1.RAG^{KO} mice of different age groups are shown on the Y-axis in B. Representative means ± SEM data from one of two independent experiments with n = 3 per each group with similar results are shown.

immuno-competent 8–10 week old female NOD mice. Rather surprisingly, CD4$^+$ BDC12-4.1 T cells expanded either in antigen-specific fashion (InsB:9-23) or with a nonspecific stimulation (a-CD3) failed to significantly protect recipient NOD mice from diabetes onset (Fig. 4B). Diabetes incidence in mice receiving Foxp3$^+$ cells mirrored that of separate sets of control mice that serve to determine cumulative diabetes incidence in our NOD colony.

Among other polarizing conditions (Th1, Th2, Th17 or Tr1), BDC12-14.1 cells could be polarized toward Th17 and Tr1, evidenced by their ability to produce IL-17 and IL-10 respectively (Fig. S2A, B). Surprisingly, the expansion of BDC12-4.1 T cells toward Th17 or Tr1 (as compared to iTreg) was very limited, which compromised their use in further *in vivo* adoptive transfer experiments. After pooling results from two experiments where we generated sufficient Tr1 cells, few NOD mice were tested for diabetes protection, and a significant fraction of them was protected from diabetes (Fig. S2C). However, given the limited

A.

B.

Figure 4. *In vitro* **polarization induces Foxp3 expression in memory BDC12-4.1 T cells but does not endow** *in vivo* **regulatory functions.** CD4$^+$CD25$^+$ cells from splenocytes of BDC12-4.1 mice polarized into Treg cells (A) *in vitro* in the presence of a-CD3 (left panel) or InsB:9-23 peptide (right panel). Expanded T cells were gated on CD4$^+$CD25$^+$ cells (not shown) and expression of CD127 and Foxp3 were determined. (B). 1×10^6 Tregs polarized with anti-CD3 (left panel) or InsB:9-23 peptide (right panel) were adoptively transferred into prediabetic 8-wk old NOD mice and diabetes development was monitored. Unmanipulated NOD mice monitored on a regular basis in our animal colony served as negative controls with cumulative diabetes incidence of ~90% by 27 wks of age. Representative results from one of three independent experiments are shown.

number of Tr1 cells that could be generated, we were unable to determine which factor(s) contributed to the differentiation of BDC12-4.1 cells into functional Tr1 cells.

Discussion

Insulin, and in particular the 15 amino acid peptide of the B-chain 9-23, is an essential autoantigen in NOD mice (reviewed in [1]). While most InsB:9-23 reactive CD4$^+$ T cell clones [5], like the BDC12-4.1 that was studied here are pathogenic [11], some, e.g., the 2H6 [12], are not. Understanding how recognition of insulin could endow pathogenic and/or regulatory roles to CD4$^+$ T cells will help us understand how organ-specific autoimmunity develops and how it can be controlled. Here, by using BDC12-4.1 Tg mice, we found that: a) few InsB:9-23-specific CD4$^+$ T cells escape negative selection and expand in the periphery, b) most peripheral BDC12-4.1 T cells are already differentiated into Teff or Treg, c) most cells that respond to InsB:9-23 peptide stimulation produce proinflammatory cytokines and d) under *in vitro* polarization conditions, peripheral BDC12-4.1 cells can be efficiently grown into phenotypic Treg (Foxp3$^+$) cells, however, they do not protect recipient NOD mice from diabetes development upon adoptive transfer.

Recent evidence suggests that the InsB:9-23 peptide binds in at least two [16,17], but likely three [15] different registers of I-A^{g7}. Such differential binding and activation identifies two different set of T cells, type A and type B. Type A cells also recognize whole insulin processed and presented by thymic APCs and thus get deleted by negative selection. Type B cells do not recognize processed peptides escape thymic negative selection and in periphery they recognize InsB:9-23 peptide in register-2 leading to the generation of autoreactive T cells [16]. While this interesting observation explains how autoreactive T cells in NOD mice reach the periphery, it does not explain how two T cells reacting against the same InsB:9-23 peptide could develop into cells of two different fates, pathogenic (BDC12-14.1) and regulatory (2H6).

Although all CD4$^+$ T cells express the same TCR in BDC12-4.1 mice, only a fraction becomes Treg *in vivo*. Consequently, a fraction of BDC12-4.1.RAG^{KO} mice are protected from diabetes, likely depending on the Teff: Treg ratio that is established *in vivo* [13]. In the present study, BDC12-4.1 T cells were induced to uniformly express Foxp3 *in vitro*, but failed to protect from diabetes. Thus, although one may be able to achieve a Treg phenotype *in vitro* over the course of days, other mechanisms probably act in vivo to lock in Tregs' full suppressive functionality. Existence of T-cells of multiple antigen specificities in recipient mice at the time of adoptive transfer (~8-10 weeks of age) could contribute to the lack of protection upon adoptive transfer of Tregs of one antigen specificity, insB:9-23. And as such, Treg transfers into younger mice with a smaller T-cell repertoire or with lesser autoantibody presence/levels may provide a different result. Various other possibilities could also account for the lack of protection; perhaps the number of transferred cells was low, the infused iTreg cell population was functionally unstable or it was contaminated by effector T cells.

Multiple lines of evidence suggest that strength of the TCR signal involving the trimolecular complex of TCR-MHC-peptide can dictate the fate of the T cell. For instance, in a different T-cell model, a two-fold increase in the concentration of MHC-antigen can make a responding CD8$^+$ T cell go from a non-dividing cell to a dividing cell [18] and similar dose responses have been described for CD4$^+$T cells [19]. Further studies are needed to address whether the location, the type of the APC or the cytokine microenvironment are responsible for dictating the fate of a naïve

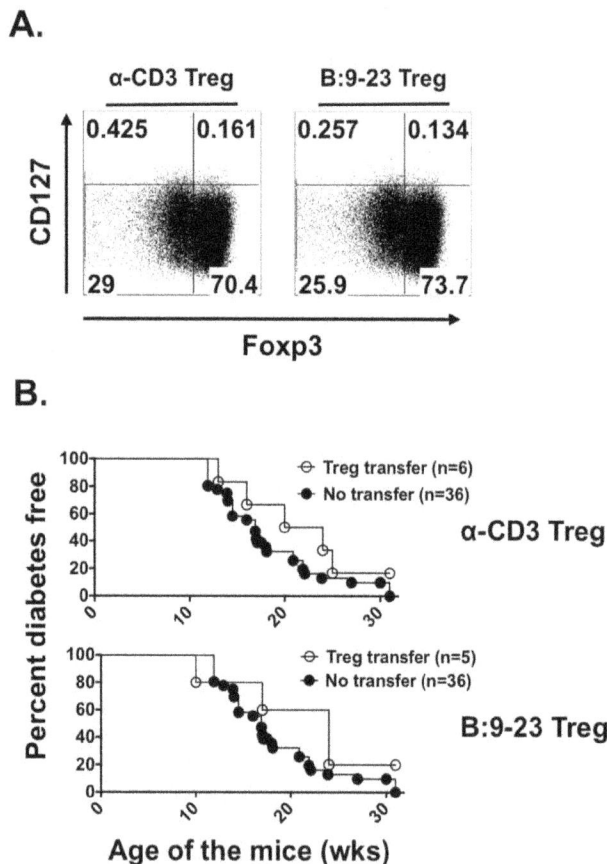

T cell or whether its fate is already predetermined in the thymus. We found that iTreg cells generated from thymocytes, analogous to splenocytes, cannot transfer protection from T1D (data not shown). Given that these studies are very preliminary (only 4 NOD mice tested), additional experiments are necessary to determine how we can drive BDC12-4.1 TCR Tg CD4+ T cells toward a stable Foxp3+ regulatory fate. Further, the fate of the *in vitro* generated BDC12-4.1 Tregs i.e., whether they retain their Treg phenotype *in vivo* and its role in protection from T1D onset could be explored. As cell therapy with *in vitro* generated Treg cells moves closer to the clinic, [20,21] it will be essential to determine whether it is feasible to alter the differentiation state of a T cell with an acquired functional phenotype.

In conclusion, we demonstrated that *in vitro* reprogramming of antigen-specific, self-reactive T cells into Foxp3-expressing, phenotypic Treg is possible. However, the resulting population was not endowed with functional suppressive capacity under our experimental conditions. Our data show that when pre-differentiated autoantigen-specific CD4+ T cells are used as a starting population, their differentiation conditions need to be optimized to enable therapeutic success.

Materials and Methods

Ethics statement

Mice were maintained in La Jolla Institute for Allergy and Immunology (LIAI) animal facility, under pathogen-free conditions following the LIAI institutional animal care and use committee (IACUC) guidelines for the use and care of laboratory animals. LIAI IACUC approved the experiments performed in this study.

Mice

BDC12-4.1 TCR transgenic mice were kindly provided by Prof. George Eisenbarth while 2H6.RAG+ mice were provided by Dr. Li Wen's group. Presence of transgenic TCR-α was determined by PCR [2], while TCR-β presence was determined by FACS analysis of Vβ2 or Vβ14 expression. BDC12-4.1/RAG+ mice were crossed into RAG^{KO} background and F1 were intercrossed to obtain BDC12-4.1/RAG.^{KO} mice. RAG^{KO} status of offspring was confirmed by PCR analysis as well as the absence of B220 positive cells by FACS.

Cytokine ELISPOT

Interferon (IFN)-γ, interleukin (IL)-4, IL-17, IL-10 and IL-2 were determined as previously described [13]. Spleen cells were prepared by homogenization in red blood cell lysis buffer and cultured at $2-4\times10^5$ cells/well in triplicate. Cells were cultured in RPMI media supplemented with 10% FBS (Life technologies). InsB:9-23 peptide (50 μg/ml) used for stimulation was high performance liquid chromatography purified (>90%) and dissolved in sterile DMSO (SynPep, Dublin, CA). 3-amino-9-ethylcarbazole (AEC) substrate and Chromogen solution (BD Biosciences) were used as the detection method, and wells were counted and analyzed using the KS ELISPOT reader, software version 4.

Proliferation assays

Purified CD4+ T cells from BDC12-4.1/RAG.^{KO} or 2H6 mice were plated in triplicate, in round-bottom 96-well plates, at 5–10×10^4 T cells per well with an equal number of mitomycin C-treated T-depleted splenocytes (TDS) from a NOD mice as APCs. The cultures were pulsed with 1 μCi of [^{3}H]-thymidine (2 Ci/mmol) on day 1 and harvested 16–24 h later using a Tomtec 96-

well harvester. The samples were then counted using a Wallac Betaplate scintillation counter. The mean proliferation and SEM of triplicate cultures are shown.

Flow cytometry

After a 2.4G2 blocking step, cells were stained for CD4, CD8, CD44, CD62L, CD69, B220, CD25, CD3, CD127, and Vβ2 or Vβ14 (eBioscience or Biolegend or BD-Pharmingen, San Diego, CA, USA). All antibody incubations were performed at 4°C for 30 minutes (isotype controls were included). Intracellular Foxp3 staining was performed using Foxp3 staining kit (eBioscience) and manufacturer's protocol. Intracellular cytokine staining was performed as described [13]. Cells were immediately acquired on a LSRII flow cytometer (BD Biosciences) and analyzed using the FlowJo software (Treestar).

CD4+CD25+/CD25- cell purification

From pooled splenocytes, CD4+CD25+ cells were purified using CD4+CD25+ Treg isolation kit (Miltenyi Biotec Inc., Auburn, CA) according to the manufacturer's protocol. CD4+CD25- cells were obtained by collecting the flow through cells during positive selection of CD4+CD25+ cells. Confirmation of >80% purity was performed by FACS before *in vitro* culture.

In vitro polarization and expansion of Foxp3+ cells

Purified CD4+CD25+ or CD4+CD25- cells were cultured in 10% FBS/RPMI medium (Life Technologies). For activation, either plate-bound anti-CD3 (1 μg/ml) or InsB:9-23 peptide (50 μg/ml) was used for *in vitro* stimulation during culture period. For each polarization, the cells were cultured in media containing various supplements as follows; for Th1 polarization, IL-2 (50 U/ml), IL-12 (5 ng/ml), anti-IL-4 (10 μg/ml) were added, for Th2 polarization IL-2 (50 U/ml), IL-4 (5 ng/ml) and anti-IFN-γ (10 μg/ml) were added. For Th17, IL-1β (5 ng/ml), TGF-β (5 ng/ml), and IL-21 (5 ng/ml) were added. For Treg cultures, IL-2 (50 U/ml) and TGF-β (5 ng/ml), were added, and finally for Tr1 cultures, IL-2 (50 U/ml), dexamethasone (50 nM) and vitamin D3 (100 nM) were added. All the cytokines except IL-2 were obtained from Peprotech while IL-2 was obtained from R&D systems. The cells were cultured for 7-10 days with fresh culture media added at regular intervals of 2-3 days. At the end of culture period, *in vitro* polarized cells were rested for 3 days by removing the stimulating agent (anti-CD3 or InB:9-23) and culturing in supplemented media.

Adoptive transfer of in vitro generated Treg cell lines

CD4+CD25+ cells were purified using Treg isolation kit (Miltenyi Biotech Inc.,), resuspended in Ca^{+2}/Mg^{+2} free PBS and 1×10^6 cells/mouse were transferred into recipient NOD mice via i.v., tail vein injection. Unmanipulated NOD mice were used as controls for these experiments.

Diabetes monitoring

Blood glucose levels were monitored weekly with OneTouch Ultra blood glucose monitoring system (LifeScan Inc., Milpitas, CA, USA) and mice were considered to be diabetic when two consecutive blood glucose values (BGV) measured above 250 mg/dl.

Statistical analysis

Data are expressed as a mean ± SD. Statistical significance of the difference between means was determined using the 2-tailed Student's *t*-test using Graphpad PRISM software (Graphpad, San

Diego, CA, USA). For diabetes incidence measurement, statistical significance was determined by Kaplan Meier analysis. *,p<0.05, **, p<0.01, ***, p<0.001.

Supporting Information

Figure S1 2H6 T cells mobilize calcium upon TCR stimulation. Purified CD4$^+$ cells from 2H6 mice were labeled with CFSE and Indo-1. TDS from a non-diabetic NOD mouse were incubated with 50 ug/mL InsB:9-23 peptide in the presence or absence of Glyphosine. 2H6 cells were stimulated with no antigen (APCs only, negative control) or a-CD3 cross-linking (positive control) or APCs incubated with InsB:9-23 peptide. Ionomycin stimulation was used as maximal strength positive control stimulation to induce Ca^{+2} flux from all cells. 2H6 cells were spun for 8 s at 8000 rpm in a microcentrifuge, right after the addition of the stimulation (APCs with or without the insB:9-23 peptide) followed by brief vortex and data acquisition on an LSR-II.

Figure S2 BDC12-4.1 T cells can be polarized into Th17 and Tr1 cells. CD4$^+$ cells from BDC12-4.1 mice cultured *in vitro* under Th17 (A) or Tr1 (B) polarizing conditions. Such polarized cells were restimulated with B:9-23 and production of TNF-α, IFN-γ, IL-4, IL-17 or IL-10 was determined by ICCS. (C) 1×10^6 Tr1's/mouse were adoptively transferred into prediabetic 8-wk old NOD mice and diabetes development was monitored.

Acknowledgments

We would like to thank Malina Mclure for managing our mouse colonies and Priscilla Colby for managerial assistance (both at LIAI).

Author Contributions

Conceived and designed the experiments: MvH. Performed the experiments: GS GF SS TJ AD JM. Analyzed the data: GS GF KTC. Contributed reagents/materials/analysis tools: MvH. Wrote the paper: GS GF KTC MvH.

References

1. Zhang L, Nakayama M, Eisenbarth GS (2008) Insulin as an autoantigen in NOD/human diabetes. Curr Opin Immunol 20: 111-118.
2. Nakayama M, Abiru N, Moriyama H, Babaya N, Liu E, et al. (2005) Prime role for an insulin epitope in the development of type 1 diabetes in NOD mice. Nature 435: 220-223.
3. Wegmann DR, Norbury-Glaser M, Daniel D (1994) Insulin-specific T cells are a predominant component of islet infiltrates in pre-diabetic NOD mice. Eur J Immunol 24: 1853-1857.
4. Wegmann DR, Gill RG, Norbury-Glaser M, Schloot N, Daniel D (1994) Analysis of the spontaneous T cell response to insulin in NOD mice. J Autoimmun 7: 833-843.
5. Daniel D, Gill RG, Schloot N, Wegmann D (1995) Epitope specificity, cytokine production profile and diabetogenic activity of insulin-specific T cell clones isolated from NOD mice. Eur J Immunol 25: 1056-1062.
6. Zekzer D, Wong FS, Wen L, Altieri M, Gurlo T, et al. (1997) Inhibition of diabetes by an insulin-reactive CD4 T-cell clone in the nonobese diabetic mouse. Diabetes 46: 1124-1132.
7. Fairchild PJ, Wildgoose R, Atherton E, Webb S, Wraith DC (1993) An autoantigenic T cell epitope forms unstable complexes with class II MHC: a novel route for escape from tolerance induction. Int Immunol 5: 1151-1158.
8. Liu GY, Fairchild PJ, Smith RM, Prowle JR, Kioussis D, et al. (1995) Low avidity recognition of self-antigen by T cells permits escape from central tolerance. Immunity 3: 407-415.
9. Mingueneau M, Jiang W, Feuerer M, Mathis D, Benoist C (2012) Thymic negative selection is functional in NOD mice. J Exp Med 209: 623-637.
10. Yu B, Gauthier L, Hausmann DH, Wucherpfennig KW (2000) Binding of conserved islet peptides by human and murine MHC class II molecules associated with susceptibility to type I diabetes. Eur J Immunol 30: 2497-2506.
11. Jasinski JM, Yu L, Nakayama M, Li MM, Lipes MA, et al. (2006) Transgenic insulin (B:9-23) T-cell receptor mice develop autoimmune diabetes dependent upon RAG genotype, H-2g7 homozygosity, and insulin 2 gene knockout. Diabetes 55: 1978-1984.
12. Du W, Wong FS, Li MO, Peng J, Qi H, et al. (2006) TGF-beta signaling is required for the function of insulin-reactive T regulatory cells. J Clin Invest 116: 1360-1370.
13. Fousteri G, Jasinski J, Dave A, Nakayama M, Pagni P, et al. (2012) Following the Fate of One Insulin-Reactive CD4 T cell: Conversion Into Teffs and Tregs in the Periphery Controls Diabetes in NOD Mice. Diabetes.
14. Daniel C, Weigmann B, Bronson R, von Boehmer H (2011) Prevention of type 1 diabetes in mice by tolerogenic vaccination with a strong agonist insulin mimetope. J Exp Med 208: 1501-1510.
15. Crawford F, Stadinski B, Jin N, Michels A, Nakayama M, et al. (2011) Specificity and detection of insulin-reactive CD4+ T cells in type 1 diabetes in the nonobese diabetic (NOD) mouse. Proc Natl Acad Sci U S A 108: 16729-16734.
16. Mohan JF, Levisetti MG, Calderon B, Herzog JW, Petzold SJ, et al. (2010) Unique autoreactive T cells recognize insulin peptides generated within the islets of Langerhans in autoimmune diabetes. Nat Immunol 11: 350-354.
17. Mohan JF, Petzold SJ, Unanue ER (2011) Register shifting of an insulin peptide-MHC complex allows diabetogenic T cells to escape thymic deletion. J Exp Med 208: 2375-2383.
18. Henrickson SE, Mempel TR, Mazo IB, Liu B, Artyomov MN, et al. (2008) T cell sensing of antigen dose governs interactive behavior with dendritic cells and sets a threshold for T cell activation. Nat Immunol 9: 282-291.
19. Obst R, van Santen HM, Mathis D, Benoist C (2005) Antigen persistence is required throughout the expansion phase of a CD4(+) T cell response. J Exp Med 201: 1555-1565.
20. Marek-Trzonkowska N, Mysliwec M, Siebert J, Trzonkowski P (2013) Clinical application of regulatory T cells in type 1 diabetes. Pediatr Diabetes 14: 322-332.
21. Marek-Trzonkowska N, Mysliwiec M, Dobyszuk A, Grabowska M, Techmanska I, et al. (2012) Administration of CD4+CD25highCD127- regulatory T cells preserves beta-cell function in type 1 diabetes in children. Diabetes Care 35: 1817-1820.

25

The C-Type Lectin OCILRP2 Costimulates EL4 T Cell Activation via the DAP12-Raf-MAP Kinase Pathway

Qiang Lou, Wei Zhang, Guangchao Liu, Yuanfang Ma*

Henan Engineering Lab of Antibody Medicine, Key Laboratory of Cellular and Molecular Immunology, Medical College of Henan University, Kaifeng 475004, China

Abstract

OCILRP2 is a typical Type-II transmembrane protein that is selectively expressed in activated T lymphocytes, dendritic cells, and B cells and functions as a novel co-stimulator of T cell activation. However, the signaling pathways underlying OCILRP2 in T cell activation are still not completely understood. In this study, we found that the knockdown of OCILRP2 expression with shRNA or the blockage of its activity by an anti-OCILRP2 antagonist antibody reduced CD3/CD28-costimulated EL4 T cell viability and IL-2 production, inhibit Raf1, MAPK3, and MAPK8 activation, and impair NFAT and NF-κB transcriptional activities. Furthermore, immunoprecipitation results indicated that OCILRP2 could interact with the DAP12 protein, an adaptor containing an intracellular ITAM motif that can transduce signals to induce MAP kinase activation for T cell activation. Our data reveal that after binding with DAP12, OCILRP2 activates the Raf-MAP kinase pathways, resulting in T cell activation.

Editor: Rajesh Mohanraj, Faculty of Medicine & Health Sciences, United Arab Emirates

Funding: This work was supported by grants from National Natural Science Foundation of China (No. 30972687) (http://www.nsfc.gov.cn) (YFM) and from 'Seed scientific research grant for talented scientist' (http://www.henu.edu.cn) (QL). The funders had no role in study design, data collection and analysis, decision to publish, or preparation of the manuscript.

Competing Interests: The authors have declared that no competing interests exist.

* Email: yuanfangma@126.com

Background

T cell activation is tightly regulated by an intricate series of signals provided by the T cell receptor/CD3 complex, cytokines, and co-stimulatory ligand/receptor systems. One of the best characterized co-stimulatory molecules expressed by T cells is CD28 [1], which interacts with CD80 (B7.1) and CD86 (B7.2) at the membrane of APCs (antigen-presenting cells). Recently, C-type lectin-like receptors (CTLRs), such as OCILRP2 [2], have emerged as a new category of T cell co-stimulatory molecules due to their ability to co-stimulate T cell proliferation and cytokine secretion. However, the signaling pathway underlying OCILRP2 is not completely understood.

Anti-CD3 or phorbol myristate acetate (PMA)-mediated MAPK activation involves the activation of Ras, leading to the activation of Raf-1 and the subsequent activation of MEK (MAPK or ERK kinase) [3]. The intracellular domain of OCILRP2 lacks the immunoreceptor tyrosine-based activation motif (ITAM) that triggers lymphocyte activation, suggesting that OCILRP2 may transmit co-stimulatory signal via adaptors, such as DAP12 [4,5], which interacts with NKG2D (natural killer group 2, member D) in activated NK cells and CD8$^+$ T cells [6]. DAP12 is a 12-kDa transmembrane protein that contains an aspartic acid residue in its transmembrane domain and a single cytoplasmic ITAM. DAP12 most likely activates SHC (Src homology 2 domain containing) transforming protein 1 via the Syk-family protein-tyrosine kinase Zap-70 [7,8]. The sequential phosphorylation of the adaptors further triggers downstream signaling events, including the activation of the MAP and JNK kinases and nuclear translocation

of transcription factors NF-AT [9], NF-κB [10], and AP-1 [11], leading to IL-2 gene expression and T cell activation. Activated T cells also produce the alpha subunit of the IL-2 receptor (CD25 or IL-2R), enabling a fully functional receptor that can bind with IL-2, which in turn activates the T cell's proliferation pathways.

OCILRP2 is a type II transmembrane CTLR that is expressed in osteoblasts, B cells, dendritic cells (DCs), and activated T cells. Splenocytes derived from OCILRP2-Ig-treated mice show a significant reduction in proliferation and level of IL-2, and the addition of OCILRP2-Ig results in a dose-dependent inhibition of CD4$^+$ T cell proliferation and IL-2 production, suggesting that OCILRP2 is required for splenocyte activation [12].

The murine T cell line EL4 produces IL-2 in the presence of appropriate signals and provides a model system for analyzing T cell activation co-stimulated by H-2 and CD3 antibodies [13]. JNK phosphorylation and c-*jun* transcription were found to be induced in EL4 cells in response to phorbol ester [14]. The EL4 cell line has also been used to explore the roles of ERK activation in downstream responses. In this study, we confirmed that OCILRP2 co-stimulates T cell activation in mouse EL4 cells, and for the first time, we identify that an adaptor protein, DAP12, interacts with OCILRP2 and is involved in this T cell activation. Mechanistic studies revealed that the re-localization of OCILRP2 from the cytoplasm to the membrane under the stimulation of CD3/CD28 antibodies might be responsible for the observed T cell activation by activating the MAPK signal transduction pathway. These results provide novel insight into the mechanisms of T cell activation.

Materials and Methods

Cell culture

EL4 (ATCC TIB 181) cells were purchased from American Type Culture Collection and cultured as described [15]. The EL4 cells were stimulated for the indicated times with combinations of anti-CD3 (sc-18871, Santa Cruz, USA) and/or anti-CD28 antibodies (sc-12727, Santa Cruz, USA). In some experiments, an anti-IL-2 antibody (H-20, Santa Cruz, USA) or anti-OCILRP2 antibody (AF3370, R&D systems, USA) was added to the culture medium. Controls were stimulated with phorbol myristate acetate (PMA) (p1585, 50 ng/mL, Sigma, USA) and ionomycin (I3909, 100 ng/mL, Sigma, USA).

Plasmid construction

The full-length OCILRP2 sequence was obtained from mouse B cells stimulated with anti-IgM (115-001-020, Jackson Immunotech, USA) in the presence of cycloheximide and then cloned into the pCDNA3-HA vector to yield pCDNA3-HA-OCILRP2. An OCILRP2 siRNA-expressing vector pEGFP-C3-siOCILRP2 was provided by Wenzhi Tian (Weill Medical College of Cornell University).

DAP12 was generated by PCR and introduced into the pDsRed-C1 vector or pGEX-4T-1 vector using the same method as that for OCILRP2. The full-length recombinant OCILRP2 protein GST-OCILRP2 and its two recombinant mutants, GST-OCILRP2e (N terminal region) and GST-OCILRP2i (C terminal region), were cloned into the pGEX-4T-1 cloning vector using standard molecular biology techniques. The pGEX-4T-1 recombinant vectors were then cloned into E. coli BL21 competent cells. GST proteins were purified over glutathione-agarose columns and stored in 50% (volume/volume) glycerol at -20°C. All constructs were sequenced and verified for accuracy, and all fusion proteins were checked for purity by SDS-PAGE and Coomassie staining.

Cytokine IL-2 determination

EL4 cells (5×10^5 cells/mL) were incubated with or without anti-CD3/CD28 antibodies or PMA (10 ng/mL) and ionomycin (100 ng/mL) for 12, 24, and 48 h. Supernatants were obtained by centrifugation for 3 min using a microcentrifuge. Cytokine IL-2 secreted into the supernatant was determined via ELISA (R&D systems, USA), and the samples were analyzed using a spectrophotometer (Beckman Coulter DU 640, USA). The IL-2 sample levels were determined by comparison to a standard curve of recombinant mouse IL-2 and are expressed as the mean ± S.E., as determined for each group from three independent experiments.

Flow cytometry analysis

EL4 cells (1×10^6 cells) were stimulated with or without anti-CD3/CD28 antibodies or PMA/ionomycin. After 48 h of stimulation, the cells were incubated with an anti-OCILRP2 antagonist antibody for 30 min on ice, followed by staining with an FITC (sc-2777)-labeled secondary antibody. The appropriate conjugated isotype-matched IgGs were used as controls. The cells were analyzed with Cellquest software using a BD FACS Calibur flow cytometer.

T cell survival assay

The number of viable EL4 cells was monitored using Cell Counting Kit-8 (CCK-8) (C0038, Beyotime, China). To assay EL4 T cell viability with OCILRP2-mediated co-stimulation, 96-well flat-bottom microtiter plates were pre-coated with an anti-CD3/CD28 antibody, anti-CD3/CD28/OCILRP2 antibody (25 μg/mL), or anti-CD3/CD28/IL-2 antibody overnight at 4°C. The

cells were also transfected with the pEGFP-siOCILRP2 plasmid and then stimulated with the anti-CD3/CD28 antibodies. 100 μL of the cell suspension (5,000 cells/well) was dispensed into each well of a 96-well plate. After incubation for 24, 48, and 72 h (37°C), 10 μL of CCK-8 solution was added to each well, and the cells were incubated for 1 h (37°C). The absorbance was measured at 450 nm using a spectrophotometer (Beckman Coulter DU 640, USA).

GST pull-down and Co-immunoprecipitation assay

GST pull-down and co-immunoprecipitation (co-IP) were performed as described previously [16]. E. coli BL21 cells were harvested by centrifugation and then resuspended in buffer (PBS, 1% Triton-X 100, and 1 mM dithiothreitol (DTT)) for sonication. After centrifugation of the sonicated lysates, the supernatants were incubated with Glutathione-Sepharose 4B beads (GE) for purification. Forty-eight hours after stimulation with CD3/CD28 antibodies, EL4 cells were washed three times with ice-cold PBS and suspended in lysis buffer (20 mM Tris-HCl (pH 8.0), 200 mM NaCl, 1 mM EDTA (pH 8.0), 0.5% Nonidet P-40, 1 mM Na$_3$VO$_4$, 25 g/mL phenylmethylsulfonyl fluoride, 1 mM β-glycerophosphate, and 1× protease inhibitor cocktail). After shaking for 30 min (4°C), the cells were centrifuged at 12,000 x g for 10 min (4°C). The resulting supernatants were divided into three parts. One-tenth of the supernatant was boiled in 40 μl 2× SDS protein loading buffer and used for input. Equal parts of the remaining supernatant were incubated with GST or GST-fused proteins. After shaking for 2 h (4°C), the beads were washed three times with washing buffer (20 mM Tris-HCl (pH 8.0), 200 mM NaCl, 1 mM EDTA (pH 8.0), and 0.5% Nonidet P-40) and boiled in 40 μl loading buffer for SDS-PAGE.

For co-immunoprecipitation, pCDNA3-HA-OCILRP2 and pDsRed-C1-DAP12 were co-transfected into 293T cells for 48 hours. The supernatant of the co-transfected cells was immunoprecipitated with 1 μg of specific antibodies or control IgG (Santa Cruz), shaken for 2 h (4°C), mixed with 30 μL protein A/G (Santa Cruz), incubated for another 2 h (4°C), and washed three times with washing buffer. Proteins bound to the beads were boiled in 40 μL loading buffer.

Immunofluorescence staining and Confocal microscopy

The procedure for immunofluorescence (IF) was performed as previously described [16]. Briefly, EL4 cells transfected overnight with pEGFP-C3-siOCILRP2 were stimulated with anti-CD3/CD28 antibodies. For the other groups, EL4 cells were stimulated with or without anti-CD3/CD28 or anti-CD3/CD28/OCILRP2 antibodies. All cells were incubated on glass cover slips and fixed with 3.5% paraformaldehyde for 15 min, which was then stopped by the addition of 30 mM glycine. After washing, the cells were permeabilized with 0.1% Triton X-100 for 15 min and blocked with 3% bovine serum albumin in PBS for at least 1 h (4°C). A polyclonal anti-OCILRP2 antibody (AF3370, R&D systems, USA) and monoclonal anti-DAP12 antibody (sc-133174, Santa Cruz, USA) were used at a 1:2000 dilution. Goat anti-mouse-IgG-PE (sc-3738, Santa Cruz, USA) and rabbit anti-goat-IgG-FITC (sc-2777, Santa Cruz, USA) secondary antibodies were used at a 1:100 dilution. Nuclei were stained with 4', 6'-diamidino-2-phenylindole dihydrochloride (DAPI) (D9542, Sigma-Aldrich, USA), and the cells were examined by confocal microscopy (98DDFR/470111CR, Bio-Rad, USA).

Western blot analysis

EL4 cells transfected overnight with pEGFP-C3-siOCILRP2 were stimulated with anti-CD3/CD28 antibodies. For the other

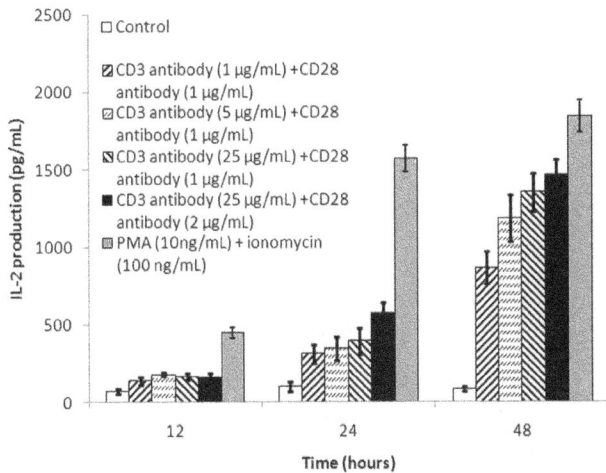

Figure 1. IL-2 secreted from EL4 cells after stimulation with an anti-CD3/CD28 mAb or PMA/ionomycin. EL4 cells were incubated with or without anti-CD3/CD28 antibodies (at various concentrations) or PMA (10 ng/mL) and ionomycin (100 ng/mL) for 12, 24, and 48 h. Supernatants were obtained by centrifugation for 3 min using a microcentrifuge. Cytokine IL-2 secreted into the supernatant was determined by ELISA.

two groups, EL4 cells were stimulated with or without anti-CD3/CD28 antibodies. Cell lysates were prepared in SDS sample buffer (Tris-HCl, SDS, and 20% glycerol) and detected using SDS-PAGE. The proteins were electrotransferred onto Immobilon-P PVDF membranes (0.45 μm, Millipore, USA) and probed with the appropriate primary antibodies against the following: p-Raf-1 (Ser 338) (sc-12358, Santa Cruz, 1:200), caspase-8 p18 (G-1) (sc-166596, Santa Cruz, 1:500), caspase-3 p17 (B-4) (sc-271028, Santa Cruz, 1:500), JNK1 (D-6) (sc-137018, Santa Cruz, 1:500), p-JNK1/2/3 (T183+Y185) pAb (BS4322, Bioworld Technology, 1:500), ERK 1/2 (H-72) (sc-292838, Santa Cruz, 1:200), p-ERK 1/2 (Thr202/Tyr204) (sc-16982, Santa Cruz, 1:200), IκB-alpha (N-terminus) mAb (MB0106, Bioworld Technology, 1:1000), β-actin (Sigma, 1:5,000), and β-tubulin (Sigma, 1:5000)). After incubation with a horseradish peroxidase-conjugated secondary antibody (Santa Cruz, 1:10,000) for 3-4 h, the membranes were washed with PBST. Immunoreactivity was visualized using an ECL system (Perkin Elmer, USA), and densitometry scanning of the intensity of the bands was quantified using ImageJ.

cDNA synthesis and Quantitative real-time PCR analysis

RNA from anti-CD3/CD28 antibody- or anti-CD3/CD28/OCILRP2 antibody-stimulated EL4 cells and normal EL4 cells were isolated using trizol reagent (15596-018, Invitrogen). A 3-μg of RNA was used for cDNA synthesis with a random primer mix, 10 mM dNTPs, M-MLV RT buffer, and M-MLV reverse transcriptase (Promega, Madison, USA). The RT reaction was performed at 42°C for 1 hour, followed by deactivation for 5 minutes at 90°C. cDNA for IL-2, NFκB, NFAT, MAPK8, and MAPK3 or the control household gene *β-actin* was amplified using SYBR Premix Ex Taq (RRO41A, TaKaRa, Shiga, Japan), and expression was monitored using an Rotor-gene 6000 real-time platform (Corbett Research, Australia). CT values were normalized for the expression of the *β-actin* gene.

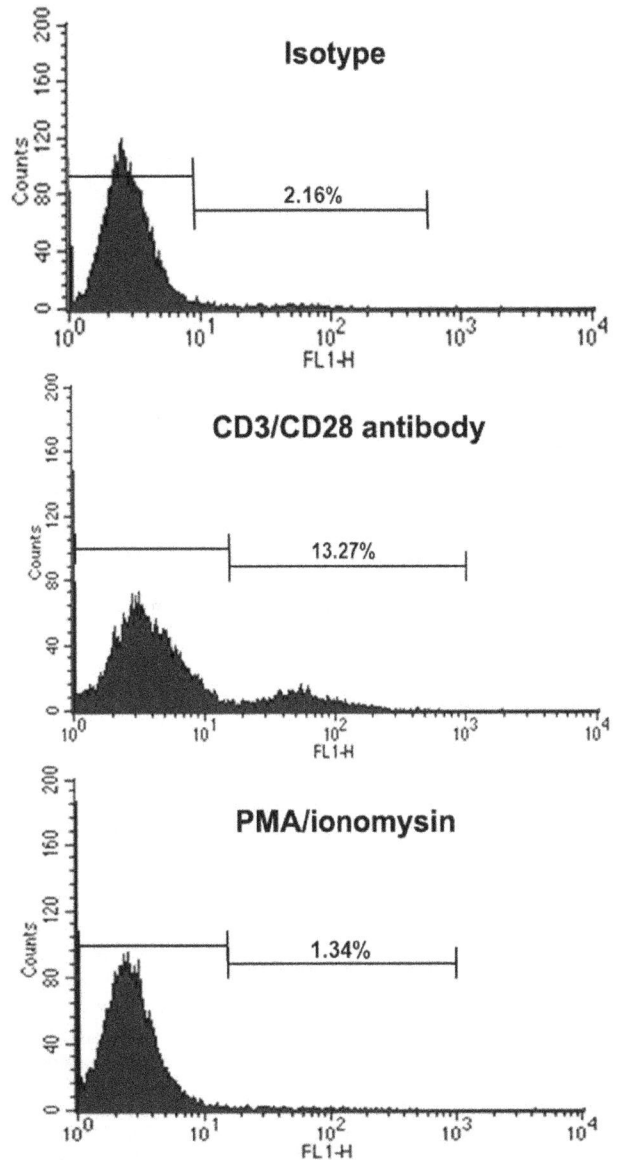

Figure 2. Membrane re-localization of OCILRP2 via treatment with an anti-CD3/CD28 mAb. EL4 cells were incubated with plate-bound CD3/CD28 antibodies, isotype-matched mIgGs, or PMA/ionomycin for 48 h. The cells (1×10^6 cells) were then incubated with an anti-OCILRP2 antagonist antibody for 30 min on ice, followed by staining with an FITC-labeled second antibody. The cells were analyzed with Cellquest software using a FACS Calibur flow cytometer.

Statistical analysis

Experimental data were analyzed with SPSS software and compared using Student's *t*-test. Differences with a P value of < 0.05 were considered statistically significant.

Results

Membrane translocation of OCILRP2 is involved in the co-stimulation of EL4 cell activation

It has been reported that OCILRP2 is expressed in B cells, dendritic cells (DCs), and activated T cells and is a novel co-stimulator of primary mouse T cell activation [12]. In the present

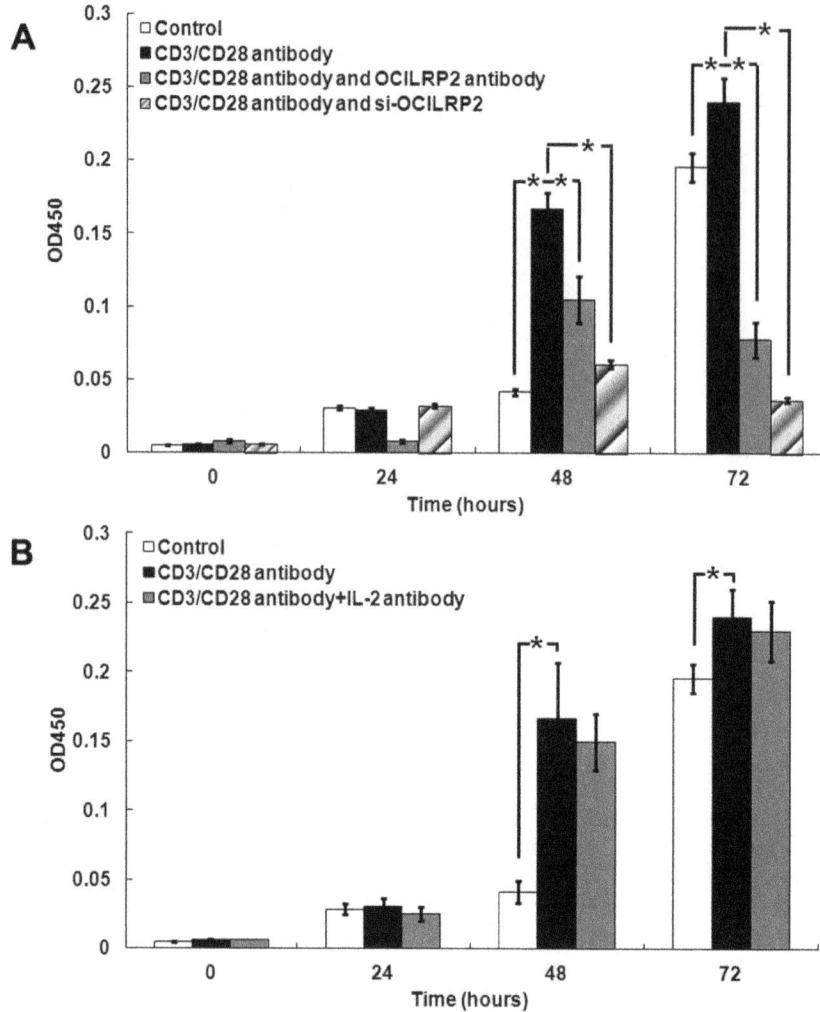

Figure 3. OCILRP2 co-stimulation affects EL4 cell viability. Six-well flat-bottom microtiter plates were pre-coated with anti-CD3/CD28 antibodies or anti-CD3/CD28/OCILRP2 antibodies (a) or anti-CD3/CD28/IL-2 antibodies (b) overnight at 4°C. Cells were transfected with pEGFP-siOCILRP2 plasmid and then stimulated with the anti-CD3/CD28 antibodies (a). Then, 100 μL of the cell suspension (5,000 cells/well) was dispensed into each well of a 96-well plate. After incubation for 24, 48, and 72 h (37°C), 10 μL of CCK-8 solution was added to each well, and the cells were incubated for 1 h (37°C). The absorbance was measured at 450 nm using a spectrophotometer (Beckman Coulter DU 640, USA). *$P < 0.05$.

study, we first investigated the effect of OCILRP2 on PMA-sensitive EL4 cell activation. EL4 cells were stimulated with PMA/ionomycin, anti-CD3/CD28 antibodies, and anti-CD3/CD28/OCILRP2 antibodies at varying concentrations pre-coated in 96-well cell plates for 12, 24, 48 h; IL-2 secretion was then analyzed by ELISA. The highest level of IL-2 secretion from EL4 cells was found after PMA/ionomycin stimulation or after combined stimulation with the anti-CD3 antibody (25 μg/mL) and anti-CD28 antibody (2 μg/mL) for 48 h (1845 ± 103.5 pg/mL and 1464 ± 98.55 pg/mL, respectively) (Fig. 1). This was used as the standard stimulating concentration for EL4 cell activation in the present study.

After the stimulation of EL4 cells by CD3/CD28 antibodies, most of the OCILRP2 proteins are transferred from the cytoplasm to the cell membrane, which was confirmed by a flow cytometric analysis. Although 2.16% of the 'resting' EL4 cells expressed OCILRP2, the percentage of EL4 cells expressing OCILRP2 increased to 13.27% at 48 h following CD3/CD28 stimulation

(Fig. 2). However, the PMA/ionomycin-treated EL4 cells did not exhibit this membrane translocation.

An antagonist OCILRP2 antibody reduces the viability of EL4 cells stimulated by CD3/CD28 antibodies

Because OCILRP2 functions in EL4 cell activation, the role of OCILRP2 in EL4 cell viability was further examined using a CCK8 cell proliferation kit. Incubation with the anti-CD3/CD28 antibody for 48 h or 72 h promoted viability. However, the simultaneous incubation with the anti-OCILRP2 antagonist antibody or the knock down of OCILRP2 expression significantly reduced viability by approximately 1.59 and 2.73 times at 48 h and 3.08 and 6.54 times at 72 h, respectively (Fig. 3a). However, the cell cycle percentages did not change notably (Fig. S1).

To determine whether the observed EL4 cell viability was caused by the direct effect of OCILRP2 or the high level of IL-2 secreted by the cells, the extent of EL4 cell viability with anti-CD3/CD28/IL-2 or anti-CD3/CD28 antibody stimulation were compared. Similar cell viability was observed (Fig. 3b).

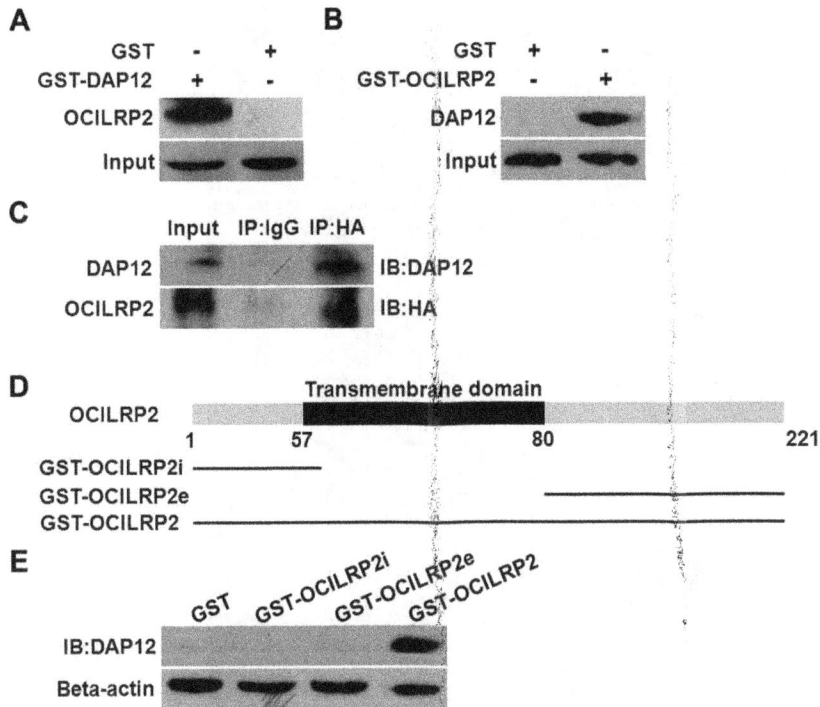

Figure 4. Interaction of OCILRP2 and DAP12 in GST pull-down and co-immunoprecipitation assays. The GST pull-down assay was carried out using purified beads that contained GST, GST-DAP12, or GST-OCILRP2. Precipitated OCILRP2 or DAP12 was detected by western blotting using an anti-OCILRP2 or anti-DAP12 antibody, respectively (a, b). 293T cells were grown in 6-cm dishes and transfected with the pCDNA3-HA-OCILRP2 and pDsRed-C1-DAP12 plasmids, respectively. OCILRP2 and DAP12 were detected by western blotting using an anti-HA antibody or an anti-DAP12 antibody (c). Schematic diagram of OCILRP2 predicted by SMART software. The green column represents the transmembrane region (amino acids 57–80) (d). The GST pull-down assay was carried out using purified beads that contained GST, full-length GST-OCILRP2, GST-OCILRP2i (aa 1–57), or GST-OCILRP2e (aa 80–221). Precipitated DAP12 was detected by western blotting using an anti-DAP12 antibody (e).

OCILRP2 interacts with DAP12 in vitro and in vivo

Because DAP12 contains an immunoreceptor tyrosine-based activation motif (ITAM) region that transmits the activation signal, we then investigated the contribution of DAP12 to membrane translocation. To determine the mechanism of the effect of OCILRP2 on T cell activation, we assessed OCILRP2 interactions with the adaptor protein DAP12, as the intracellular region of OCILRP2 is relatively short and may be insufficient to transmit a signal. A GST pull-down assay was performed to verify the OCILRP2/DAP12 interaction. GST-fused OCILRP2 was expressed in *E. coli* (BL21/DE3) and purified on glutathione-Sepharose 4B beads. After incubation with EL4 cell lysates, the precipitated proteins were separated by SDS-PAGE and detected by western blotting using an anti-DAP12 antibody. The results showed that DAP12 bound to GST-OCILRP2 but not to GST alone (Fig. 4a). A reciprocal experiment using GST-DAP12 and OCILRP2 gave a similar result (Fig. 4b). To show that OCILRP2 also interacts with DAP12 in cells, 293T cells were co-transfected with the pCDNA3-HA-OCILRP2 and pDsRed-C1-DAP12 plasmids, and interaction between OCILRP2 and DAP12 was observed by co-immunoprecipitation with an anti-HA or anti-DAP12 antibody (Fig. 4c).

To better understand the function of the association between OCILRP2 and DAP12, it was necessary to map the amino acid sequences required for their binding. Thus, a protein truncation assay was performed to identify the region of OCILRP2 that interacts with DAP12. Because OCILRP2 has a transmembrane region and a C-type lectin-like cytoplasmic domain structure (predicted by SMART software), OCILRP2 was truncated at its

N-terminal (aa 1–57) and C-terminal (aa 80–221) regions based on a prediction model (Fig. 4d) and fused with GST. The GST pull-down results showed that only the full-length, but not the N-terminal region or C-terminal region, of OCILRP2 bound to DAP12 (Fig. 4e), indicating that the interaction of OCILRP2 with DAP12 maps to the transmembrane region: aa 58–79.

To investigate in detail the mechanism responsible for T cell activation upon OCILRP2 stimulation, we tested the OCILRP2/DAP12 interaction in EL4 cells by confocal laser microscopy (CLSM) after immunological staining with PE- or FITC-labeled antibodies. EL4 cells were stimulated with CD3/CD28 antibodies, CD3/CD28/OCILRP2 antibodies, or CD3/CD28 antibodies and then transfected with an OCILRP2-interfering plasmid. Our data showed a cell membrane colocalization of OCILRP2 with DAP12 (Fig. 5). OCILRP2 trafficked from the cell cytoplasm to the cell membrane, and strong merge signals were observed in the cell membrane regions in EL4 cells.

OCILRP2 participates in anti-CD3/CD28 antibody-induced EL4 cell activation by promoting Erk and Jnk phosphorylation

Because OCILRP2 was demonstrated to participate in anti-CD3/CD28 antibody-induced activation as well as in the secretion of IL-2 by EL4 cells, the effects of anti-CD3/CD28 antibodies and si-OCILRP2 on the expressions of the MAPK and PI3K/Akt pathways were investigated by western blotting to clarify the underlying mechanisms. The results of western blotting showed that anti-CD3/CD28 antibodies induced the phosphorylation of ERK1/2 and JNK (Fig. 6a). In contrast, knock-down of

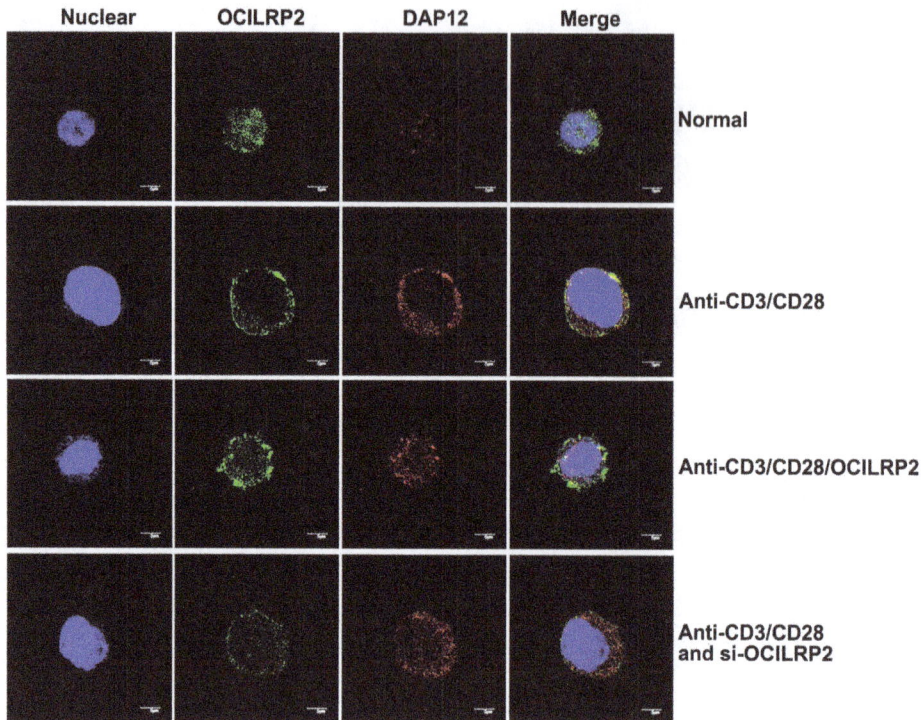

Figure 5. Membrane co-localization of OCILRP2 and DAP12 under anti-CD3/CD28 mAb treatment in EL4 T cells. EL4 T cells pre-transfected with pEGFP-siOCILRP2 or pre-coated with the OCILRP2 Ab were cultured overnight in the presence or absence of an anti-CD3/CD28 mAb and then stained for OCILRP2 (green) and nuclear stained with DAPI (blue) and DAP12 (red) to study OCILRP2 and DAP12 protein expression and localization. Unstimulated EL4 T cells exhibited OCILRP2 protein expression in the cytoplasm (upper panels). In contrast, CD3/CD28-activated EL4 T cells showed intracellular and membrane OCILRP2. OCILRP2/DAP12 co-localization appears in yellow. Each picture is representative of the vast majority of the observed cells on the slides.

OCILRP2 inhibited the anti-CD3/CD28 antibody-induced phosphorylation of ERK1/2 and JNK in EL4 cells. However, anti-CD3/CD28 antibodies did not significantly affect the phosphorylation of Akt (Fig. 6b).

Because ERK1 and JNK are involved in EL4 cell IL-2 expression, Raf was examined to determine whether it is involved in this signaling pathway. The results showed that the phosphorylation of Raf was inhibited by si-OCILRP2 (Fig. 6b).

An anti-OCILRP2 antagonist antibody decreased the transcriptional levels of NF-κB, NFAT, MAPK3, MAPK8, and IL-2

The NF-κB and NFAT (nuclear factor of activated T cells) proteins are key regulators of T cell development and function [17]. Changes in the levels of NF-κB and NFAT transcription were compared after stimulation by CD3/CD28 antibodies with or without the anti-OCILRP2 antagonist antibody. NF-κB and NFAT transcripts were preferentially expressed (up-regulated 3.6 and 10.9 times, respectively) in the EL4 cells stimulated with CD3/CD28 antibodies. Additionally, after CD3/CD28 antibody stimulation, the expression of Interleukin-2 (IL-2), MAPK3 (coding for ERK1/2), and MAPK8 (coding for JNK1) were also increased by approximately 1.9, 23.6, and 7.3 times (P<0.05), respectively (Fig. 7).

Discussion

In the present study, the costimulation of mouse T cell activation by the C-type lectin-like molecule OCILRP2 was confirmed in the EL4 cell line. In addition, OCILRP2 redistribution to the cell membrane and its interaction with the adaptor protein DAP12 was likely the cause of EL4 cell activation.

Wenzhi Tian et al. [12] first reported the effects of OCILRP2 on primary human T cell proliferation and IL-2 production. These authors found that silencing OCILRP2 leads to intrinsic defects in T cell survival as well as cell cycle progression in response to TCR and CD28 signaling. Recently, further studies on the possible mechanism of T cell activation have been reported. Thebault P et al. demonstrated that the C-type lectin-like receptor CLEC-1, expressed by myeloid cells and endothelial cells, is up-regulated by immunoregulatory mediators and moderates T cell activation [18]. Another study by Clifford S. Guy et al. reported that T cell proliferation requires the recruitment of Vav1 to the CD3 complex and activation of the Notch signaling pathway [19]. However, due to the lack of signaling motifs in its intracellular domain, the mechanism underlying OCILRP2-mediated T cell co-stimulation has remained undefined.

OCILRP2 lacks cytoplasmic signaling motifs but contains charged residues in its transmembrane domains, which may allow associations with signaling partners, such as homodimers DAP12 or DAP10 (Fig. 8?). The 2 homodimers initiate distinct signaling cascades: DAP12 activates the Syk/ZAP70 pathway, and DAP10 signals through the PI3K pathway [20–24]. Western blot analyses with antibodies against phosphorylated Akt revealed equal protein levels in EL4 cells treated with CD3/CD28 antibodies or CD3/CD28/OCILRP2 antibodies, thus demonstrating that the co-stimulatory activation of OCILRP2 may not occur via the DAP10 signaling pathway. DAP12 homodimers associate with a variety of

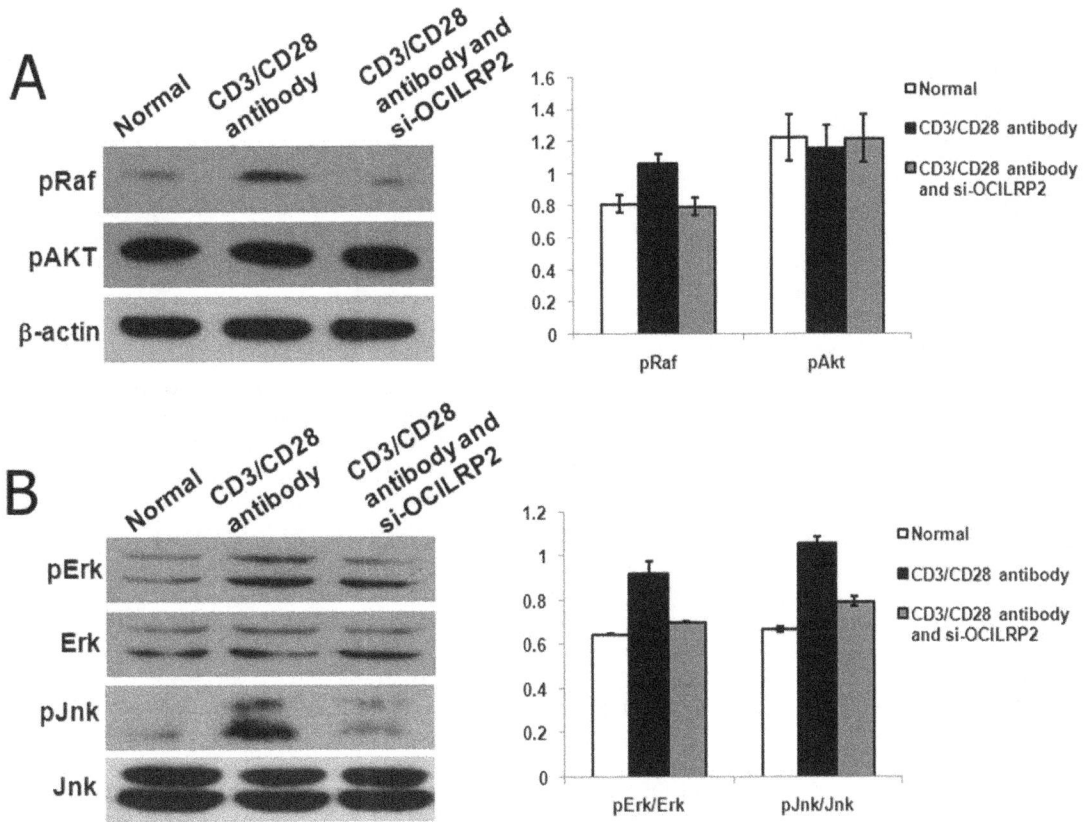

Figure 6. Western blot analysis of Raf, Erk, Jnk, and Akt phosphorylation in EL4 cells. EL4 T cells were incubated in DMEM medium with an immobilized anti-CD3/CD28 mAb in the presence or absence of si-OCILRP2. After incubation at 37°C for 48 h, the T cells were lysed, and aliquots of 20 µg of the whole-cell lysate were analyzed by western blotting using antibodies against phospho-Erk, Erk, phospho-Jnk, and Jnk (a) and phospho-Raf and phosphor-Akt (b). The data are expressed as a percentage of the level of active Erk or Jnk of the total Erk or Jnk. Each data point represents the mean ± S.E. from three separate experiments.

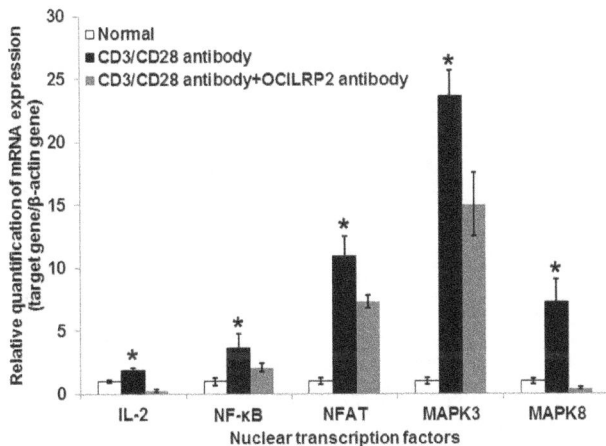

Figure 7. mRNA expression in EL4 cells stimulated with or without anti-CD3/CD28 antibodies or anti-CD3/CD28/OCILRP2 antibodies. RNA from un-stimulated or CD3/CD28 antibody- or CD3/CD28/OCILRP2 antibody-stimulated EL4 cells was isolated using the RNeasy kit (Qiagen). cDNA of IL-2, NF-κB, NFAT, MAPK3, and MAPK8 or the control household gene β-actin was amplified using SYBR Premix Ex Taq (RRO41A, TaKaRa, Shiga, Japan), and expression was monitored using an Rotor-gene 6000 real-time platform (Corbett Research, Australia). Ct values were normalized for the expression of the β-actin gene. *$P < 0.05$.

receptors expressed by macrophages, monocytes and myeloid cells including TREM2 [25], Siglec H [26] and SIRP-beta [27], as well as activating KIR [28] and the NKG2C proteins [29] expressed by NK cells. In this study, an interaction between OCILRP2 and DAP12 was demonstrated, and the interactions can be mediated by transmembrane domain of OCILRP2. OCILRP2 has a short cytoplasmic tail (57 amino acids) that lacks an ITAM or other tyrosine motif, may recruit adaptor protein to activate downstream signaling pathways during T cell activation. DAP12 may be playing a role in enhancing the maturation and stabilization of OCILRP2 or that DAP12 has a role in impacting the trafficking of OCILRP2 to the cell surface. In NK cells, spleen tyrosine kinase (SYK) and ζ-chain-associated protein kinase of 70 kDa (ZAP70) are recruited to the plasma membrane following DAP12 phosphorylation, leading to the activation of phosphatidylinositol 3-kinase (PI3K) and tyrosine phosphorylation of the scaffolding proteins LAT (linker for activation of T cells) and LcK (Leukocyte C-terminal Src kinase) [30]. Interestingly, Wenzhi Tian et al. [2] recently identified reduced LcK tyrosine phosphorylation in OCILRP2-silenced T cells, whereas the tyrosine phosphorylation of LAT was unchanged, suggesting that DAP12 may transmit the OCILRP2 co-stimulatory signal via the DAP12-Lck pathway.

Our laboratory has utilized EL4, a murine thymoma cell line, as a model system in which to explore the intracellular signaling pathways that are activated upon ligation of the co-stimulatory receptor OCILRP2. The anti-CD3 antibody-induced activation of EL4 cells was enhanced in the presence of an immunologically cross-linked and immobilized anti-H2 antibody [13]. In the present study, our results demonstrate that OCILRP2 does not cooperate with either anti-CD3 or -CD28 antibodies to enhance IL-2 release; rather, the effect of OCILRP2 was observed only when the cells were stimulated with a combination of both antibodies. Therefore, OCILRP2 overexpression or translocation does not replace signaling by either of the two receptor and does not appear to be uniquely coupled to TCR or CD28. In addition, an anti-IL-2 antibody did not affect OCILRP2-mediated viability, suggesting that IL-2 is not the primary stimulus driving the expansion of anti-CD3 plus anti-CD28-stimulated T cells.

The mechanism by which OCILRP2 co-stimulation enhances TCR signals is not clear. CD28 enhances TCR signaling by stimulating lipid raft redistribution at the site of TCR engagement [31]. Moreover, there is evidence demonstrating that CD28 can translocate to lipid rafts upon cross-linking and that this correlates with its co-stimulation of IL-2 production [32]. OCILRP2 may play a role similar to that of CD28 by facilitating TCR-mediated raft microdomain formation. T cell receptor signal transduction is initiated by the assembly and aggregation of signaling complexes including the adaptor molecule LAT [33], the Src homology 2 domain-containing leukocyte protein of 76 kDa (SLP-76) [34], Lck [35], and Fyn [36]. OCILRP2 may be recruited to lipid rafts and facilitate Lck tyrosine phosphorylation. Because human DAP12 reportedly binds the SH2 domains of Syk and Zap-70 [7], the ligation of OCILRP2 may lead to the activation of Syk and Zap-70.

MAPKs are regarded as key switches of cellular activation and proliferation [37]. Within the context of co-stimulatory OCILRP2 signaling, an increase in Jnk or Erk phosphorylation was observed. The phosphorylation of Raf was inhibited by si-OCILRP2, suggesting that Raf might be essential for the regulation of CD3/CD28 antibody-induced IL-2 expression.

The pathway revealed by our findings provides a molecular basis for the defective TCR-mediated activation of OCILRP2-silenced mouse T lymphocytes (Fig. S3). Therefore, selective pharmacological strategies designed to modulate the recruitment of OCILRP2 to the cell membrane may prove therapeutically useful for modulating T cell co-stimulatory signals in immunological diseases.

Conclusions

In the present study of anti-CD3/CD28 antibodies, OCILRP2 re-localized to the EL4 T cell membrane and interacted with the adaptor protein DAP12 to transmit the T cell activation signal, leading to the activation of the downstream MAPK signaling pathway and nuclear transcription factors in the murine EL4 T cell line.

Supporting Information

Figure S1 Analysis of cell cycle progression. EL4 cells were untreated or treated with anti-CD3/CD28 antibodies, an anti-OCILRP2 antagonist antibody, or si-OCILRP2. The cells were harvested after 48 h, fixed, stained, and analyzed for DNA content. The distribution and percentage of cells in pre-phase and G1, S, and G2/M phases of the cell cycle are indicated.

Figure S2 Postulated schematic diagram of OCILRP2 and DAP12 interaction.

Figure S3 Schematic model for the mechanism of OCILRP2-stimulated T cell activation.

Acknowledgments

We appreciate Prof. Youhai H. Chen at University of Pennsylvania School of Medicine and Dr. Wenzhi Tian at Weill Medical College of Cornell University for their advice on this manuscript.

Author Contributions

Conceived and designed the experiments: QL YFM. Performed the experiments: QL WZ GCL. Analyzed the data: QL. Contributed reagents/materials/analysis tools: QL. Wrote the paper: QL.

References

1. Nunes JA, Truneh A, Olive D, Cantrell DA (1996) Signal transduction by CD28 costimulatory receptor on T cells. B7-1 and B7-2 regulation of tyrosine kinase adaptor molecules. J Biol Chem 271: 1591–1598.
2. Tian W, Feng B, Liou HC (2005) Silencing OCILRP2 leads to intrinsic defects in T cells in response to antigenic stimulation. Cell Immunol 235: 72–84.
3. Franklin RA, Tordai A, Patel H, Gardner AM, Johnson GL, et al. (1994) Ligation of the T cell receptor complex results in activation of the Ras/Raf-1/MEK/MAPK cascade in human T lymphocytes. The Journal of clinical investigation 93: 2134–2140.
4. Lanier LL, Corliss BC, Wu J, Leong C, Phillips JH (1998) Immunoreceptor DAP12 bearing a tyrosine-based activation motif is involved in activating NK cells. Nature 391: 703–707.
5. Mason LH, Willette-Brown J, Anderson SK, Gosselin P, Shores EW, et al. (1998) Cutting edge: characterization of an associated 16-kDa tyrosine phosphoprotein required for Ly-49D signal transduction. The Journal of Immunology 160: 4148–4152.
6. Groh V, Rhinehart R, Randolph-Habecker J, Topp MS, Riddell SR, et al. (2001) Costimulation of CD8alphabeta T cells by NKG2D via engagement by MIC induced on virus-infected cells. Nat Immunol 2: 255–260.
7. McVicar DW, Taylor LS, Gosselin P, Willette-Brown J, Mikhael AI, et al. (1998) DAP12-mediated signal transduction in natural killer cells. A dominant role for the Syk protein-tyrosine kinase. J Biol Chem 273: 32934–32942.
8. Lin J, Weiss A (2001) T cell receptor signalling. Journal of cell science 114: 243–244.
9. Shaw JP, Utz PJ, Durand DB, Toole JJ, Emmel EA, et al. (1988) Identification of a putative regulator of early T cell activation genes. Science 241: 202–205.
10. Ruan Q, Chen YH (2012) Nuclear factor-kappaB in immunity and inflammation: the Treg and Th17 connection. Advances in experimental medicine and biology 946: 207–221.
11. Minden A, Lin A, Claret FX, Abo A, Karin M (1995) Selective activation of the JNK signaling cascade and c-Jun transcriptional activity by the small GTPases Rac and Cdc42Hs. Cell 81: 1147–1157.
12. Tian W, Nunez R, Cheng S, Ding Y, Tumang J, et al. (2005) C-type lectin OCILRP2/Clr-g and its ligand NKRP1f costimulate T cell proliferation and IL-2 production. Cell Immunol 234: 39–53.
13. Brams P, Claesson MH (1989) T-cell activation. I. Evidence for a functional linkage between class I MHC antigens and the Tc-Ti complex. Immunology 66: 348–353.
14. Jain J, Loh C, Rao A (1995) Transcriptional regulation of the IL-2 gene. Current opinion in immunology 7: 333–342.
15. Sansbury HM, Wisehart-Johnson AE, Qi C, Fulwood S, Meier KE (1997) Effects of protein kinase C activators on phorbol ester-sensitive and -resistant EL4 thymoma cells. Carcinogenesis 18: 1817–1824.
16. Wang Y, Xu Y, Tong W, Pan T, Li J, et al. (2011) Hepatitis C virus NS5B protein delays s phase progression in human hepatocyte-derived cells by relocalizing cyclin-dependent kinase 2-interacting protein (CINP). J Biol Chem 286: 26603–26615.
17. Macian F (2005) NFAT proteins: key regulators of T-cell development and function. Nature reviews Immunology 5: 472–484.
18. Thebault P, Lhermite N, Tilly G, Le Texier L, Quillard T, et al. (2009) The C-type lectin-like receptor CLEC-1, expressed by myeloid cells and endothelial cells, is up-regulated by immunoregulatory mediators and moderates T cell activation. J Immunol 183: 3099–3108.
19. Guy CS, Vignali KM, Temirov J, Bettini ML, Overacre AE, et al. (2013) Distinct TCR signaling pathways drive proliferation and cytokine production in T cells. Nat Immunol 14: 262–270.
20. Billadeau DD, Upshaw JL, Schoon RA, Dick CJ, Leibson PJ (2003) NKG2D-DAP10 triggers human NK cell-mediated killing via a Syk-independent regulatory pathway. Nat Immunol 4: 557–564.

21. Upshaw JL, Arneson LN, Schoon RA, Dick CJ, Billadeau DD, et al. (2006) NKG2D-mediated signaling requires a DAP10-bound Grb2-Vav1 intermediate and phosphatidylinositol-3-kinase in human natural killer cells. Nat Immunol 7: 524–532.

22. Raulet DH (2003) Roles of the NKG2D immunoreceptor and its ligands. Nature reviews Immunology 3: 781–790.

23. Lanier LL (2005) NK cell recognition. Annual review of immunology 23: 225–274.

24. Wu J, Cherwinski H, Spies T, Phillips JH, Lanier LL (2000) DAP10 and DAP12 form distinct, but functionally cooperative, receptor complexes in natural killer cells. J Exp Med 192: 1059–1068.

25. Humphrey MB, Daws MR, Spusta SC, Niemi EC, Torchia JA, et al. (2006) TREM2, a DAP12-associated receptor, regulates osteoclast differentiation and function. Journal of bone and mineral research: the official journal of the American Society for Bone and Mineral Research 21: 237–245.

26. Ishida-Kitagawa N, Tanaka K, Bao X, Kimura T, Miura T, et al. (2012) Siglec-15 protein regulates formation of functional osteoclasts in concert with DNAX-activating protein of 12 kDa (DAP12). J Biol Chem 287: 17493–17502.

27. Dietrich J, Cella M, Seiffert M, Buhring HJ, Colonna M (2000) Cutting edge: signal-regulatory protein beta 1 is a DAP12-associated activating receptor expressed in myeloid cells. J Immunol 164: 9–12.

28. Mulrooney TJ, Posch PE, Hurley CK (2013) DAP12 impacts trafficking and surface stability of killer immunoglobulin-like receptors on natural killer cells. J Leukoc Biol 94: 301–313.

29. Wei P, Xu L, Li CD, Sun FD, Chen L, et al. (2014) Molecular dynamic simulation of the self-assembly of DAP12-NKG2C activating immunoreceptor complex. PLoS One 9: e105560.

30. Turnbull IR, Colonna M (2007) Activating and inhibitory functions of DAP12. Nature reviews Immunology 7: 155–161.

31. Viola A, Schroeder S, Sakakibara Y, Lanzavecchia A (1999) T lymphocyte costimulation mediated by reorganization of membrane microdomains. Science 283: 680–682.

32. Tavano R, Gri G, Molon B, Marinari B, Rudd CE, et al. (2004) CD28 and lipid rafts coordinate recruitment of Lck to the immunological synapse of human T lymphocytes. J Immunol 173: 5392–5397.

33. Zhang W, Sloan-Lancaster J, Kitchen J, Trible RP, Samelson LE (1998) LAT: the ZAP-70 tyrosine kinase substrate that links T cell receptor to cellular activation. Cell 92: 83–92.

34. Yokosuka T, Sakata-Sogawa K, Kobayashi W, Hiroshima M, Hashimoto-Tane A, et al. (2005) Newly generated T cell receptor microclusters initiate and sustain T cell activation by recruitment of Zap70 and SLP-76. Nat Immunol 6: 1253–1262.

35. Straus DB, Weiss A (1992) Genetic evidence for the involvement of the lck tyrosine kinase in signal transduction through the T cell antigen receptor. Cell 70: 585–593.

36. Samelson LE, Phillips AF, Luong ET, Klausner RD (1990) Association of the fyn protein-tyrosine kinase with the T-cell antigen receptor. Proc Natl Acad Sci U S A 87: 4358–4362.

37. Li W, Whaley CD, Mondino A, Mueller DL (1996) Blocked signal transduction to the ERK and JNK protein kinases in anergic CD4+ T cells. Science (New York, NY) 271: 1272–1276.

26

Coincident Pre-Diabetes Is Associated with Dysregulated Cytokine Responses in Pulmonary Tuberculosis

Nathella Pavan Kumar[1,2], Vaithilingam V. Banurekha[2], Dina Nair[2], Rathinam Sridhar[3], Hardy Kornfeld[4], Thomas B. Nutman[5], Subash Babu[1,5]*

1 National Institutes of Health—International Center for Excellence in Research, Chennai, India, **2** National Institute for Research in Tuberculosis, Chennai, India, **3** Government Stanley Medical Hospital, Chennai, India, **4** Department of Medicine, University of Massachusetts Medical School, Worcester, Massachusetts, United States of America, **5** Laboratory of Parasitic Diseases, National Institute of Allergy and Infectious Diseases, National Institutes of Health, Bethesda, Maryland, United States of America

Abstract

Background: Cytokines play an important role in the pathogenesis of pulmonary tuberculosis (PTB) - Type 2 diabetes mellitus co-morbidity. However, the cytokine interactions that characterize PTB coincident with pre-diabetes (PDM) are not known.

Methods: To identify the influence of coincident PDM on cytokine levels in PTB, we examined circulating levels of a panel of cytokines in the plasma of individuals with TB-PDM and compared them with those without PDM (TB-NDM).

Results: TB-PDM is characterized by elevated circulating levels of Type 1 (IFNγ, TNFα and IL-2), Type 17 (IL-17A and IL-17F) and other pro-inflammatory (IL-1β, IFNβ and GM-CSF) cytokines. TB-PDM is also characterized by increased systemic levels of Type 2 (IL-5) and regulatory (IL-10 and TGFβ) cytokines. Moreover, TB antigen stimulated whole blood also showed increased levels of pro-inflammatory (IFNγ, TNFα and IL-1β) cytokines as well. However, the cytokines did not exhibit any significant correlation with HbA1C levels or with bacterial burdens.

Conclusion: Our data reveal that pre-diabetes in PTB individuals is characterized by heightened cytokine responsiveness, indicating that a balanced pro and anti - inflammatory cytokine milieu is a feature of pre-diabetes - TB co-morbidity.

Editor: Katalin Andrea Wilkinson, University of Cape Town, South Africa

Funding: This work was funded by the Division of Intramural Research, National Institute of Allergy and Infectious Diseases (NIAID), National Institutes of Health (NIH). The funders had no role in study design, data collection and analysis, decision to publish or preparation of the manuscript.

Competing Interests: The authors have declared that no competing interests exist.

* Email: sbabu@mail.nih.gov

Introduction

Pre-diabetes (PDM) or intermediate hyperglycemia is a high risk state for diabetes that is defined by glycemic variables that are higher than normal, but lower than diabetic thresholds [1]. The prevalence of PDM is increasing worldwide, and it is estimated that over 470 million people will have PDM by 2030 [2]. PDM is associated with the simultaneous presence of insulin resistance and pancreatic beta-cell dysfunction - abnormalities that start before changes in glycemic control are detectable [1,3]. Observational evidence shows associations between PDM and early forms of complications known to occur in typical diabetes including nephropathy, small fiber neuropathy, retinopathy and macro-vascular disease [1,3]. Typically 5–10% of individuals with PDM become diabetic every year, although the conversion rates vary with population characteristics and definition of PDM [4,5].

Type 2 DM is one of the major risk factors for the development of active pulmonary tuberculosis (PTB) and this interaction is typically characterized by elevated systemic levels of pro-inflammatory cytokines especially Type 1 and Type 17 cytokines [6,7],

cytokines that appear to play an important role in pathogenesis. Whether PDM is also associated with increased susceptibility to active PTB or whether this interaction is associated with a dysregulated cytokine environment is not known. Epidemiological studies have shown a high prevalence of PDM in PTB [8,9]. In one study from India, a country with extremely high burdens of both TB and DM, it was shown that among newly diagnosed TB patients, 25% had DM while another 25% had PDM, numbers that are in stark contrast to DM and PDM in the general population where the prevalences are 10% and 8%, respectively [8]. Since DM is not only associated with an increased risk of developing active TB but also with TB disease severity and treatment outcomes [10], it stands to reason that PDM might also potentially have an impact on the outcome of PTB.

In this study, we sought to delineate the influence of PDM on the systemic and antigen -specific cytokine response in patients newly diagnosed with active PTB. We focused on a large panel of Type 1, Type 2, Type 17, regulatory and other pro – inflammatory cytokines in plasma and TB antigen-stimulated whole blood from individuals with active TB and coincident PDM (TB-PDM) and compared these to those with active TB but without pre-diabetes (TB-NDM). We show that the pre-diabetic state at the time of PTB causes systemic increases in the levels of most of the pro – and anti – inflammatory cytokines, some appearing to be TB antigen-induced. Thus, our data suggest that heightened cytokine levels in active PTB may be associated with even moderate glycemic control.

Materials and Methods

Ethics statement

All individuals were examined as part of a natural history study protocol approved by the Institutional Review Board of the National Institute of Research in Tuberculosis (NCT01154959), and informed written consent was obtained from all participants.

Study Population

We studied a group of 90 individuals with active PTB attending the TB Clinic at Stanley Medical Hospital, Chennai, India. Patients were prospectively/consecutively enrolled with 48 having PDM and 42 having normal HbA1c levels (NDM). PTB was diagnosed on the basis of sputum smear and culture positivity. Bacterial burdens were assessed by measuring smear grades following Ziehl-Nielsen staining of sputum smears. PDM was diagnosed on the basis of glycated hemoglobin (HbA1c) levels, according to the American Diabetes Association criteria (all PDM individuals had HbA1c levels between 5.7 and 6.4%). All the individuals were HIV seronegative. The two groups did not differ significantly in terms of the sputum smear grade. All individuals were anti-tuberculous treatment naïve. Anthropometric measurements, including height, weight, and waist circumference, and biochemical parameters, including random plasma glucose, fasting lipid profile and HbA1c were obtained using standardized techniques as detailed elsewhere [11].

ELISA

Plasma cytokines and chemokines were measured using a Bioplex multiplex cytokine assay system (Bio-Rad, Hercules, CA). The parameters analyzed were IFNγ, TNFα, IL-2, IL-17A, IL-4, IL-5, IL-10, IL-6, IL-12 and GM-CSF. Plasma levels of TGFβ, IL-1α, IL-1β (all R& D Systems); IL-17F (Biolegend); IL-22 (eBioscience); Type 1 interferons (IFNs) - IFNα (multiple subtypes) and IFNβ (PBL Interferon Source) were measured by ELISA.

Quantiferon supernatant ELISA

Whole blood from a subset of TB-PDM and TB-NDM individuals (n = 22 each) was incubated with either no antigen or TB antigen (ESAT-6, CFP-10, TB 7.7) according to the manufacturers instructions using the Quantiferon in Tube Gold kit. The unstimulated or TB antigen stimulated whole blood supernatants were then used to analyze the levels of IFNγ, TNFα, IL-17A and IL-1β using the Duo-set ELISA kits from R& D systems.

Ex vivo analysis

All antibodies used in the study were from BD Biosciences/BD Pharmingen/eBioscience/R&D systems. Whole blood was used for ex vivo phenotyping and it was performed on all 90 individuals. Naïve and memory T cell phenotyping was performed using CD45RA and CCR7 staining on CD4$^+$ and CD8$^+$ T cells and natural regulatory T cell (nTregs) phenotyping using CD25, Foxp3 and CD127. A representative graph showing the gating strategy for CD4$^+$ and CD8$^+$ T cell subsets is depicted in Figure S1.

Statistical Analysis

Geometric means (GM) were used for measurements of central tendency. Statistically significant differences between two groups were analyzed using the nonparametric Mann-Whitney U test followed by Holm's correction for multiple comparisons. Correlations were calculated using Spearman rank correlation. Analyses were performed using GraphPad PRISM Version 5.01.

Results

Study population characteristics

The baseline characteristics including demographic and biochemical features of the study population are shown in Table 1. As can be seen, compared to subjects without pre-diabetes (TB-NDM), those with pre-diabetes and TB (TB-PDM) had higher glycated hemoglobin but did not differ significantly in other biochemical parameters including random blood glucose, serum cholesterol, HDL, LDL and triglycerides levels. In addition, the baseline immunological profile reveals significantly lower frequencies of CD4$^+$ regulatory T cells (p = 0.0009) and significantly higher frequencies of CD8$^+$ effector memory T cells (p = 0.0047) in TB-PDM individuals.

TB-PDM is associated with increased circulating levels of Type 1 and Type 17 cytokines

To determine the influence of PDM on Type 1 and Type 17 cytokines in active PTB, we measured the circulating levels of IFN-γ, TNFα and IL-2 as well as IL-17A, IL-17F and IL-22 in TB-PDM and TB-NDM individuals (Figure 1). As shown in Figure 1A, the systemic levels of all three Type 1 cytokines – IFNγ (Geometric Mean of 335.9 pg/ml in TB-PDM versus 169.2 pg/ml in TB-NDM), TNFα (GM of 338.4 pg/ml vs. 252.4 pg/ml) and IL-2 (GM of 25.1 pg/ml vs. 13.9 pg/ml) were significantly higher in TB-PDM compared to TB-NDM individuals. Similarly, the systemic levels of the prototypical Type 17 cytokines – IL-17A (GM of 106.3 pg/ml vs. 90.6 pg/ml) and IL-17F (GM of 202.8 pg/ml vs. 138.1 pg/ml) were also significantly higher in TB-PDM compared to TB-NDM individuals. In contrast, no significant differences in IL-22 levels were found between the two groups. Thus, TB-PDM is associated with heightened levels of Type 1 and Type 17 at the time of presentation of active PTB.

TB-PDM is associated with increased circulating levels of Type 2 and regulatory cytokines

To determine the influence of PDM on Type 2 and regulatory cytokines in active TB, we measured the circulating levels of IL-4 and IL-5 as well as IL-10 and TGFβ in TB-PDM and TB-NDM individuals (Figure 1). As shown in Figure 1B, the systemic levels of IL-5 (GM of 72.1 pg/ml vs. 46.1 pg/ml) were significantly higher in TB-PDM compared to TB-NDM individuals. Similarly, the systemic levels of the regulatory cytokines - IL-10 (GM of 61.6 pg/ml vs. 36.3 pg/ml) and TGFβ (GM of 398.2 pg/ml vs. 295.6 pg/ml) were also significantly higher in TB-PDM compared to TB-NDM individuals. Thus, TB-PDM is not associated with a concomitant decrease of Type 2 or regulatory cytokine levels at the time of presentation with active PTB.

TB-PDM is associated with increased circulating levels of other pro-inflammatory cytokines

To determine the influence of PDM on the IL-1 family and other pro-inflammatory cytokines as well as Type 1 IFNs in active TB, we measured circulating levels of these in TB-PDM and

Table 1. Demographics, biochemistry and immunology profile of TB-PDM and TB-NDM individuals.

Study Demographics	PTB-PDM	PTB-NDM	P value
Age (yrs)	42.5 (18–65)	39.5 (20–65)	NS
Sex M/F	38/10	36/6	NS
BMI (kg/m^2)	22.5 (16.4–24.5)	20.4 (14.6–22.3)	NS
Glycated Hemoglobin(%)	5.92 (5.71–6.44)	5.25 (4.04–5.65)	NS
Random glucose (mg/dl)	99 (66–161)	100 (78–156)	NS
Total cholesterol (mg/dl)	168 (142–202)	146 (124–205)	NS
Serum triglycerides (mg/dl)	102 (64–424)	98 (56–384)	NS
High density lipoprotein cholesterol (ml/dl)	37 (29–59)	42 (25–66)	NS
Low density lipoprotein cholesterol (ml/dl)	104 (44–180)	96 (52–146)	NS
Immunological Parameters			
CD4$^+$ Naïve Cells (CD45RA$^+$CCR7$^+$)	37.5(10–77)	34(11–67)	NS
CD4$^+$ Central Memory Cells (CD45RA-CCR7$^+$)	32(11–86)	27.5(15–64)	NS
CD4$^+$ Effector Memory Cells (CD45RA-CCR7-)	24.05(10–55)	29.5(9–62)	NS
CD4$^+$ Regulatory T Cells (CD25$^+$FoxP3$^+$CD127^{dim})	3.3015(2.129–7.798)	4.659(1.968–9.295)	p = 0.0009
CD8$^+$ Naïve Cells (CD45RA$^+$CCR7$^+$)	28(18–48)	25(10–69)	NS
CD8$^+$ Central Memory Cells (CD45RA-CCR7$^+$)	1.75(0.9–7.9)	1.1(0.5–7.1)	p = 0.0047
CD8$^+$ Effector Memory Cells (CD45RA-CCR7-)	34.5(10–81)	30(11–79)	NS

The values represent geometric means and range (except for age where median and range are shown). P values were calculated using the Mann-Whitney test (except for sex which was tested by Fishers exact test).

TB-NDM individuals (Figure 1). As shown in Figure 1C, the systemic levels of IL-1β (GM of 195 pg/ml vs. 140.1 pg/ml) and GM-CSF (GM of 61.8 pg/ml vs. 50.9 pg/ml) were significantly higher in TB-PDM compared to TB-NDM individuals. In contrast, the systemic levels of IL-1α, IL-6 and IL-12 were not significantly different between the two groups. Similarly, the levels of IFNβ (GM of 488.3 pg/ml vs. 220.5 pg/ml) but not IFNα were found be present at significantly higher levels in TB-PDM compared to TB-NDM individuals. Thus, TB-PDM is associated with heightened levels of pro-inflammatory cytokines at the time of presentation.

TB-PDM is associated with increased TB antigen stimulated levels of pro-inflammatory cytokines

To determine the influence of PDM on TB antigen stimulated cytokine production in active PTB, we measured circulating levels of these cytokines following stimulation of whole blood with no antigen or a cocktail of TB antigens (ESAT-6, CFP-10, TB 7.7) in a subset (n = 22 each) of TB-PDM and TB-NDM individuals (Figure 2). As shown in Figure 2A, the spontaneously produced levels of the IFNγ (GM of 70.1 pg/ml vs. 34.8 pg/ml), TNFα (GM of 69.7 pg/ml vs. 35.6 pg/ml) and IL-1β (GM of 64.4 pg/ml vs. 44.5 pg/ml) were significantly higher in TB-PDM compared to TB-NDM individuals. Similarly, as shown in Figure 2B, the TB antigen stimulated levels of IFNγ (GM of 278.8 pg/ml vs. 120.1 pg/ml), TNFα (GM of 67.2 pg/ml vs. 42.5 pg/ml) and IL-1β (GM of 65.9 pg/ml vs. 43.1 pg/ml) were also significantly higher in TB-PDM compared to TB-NDM individuals. Thus, TB-PDM is associated with heightened levels of TB antigen stimulated pro-inflammatory cytokines.

No relationship between systemic cytokines and HbA1c levels or with bacterial burdens

Since HbA1c is an accurate indicator of the level of glycemic control and increased values reflect poor control, we sought to examine the relationship between the systemic levels of Type 1, Type 17 and other pro-inflammatory cytokines with the degree of glycemic control. To this end, we assessed the association of IFNγ, TNFα, IL-2, IL-17A, IL-17F, IL-22, IL-1β, GM-CSF and IL-12 with HbA1C levels (in %) in the PDM individuals in the study. As shown in Figure 3, we observed no significant correlation between systemic cytokine levels and the HbA1c levels in TB-PDM individuals.

Since smear grades are an accurate reflection of bacterial burdens, we also sought to examine the relationship between the systemic levels of Type 1, Type 17 and other pro-inflammatory cytokines with the bacterial burdens in the TB-PDM individuals. As shown in Figure 4, we observed no significant correlation between the circulating levels of IFNγ, TNFα, IL-2, IL-17A, IL-17F, IL-10, IL-1β, IFNβ and TGFβ.

Thus, systemic levels of cytokines in TB-PDM do not reflect poor glycemic controls or increased bacterial burdens.

Discussion

PDM prevalence is increased in TB – it is presently unknown whether TB is causing PDM in susceptible individuals, or if PDM increases susceptibility to TB. Either possibility would have significant public health implications [12,13]. If PDM impairs host defense and increases the risk for progression from LTBI to active TB, then the TB burden attributable to metabolic syndromes would be far greater than current estimates. It would also imply the existence of distinct susceptibility mechanisms

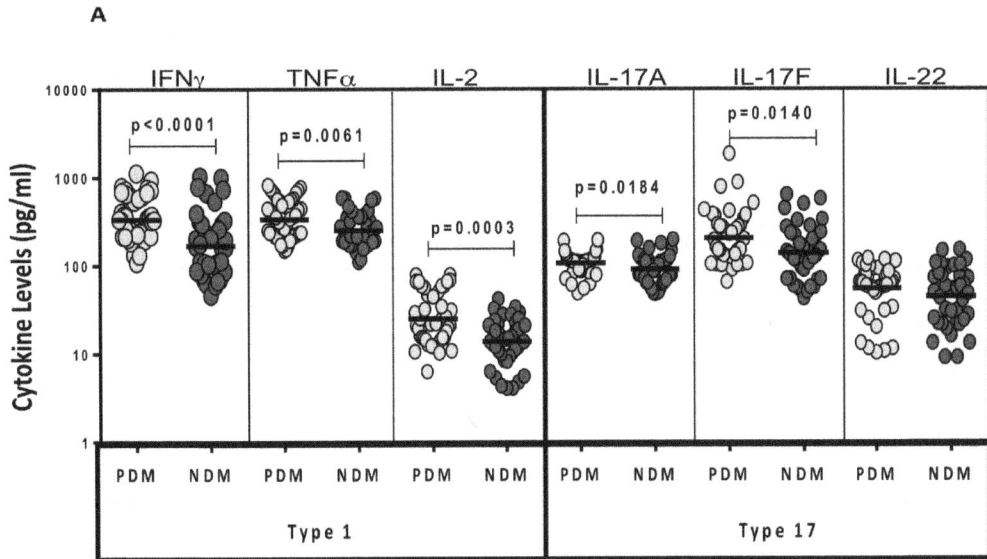

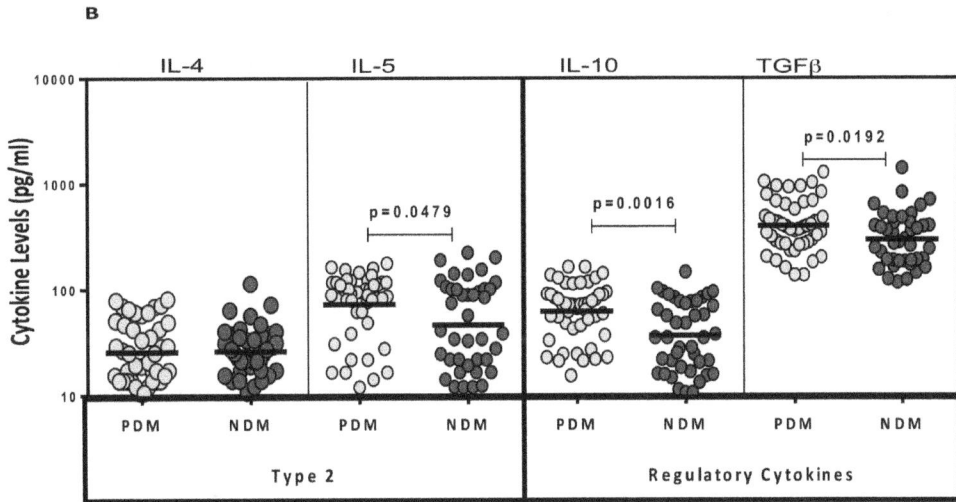

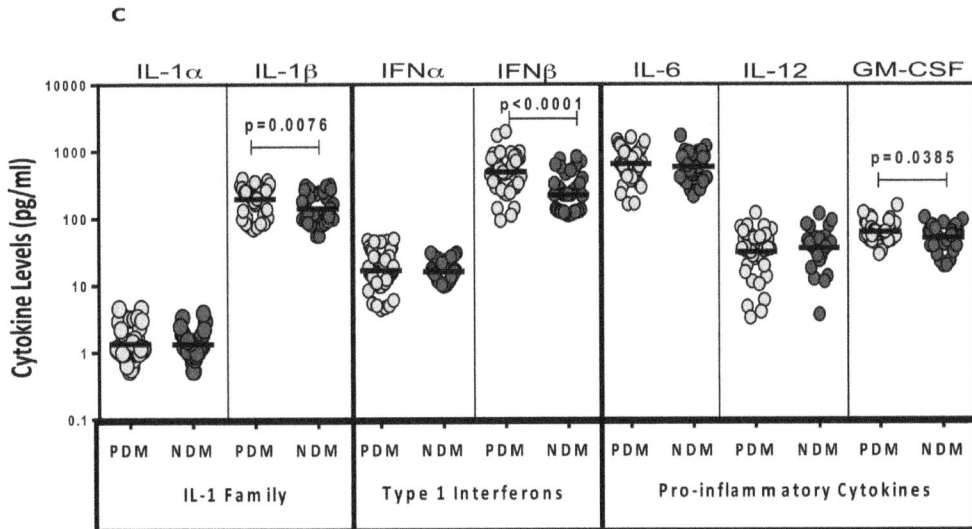

Figure 1. Elevated systemic levels of Type 1, Type 2 and other pro-inflammatory and regulatory cytokines in TB-PDM. The plasma levels of Type 1 (IFNγ, TNFα, IL-2); Type 17 (IL-17A, IL-17F and IL-22) cytokines (A) and Type 2 (IL-4, IL-5, IL-13); regulatory (IL-10 and TGFβ) cytokines (B) and other pro-inflammatory (IL-1α, IL-1β, IFNα, IFNβ, IL-6, IL-12 and GM-CSF) were measured by ELISA in TB-PDM (n = 48) and TB-NDM (n = 42) individuals. The data are represented as scatter plots with each circle representing a single individual (light grey – PDM and dark grey – NDM). P values were calculated using the Mann-Whitney test.

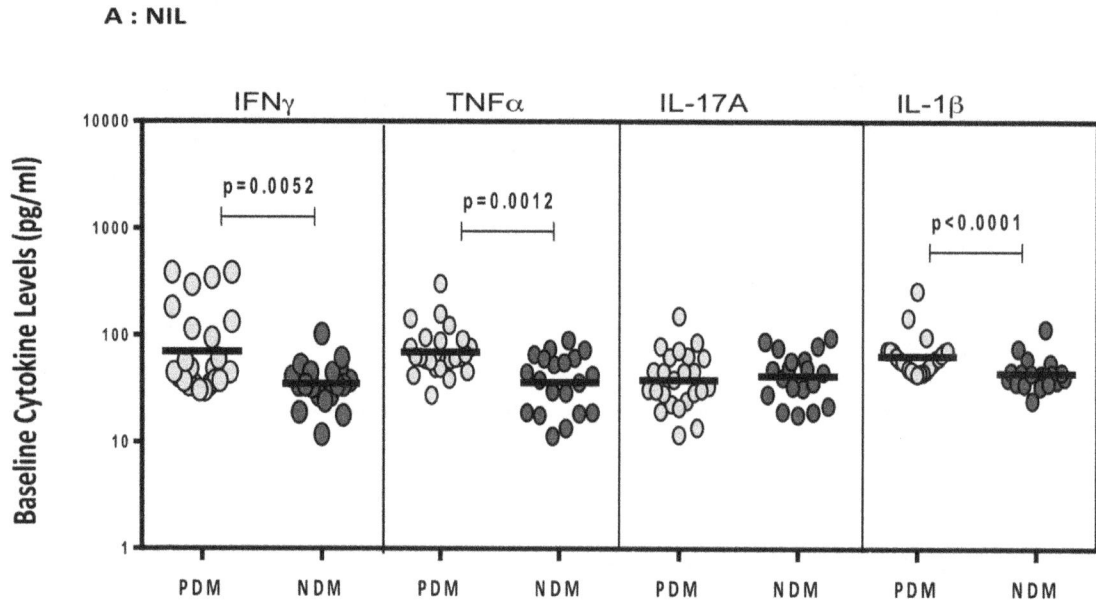

A : NIL

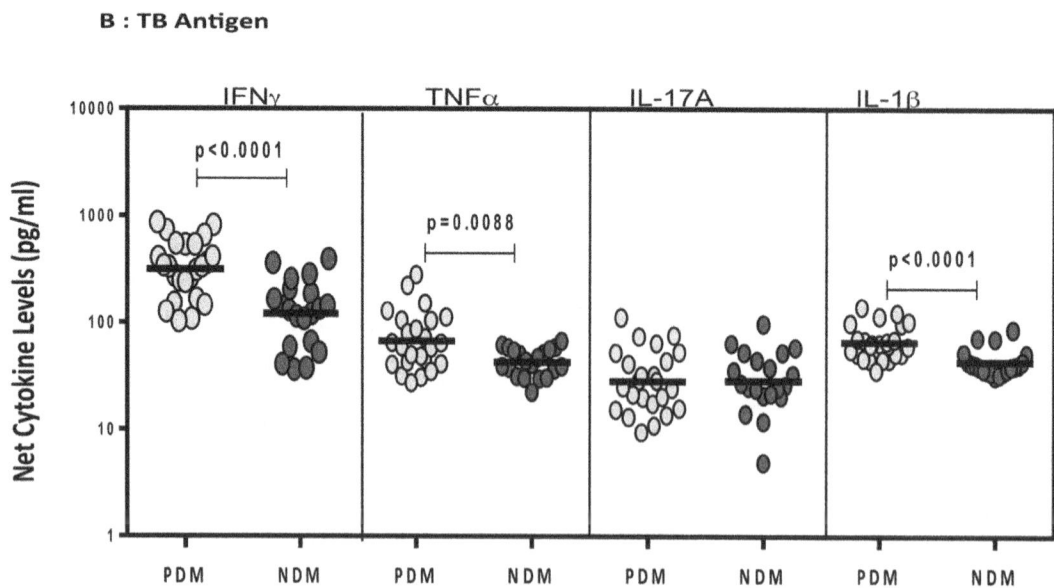

B : TB Antigen

Figure 2. Elevated TB antigen stimulated and unstimulated levels of IFNγ, TNFα, IL-17A and IL-1β in TB-PDM. The unstimulated (A) or TB antigen stimulated (B) levels of IFNγ, TNFα, IL-17A and IL-1β were measured by ELISA in whole blood of a subset of TB-PDM (n = 22) and TB-NDM (n = 22) individuals. The data are represented as scatter plots with each circle representing a single individual (light grey – PDM and dark grey – NDM). P values were calculated using the Mann-Whitney test.

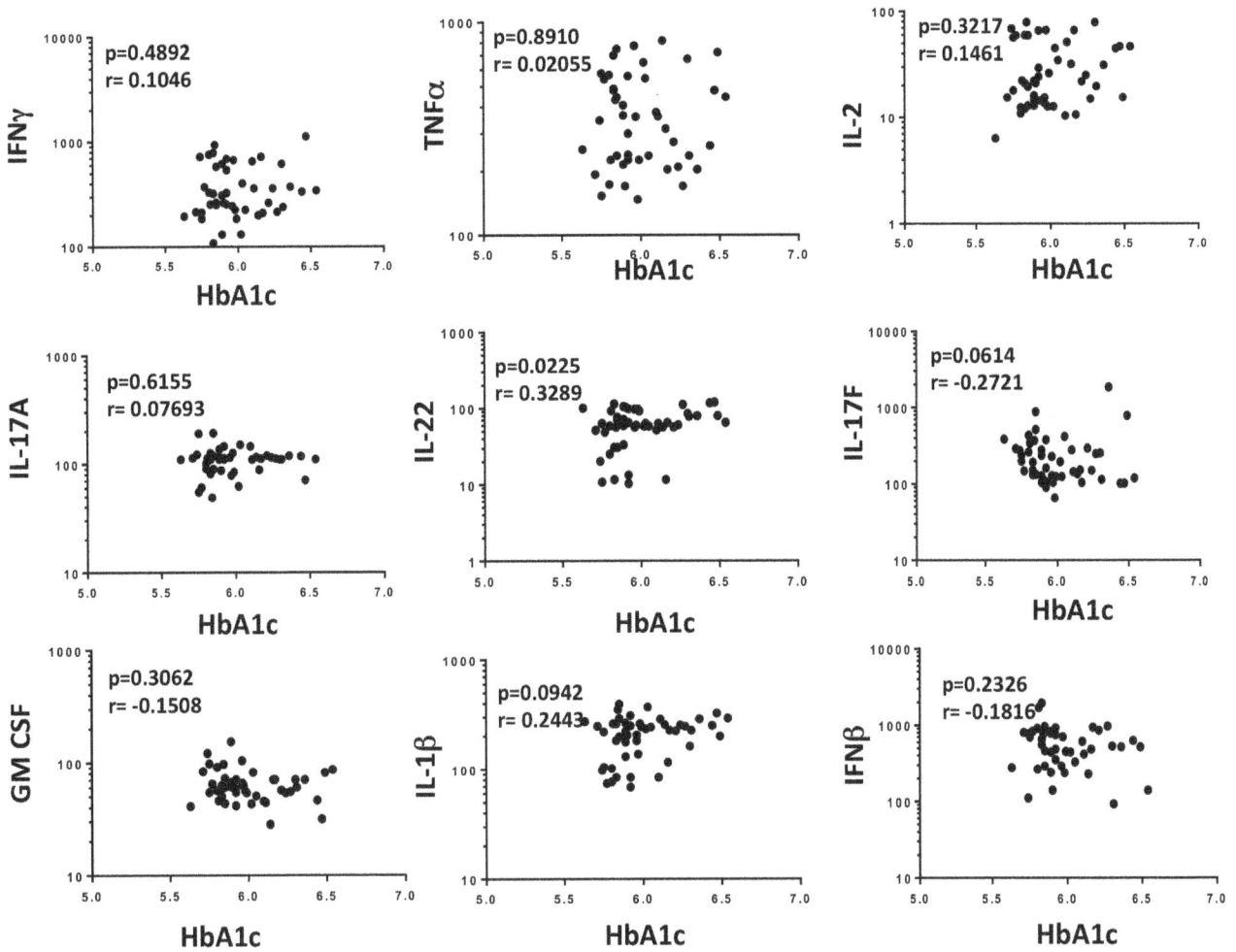

Figure 3. No relationship between systemic levels of cytokines and HbA1c levels in TB – PDM individuals. The relationship between the plasma levels of IFNγ, TNFα, IL-2, IL-17A, IL-17F, IL-22, GM-CSF, IL-1β and IFNβ and HbA1c levels was examined in TB - PDM (n = 48) individuals. The data are represented as scatter plots with each circle representing a single individual. P values were calculated using the Spearman rank correlation.

unrelated to hyperglycemia but likely shared in PDM and type 2 DM. Alternatively, TB disease might promote insulin resistance and induce PDM as a consequence of inflammatory stress. In that scenario, TB would represent a significant factor contributing to disordered glucose metabolism with implications for bidirectional screening [14,15]. It would then be important to learn whether this is a transient or persistent effect and whether TB can push pre-diabetics to full DM with all of its negative consequences.

Inflammation - induced inhibition of the insulin signaling pathway can lead to insulin resistance and contribute to the development of Type 2 DM [16]. Pre-diabetes and insulin resistance are associated with a chronic but subclinical inflammatory process that impairs insulin action in most tissues and could also hamper pancreatic beta-cell function [17]. The involvement of cytokines induced by this inflammation suggest an innate immune response [18]. Moreover, components of the immune system are altered in PDM, including altered levels of specific cytokines and chemokines, changes in the number and activation state of various immune cell subsets and increased apoptosis and tissue fibrosis [17]. Together, these changes suggest that inflammation participates in the pathogenesis of PDM but how these changes affect the immune response to bystander antigens or newly acquired infections remains unclear [19]. One possible

mechanism is that an impaired immune response in PDM facilitates either primary infection with tuberculosis or reactivation of latent tuberculosis [20,21].

Cytokines are known to play a major role in determining the outcome of mycobacterial infections [22]. However, unbalanced cytokine responses can also play an important role in promoting pathology in TB disease [23]. Thus, while Type 1 and Type 17 cytokines typically impart protection against TB infection [24], excess of TNFα [25] or IL-17 [26] are known to be associated with deleterious effects in TB disease. Moreover, Type 1 IFN driven gene expression signatures are considered a characteristic feature of active TB disease [27] and Type 1 IFNs are known to promote pathology in both animal models and human disease [28,29]. Our data clearly reveal that the PDM - TB nexus is characterized by heightened circulating levels of most of the pro-inflammatory cytokines. So, contrary to their expected role in host protection, these cytokines are more likely to be associated with promotion of pathology in PTB. This is very similar to our previous findings in overt DM and PTB, where we had observed not only elevated plasma levels of pro-inflammatory cytokines but also increased TB antigen - specific Th1 and Th17 cellular and cytokine responses [6,30].

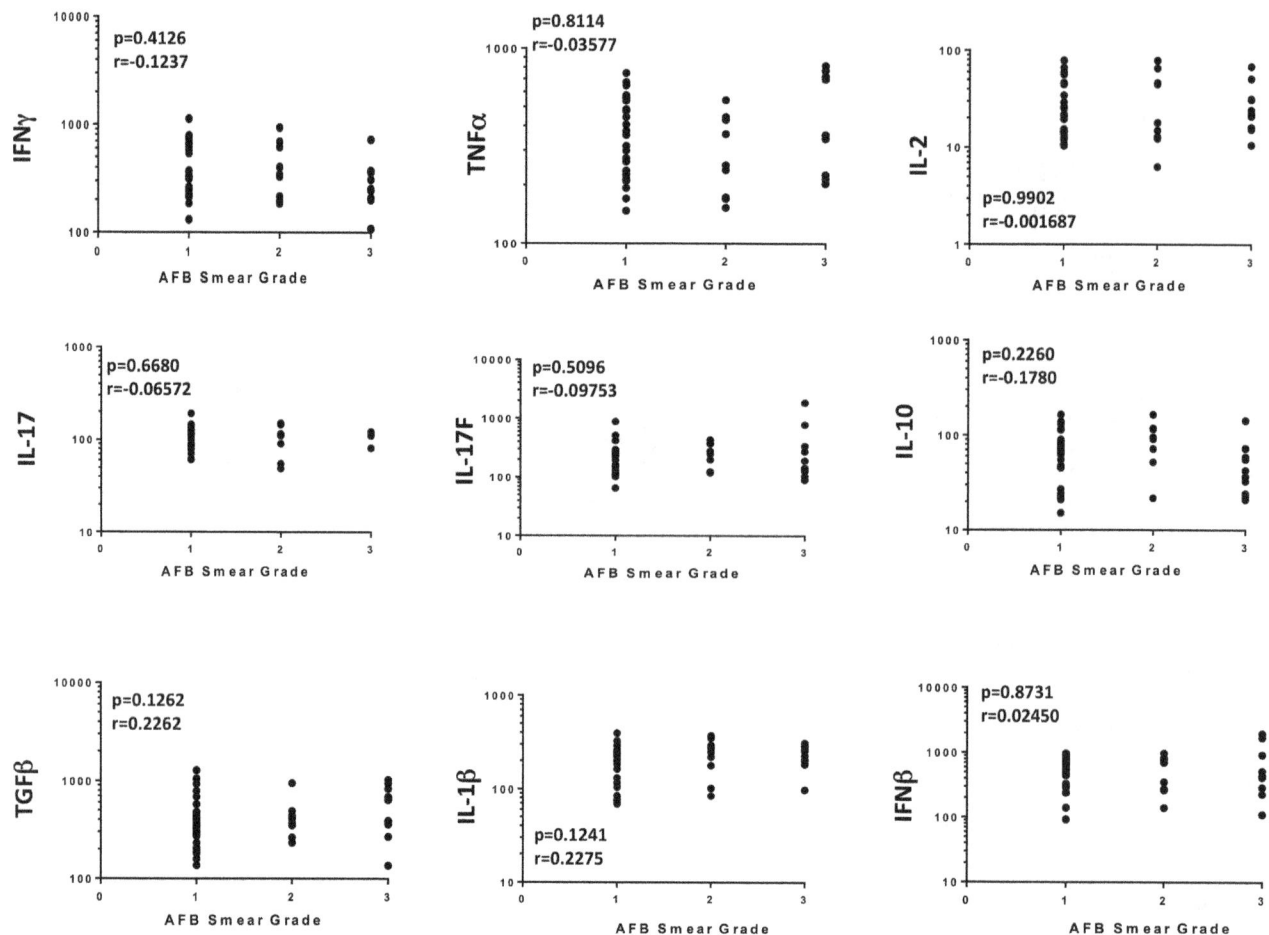

Figure 4. No relationship between systemic levels of cytokines and bacterial burdens in TB – PDM individuals. The relationship between the plasma levels of IFNγ, TNFα, IL-2, IL-17A, IL-17F, IL-10, IL-1β, IFNβ, TGFβ and bacterial burdens (as assessed by smear grades - 1[+], 2[+] and 3[+]) was examined in TB - PDM (n = 48) individuals. The data are represented as scatter plots with each circle representing a single individual. P values were calculated using the Spearman rank correlation.

One potential mechanism for the increase in levels of pro-inflammatory cytokines in TB-PDM individuals could be a concomitant decrease in the levels of systemic Type 2 or regulatory cytokines. However, as revealed by the increased systemic levels of IL-5, IL-10 and TGFβ, our data show that even regulatory cytokines are present at elevated levels in PDM individuals. Since Type 2 cytokines, IL-10 and TGFβ are known down modulators of inflammatory responses in TB [31,32], this suggests that there is a compensatory mechanism in place to regulate inflammation in the setting of PDM. Another possibility is that there is a broad and possibly unrelated increase in T cell activation responses (reflected by cytokines) in PDM. Thus, PDM in the context of active PTB is characterized by a predominantly balanced network of pro - and anti - inflammatory cytokines, accounting for the lack of differences in bacterial loads between the 2 groups studied. Moreover, systemic levels of cytokines do not exhibit any significant association with bacterial burdens, suggesting that this dysregulation of cytokine levels is not solely driven by differences in bacterial burdens.

The major limitation in analyzing the immune parameters in the circulation is the non – specific nature of the analysis. We have therefore, sought to corroborate the plasma cytokine results by measuring the levels of a subset of cytokines in TB antigen stimulated whole blood supernatants. Our data on the cytokine

responses following TB antigen stimulation clearly show that PDM has a profound effect and that elevation in circulating levels of Type 1 cytokines as well as IL-1β is reflected by similar elevations of in vitro measured cytokines following stimulation with mycobacterial antigens in TB-DM. Whether the heightened responsiveness observed in the TB-PDM individuals is specific to TB infection or is a general phenomenon applicable to different infections remains to be determined. While our data clearly provide descriptive data on the interaction between PDM and TB, future studies are needed to explore the mechanism governing this important interaction. Our data on the lack of differences in BMI and lipid metabolism appears to exclude these parameters as potential confounders (see Table 1). However, other metabolic mediators including free fatty acids that are known to be induced in insulin resistance could also play a role in this interaction. In addition, our data also reveal that the baseline frequencies of nTregs and CD8[+] effector memory T cells are significantly different between the two groups, thereby making highly unlikely that significant perturbations in CD4[+] or CD8[+] T cell numbers are responsible for the differential cytokine profiles. The cellular sources of the cytokines produced should provide us clues to the mechanism behind this differential response. Finally our data argue that the interaction of active TB with pre-diabetes is in contrast to that of latent TB with diabetes, since in the latter scenario, impairment of cytokine secretion is the major finding [33]. Hence, pre-diabetes interaction with latent TB potentially enhances susceptibility to TB disease by compromising the production of protective cytokines, while pre-diabetes interaction with active TB potentially promotes pathology by enhancing the production of cytokines.

Our study provides important insights into the influence of pre-diabetes on the pathogenesis of TB disease. Our data also suggest that this interaction might also have an effect on TB disease potentially shifting the balance of metabolic regulation from pre-diabetes to overt diabetes. These data underlie the need to assess more systematically – using epidemiological, clinical and immunological studies – the interaction between pre-diabetes and tuberculosis and suggests that intervention that targets important innate and adaptive responses may provide new clues to pursue immunological alternatives as therapeutics for dealing with the global menace of coincident diabetes and TB.

Supporting Information

Figure S1 Gating strategy for estimating frequencies of CD4$^+$ and CD8$^+$ naïve, central memory and effector memory T cells and natural regulatory T cells. (A) A representative flow cytometry plot showing the gating strategy for estimation of naïve, central memory and effector memory cells from CD4$^+$ and CD8$^+$ T cells. Naïve cells were classified as CD45RA$^+$ CCR7$^+$; effector memory cells as CD45RA- CCR7-; and central memory cells as CD45RA- CCR7$^+$. (B) A representative flow cytometry plot showing the gating strategy for estimation of nTregs from CD4$^+$ T cells. Natural T regulatory T cells (nTregs) were classified as CD4$^+$, CD25$^+$, Foxp3$^+$, CD127dim.

Acknowledgments

We thank the staff of Department of Clinical Research and the Department of Social Work, NIRT especially Ms Kalaiselvi and Government Stanley Hospital, Chennai, for valuable assistance in recruiting the patients for this study. We would like to thank R. Anuradha, M. Saravanan, Kadar Moideen and Jovvian George of the NIH-ICER for technical assistance.

Author Contributions

Conceived and designed the experiments: TBN SB. Performed the experiments: NPK. Analyzed the data: NPK SB. Contributed reagents/materials/analysis tools: VVB DN RS HK. Wrote the paper: TBN SB.

References

1. Tabak AG, Herder C, Rathmann W, Brunner EJ, Kivimaki M (2013) Prediabetes: a high-risk state for diabetes development. Lancet 379: 2279–2290.
2. Whiting DR, Guariguata L, Weil C, Shaw J (2011) IDF diabetes atlas: global estimates of the prevalence of diabetes for 2011 and 2030. Diabetes Res Clin Pract 94: 311–321.
3. Abdul-Ghani MA, DeFronzo RA (2009) Pathophysiology of prediabetes. Curr Diab Rep 9: 193–199.
4. Forouhi NG, Luan J, Hennings S, Wareham NJ (2007) Incidence of Type 2 diabetes in England and its association with baseline impaired fasting glucose: the Ely study 1990–2000. Diabet Med 24: 200–207.
5. Nathan DM, Davidson MB, DeFronzo RA, Heine RJ, Henry RR, et al. (2007) Impaired fasting glucose and impaired glucose tolerance: implications for care. Diabetes Care 30: 753–759.
6. Kumar NP, Sridhar R, Banurekha VV, Jawahar MS, Fay MP, et al. (2013) Type 2 diabetes mellitus coincident with pulmonary tuberculosis is associated with heightened systemic type 1, type 17, and other proinflammatory cytokines. Ann Am Thorac Soc 10: 441–449.
7. Restrepo BI, Fisher-Hoch SP, Pino PA, Salinas A, Rahbar MH, et al. (2008) Tuberculosis in poorly controlled type 2 diabetes: altered cytokine expression in peripheral white blood cells. Clin Infect Dis 47: 634–641.
8. Viswanathan V, Kumpatla S, Aravindalochanan V, Rajan R, Chinnasamy C, et al. (2012) Prevalence of diabetes and pre-diabetes and associated risk factors among tuberculosis patients in India. PLoS One 7: e41367.
9. Wang Q, Ma A, Han X, Zhao S, Cai J, et al. (2013) Prevalence of type 2 diabetes among newly detected pulmonary tuberculosis patients in China: a community based cohort study. PLoS One 8: e82660.
10. Dooley KE, Chaisson RE (2009) Tuberculosis and diabetes mellitus: convergence of two epidemics. Lancet Infect Dis 9: 737–746.
11. Deepa M, Pradeepa R, Rema M, Mohan A, Deepa R, et al. (2003) The Chennai Urban Rural Epidemiology Study (CURES) –study design and methodology (urban component) (CURES-I). J Assoc Physicians India 51: 863–870.
12. Harries AD, Lin Y, Satyanarayana S, Lonnroth K, Li L, et al. (2011) The looming epidemic of diabetes-associated tuberculosis: learning lessons from HIV-associated tuberculosis. Int J Tuberc Lung Dis 15: 1436–1444.
13. Kapur A, Harries AD (2013) The double burden of diabetes and tuberculosis - Public health implications. Diabetes Res Clin Pract.
14. Marais BJ, Lonnroth K, Lawn SD, Migliori GB, Mwaba P, et al. (2013) Tuberculosis comorbidity with communicable and non-communicable diseases: integrating health services and control efforts. Lancet Infect Dis 13: 436–448.
15. Sullivan T, Ben Amor Y (2012) The co-management of tuberculosis and diabetes: challenges and opportunities in the developing world. PLoS Med 9: e1001269.
16. Velloso LA, Eizirik DL, Cnop M (2013) Type 2 diabetes mellitus–an autoimmune disease? Nat Rev Endocrinol 9: 750–755.
17. Donath MY, Shoelson SE (2011) Type 2 diabetes as an inflammatory disease. Nat Rev Immunol 11: 98–107.
18. McNelis JC, Olefsky JM (2014) Macrophages, Immunity, and Metabolic Disease. Immunity 41: 36–48.
19. Martinez N, Kornfeld H (2014) Diabetes and immunity to tuberculosis. Eur J Immunol 44: 617–626.
20. Restrepo BI, Schlesinger LS (2013) Host-pathogen interactions in tuberculosis patients with type 2 diabetes mellitus. Tuberculosis (Edinb) 93 Suppl: S10–14.
21. Restrepo BI, Schlesinger LS (2014) Impact of diabetes on the natural history of tuberculosis. Diabetes Res Clin Pract.
22. Cooper AM, Mayer-Barber KD, Sher A (2011) A Role of innate cytokines in mycobacterial infection. Mucosal Immunol 4: 252–260.
23. Torrado E, Cooper AM (2013) Cytokines in the balance of protection and pathology during mycobacterial infections. Adv Exp Med Biol 783: 121–140.
24. O'Garra A, Redford PS, McNab FW, Bloom CI, Wilkinson RJ, et al. (2013) The immune response in tuberculosis. Annu Rev Immunol 31: 475–527.
25. Dorhoi A, Kaufmann SH (2014) Tumor necrosis factor alpha in mycobacterial infection. Semin Immunol 26: 203–209.
26. Torrado E, Robinson RT, Cooper AM (2011) Cellular response to mycobacteria: balancing protection and pathology. Trends Immunol 32: 66–72.
27. Berry MP, Graham CM, McNab FW, Xu Z, Bloch SA, et al. (2010) An interferon-inducible neutrophil-driven blood transcriptional signature in human tuberculosis. Nature 466: 973–977.
28. Mayer-Barber KD, Andrade BB, Barber DL, Hieny S, Feng CG, et al. (2011) Innate and adaptive interferons suppress IL-1alpha and IL-1beta production by distinct pulmonary myeloid subsets during Mycobacterium tuberculosis infection. Immunity 35: 1023–1034.
29. Mayer-Barber KD, Andrade BB, Oland SD, Amaral EP, Barber DL, et al. (2014) Host-directed therapy of tuberculosis based on interleukin-1 and type I interferon crosstalk. Nature 511: 99–103.
30. Kumar NP, Sridhar R, Banurekha VV, Jawahar MS, Nutman TB, et al. (2013) Expansion of pathogen-specific T-helper 1 and T-helper 17 cells in pulmonary tuberculosis with coincident type 2 diabetes mellitus. J Infect Dis 208: 739–748.
31. Ellner JJ (2010) Immunoregulation in TB: observations and implications. Clin Transl Sci 3: 23–28.
32. Rook GA (2007) Th2 cytokines in susceptibility to tuberculosis. Curr Mol Med 7: 327–337.
33. Kumar NP, George PJ, Kumaran P, Dolla CK, Nutman TB, et al. (2014) Diminished Systemic and Antigen-Specific Type 1, Type 17, and Other Proinflammatory Cytokines in Diabetic and Prediabetic Individuals With Latent Mycobacterium tuberculosis Infection. J Infect Dis.

Effects of Increased Von Willebrand Factor Levels on Primary Hemostasis in Thrombocytopenic Patients with Liver Cirrhosis

Andreas Wannhoff[1], Oliver J. Müller[2], Kilian Friedrich[1], Christian Rupp[1], Petra Klöters-Plachky[1], Yvonne Leopold[1], Maik Brune[3], Mirja Senner[1], Karl-Heinz Weiss[1], Wolfgang Stremmel[1], Peter Schemmer[4], Hugo A. Katus[2], Daniel N. Gotthardt[1]*

1 Department of Internal Medicine IV, University Hospital Heidelberg, Heidelberg, Germany, 2 Department of Internal Medicine III, University Hospital Heidelberg, Heidelberg, Germany, 3 Department of Internal Medicine I and Clinical Chemistry, University Hospital Heidelberg, Heidelberg, Germany, 4 Department of General and Transplant Surgery, University Hospital Heidelberg, Heidelberg, Germany

Abstract

In patients with liver cirrhosis procoagulant and anticoagulant changes occur simultaneously. During primary hemostasis, platelets adhere to subendothelial structures, via von Willebrand factor (vWF). We aimed to investigate the influence of vWF on primary hemostasis in patients with liver cirrhosis. Therefore we assessed in-vitro bleeding time as marker of primary hemostasis in cirrhotic patients, measuring the Platelet Function Analyzer (PFA-100) closure times with collagen and epinephrine (Col-Epi, upper limit of normal $\leq$165 s) or collagen and ADP (Col-ADP, upper limit of normal $\leq$118 s). If Col-Epi and Col-ADP were prolonged, the PFA-100 was considered to be pathological. Effects of vWF on primary hemostasis in thrombocytopenic patients were analyzed and plasma vWF levels were modified by adding recombinant vWF or anti-vWF antibody. Of the 72 included cirrhotic patients, 32 (44.4%) showed a pathological result for the PFA-100. They had mean closure times ($\pm$ SD) of 180$\pm$62 s with Col-Epi and 160$\pm$70 s with Col-ADP. Multivariate analysis revealed that hematocrit ($P = 0.027$) and vWF-antigen levels ($P = 0.010$) are the predictors of a pathological PFA-100 test in cirrhotic patients. In 21.4% of cirrhotic patients with platelet count $\geq$150/nL and hematocrit $\geq$27.0%, pathological PFA-100 results were found. In thrombocytopenic (<150/nL) patients with cirrhosis, normal PFA-100 results were associated with higher vWF-antigen levels (462.3$\pm$235.9% vs. 338.7$\pm$151.6%, $P = 0.021$). These results were confirmed by multivariate analysis in these patients as well as by adding recombinant vWF or polyclonal anti-vWF antibody that significantly shortened or prolonged closure times, respectively. In conclusion, primary hemostasis is impaired in cirrhotic patients. The effect of reduced platelet count in cirrhotic patients can at least be partly compensated by increased vWF levels. Recombinant vWF could be an alternative to platelet transfusions in the future.

Editor: Ferruccio Bonino, University of Pisa, Italy

Funding: AW received a grant from the Dekanat der Medizinischen Fakultät Heidelberg (Medical faculty Heidelberg). DNG was supported by a grant from Deutsche Forschungsgemeinschaft (German Research Foundation). The funders had no role in study design, data collection and analysis, decision to publish, or preparation of the manuscript.

Competing Interests: The authors have declared that no competing interests exist.

* Email: Daniel_Gotthardt@med.uni-heidelberg.de

Introduction

Patients with liver cirrhosis suffer from complex abnormalities of the hemostatic system that affect primary and secondary hemostasis and fibrinolysis. Changes in procoagulant and anticoagulant proteins occur simultaneously [1,2], and yet it has not been understood if an individual patient currently is in favor of bleeding or thrombosis. Thus, these patients can clinically present with an increased bleeding risk or an increased rate of venous thrombosis as well as develop portal vein thrombosis [3,4].

During primary hemostasis, platelets adhere to the subendothelium via the von Willebrand factor (vWF) [5]. Thrombocytopenia, thrombocytopathy, or impaired function of vWF can disrupt primary hemostasis. Thrombocytopenia is common in liver cirrhosis, occurring in up to 70% of patients even though the underlying pathomechanisms are most likely multifactorial and not yet fully understood [6]; it is assumed that an imbalance between the production and survival of platelets is its most likely cause. Thrombocytopenia can be due to bone marrow suppression or decreased thrombopoietin levels. Hypersplenism, platelet consumption, and platelet autoantibody action might decrease survival of platelets in cirrhotic patients [7]. Data on concomitant thrombocytopathy is not clear and in part controversial. As an example of thrombocytopathy, impaired platelet activation has been reported, while other results indicate hyperactivation of platelets in end-stage liver disease [7]. Levels of vWF are elevated in cirrhosis, which may be due to different causes. Endotoxemia in patients with liver cirrhosis has shown to increase vWF-levels [8].

Further, vWF mRNA levels in hepatic tissue are increased as well, indicating increased hepatic synthesis of vWF [9].

In hemostasis, von Willebrand factor binds to glycoprotein Ib on the platelet surface and to the subendothelial matrix. Besides this, vWF was recently recognized as playing important roles during angiogenesis, inflammation, cell proliferation and tumor cell growth [10]. Further, vWF levels were shown to correlate with the degree of portal hypertension as measured by hepatic venous pressure gradient and vWF levels were predictive of survival free of portal hypertension-related events and liver transplantation [11]. They were as well associated with development of hepatopulmonary syndrome [12] and in a further study prediction of mortality in patients with end-stage liver disease was equal to MELD score [13]. vWF is cleaved by the protease ADAMTS13 (a disintegrin-like and metalloprotease with thrombospondin type 1 motif 13), which is mainly synthesized in the liver and found to be reduced in cirrhosis [14,15].

Measurement of the in-vitro bleeding time using the Platelet Function Analyzer (PFA-100) is an established method for assessing primary hemostasis. It shows almost no intra-assay variability and has a high accuracy for detection of platelet function defects with an area under the ROC curve of 0.977 [16]. It successfully aids detection of patients with platelet function defects or von Willebrand's disease [17].

We assessed the PFA-100, a test that closely represents the in-vivo setting, in cirrhotic patients to investigate primary hemostasis. Therefore, we aimed to study the effect of increased levels of vWF on the in-vitro bleeding time in thrombocytopenic patients.

Materials and Methods

Patients

Patients with end-stage liver disease on the waiting list for liver transplantation at the Heidelberg University Hospital (Germany) were eligible for inclusion, regardless of etiology, platelet count, or hematocrit levels. Patients who had taken either antiplatelet drugs, non-steroidal anti-inflammatory drugs (NSAID), or other anticoagulant agents within the last ten days were excluded; patients were also excluded if no information on these drugs was available.

We measured a complete blood count as well as PFA-100 closure-times after stimulation with epinephrine or ADP, vWF-antigen, and vWF-activity as well as the ratio vWF-activity:vWF-antigen and ADAMTS13 activitiy. Analyses were separately conducted for the whole study cohort, for patients without thrombocytopenia and without anemia (defined as platelet count ≥ 150/nL and hematocrit $\geq 27\%$) and for patients with thrombocytopenia (<150/nL). Analysis was as well performed for patients with a platelet count <60/nL, which is an accepted cut-off for performing invasive procedures, such as transcutaneous liver biopsy. A platelet concentration of 50–0/nL in cirrhotic patients is sufficient to preserve thrombin generation at a level equivalent to the lower 10% of the normal range [18]. To investigate the effect of vWF-levels on platelet aggregation further, we measured vWF levels within a subset of cirrhotic patients as described below. Data on patient demographic and health characteristics, including age, sex, etiology of liver disease, Child-Turcotte-Pugh (CTP) score, and MELD score were obtained.

Ethics Statement

All patients provided written informed consent, and the study was previously approved by the local ethics committee of the medical faculty of the University Hospital Heidelberg and the study was performed in accordance with the Declaration of Helsinki.

Blood samples

Blood was drawn from the cubital or antecubital vein with a 21-gauge butterfly needle. The first milliliters of blood was collected into an EDTA-tube (ethylenediaminetetraacetic acid) and used for complete blood count. Then, citrated blood was collected for analysis of vWF. Finally, 3.8 ml of blood was collected into a tube containing 0.129 mol/l citrate (S-Monovette for PFA 100, Sarstedt AG & Co., Germany) for analysis of PFA-100 closure times.

Modification of vWF

In patients with thrombocytopenia (platelet count <150/nL), vWF levels were modified as follows to proof the hypothesis that increased vWF can compensate for reduced platelet count in patients with liver cirrhosis: Four tubes containing 0.129 mol/l citrate (S-Monovette for PFA 100) were collected per patient. Immediately after collection, 66 µg or 165 µg of a polyclonal anti-human vWF antibody (Haematologic Technologies, Inc., U.S.A.) was added to two tubes, respectively. A third tube was prepared with 25 µg of recombinant vWF (r-vWF) (Haematologic Technologies, Inc.). We aimed to add the amount of vWF that usually is found in healthy individuals and which thus would increase vWF in healthy individuals by 100%. Based on a concentration of 10µg vWF in 1 mL plasma of healthy controls [19] and an estimated hematocrit of 35% in cirrhotic patients, 25µg r-vWF are needed to meet these assumptions. A fourth tube was used as a control. All tubes were then incubated for 60 min at 37°C in a water bath. Next, PFA-100 was performed in all samples to measure closure times using collagen-epinephrine (Col-Epi) and collagen-ADP (Col-ADP). Additionally, plasma from these same samples was used to measure vWF-antigen levels.

Use of PFA-100 and determination of closure time

Without shaking, the samples were immediately brought to the central laboratory of the Heidelberg University Hospital, and were analyzed within 3 h after being drawn. Samples that underwent modification of vWF were analyzed immediately after incubation in a water bath.

For PFA-100 closure time analysis, a whole blood sample, collected in a tube with 3.8% sodium citrate, was used for input. It is aspirated through a capillary tube and exposed to a collagen membrane, coated with either epinephrine or ADP, at a shear rate of 5000–6000/s. Activation of platelets is caused by shear stress and exposure to the coated membrane, thus initiating the formation of a platelet plug. The time until full occlusion (and blood flow discontinuation) is measured; this is called the closure time and is a parameter for primary hemostasis [20].

PFA-100 (Siemens Healthcare, Germany) was performed using standard cartridges containing Col-Epi and Col-ADP (both Siemens Healthcare) and results for closure times were measured in seconds. Closure time >165 s with Col-Epi and that >118 s with Col-ADP were considered pathological. The test was stopped, if no clotting was achieved after 300 s; in this case, 300 s was recorded as closure time. According to recommendations and clinical practice, the PFA-100 was analyzed as following[16]: If the test with Col-Epi was prolonged, than Col-ADP was as well included for analysis. Only if this was prolonged as well, the PFA-100 was considered to be pathological.

Analysis of vWF and ADAMTS13

vWF-antigen levels and vWF-activity were determined turbidimetric assays on a Siemens BCS XP system applying appropriate reagents (vWF Ag and INNOVANCE vWF Ac kits, respectively,

Table 1. Characteristics of patients with liver cirrhosis.

	Child A	Child B	Child C	Total
Patients, n (%)	19 (26.4%)	31 (43.1%)	22 (30.6%)	72
Female, n (%)	6 (31.6%)	11 (35.5)	11 (50.0%)	28 (38.9%)
Age, yrs. (±SD)	48.5 (±8.9)	51.3 (±11.1)	52.8 (±9.4)	51.0 (±10.1)
Etiology of cirrhosis				
Cryptogenic, n (%)	1 (5.3%)	4 (12.9%)	3 (13.6%)	8 (11.1%)
Alcoholic, n (%)	8 (42.1%)	14 (45.2%)	13 (59.1%)	35 (48.6%)
Viral hepatitis, n (%)	5 (26.3%)	6 (19.4%)	5 (22.7%)	16 (22.2%)
Autoimmune hepatitis, n (%)	0	3 (9.7%)	0	3 (4.2%)
Cholestatic[a], n (%)	3 (15.8%)	4 (12.9%)	0	7 (9.7%)
Other[b], n (%)	2 (10.5%)	0	1 (4.5%)	3 (4.2%)
LabMELD, median (range)	8 (7–12)	12 (7–21)	19 (13–37)	12 (7–37)

Description of baseline parameters such as age, sex, and etiology of patients with liver cirrhosis and labMELD-score; grouped by Child-Turcotte-Pugh score.
[a]Including primary sclerosing cholangitis and biliary atresia.
[b]Including Wilson disease and polycystic liver disease.

all by Siemens Healthcare). Normal ranges of vWF-antigen and vWF-activity were 70–120% and 61–179%, respectively, in patients with all blood types; normal vWF-activity was 46–146% in patients with blood type O.

For measurement of ADAMTS13 activity, citrate plasma samples of 50 patients were kept in aliquots at −20°C before analysis in the central laboratory. ADAMTS13 activity was determined applying the Technozym ADAMTS-13 Activity ELISA kit (Technoclone, Heidelberg, Germany) on a Biochrom EZ Read 400 ELISA Microplate Reader at 450 nm according to the manufacturer's instructions.

Statistical analysis

Results for closure times, vWF-antigen, vWF-activity, ADAMTS13, hematocrit, and platelet counts are reported as means with standard deviations (SD). Student's t-test and one way ANOVA were used to compare results of parametric data. For comparison of categorical variables, Fisher's exact test was used. Closure times, hematocrit, platelet count, vWF, and ADAMTS13 were evaluated on the basis of CTP and MELD scores. Multivariate analysis was done using a logistic regression model. Only variables showing a $P<0.1$ in univariate analysis were included for multivariate analysis. Results of the vWF-modification experiments were analyzed using the t-test for paired samples. Statistical analyses were performed using IBM SPSS version 21 (IBM Corp, Armonk, NY). Significance was defined as $P<0.05$. Original data can be found in Tables S1 and S2.

Results

Study cohort

A total of 95 patients with liver cirrhosis were screened between January 2012 and October 2013; of these, 23 were excluded because of anti-platelet drugs or NSAIDs intake. PFA-100 closure time using Col-Epi was determined in the remaining 72 patients; of these, Col-ADP was available in 62 patients.

Among the included 72 cirrhotic patients, 19 (26.4%) had Child A cirrhosis, 31 (43.1%), Child B cirrhosis, and 22 (30.6%), Child C cirrhosis; labMELD score ranged from 7 to 37 (median: 12). Further details on patient characteristics are given in Table 1. Enrolment details of the study population are shown in Figure 1.

PFA-100 closure times and basic laboratory values in cirrhotic patients

The mean PFA-100 closure time with Col-Epi in cirrhotic patients was 180±62 s and that with Col-ADP was 160±70 s. Of the 72 samples tested with Col-Epi, 35 (48.6%) had results within the normal range, while 37 (51.4%) had pathological results. Of the 62 samples tested with Col-ADP, 22 (35.5%) had results within the normal range and 40 (64.5%) had pathological results. Of the patients with prolonged Col-Epi, measurement of Col-ADP was pathological in 32 (86.5%), thus a total of 32 of the 72 patients (44.4%) were classified as having a pathological test results for the PFA-100.

All patients had a mean platelet count of 109/nL (±63) and mean hematocrit of 34.2% (±6.9). Mean vWF-antigen was

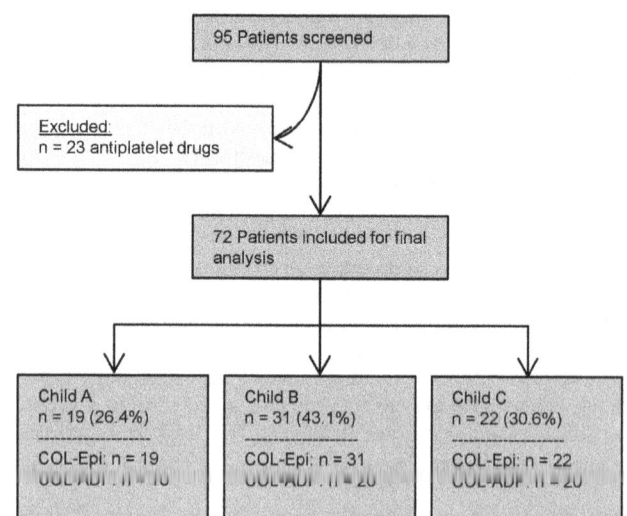

Figure 1. Selection of the study population. The enrolment details of the study population are shown, including the number of patients excluded because of the use of antiplatelet drugs or because there was no information on use of these drugs. For all subgroups, the number of available test results for PFA-100 with Col-Epi and Col-ADP is given.

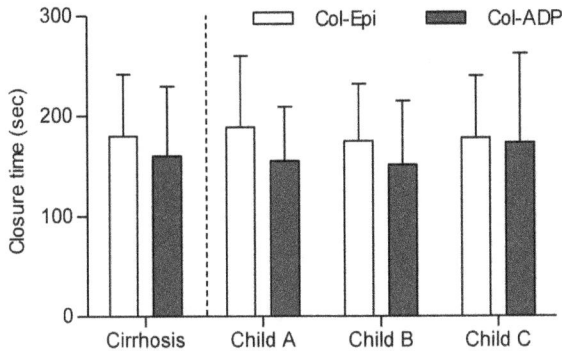

Figure 2. Results for PFA-100 in cirrhotic patients. Overall, mean closure times were above the upper limit of normal for Col-Epi (>165 s) and Col-ADP (>118 s) in cirrhotic patients. There were no significant differences between patients with different Child-Turcotte-Pugh scores.

383.9% (±200.6) mean vWF-activity was 313.5% (±168.7) and mean vWF-activity:vWF-antigen ratio was 0.83 (±0.14). Mean ADAMTS13 activity was 67.9% (±24.0).

Analysis by Child-Turcotte-Pugh score revealed no significant differences for mean closure times after induction with either Col-Epi or Col-ADP (Figure 2) nor in the rate of pathological PFA-100 test results. Yet there were significant differences in hematocrit, vWF-antigen and vWF-activity and a strong trend towards reduced ADAMTS13 activity in CTP B ($P = 0.050$) and CTP C ($P = 0.070$) compared to CTP A patients was observed (Table 2). Additionally, there were no significant differences in PFA-100 closure times between patients with Child-Turcotte-Pugh A, B, and C, if only patients with a platelet count ≥150/nL and hematocrit ≥27.0% were included (data not shown).

Analysis of PFA-100 closure times in thrombocytopenic patients with liver cirrhosis

A total of 58 patients with thrombocytopenia (<150/nL) were included, among which were 29 (50.0%) with a pathological result for the PFA-100 test. This resembles a strong trend towards an increased rate of pathological results in these patients compared to the non-thrombocytopenic group (3 out of 11, $P = 0.053$). Compared to the 14 non-thrombocytopenic patients, patients with a platelet count <150/nL had prolonged closure times for Col-Epi (187 ± 62 s vs. 149 ± 53 s; $P = 0.037$) and Col-ADP (164 ± 70 s vs. 140 ± 70 s; $P = 0.281$). There were significantly more pathological results for Col-ADP (58.1% vs. 6.5%; $P = 0.019$) in the thrombocytopenic group compared to the non-thrombocytopenic patients, but this was not significant for Col-Epi (44.4% vs. 6.9%; $P = 0.240$).

Thrombocytopenic patients had significantly more advanced liver cirrhosis (median MELD 13 [range 7–37] vs. 11 [range 7–20]; $P = 0.040$ according to Mann-Whitney-U test), but did not show a significant difference in hematocrit ($33.7 \pm 6.9\%$ vs. $36.4 \pm 6.5\%$; $P = 0.184$). Levels of vWF-antigen were higher in the thrombocytopenic group ($400.5 \pm 206.2\%$ vs. $310.0 \pm 160.0\%$; $P = 0.143$) as were levels of vWF-activity ($333.6 \pm 176.5\%$ vs. $223.7 \pm 86.0\%$, $P = 0.033$).

In patients with a platelet count of less 60/nL (n = 12) closure time was 201 ± 66 s for Col-Epi. After performing Col-ADP in the 8 (66.7%) patients with prolonged results for Col-Epi, all these patients were diagnosed with a pathological PFA-100. There was no statically significant difference in PFA closure times compared to patients with a platelet count ≥60/nL (Col-Epi: $P = 0.203$, Col-ADP: $P = 0.341$), but there was a trend towards a higher rate of pathological PFA-100 test in these patients compared to those with a platelet count ≥60/nL ($P = 0.090$).

Analysis of vWF in thrombocytopenic patients

Analysis of vWF in thrombocytopenic patients (defined as platelet count <150/nL) revealed an association with closure times: vWF-antigen was significantly higher in those thrombocy-

Table 2. Results for PFA-100, full blood count, and vWF.

	Child A	Child B	Child C	P<0.05
Col-Epi, n (%)	19	31	22	
Closure time, s (±SD)	189 (±71)	175 (±57)	178 (±62)	n.s.
Pathological, n (%)	10 (52.6%)	15 (48.4%)	12 (54.5%)	n.s.
Col-ADP n (%)	16	26	20	
Closure time, s (±SD)	155 (±54)	151 (±64)	173 (±89)	n.s.
Pathological, n (%)	12 (75.0%)	15 (57.7%)	13 (65.0%)	n.s.
PFA-100 test result				
Pathological, n (%)	8 (42.1%)	13 (41.9%)	11 (50.0%)	n.s.
Laboratory values				
Platelet count,/nL (±SD)	122 (±50)	115 (±80)	91 (±40)	n.s.
Hematocrit, % (±SD)	38.9 (±5.9)	34.0 (±5.9)	30.4 (±6.8)	A/B, A/C
vWF-antigen, % (±SD)	274.1 (±111.1)	358.5 (±148.6)	513.5 (±252.3)	A/C, B/C
vWF-activity, % (±SD)	223.1 (±101.7)	301.9 (±132.2)	407.3 (±212.3)	A/C
vWF-activity:vWF-antigen ratio (±SD)	0.81 (±0.11)	0.85 (±0.14)	0.83 (±0.14)	n.s.
ADAMTS13, % (SD)	81.0 (±18.9)	64.5 (±23.2)	63.7 (±26.2)	n.s.

Results for PFA-100 and basic laboratory values are grouped by Child-Turcotte-Pugh classification. The 'P<0.05'-column indicates significant differences between groups according to one-way ANOVA or Fisher's exact test. For example, A/C indicates a significant difference between CTP groups A and C.

topenic patients with a normal PFA-100 (462.3±235.9%) compared to those with pathological results (338.7±151.6%, $P=0.021$). A similar trends was as well found for vWF-activity (376.2±209.7% vs. 291.0±125.1%, $P=0.065$). Regarding vWF-activity:vWF-antigen ratio and ADAMTS13 activity no differences were found ($P=0.161$ and $P=0.628$, respectively). These results on the differences in vWF-antigen and vWF-activity were as well present when separately analyzed for Col-Epi and Col-ADP (Table 3, Figure 3A).

Results after modification of vWF

In 21 patients with a platelet count <150/nL, plasma vWF levels were modified with a polyclonal antibody or with recombinant vWF. Mean closure times were 197±60 s (Col-Epi) and 159±61 s (Col-ADP) in the unmodified samples. Compared to these, closure times were 178±57 s (Col-Epi; $P=0.019$) and 149±60 s (Col-ADP; $P=0.189$) after addition of recombinant vWF and we found a significant increase in vWF antigen levels in all 21 samples ($P<0.001$). Addition of 66 µg of anti-vWF-antibody resulted in closure times of 247±49 s for Col-Epi ($P=0.016$) and 213±45 s for Col-ADP ($P=0.091$); addition of 165 µg resulted in closure times of 274±33 s for Col-Epi ($P=0.005$) and 277±32 s for Col-ADP ($P=0.006$). Results are shown in Figure 3B-D and summarized in Table 4.

Detection of thrombocytopathy in patients with normal platelet count and hematocrit

Overall, 14 patients with liver cirrhosis had a platelet count ≥ 150/nL and hematocrit ≥27%. Mean closures time were 149±53 s for Col-Epi. Pathological results for Col-Epi were found in 5 (35.7%) patients and after measurement of Col-ADP in these patients, a total of 3 (21.4%) patients were diagnosed with a pathological PFA-100 test. There were no differences regarding platelet count, hematocrit, or vWF between patients with normal and pathological results.

Analysis of independent predictors of pathologic results for the PFA-100 test

The influence of the following variables on the outcome of the PFA-100 was investigated: age, sex, labMELD score, serum albumin, platelet count, hematocrit, vWF-antigen, vWF-activity:vWF-antigen ratio, and ADAMTS13. In univariate analysis only platelet count ($P=0.086$), hematocrit ($P=0.054$) and vWF-antigen ($P=0.064$) levels were associated ($P<0.1$) with the outcome of the PFA-100. In a multivariate analysis including these three variables, only hematocrit ($P=0.027$) and vWF-antigen ($P=0.010$) turned out to significantly influence the PFA-100 test results, yet there was a strong trend for platelet count as well ($P=0.069$). The same analysis was performed in thrombocytopenic patients (<150/nL), which revealed again hematocrit ($P=0.026$) and vWF-antigen ($P=0.013$) as independent predictors of the test outcome (Table 5 and 6).

Discussion

Over the past years, knowledge about hemostasis in patients with cirrhosis has greatly expanded and revealed that conventional coagulation parameters as International Normalized Ratio (INR), prothrombin time, or platelet count are not as reliable to indicate an increased risk of bleeding as assumed previously. Especially with regard to platelet transfusions or supplementation with coagulation factors, clinicians are in need of tests that determine the actual hemostatic balance in these patients more accurately [21]. Therefore, we conducted a study to evaluate primary

Table 3. Analysis of the effect of vWF on results of PFA-100 in thrombocytopenic patients.

	PFA-100			Col-Epi			Col-ADP		
	norm.	path.	P	norm.	path.	P	norm.	path.	P
vWF-antigen, % (±SD)	462.3 (±235.9)	338.7 (±151.6)	0.021	467.8 (±248.7)	345.8 (±146.3)	0.033	470.6 (±252.3)	358.3 (±171.8)	0.077
vWF-activity, % (±SD)	376.2 (±209.7)	291.0 (±125.1)	0.065	383.7 (±220.7)	292.9 (±119.1)	0.067	401.2 (±241.3)	300.9 (±135.8)	0.068
vWF-activity:vWF- antigen ratio	0.82 (±0.13)	0.87 (±0.14)	0.161	0.83 (±0.14)	0.86 (±0.14)	0.372	0.84 (±0.11)	0.86 (±0.14)	0.712

Comparison of vWF-antigen and vWF-activity in thrombocytopenic (<150/nL) patients with liver cirrhosis and the effect of vWF on results of PFA-100 measured with Col-Epi and Col-ADP (norm. = normal test result, path. = pathological test result).

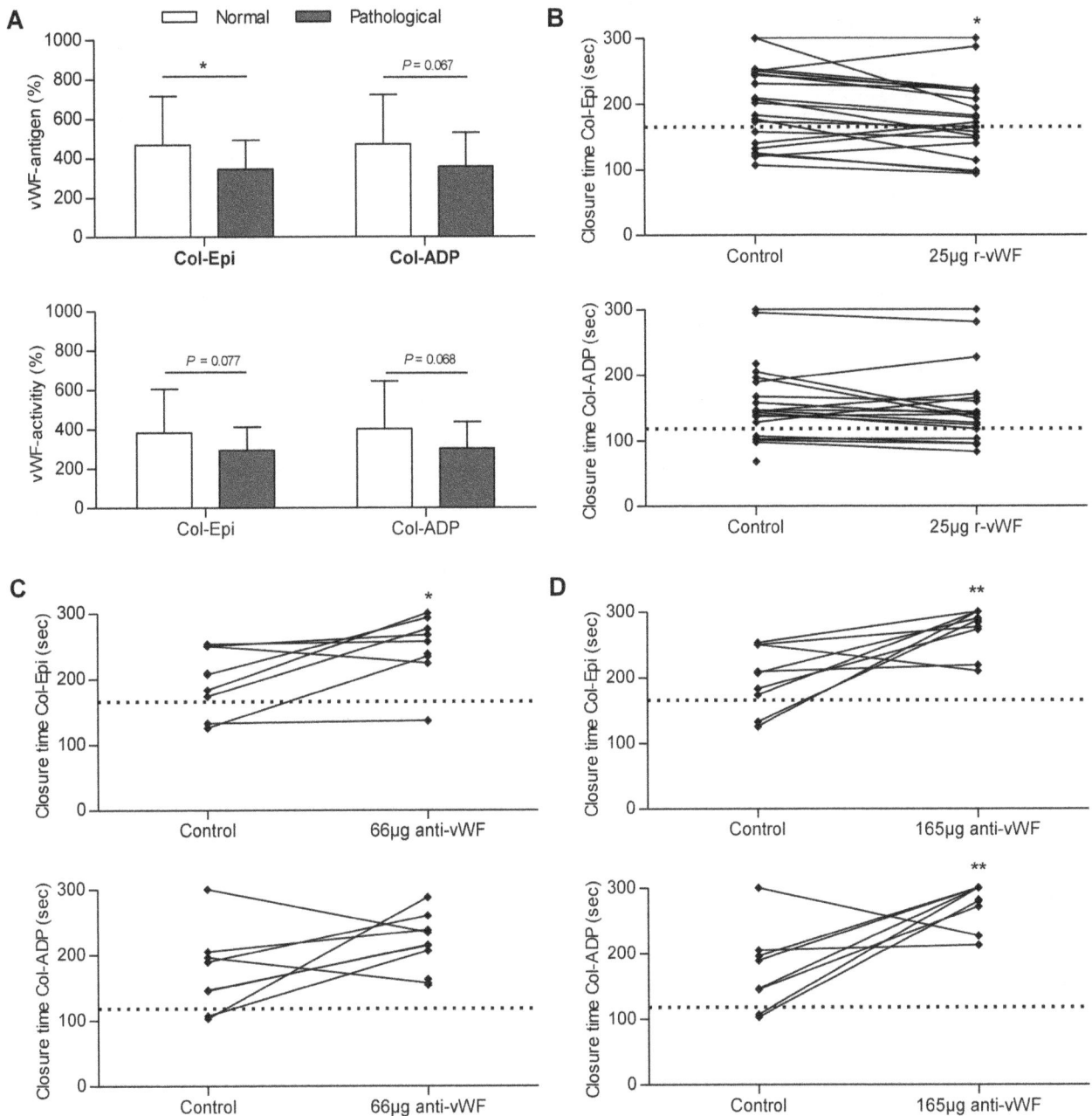

Figure 3. Effect of von Willebrand factor on primary hemostasis in thrombocytopenic patients with liver cirrhosis. Increased levels of vWF were associated with maintained normal primary hemostasis in patients with liver cirrhosis and reduced platelet count (<150/nL). vWF-antigen and vWF-activity were higher in patients with normal results for PFA-100 after measuring with Col-Epi and Col-ADP (A+B). Substitution of recombinant vWF (r-vWF) resulted in improved primary hemostasis as compared to unmodified samples (C). Addition of a 66-µg or 165-µg polyclonal anti-vWF-antibody levels led to prolonged closure times compared to unmodified control samples (D+E). Horizontal lines represent the upper limit of normal for closure times with Col-Epi or Col-ADP [**: $P<0.01$, *: $P<0.05$].

hemostasis in patients with liver cirrhosis by means of PFA-100 closure times. On the one hand side our results indicate that primary hemostasis is impaired in a large number of patients and we found a high rate of results indicating thrombocytopathy. On the other hand side we also demonstrated that increased vWF levels can compensate for reduced platelet count.

PFA-100 is a validated test for screening of platelet function disorders and von Willebrand's disease [17,22] and has been used to detect platelet-related defects of primary hemostasis in dialysis

patients as well [23]. Until now, data on its use in patients with liver cirrhosis is only available from two smaller studies. The first study reported increased closure times in 20 patients with Child A or B cirrhosis. An improvement of closure times was shown after experimentally increasing hematocrit [24]. Since we found pathological results in patients with a hematocrit ≥27% in the present study, we esteem that transfusion of packed red blood cells may only improve primary hemostasis in some patients. The second study focused on differences between cholestatic and non-

Table 4. Effect of vWF levels on primary hemostasis in thrombocytopenic patients with cirrhosis.

	25 µg r-vWF	66 µg anti-vWF	156 µg anti-vWF
Col-Epi	↓	↑	↑
Col-ADP	↔	↑	↑

Overview of the main results: changes in closure times after addition of either recombinant vWF or anti-vWF-antibody (↔: no change, ↓: improved, ↑: worsened).

cholestatic causes of liver diseases. Closure times for patients with primary biliary cirrhosis and primary sclerosing cholangitis were less compared to patients with non-cholestatic causes of cirrhosis [25]. Despite including more patients, especially with end-stage liver disease, to our knowledge, this is the first study to acknowledge platelet count, hematocrit, and vWF in the analysis. The latter two were as well identified as independent predictors of maintained primary hemostasis in multivariate analysis, yet a strong trend was found for platelet count as well. Our study results support the hypothesis that cirrhosis disrupts primary hemostasis, which does seem independent on the stage of cirrhosis.

Within our samples of non-thrombocytopenic, non-anemic patients, we obtained pathological results for the PFA-100 in 21.4% of cases. Platelet dysfunction is the most likely reason for these pathological results, since patients with low hematocrit and low platelet count were not included in this analysis and vWF-antigen and vWF-activity were increased. Until now, data on the presence of thrombocytopathy in cirrhotic patients is still controversial [7]. Possible causes of thrombocytopathy in liver cirrhosis are signal transduction defects, storage pool disorders, or impaired thromboxane A2 synthesis [26,27,28]. According to our

findings, in a system closely mimicking in-vivo primary hemostasis, platelet function defects are present in cirrhotic patients and might contribute to prolonged primary hemostasis.

Analysis of the PFA-100 test results and results for Col-Epi and Col-ADP in thrombocytopenic patients only revealed a higher rate of pathological results in some of the analysis in these patients with reduced platelet count, but results did show no differences for the other analyses. This was true for either of two cut-offs used in our analysis, namely 150/nL and 60/nL. This strengthens the hypothesis that platelet count alone as a static parameter does not resemble of the current state of coagulation in cirrhotic patients. This is further supported by a ROC (receiver operating characteristic) analysis performed to analyze whether platelet count predicts PFA-100 results. This revealed an area under the curve of 0.716 and thus showing only moderate capability of discriminating between normal and pathological PFA-100 results. The assessment of bleeding risk before medical interventions probably is not well predicted based upon a static parameter, such as platelet count [29]. Therefore tests globally and dynamically assessing primary hemostasis should be further investigated, especially since other factors, as vWF or hematocrit, might

Table 5. Results for univariate analysis of predictors of a pathological PFA-100 test result.

Variable	Exp(B)	95% KI für Exp(B)	P
All patients			
Age	0.981	0.936–1.028	0.418
Sex	0.900	0.346–2.339	0.829
MELD	1.019	0.943–1.101	0.627
Albumin	0.984	0.916–1.057	0.661
Platelet count	0.992	0.983–1.001	0.086
Hematocrit	0.930	0.864–1.001	0.054
vWF-antigen	0.997	0.994–1.000	0.064
vWF-activity:vWF-antigen ratio	13.528	0.409–447.335	0.145
ADAMTS13	0.991	0.967–1.014	0.437
Platelets <150/nL			
Age	0.969	0.920–1.022	0.246
Sex	1.161	0.398–3.392	0.785
MELD	0.998	0.920–1.083	0.967
Albumin	0.994	0.916–1.079	0.888
Platelet count	0.990	0.974–1.006	0.223
Hematocrit	0.932	0.860–1.010	0.086
vWF-antigen	0.996	0.993–1.000	0.032
vWF-activity:vWF-antigen ratio	17.371	0.309–967.333	0.165
ADAMTS13	0.994	0.969–1.019	0.619

Univariate analysis of the following variables was performed to identify predictors of a pathological PFA-100 test results in the whole study cohort and in thrombocytopenic cirrhotic patients. Multivariate analysis was then performed with variables showing a P-value ≤0.1 in univariate analysis.

Table 6. Results for multivariate analysis of predictors of a pathological PFA-100 test result.

Variable	Exp(B)	95% KI für Exp(B)	P
All patients			
Platelet count	0.990	0.980–1.001	0.069
Hematocrit	0.909	0.834–0.989	0.027
vWF-antigen	0.995	0.992–0.999	0.010
Platelets <150/nL			
Hematocrit	0.901	0.822–0.987	0.026
vWF-antigen	0.995	0.992–0.999	0.013

Variables with a P≤0.1 in univariate analysis were included in multivariate analysis, which was separately performed for the whole study cohort and for patients with a platelet count y 150/nL.

compensate for a reduced platelet count. These studies should as well evaluate if bleeding complications are related to pathological test result. Our study indicates that the PFA-100 might be useful to characterize the interplay of increased vWF and reduced platelet count in cirrhotic patients. Thus, PFA-100 should be examined in cirrhotic patients undergoing medical interventions.

In patients with cirrhosis and thrombocytopenia, maintenance of normal primary hemostasis seems to depend greatly on concomitantly increased vWF levels and reduced levels of the vWF cleaving protease ADAMTS13 [15,30]. Evidence for this was first reported by Lisman et al. [31] and is supported by our analysis of thrombocytopenic patients and the vWF-modification experiment. In addition to the important work by Lisman et al., who used pooled plasma from healthy controls and patients with liver cirrhosis we further decided to directly modify plasma vWF levels. We were thus able to directly identify vWF as the important coagulation factor responsible for maintained primary hemostasis. We found that higher vWF-antigen and higher vWF-activity in thrombocytopenic patients were associated with normal closure times. Since there were no differences in vWF-activity:vWF-antigen ratio, we conclude that the difference is due to an increase in vWF-antigen and not due to differences in functionality of vWF. Further no influence of ADAMTS13 was noted in this setting and in the multivariate analysis performed. A decrease of ADAMTS13 in decompensated cirrhosis is in line with previous results [15]. Further, in Line with Lisman et al., we found a negative correlation between ADAMTS13 and the vWF-activity:vWF-antigen ratio (Pearson's r = −0.350, P = 0.013), indicating increased vWF proteolysis in some patients with consequently reduced vWF activity [31]. Yet neither ADAMTS13 nor the vWF-activity:vWF-antigen ratio were predictive of the PFA-100 test results, which was only true for vWF-antigen, which did not correlate to ADAMTS13. We thus suspect that a decrease in ADAMTS13 is not the solitary reason for increased vWF levels and thereby maintained normal primary hemostasis in cirrhotic patients. In thrombocytopenic patients, the addition of r-vWF significantly improvement closure times while addition of an anti-vWF-antibody yielded significantly prolonged closure times. Yet, it remains unclear whether there is physiological connection between increased vWF and decrease platelet count or not, but most interestingly both changes are commonly found in portal hypertension [11]. PFA-100 has previously been shown to correlate well with vWF [32]; therefore, we assume that it is an appropriate test to measure the effect of different vWF levels. Whether measurement of the PFA-100 or supplementation of

vWF could be an option in clinical practice needs to be further evaluated. The test could be used to identify patients with impaired primary hemostasis who might benefit from increased platelet counts or vWF levels and to differentiate them from patients with risk of thrombosis due to use of pro-coagulant drugs. This is of importance, since the substitution of thrombopoietin is associated with increased rate of thrombosis [33] and platelet transfusion during liver transplantation is associated with increased mortality [21]. With regard to the supplementation of vWF, previous studies on the administration of desmopressin, able to induce vWF release from the endothelium, resulted in an improved in-vivo bleeding time, thereby supporting this approach [34,35]. Yet, before this can be implemented in clinical practice further studies are needed to determine the optimal dose of r-vWF and to actually show an improvement compared to platelet transfusion in a clinical trial.

In conclusion, we found that primary hemostasis is impaired in cirrhotic patients probably because of reduced platelet count or hematocrit, but also because of thrombocytopathy. Increased vWF levels can partially compensate for reduced platelet count and the supplementation with r-vWF should further be investigated and compared with platelet transfusion.

Supporting Information

Table S1 Results for PFA-100 in patients with liver cirrhosis.

Table S2 Results of the vWF modification experiment.

Acknowledgments

We would like to thank Bärbel Calvo for her assistance with PFA-100 analyses.

Author Contributions

Conceived and designed the experiments: AW OJM KHW WS PS HAK DNG. Performed the experiments: AW KF CR PK YL MB MS DNG. Analyzed the data: AW OJM KF CR PK YL MB MS KHW DNG. Contributed reagents/materials/analysis tools: AW OJM MB WS DNG. Wrote the paper: AW OJM KF CR MS DNG. Critically revised the manuscript for important intellectual content: MB KHW WS PS HAK. Approved the final version of the article: AW OJM KF CR PK YL MB MS KHW WS PS HAK DNG.

References

1. Tripodi A, Mannucci PM (2011) The coagulopathy of chronic liver disease. N Engl J Med 365: 147–156.
2. Lisman T, Porte RJ (2010) The role of platelets in liver inflammation and regeneration. Semin Thromb Hemost 36: 170–174.
3. Sogaard KK, Horvath-Puho E, Gronbaek H, Jepsen P, Vilstrup H, et al. (2009) Risk of venous thromboembolism in patients with liver disease: a nationwide population-based case-control study. Am J Gastroenterol 104: 96–101.
4. Amitrano L, Guardascione MA, Brancaccio V, Margaglione M, Manguso F, et al. (2004) Risk factors and clinical presentation of portal vein thrombosis in patients with liver cirrhosis. J Hepatol 40: 736–741.
5. Sakariassen KS, Bolhuis PA, Sixma JJ (1979) Human blood platelet adhesion to artery subendothelium is mediated by factor VIII-Von Willebrand factor bound to the subendothelium. Nature 279: 636–638.
6. Giannini EG, Savarino V (2008) Thrombocytopenia in liver disease. Curr Opin Hematol 15: 473–480.
7. Violi F, Basili S, Raparelli V, Chowdary P, Gatt A, et al. (2011) Patients with liver cirrhosis suffer from primary haemostatic defects? Fact or fiction? J Hepatol 55: 1415–1427.
8. Ferro D, Quintarelli C, Lattuada A, Leo R, Alessandroni M, et al. (1996) High plasma levels of von Willebrand factor as a marker of endothelial perturbation in cirrhosis: relationship to endotoxemia. Hepatology 23: 1377–1383.
9. Hollestelle MJ, Geertzen HG, Straatsburg IH, van Gulik TM, van Mourik JA (2004) Factor VIII expression in liver disease. Thromb Haemost 91: 267–275.
10. Lenting PJ, Casari C, Christophe OD, Denis CV (2012) von Willebrand factor: the old, the new and the unknown. J Thromb Haemost 10: 2428–2437.
11. La Mura V, Reverter JC, Flores-Arroyo A, Raffa S, Reverter E, et al. (2011) Von Willebrand factor levels predict clinical outcome in patients with cirrhosis and portal hypertension. Gut 60: 1133–1138.
12. Horvatits T, Drolz A, Roedl K, Herkner H, Ferlitsch A, et al. (2014) vWF, a screening tool for detection of hepatopulmonary syndrome in patients with liver cirrhosis. J Hepatol.
13. Ferlitsch M, Reiberger T, Hoke M, Salzl P, Schwengerer B, et al. (2012) von Willebrand factor as new noninvasive predictor of portal hypertension, decompensation and mortality in patients with liver cirrhosis. Hepatology 56: 1439–1447.
14. Levy GG, Motto DG, Ginsburg D (2005) ADAMTS13 turns 3. Blood 106: 11–17.
15. Mannucci PM, Canciani MT, Forza I, Lussana F, Lattuada A, et al. (2001) Changes in health and disease of the metalloprotease that cleaves von Willebrand factor. Blood 98: 2730–2735.
16. Mammen EF, Comp PC, Gosselin R, Greenberg C, Hoots WK, et al. (1998) PFA-100 system: a new method for assessment of platelet dysfunction. Semin Thromb Hemost 24: 195–202.
17. Harrison P, Robinson MS, Mackie IJ, Joseph J, McDonald SJ, et al. (1999) Performance of the platelet function analyser PFA-100 in testing abnormalities of primary haemostasis. Blood Coagul Fibrinolysis 10: 25–31.
18. Tripodi A, Primignani M, Chantarangkul V, Clerici M, Dell'Era A, et al. (2006) Thrombin generation in patients with cirrhosis: the role of platelets. Hepatology 44: 440–445.
19. Mannucci PM (1998) von Willebrand factor: a marker of endothelial damage? Arterioscler Thromb Vasc Biol 18: 1359–1362.
20. Kundu SK, Heilmann EJ, Sio R, Garcia C, Davidson RM, et al. (1995) Description of an in vitro platelet function analyzer—PFA-100. Semin Thromb Hemost 21 Suppl 2: 106–112.
21. Saner FH, Gieseler RK, Akiz H, Canbay A, Görlinger K (2013) Delicate Balance of Bleeding and Thrombosis in End-Stage Liver Disease and Liver Transplantation. Digestion 88: 135–144.
22. Buyukasik Y, Karakus S, Goker H, Haznedaroglu IC, Ozatli D, et al. (2002) Rational use of the PFA-100 device for screening of platelet function disorders and von Willebrand disease. Blood Coagul Fibrinolysis 13: 349–353.
23. Zupan IP, Sabovic M, Salobir B, Ponikvar JB, Cernelc P (2003) Utility of in vitro closure time test for evaluating platelet-related primary hemostasis in dialysis patients. Am J Kidney Dis 42: 746–751.
24. Escolar G, Cases A, Vinas M, Pino M, Calls J, et al. (1999) Evaluation of acquired platelet dysfunctions in uremic and cirrhotic patients using the platelet function analyzer (PFA-100): influence of hematocrit elevation. Haematologica 84: 614–619.
25. Pihusch R, Rank A, Gohring P, Pihusch M, Hiller E, et al. (2002) Platelet function rather than plasmatic coagulation explains hypercoagulable state in cholestatic liver disease. J Hepatol 37: 548–555.
26. Laffi G, La Villa G, Pinzani M, Ciabattoni G, Patrignani P, et al. (1986) Altered renal and platelet arachidonic acid metabolism in cirrhosis. Gastroenterology 90: 274–282.
27. Laffi G, Marra F, Failli P, Ruggiero M, Cecchi E, et al. (1993) Defective signal transduction in platelets from cirrhotics is associated with increased cyclic nucleotides. Gastroenterology 105: 148–156.
28. Laffi G, Marra F, Gresele P, Romagnoli P, Palermo A, et al. (1992) Evidence for a storage pool defect in platelets from cirrhotic patients with defective aggregation. Gastroenterology 103: 641–646.
29. Vieira da Rocha EC, D'Amico EA, Caldwell SH, Flores da Rocha TR, Soares ESCS, et al. (2009) A prospective study of conventional and expanded coagulation indices in predicting ulcer bleeding after variceal band ligation. Clin Gastroenterol Hepatol 7: 988–993.
30. Lisman T, Porte RJ (2010) Rebalanced hemostasis in patients with liver disease: evidence and clinical consequences. Blood 116: 878–885.
31. Lisman T, Bongers TN, Adelmeijer J, Janssen HL, de Maat MP, et al. (2006) Elevated levels of von Willebrand Factor in cirrhosis support platelet adhesion despite reduced functional capacity. Hepatology 44: 53–61.
32. Haubelt H, Anders C, Vogt A, Hoerdt P, Seyfert UT, et al. (2005) Variables influencing Platelet Function Analyzer-100 closure times in healthy individuals. Br J Haematol 130: 759–767.
33. Tripodi A, Primignani M (2013) Nontransfusional approach to increased platelet count in patients with cirrhosis and thrombocytopenia. Hepatology 58: 1177–1180.
34. Burroughs AK, Matthews K, Qadiri M, Thomas N, Kernoff P, et al. (1985) Desmopressin and bleeding time in patients with cirrhosis. Br Med J (Clin Res Ed) 291: 1377–1381.
35. Mannucci PM, Vicente V, Vianello L, Cattaneo M, Alberca I, et al. (1986) Controlled trial of desmopressin in liver cirrhosis and other conditions associated with a prolonged bleeding time. Blood 67: 1148–1153.

Permissions

The contributors of this book come from diverse backgrounds, making this book a truly international effort. This book will bring forth new frontiers with its revolutionizing research information and detailed analysis of the nascent developments around the world.

We would like to thank all the contributing authors for lending their expertise to make the book truly unique. They have played a crucial role in the development of this book. Without their invaluable contributions this book wouldn't have been possible. They have made vital efforts to compile up to date information on the varied aspects of this subject to make this book a valuable addition to the collection of many professionals and students.

This book was conceptualized with the vision of imparting up-to-date information and advanced data in this field. To ensure the same, a matchless editorial board was set up. Every individual on the board went through rigorous rounds of assessment to prove their worth. After which they invested a large part of their time researching and compiling the most relevant data for our readers.

The editorial board has been involved in producing this book since its inception. They have spent rigorous hours researching and exploring the diverse topics which have resulted in the successful publishing of this book. They have passed on their knowledge of decades through this book. To expedite this challenging task, the publisher supported the team at every step. A small team of assistant editors was also appointed to further simplify the editing procedure and attain best results for the readers.

Apart from the editorial board, the designing team has also invested a significant amount of their time in understanding the subject and creating the most relevant covers. They scrutinized every image to scout for the most suitable representation of the subject and create an appropriate cover for the book.

The publishing team has been an ardent support to the editorial, designing and production team. Their endless efforts to recruit the best for this project, has resulted in the accomplishment of this book. They are a veteran in the field of academics and their pool of knowledge is as vast as their experience in printing. Their expertise and guidance has proved useful at every step. Their uncompromising quality standards have made this book an exceptional effort. Their encouragement from time to time has been an inspiration for everyone.

The publisher and the editorial board hope that this book will prove to be a valuable piece of knowledge for researchers, students, practitioners and scholars across the globe.

List of Contributors

Yoshikuni Kawaguchi, Yasuhiko Sugawara, Nobuhisa Akamatsu, Junichi Kaneko, Takeaki Ishizawa, Sumihito Tamura, Taku Aoki, Yoshihiro Sakamoto, Kiyoshi Hasegawa, Norihiro Kokudo
Artificial Organ and Transplantation Surgery Division, Department of Surgery, Graduate School of Medicine, University of Tokyo, Tokyo, Japan

Tsuyoshi Hamada
Department of Gastroenterology, Graduate School of Medicine, University of Tokyo, Tokyo, Japan

Tomohiro Tanaka
Organ Transplantation Service, University of Tokyo, Tokyo, Japan

Gamze Günal-Sadık and Rolf Jessberger
Institute of Physiological Chemistry, Faculty of Medicine Carl Gustav Carus, Dresden University of Technology, Dresden, Germany

Maciej Paszkowski-Rogacz and Frank Buchholz
Department of Medical Systems Biology, University Hospital and Medical Faculty Carl Gustav Carus, Dresden University of Technology, Dresden, Germany

Kalaimathy Singaravelu
Cellular Networks and Systems Biology, Biotechnology Center, Dresden University of Technology, Dresden, Germany

Andreas Beyer
Cellular Networks and Systems Biology, Biotechnology Center, Dresden University of Technology, Dresden, Germany
CECAD, Universität zu Köln, Köln, Germany

Peter Willeit
Department of Neurology, Innsbruck Medical University, Innsbruck, Austria
Department of Public Health and Primary Care, University of Cambridge, Cambridge, United Kingdom

Julia Raschenberger, Margot Haun and Florian Kronenberg
Division of Genetic Epidemiology, Innsbruck Medical University, Innsbruck, Austria

Emma E. Heydon and Adam S. Butterworth
Department of Public Health and Primary Care, University of Cambridge, Cambridge, United Kingdom

Sotirios Tsimikas and Joseph L. Witztum
Department of Medicine, University of California San Diego, La Jolla, United States of America

Agnes Mayr
Department of Laboratory Medicine, Bruneck Hospital, Bruneck, Italy

Siegfried Weger
Department of Internal Medicine, Bruneck Hospital, Bruneck, Italy

Johann Willeit and Stefan Kiechl
Department of Neurology, Innsbruck Medical University, Innsbruck, Austria

Hao K. Lu, Lachlan R. Gray, Fiona Wightman, Paula Ellenberg and Gabriela Khoury
Department of Infectious Diseases, Monash University, Melbourne, Victoria, Australia
Centre for Biomedical Research, Burnet Institute, Melbourne, Victoria, Australia

Wan-Jung Cheng
Centre for Biomedical Research, Burnet Institute, Melbourne, Victoria, Australia

Talia M. Mota and Paul R. Gorry
Department of Infectious Diseases, Monash University, Melbourne, Victoria, Australia
Centre for Biomedical Research, Burnet Institute, Melbourne, Victoria, Australia
Department of Microbiology and Immunology, University of Melbourne, Melbourne, Victoria, Australia

Steve Wesselingh
Centre for Biomedical Research, Burnet Institute, Melbourne, Victoria, Australia
South Australian Health and Medical Research Institute, Adelaide, Australia

Paul U. Cameron
Department of Infectious Diseases, Monash University, Melbourne, Victoria, Australia
Centre for Biomedical Research, Burnet Institute, Melbourne, Victoria, Australia
Infectious Disease Unit, Alfred Hospital, Melbourne, Victoria, Australia

Melissa J. Churchill
Centre for Biomedical Research, Burnet Institute, Melbourne, Victoria, Australia
Department of Microbiology, Monash University, Clayton, Victoria, Australia
Department of Medicine, Monash University, Clayton, Victoria, Australia

Sharon R. Lewin
Department of Infectious Diseases, Monash University, Melbourne, Victoria, Australia
Centre for Biomedical Research, Burnet Institute, Melbourne, Victoria, Australia
Infectious Disease Unit, Alfred Hospital, Melbourne, Victoria, Australia
Peter Doherty Institute, Melbourne University, Melbourne, Victoria, Australia

Hideki Sugimoto, Shingo Konno, Nobuatsu Nomoto, Hiroshi Nakazora, Mayumi Murata, Hisao Kitazono, Tomomi Imamura, Masashi Inoue, Miyuki Sasaki, Akihisa Fuse, Wataru Hagiwara, Mari Kobayashi and Toshiki Fujioka
Division of Neurology, Department of Internal Medicine, Toho University Ohashi, Tokyo, Japan

Rajshekhar Gannavarpu, Basanta Bhaduri and Gabriel Popescu
Quantitative Light Imaging Laboratory, Department of Electrical and Computer Engineering, Beckman Institute for Advanced Science and Technology, University of Illinois at Urbana-Champaign, Urbana, Illinois, United States of America

Krishnarao Tangella
Department of Pathology, Christie Clinic, and University of Illinois at Urbana-Champaign, Urbana, Illinois, United States of America

Tomoya Hirose, Naoya Matsumoto, Taro Irisawa, Hideo Hosotsubo and Takeshi Shimazu
Department of Traumatology and Acute Critical Medicine, Osaka University Graduate School of Medicine, Osaka, Japan

Shigeto Hamaguchi, Masafumi Seki, Norihisa Yamamoto and Kazunori Tomono
Division of Infection Control and Prevention, Osaka University Graduate School of Medicine, Osaka, Japan

Osamu Tasaki
Department of Emergency Medicine, Unit of Clinical Medicine, Nagasaki University Graduate School of Biomedical Sciences, Nagasaki, Japan

Kouji Yamamoto
Department of Medical Innovation, Osaka University Hospital, Osaka, Japan

Yukihiro Akeda and Kazunori Oishi
International Research Center for Infectious Diseases, Research Institute for Microbial Diseases, Osaka University, Osaka, Japan

Hiromichi Takahashi and Masaru Nakagawa
Division of Biochemistry, Department of Biomedical Sciences, Nihon University School of Medicine, Tokyo, Japan
Division of Hematology and Rheumatology, Department of Medicine, Nihon University School of Medicine, Tokyo, Japan

Yoshihiro Hatta, Noriyoshi Iriyama, Jin Takeuchi and Masami Takei
Division of Hematology and Rheumatology, Department of Medicine, Nihon University School of Medicine, Tokyo, Japan

Yuichiro Hasegawa, Hikaru Uchida and Makoto Makishima
Division of Biochemistry, Department of Biomedical Sciences, Nihon University School of Medicine, Tokyo, Japan

Xi Zhang
Department of Medical Oncology, Shanghai Tenth People's Hospital, Tongji University, School of Medicine, Shanghai, China

Wei Zhang and Li-jin Feng
Department of Pathology, Shanghai Tenth People's Hospital, Tongji University, School of Medicine, Shanghai, China

Florian Noulin, Anna Rosanas-Urgell, Annette Erhart and Céline Borlon
Unit of Malariology, Institute of Tropical Medicine, Antwerp, Belgium

Javed Karim Manesia and Catherine M. Verfaillie
Department of development and regeneration, Stem Cell Institute, Leuven, Belgium

Jan Van Den Abbeele
Unit ofVeterinary Protozoology, Institute of Tropical Medicine, Antwerp, Belgium

Umberto d'Alessandro
Medica l Research Council Unit, Fajara, The Gambia

Shu-Ching Chen and Pei-Yu Chang
Department of Medical Research, National Taiwan University Hospital, Taipei, Taiwan

Yu-Chia Su
National Laboratory Animal Center, National Applied Research Laboratories, Taipei, Taiwan

Ya-Ting Lu, Hung-Ju Lin and Yo-Ping Lai
Department of Internal Medicine, National Taiwan University Hospital, Taipei, Taiwan

Patrick Chow-In Ko
Department of Emergency Medicine, National Taiwan University Hospital, Taipei, Taiwan

Hong-Nerng Ho
Department of Obstetrics and Gynecology, National Taiwan University, College of Medicine, Taipei, Taiwan

Michiel B. Haeseker and Cathrien A. Bruggeman
Department of Medical Microbiology, Maastricht University Medical Center, Maastricht, the Netherlands
Care and Public Health Research Institute (CAPHRI), Maastricht, the Netherlands

Sander Croes, Cees Neef and Leo M. L. Stolk
Department of Clinical Pharmacy and Toxicology, Maastricht University Medical Center, Maastricht, the Netherlands

Annelies Verbon
Department of Internal Medicine, Erasmus Medical Center, Rotterdam, the Netherlands

Daniele Saverino
Department of Experimental Medicine – Section of Human Anatomy, University of Genova, Genova, Italy

Giampaola Pesce, Princey Antola and Marcello Bagnasco
Autoimmunity Unit, Department of Internal Medicine, University of Genova, Genova, Italy

Brunetta Porcelli
Department of Internal Medicine, University of Siena, Siena, Italy

Ignazio Brusca
Department of Clinical Pathology, Buccheri La Ferla Hospital, Palermo, Italy

Danilo Villalta
Allergology and Clinical Immunology, S. Maria degli Angeli Hospital, Pordenone, Italy

Marilina Tampoia
Laboratory of Clinical Pathology, University Hospital, Bari, Italy

Renato Tozzoli
Clinical Pathology, Department of Laboratory Medicine, S. Maria degli Angeli Hospital, Pordenone, Italy

Elio Tonutti
Immunopathology and Allergology Unit, S. Maria della Misericordia Hospital, Udine, Italy

Maria Grazia Alessio
Department of Laboratory Medicine, Biochemistry Laboratory, Riuniti Hospital, Bergamo, Italy

Nicola Bizzaro
Laboratory of Clinical Pathology, San Antonio Hospital, Tolmezzo, Udine, Italy

Kevin H. Eng
Department of Biostatistics and Bioinformatics, Roswell Park Cancer Institute, Buffalo, NY, United States of America

Takemasa Tsuji
Center for Immunotherapy, Roswell Park Cancer Institute, Buffalo, NY, United States of America

I-Ting Chow, Junbao Yang, Theresa J. Gates, Eddie A. James, Duy T. Mai and Carla Greenbaum
Benaroya Research Institute at Virginia Mason, Seattle, WA, United States of America

William W. Kwok
Benaroya Research Institute at Virginia Mason, Seattle, WA, United States of America

Department of Medicine, University of Washington, Seattle, WA, United States of America

Yoko Nagumo
Faculty of Life and Environmental Sciences, University of Tsukuba, Tsukuba, Japan
Department of Immunology, Faculty of Medicine, University of Tsukuba, Tsukuba, Japan

Akiko Iguchi-Manaka
Department of Immunology, Faculty of Medicine, University of Tsukuba, Tsukuba, Japan
Department of Breast and Endocrine Surgery, Faculty of Medicine, University of Tsukuba, Tsukuba, Japan

Yumi Yamashita-Kanemaru and Fumie Abe
Department of Immunology, Faculty of Medicine, University of Tsukuba, Tsukuba, Japan
Japan Science and Technology Agency, Core Research for Evolutional Science and Technology (CREST), University of Tsukuba, Tsukuba, Japan

Günter Bernhardt
Institute of Immunology, Hannover Medical School, Hannover, Germany

Akira Shibuya
Department of Immunology, Faculty of Medicine, University of Tsukuba, Tsukuba, Japan
Japan Science and Technology Agency, Core Research for Evolutional Science and Technology (CREST), University of Tsukuba, Tsukuba, Japan
Life Science Center of Tsukuba Advanced Research Alliance (TARA), University of Tsukuba, Tsukuba, Japan

Kazuko Shibuya
Department of Immunology, Faculty of Medicine, University of Tsukuba, Tsukuba, Japan

Kelly A. Fimlaid and Beth D. Kirkpatrick
Department of Microbiology and Molecular Genetics, University of Vermont, Burlington, Vermont, 05405, United States of America
University of Vermont College of Medicine, Vaccine Testing Center and Unit of Infectious Diseases, Burlington, Vermont, United States of America

Janet C. Lindow
University of Vermont College of Medicine, Vaccine Testing Center and Unit of Infectious Diseases, Burlington, Vermont, United States of America

David R. Tribble
Infectious Disease Clinical Research Program, Uniformed Services University of the Health Sciences, Bethesda, Maryland, United States of America

Janice Y. Bunn
University of Vermont College of Mathematics, Burlington, Vermont, United States of America

Alexander C. Maue,
5 Naval Medical Research Center, Enteric Diseases Department, Silver Spring, Maryland, United States of America

Xiaofan Huang, Lingyun Ren, Chao Cheng, Jie Wu, Yuan Sun and Zheng Liu
Department of Cardiovascular Surgery, Union Hospital, Tongji Medical College, Huazhong University of Science and Technology, Wuhan, People's Republic of China

Ping Ye
Department of Cardiology, Central Hospital of Wuhan, Wuhan, People's Republic of China

Sihua Wang
Department of Thoracic Surgery, Union Hospital, Tongji Medical College, Huazhong University of Science and Technology, Wuhan, People's Republic of China

Aini Xie
Division of Diabetes, Endocrinology and Metabolism, Department of Medicine, Baylor College of Medicine, Houston, Texas, United States of America

Jiahong Xia
Department of Cardiovascular Surgery, Union Hospital, Tongji Medical College, Huazhong University of Science and Technology, Wuhan, People's Republic of China
Department of Cardiovascular Surgery, Central Hospital of Wuhan, Wuhan, People's Republic of China

Tobias Eggert, José Medina-Echeverz, Firouzeh Korangy and Tim F. Greten
1 Gastrointestinal Malignancy Section, Center for Cancer Research, National Cancer Institute, National Institutes of Health, Bethesda, Maryland, United States of America

Tamar Kapanadze
Gastrointestinal Malignancy Section, Center for Cancer Research, National Cancer Institute, National Institutes of Health, Bethesda, Maryland, United States of America
Department of Gastroenterology, Hepatology and Endocrinology, Hannover Medical
School, Hannover, Germany

Michael J. Kruhlak
Experimental Immunology Branch, Center for Cancer Research, National Cancer Institute, National Institutes of Health, Bethesda, Maryland, United States of America

Ying Wang, Yan-Chao Shi and Ming Shi
Research Center for Liver Transplantation, Beijing 302 Hospital, Peking University Health Science Center, Beijing, China
Research Centre for Liver Transplantation, Beijing 302 Hospital, Beijing, China

Min Zhang, Zhen-Wen Liu, Yan-Ling Sun and Hong-Bo Wang
Research Centre for Liver Transplantation, Beijing 302 Hospital, Beijing, China

Wei-Guo Ren
The Third Xiangya Hospital of Central South University, Changsha, China

Lei Jin and Fu-Sheng Wang
Research Center for Biological Therapy, Beijing 302 Hospital, Beijing, China

Alexander Wehr, Christer Baeck, Christian Trautwein, Frank Tacke and Tom Luedde
Department of Medicine III, RWTH University-Hospital, Aachen, Germany

Florian Ulmer and Ulf Peter Neumann
Department of General, Visceral and Transplant Surgery, RWTH University-Hospital, Aachen, Germany

Nikolaus Gassler
Institute of Pathology, RWTH University-Hospital, Aachen, Germany

Kanishka Hittatiya
Department of Pathology, Rheinische Friedrich-Wilhelms-University, Bonn, Germany

Elena G. Kamburova, Hans J. P. M. Koenen and Irma Joosten
Department of Laboratory Medicine - Medical Immunology, Radboud University Medical Centre, Nijmegen, The Netherlands

Martijn W. F. van den Hoogen, Marije C. Baas and Luuk B. Hilbrands
Department of Nephrology, Radboud University Medical Centre, Nijmegen, The Netherlands

Nathalie Muls and Hong Anh Dang
Neurochemistry Unit, Institute of Neuroscience, Université catholique de Louvain, Brussels, Belgium

Christian J. M. Sindic and Vincent van Pesch
Neurochemistry Unit, Institute of Neuroscience, Université catholique de Louvain, Brussels, Belgium
Cliniques Universitaires Saint-Luc, Brussels, Belgium

Ghanashyam Sarikonda, Georgia Fousteri, Sowbarnika Sachithanantham, Jacqueline F. Miller, Amy Dave and Therese Juntti
Diabetes Center, La Jolla Institute for Allergy and Immunology, La Jolla, California, USA

Ken T. Coppieters
Type 1 Diabetes R&D center, Novo Nordisk Inc., Seattle, Washington, USA

Matthias von Herrath
Diabetes Center, La Jolla Institute for Allergy and Immunology, La Jolla, California, USA
Type 1 Diabetes R&D center, Novo Nordisk Inc., Seattle, Washington, USA

Qiang Lou, Wei Zhang, Guangchao Liu and Yuanfang Ma
Henan Engineering Lab of Antibody Medicine, Key Laboratory of Cellular and Molecular Immunology, Medical College of Henan University, Kaifeng 475004, China

Nathella Pavan Kumar
National Institutes of Health—International Center for Excellence in Research, Chennai, India
National Institute for Research in Tuberculosis, Chennai, India

Vaithilingam V. Banurekha and Dina Nair
National Institute for Research in Tuberculosis, Chennai, India

Rathinam Sridhar
Government Stanley Medical Hospital, Chennai, India

Hardy Kornfeld
Department of Medicine, University of Massachusetts Medical School, Worcester, Massachusetts, United States of America

Thomas B. Nutman
Laboratory of Parasitic Diseases, National Institute of Allergy and Infectious Diseases, National Institutes of Health, Bethesda, Maryland, United States of America

Subash Babu
National Institutes of Health—International Center for Excellence in Research, Chennai, India
Laboratory of Parasitic Diseases, National Institute of Allergy and Infectious Diseases,
National Institutes of Health, Bethesda, Maryland, United States of America

Andreas Wannhoff, Kilian Friedrich, Christian Rupp, Petra Klöters-Plachky, Yvonne Leopold, Mirja Senner, Karl-Heinz Weiss, Wolfgang Stremmel and Daniel N. Gotthardt
Department of Internal Medicine IV, University Hospital Heidelberg, Heidelberg, Germany

Oliver J. Müller and Hugo A. Katus
Department of Internal Medicine III, University Hospital Heidelberg, Heidelberg, Germany

Maik Brune
Department of Internal Medicine I and Clinical Chemistry, University Hospital Heidelberg, Heidelberg, Germany

Peter Schemmer
Department of General and Transplant Surgery, University Hospital Heidelberg, Heidelberg, Germany

Index

A

Acute Rejection, 136, 154-160, 170-171
Alloreactive Responses, 154, 158
Anti-tumor Immunity, 81, 85
Autoantigen, 119, 185, 188-190

B

Biological Parameters, 49-52
Blood Cells, 43, 46, 50, 52, 74-75, 79-80, 207, 213
Blood Coagulation, 42
Blood Plasma, 42, 46
Blood Smears, 49-50, 52-54
Bloodstream, 49, 52-57

C

C-reactive Protein, 18, 20-23, 36, 39, 67
Cancer Testis, 103, 109-110
Cancer Testis Antigens, 109
Cardiopulmonary Arrest, 49, 52-53
Cd8z T-cell, 103
Cell Preparation, 15, 83
Cell Proliferation, 82-83, 85, 151, 158, 169, 177, 191, 194, 196, 198, 209
Cellular Tomography, 42
Cfse Labeling, 81
Chromatin, 9-10, 13, 15, 17, 27-29, 34-35, 50, 53-54, 57
Chromosomal Interactions, 9-10
Chronic Hyperglycemia, 81
Citrullinated Histone H3, 49-51, 53-57
Clot Rheology, 46-47
Clotting Process, 42, 44
Co-morbidity, 200
Cohesin, 9-13, 15-17
Cohesin Binding, 10-13, 15-16
Costimulatory Molecules, 102, 121
Cytokine Production, 81, 87, 113, 121, 128-129, 132, 134-135, 171, 174, 177, 186-187, 198, 202
Cytokines, 55, 59, 64, 66, 72, 121, 123, 125-134, 136, 138, 140, 142, 145, 149-152, 160-163, 166-168, 171-172, 176-177, 181, 186, 188-189, 191, 200-202, 204-207
Cytotoxicity, 28-29, 87, 121, 126-127

D

Diabetes, 18-26, 37, 42, 81, 83, 87-88, 97, 112-114, 116, 119-120, 136, 142-143, 161, 185-190, 200-201, 205-207

Diabetic Hosts, 81, 87
Diabetic Mice, 81, 85
Disease-free Survival, 67-68, 70-71, 73
Dna Repair, 9

F

Fibrin Clot, 42, 44-47
Fibrin Fibers, 42, 45-47
Fibrin Polymerization, 42, 44-46
Fractal Nature, 42, 44, 46-47

G

Gastric Cancer, 67-68, 70, 72-73, 126
Gene Loci, 9, 12-14, 26

H

Haematological Malignancy, 91-92, 94
Heart Disease, 25, 41, 49, 52-54, 136
Hematopoietic Cell, 89
Hyperglycemia, 81, 87, 200, 205
Hypoalbuminemia, 89

I

Ig Molecule, 9
Immune Cells, 55, 85, 103, 125-126, 134, 136-137, 147-149, 151-152, 163, 168, 177, 181
Immune Mechanism, 49, 136
Immune-related Genes, 103-104, 106, 108
Immunoglobulin, 9, 16-17, 20, 97, 102, 176, 199
Immunoreactive, 52, 103, 105, 107, 109-110
Immunotherapeutic Strategy, 185
Infected Patients, 27-29, 32-33, 35, 49, 54, 56, 75, 98-99
Insulin Deficiency, 81
Intracellular Cytokine Staining, 83, 113, 117, 119, 172, 189
Intraperitoneal Injection, 81-83, 137

L

Liver Alloresponse, 154
Liver Resection, 1, 8
Liver Transplantation, 1, 3-8, 102, 154-158, 160-161, 209, 215
Lymphocytes, 9, 17, 65, 72-73, 85, 87-88, 103, 105-106, 110, 112-113, 119, 121, 124, 126-129, 134, 137, 143, 154, 160, 163, 167, 169, 177-179, 181, 184, 187, 191, 198-199

M

Maturation, 9, 12-13, 15, 66, 78, 87-88, 132, 135, 154-155, 197

Mca-induced Tumors, 121, 123, 127

Myeloperoxidase, 49

N

Neutropenia, 89-92, 94

Neutrophil Extracellular Traps, 49, 53-57

Neutrophil Lymphocyte Ratio, 67-68, 73

Non-homologous, 10, 15

Non-reoperation, 1-4, 6

O

Organ Transplantation, 154, 156, 160, 177

Ovarian Cancer, 103-104, 110

P

P14-tcr Transgenic Mice, 81

Pathogenesis, 23, 58, 96, 112-113, 135, 161, 169-170, 178, 200, 205, 207

Pathogens, 35, 49-50, 54-55, 128-129

Peak Plasma, 89

Peripheral Lymphoid Tissues, 85

Pharmacokinetic, 89-91, 94

Plasma Cells, 12, 15, 132

Polarization, 66, 88-90, 119, 129, 136-143, 185-186, 188-189

Power Spectrum, 42, 44-47

Pulmonary Tuberculosis, 200, 207

R

Recipient Survival, 1-2, 4, 6

Recombination, 9-11, 13, 15, 17

Rejection Activity Index, 154, 156

Reoperation Rate, 1, 6

S

Streptozotocin-induced Diabetic, 81

Stz-diabetic Hosts, 81

T

T Cell Receptor, 81, 87, 103, 167, 191, 198-199

T-cell Receptor, 104, 185, 190

Thromboembolic Disorders, 42

Tracheal Aspirate, 49-52, 54-57

Tumor Microenvironment, 103, 105, 109-110, 153

Tumor-bearing Mice, 81, 85, 145-153

Tumor-killing, 81, 85

V

Vancomycin, 89-94

Vigilant Surveillance, 1, 6, 8

X

X-ray Scattering, 42

www.ingramcontent.com/pod-product-compliance
Lightning Source LLC
Chambersburg PA
CBHW082100190326
41458CB00010B/3534